For Instructors

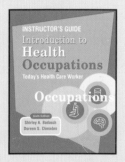

Instructor's Guide
ISBN: 0-13-110267-2

This manual contains a wealth of material to help faculty plan and manage the course. It includes chapter overviews, detailed lecture suggestions and outlines, learning objectives, teaching tips, and more for each chapter. Selected Transparency Masters are provided in the manual; more masters are provided on the Companion Website www.prenhall.com/badasch.

Instructor's Resource CD-ROM
ISBN: 0-13-110268-0

This cross-platform CD-ROM provides illustrations in PowerPoint from this textbook for use in classroom lectures. It also contains the Test-Gen electronic test bank. This supplement is available to faculty free upon adoption of the textbook.

Companion Website Syllabus Manager
www.prenhall.com/badasch

Faculty adopting this textbook have **free** access to the online **Syllabus Manager** feature of the Companion Website, www.prenhall.com/badasch. Syllabus Manager offers a whole host of features that facilitate the students' use of the Companion Website, and allows faculty to post syllabi and course information online for their students. For more information or a demonstration of Syllabus Manager, please contact a Prentice Hall Sales Representative.

BRIEF TABLE OF CONTENTS

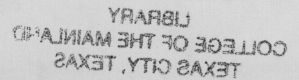

Introduction to
Health Occupations

Today's Health Care Worker

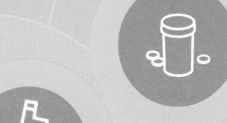

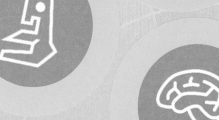

Sixth Edition

Shirley A. Badasch, M.Ed, RN

Doreen S. Chesebro, B.Ed, LVN

Prentice
Hall

Upper Saddle River, New Jersey 07458

Library of Congress Cataloging-in-Publication Data
Badasch, Shirley A., (date)
Introduction to health occupations: today's health care
    worker/Shirley A. Badasch,
Doreen S. Chesebro.—6th ed. p. cm.
Includes index.
ISBN 0-13-045745-0
1. Allied health personnel—Vocational guidance. I. Title: Health
    occupations. II. Chesebro, Doreen S., (date) III. Title.
R697.A4.B33 2004
610.69—dc21

2002038100

Publisher: *Julie Levin Alexander*
Assistant to Publisher: *Regina Bruno*
Executive Editor: *Maura Connor*
Acquisitions Editor: *Barbara Krawiec*
Development Editor: *Maureen Muncaster*
Editorial Assistant: *Sheba Jalaluddin*
Director of Manufacturing and Production: *Bruce Johnson*
Managing Production Editor: *Patrick Walsh*
Production Liaison: *Mary C. Treacy*
Production Editor: *Emily Bush, Carlisle Publishers Services*
Manufacturing Manager: *Ilene Sanford*
Manufacturing Buyer: *Pat Brown*
Design Director: *Cheryl Asherman*
Senior Design Coordinator: *Maria Guglielmo Walsh*
Manager of Media Production: *Amy Peltier*
New Media Project Manager: *Lisa Rinaldi*
Senior Marketing Manager: *Nicole Benson*
Marketing Coordinator: *Janet Ryerson*
Product Information Manager: *Rachele Strober*
Composition: *Carlisle Communications, Ltd.*
Cover Printer: *Lehigh Press*
Printer/Binder: *Von Hoffman Press*

For co-writing Chapter 19, "Medical Clerical Worker,"
acknowledgments go to Monica Maldonado-Puertas, Education
Coordinator, Business Bristol Park Medical Group, Inc., Costa
Mesa, California.
For co-writing Chapter 21, "Dental Assistant,"
acknowledgments go to Vivian Muensterman, Baldy View ROP.

Printed in the United States of America

Prentice-Hall International (UK) Limited, *London*
Prentice-Hall of Australia Pty. Limited, *Sydney*
Prentice-Hall Canada Inc., *Toronto*
Prentice-Hall Hispanoamericana, S.A., *Mexico*
Prentice-Hall of India Private Limited, *New Delhi*
Prentice-Hall of Japan, Inc., *Tokyo*
Prentice-Hall (Singapore) Pte. Ltd.
Editora Prentice-Hall do Brasil, Ltda., *Rio de Janeiro*
Pearson Education, Upper Saddle River

DEDICATION
**This revision is dedicated: To our many friends
and especially our families, who loved us and
waited.**

Notice: Care has been taken to confirm the accuracy of the information presented in this book. The authors, editors, and the publisher, however, cannot accept any responsibility for errors or omissions or for consequences from application of the information in this book and make no warranty, express or implied, with respect to its contents.

The authors and publishers have exerted every effort to ensure that drug selections and dosages set forth in this text are in accord with current recommendations and practice at time of publication. However, in view of ongoing research, changes in government regulations, and the constant flow of information relating to drug therapy and drug reactions, the reader is urged to check the package inserts of all drugs for any change in indications of dosage and for added warnings and precautions. This is particularly important when the recommended agent is a new and/or infrequently employed drug.

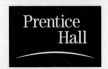

10 9 8 7 6 5 4 3 2 1

ISBN 0-13-045745-0

CONTENTS

Chapter 14

Employability and Leadership 308

Part 2

Multidisciplinary Skills 325

Chapter 15

Nurse Assistant/Patient Caregiver 326

PROCEDURES

PREFACE

The increase in longevity and changes in the health care system create an increased need for educated and skilled health care workers. This need for health care workers is expected to continue its growth well into the twenty-first century. Gerontology, rehabilitation, ambulatory care, outpatient services, and managed care are expected to show the greatest growth. The occupations that service these high growth areas include: dental assistants, long-term care nursing assistants, nursing assistants with advanced skills, assistive personnel, home health care aides, medical assistants, laboratory assistants/phlebotomists, physical therapy aides, food service workers, environmental service workers, electrocardiogram technicians, and central supply/central processing workers. Demand for multidisciplinary health care workers is high due to the increasing need to provide appropriate care and customer service that meet patient/client needs and new budgetary restraints. These multiskilled workers may work under a variety of job titles ranging from Unlicensed Assistive Personnel to Assistive Caregivers to Patient Care Partners.

Because preventive health is a key component in twenty-first century health care, preventive health care and patient teaching are emphasized throughout the text. The qualities and values required to become an outstanding health care worker are also interwoven throughout the text and learning system materials. All of the information in this textbook has been carefully reviewed and updated. New areas of emphasis address the continuing changes in healthcare, such as subacute care and assistive caregiving for acute care.

A unique **learning system** divides the text into two parts. The first part, Basic Knowledge and Skills, chapters one through fourteen, includes the basic information all health care workers must have to work in any department within the health care environment. The second part, Multidisciplinary Skills, chapters fifteen through twenty-four, spans a variety of entry-level occupations. Students can select one occupational area or several occupational areas in Part Two, allowing them an opportunity to become a multiskilled health worker. This **learning system** also provides all areas of training required by the 1987 Omnibus Budget Reconciliation Act (OBRA), it addresses the National Standards, and allows for state differences in curriculum and JACHO Standards such as age-specific communication.

The changing requirements for health care presents educators and students alike with ever-changing challenges. *Introduction to Health Occupations, Sixth Edition,* helps meet the needs of not only the health care system, but all levels of students, from secondary and postsecondary to English as a second language (ESL) students.

New to the Sixth Edition

New features have been added to strengthen student instruction with more practice in hands-on exercises and enhanced visual learning, team building, communication, multicultural competence and familiarity with new technology. These features

- Provide auditory learners with an **audio glossary** on the **free CD-ROM and the Companion Website (www.prenhall.com/badasch)**
- Increase hands-on opportunities with a new **"Learn by Doing"** component at the end of each unit
- Help visual learners with **new tables, charts and boxes**
- Add clarity by opening every procedure with a **rationale**
- Give enhanced documentation exposure with **charting examples**
- Enhance the "Thinking Critically" segment at the end of each chapter with new kinds of activities, including those related to **patient satisfaction, patient advocacy, time management, and safety**
- Strengthen portfolios by adding a **"Portfolio Tip"** at the end of every chapter
- Broaden the scope of activities away from written reports and toward **group role-playing, and participatory practice and peer interactions**
- Include **computer- and Web-oriented learning**
- Update content by adding new topics, such as **bioterrorism** in the disaster-preparedness unit
- Expand career overviews by addressing additional careers such as **veterinary medicine**

These new features enhance the basic, time-tested structure and features that include:

- *Easy readability* meets the learning needs of all students.
- *Margin Glossary* provides immediate feedback and understanding of vocabulary.
- *Student Workbook* provides additional reinforcement to help in the retention of content and works in tandem with *Steps to Success* activities at the beginning of each unit to help guide students through new material.

- **Skills Check-off Sheets** are designed for both practice and competency assessment. These check-off sheets provide step-by-step instructions to help students perform procedures correctly and competently.

- **Portfolio Connection** helps students develop a vocational portfolio to demonstrate job or higher education readiness.

- **Your Link to Success** encourages students to think critically and apply unit concepts to real life situations.

- **Age-Specific Communication Skills** are addressed throughout.

- **Medical Math Chapter** reviews the basic math concepts which students will need to succeed, such as multiplication, division, percentages, and fractions.

- **Medical Terminology** is addressed throughout the text and workbook.

- **Standard Precautions** are highlighted throughout to safeguard the health of both students and patients.

Instructors and students alike will benefit from our complete learning package, which like the text has been updated and expanded with new activities. This package includes:

■ Instructor's Guide

Our instructor's guide is loaded with content, teaching hints, and resources to help make your job as instructor easier. It contains presentation content, suggested activities, points of interest, advance preparation hints, examples, additional discussion topics, and guidelines, as well as resources for program enhancement. These resources include

- transparency masters to add interest and facilitate learning
- worksheet keys
- evaluations with keys
- detailed activities and instructions that promote critical thinking.
- Additional chapters and skills are included for Radiology Aide/Darkroom Attendant, Nursing Assistant–Acute Care Specialists, Assistive Caregiver, and Food Service Worker. In addition, a Test Item File (printed test questions) is also available as part of our complete learning package.

■ Instructor's Guide CD-ROM

Our Instructor's Guide CD-ROM provides an electronic test bank and Power Point images. In addition, the print Instructor's Guide is available on the CD-ROM for your customization.

■ Student Workbook

Our student workbook provides students with a variety of practice activities that include worksheets, scenarios, activities, and selected check-off sheets designed for both practice and competency assessment. These check-off sheets provide step-by-step instructions to help students perform procedures correctly and competently. A complete set of check-off sheets can be obtained through the Companion Website described below. All of these Workbook activities will help students successfully learn the skills required for their respective career choices.

■ Companion Website www.prenhall.com/badasch

The Companion Website, tied chapter-by-chapter to the text, gives students an on-line study guide that provides immediate feedback, guides them step-by-step through procedures with skill check-off sheets, and provides links to interesting and relevant sites on the World Wide Web. The Companion Website shell also enables instructors to create a customized syllabus and download Power Point slides and transparency masters.

■ Student CD-ROM

Packaged *free* with the textbook, the CD-ROM provides an interactive program that allows students to practice answering questions. It also contains an audio glossary and a link to the Companion II Website (an Internet connection is required).

Health care workers provide a valuable service to society. They are responsible for people of all ages and cultures who require a wide array of services. Today's health care worker must fill a variety of roles from caregiver to patient educator and beyond. *Introduction to Health Occupations, Sixth Edition,* prepares students for all these roles by providing the skills information they need to be effective health care workers.

Organization of the Book

Part 1

Part One of this book provides the core knowledge that all health care workers must learn before entering a health care occupation. Part One consists of chapters 1 through 14.

Part 2

Part Two provides students the knowledge, tasks, and skills for the health care area of your choice. The step-by-step procedures enhance the text's content and reinforce student learning. The procedures prepare you to perform the skills necessary in your chosen health career area. If you cannot complete the objectives or demonstrate the procedures successfully, you are not adequately prepared for work, internship, or the community classroom. When you successfully complete the objectives in Part One and the Objectives for the health career chosen in Part Two, you are prepared for an entry-level position in a health care setting. You may choose to complete one area and then move into another area. Many of the skills are transferable. The emphasis in the workplace today is on multidisciplinary trained workers. The more areas in which you are proficient, the more marketable you are.

List of Occupations in Part Two

- Nurse Assistant/Patient Caregiver
- Home Health Aide
- Electrocardiogram Technician
- Laboratory Assistant/Medical Assistant Laboratory Skills; Phlebotomist
- Physical Therapy Aide
- Central Supply/Central Processing Worker
- Environmental Services Technician/Housekeeper
- Health Information Technician
- Clinical Medical Assistant
- Dental Assistant

Note: Nurse Assistant—Acute Care Specialties/Assistive Personnel, Food Service Worker, and Radiology Aide/Darkroom Attendant chapters are located in the Instructor's Guide. If you are interested in one of these areas, ask your teacher for the chapter.

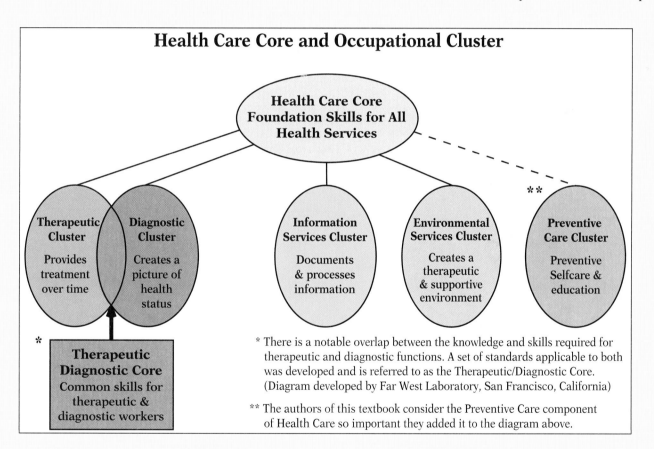

Health Care Core and Occupational Cluster

Health Care Core Foundation Skills for All Health Services

Therapeutic Cluster
Provides treatment over time

Diagnostic Cluster
Creates a picture of health status

Information Services Cluster
Documents & processes information

Environmental Services Cluster
Creates a therapeutic & supportive environment

Preventive Care Cluster
Preventive Selfcare & education

* **Therapeutic Diagnostic Core**
Common skills for therapeutic & diagnostic workers

* There is a notable overlap between the knowledge and skills required for therapeutic and diagnostic functions. A set of standards applicable to both was developed and is referred to as the Therapeutic/Diagnostic Core. (Diagram developed by Far West Laboratory, San Francisco, California)

** The authors of this textbook consider the Preventive Care component of Health Care so important they added it to the diagram above.

We reviewed the National Health Care Skill Standards to guide us in determining what information meets the needs of future health care workers: "Health care skill standards are statements which answer the question, 'What does a worker need to know and be able to do to contribute to the safe and effective delivery of health care?' The standards will inform current and future health care workers, employers, and educators what skills and knowledge workers need to succeed—in a job and in a career. It is envisioned that these standards will help provide the foundation for better worker preparation, both in school and on the job" (*Quality & Excellence Health Care Skill Standards*). We continued to ask the question: What does a worker need to know and be able to do to contribute to the safe and effective delivery of health care? When the authors ask this question about each topic in the text, it focuses the information on key material needed by an entry-level health care worker and eliminates unnecessary material.

Note: State standards/guidelines may divide the health care services differently than the National Standards. For example, Preventive Health Care may be a state cluster (see above figure).

1987 Omnibus Budget Reconciliation Act (OBRA)

To ensure quality care in long-term care (Skilled Nursing) facilities new guidelines were adopted by the Federal Government. These guidelines are known as OBRA. The OBRA Act of 1987 requires that individuals employed in skilled nursing facilities receive training and be evaluated on their skills. OBRA requires a minimum of 16 hours of instruction before resident contact. These are classroom hours and are identified on the following table with an asterisk.

Omnibus Budget Reconciliation Act of 1987 Requirements Health Care Worker Subject Areas That Satisfy All OBRA Requirements		
1. Communication and Interpersonal Communications	Chapter 4:	Meeting Your Needs and the Needs of Others
	Unit 2:	Understanding Human Needs
	Topic:	Meeting the Needs of Co-workers and Other Staff
	Unit 3:	Cultural Competency
	Topics:	Culture and Behavior
		Gestures and Body Language
		Communicating Effectively with Other Cultures
		Folk Medicine
	Chapter 5:	Effective Communications
	Unit 1:	Interpersonal Communication for All Ages
	Topics:	Elements That Influence Your Relationships with Others
		Barriers to Communication
		Elements of Communication
		Good Listening Skills
		Verbal Communication
		Nonverbal Communication
2. Infection Control[*]	Chapter 12:	Controlling Infection
	Unit 1:	The Nature of Microorganisms
	Topics:	Introduction to Microorganisms
		How Microorganisms Affect the Body
		How Microorganisms Spread
		Signs and Symptoms of Infection
	Unit 2:	Asepsis
	Topics:	Standard Precautions
		Controlling the Spread of Infection
	Unit 3	Standard Precautions
	Topics:	Introduction to Standard Precautions
		Transmission-Based Precaution Rooms
3. Safety and Emergency Procedures[*]	Chapter 13	Patient and Employee Safety
	Unit 1:	General Safety and Injury and Illness Prevention
	Topics:	OSHA Standards
		General Safety
	Unit 2:	Patient Safety
	Topics:	Identifying the Patient
		Ambulation Devices
		Transporting Devices
		Postural Supports
		Side Rails
	Unit 3:	Disaster Preparedness
	Topics:	Disaster Plan
		Fire Causes and Prevention
	Unit 4:	Principles of Body Mechanics
	Topic:	Body Mechanics
	Unit 5:	First Aid
	Topics:	General Principles of First Aid
		Life-Threatening Situations

Omnibus Budget Reconciliation Act of 1987 Requirements Health Care Worker Subject Areas That Satisfy All OBRA Requirements (continued)

4. Promoting Residents' Independence*	Chapter 9:	Human Growth and Development
	Unit 3:	Disabilities and Role Changes
	Topics:	Importance of Independence
		Physical Disabilities
		Role Changes in the Disabled

5. Respecting Resident Rights*	Chapter 3:	Medical Ethics and Law
	Unit 2:	Legal Roles and Responsibilities of a Health Care Worker
	Topics:	Legal Responsibilities
		Confidentiality

6. Basic Nursing Skills	Chapter 11:	Measuring Vital Signs
	Unit 1:	Temperature, Pulse, and Respiration
	Unit 2:	Blood Pressure
		Abnormal signs (integrated into chapter when indicated)
	Chapter 15:	Nurse Assistant/Patient Caregiver
	Unit 1:	Basic Care Skills/OBRA Standards/Long-Term Care
	Topics:	Height and Weight
		Measuring Intake and Output
		Abnormal signs (integrated into chapter where appropriate)

7. Personal Care Skills	Chapter 15:	Nurse Assistant/Patient Caregiver
	Unit 1:	Basic Care Skills/OBRA Standards/Long-Term Care
	Topics:	Morning and Evening Care (AM and PM Care)
		Skin Management
		Oral Hygiene
		Offering the Urinal and/or Bedpan
		Movement and Ambulation of the Resident
		Positioning and Body Alignment
		Range of Motion
		Bathing the Resident
		Care of Hair and Nails
		Shaving the Resident
		Dressing and Undressing the Resident
		Bedmaking
		Feeding the Resident
		Incontinent Resident

8. Mental Health and Social Service Needs	Chapter 3:	Medical Ethics and Law
	Unit 2:	Legal Roles and Responsibilities of a Health Care Worker
	Topic:	Legal Responsibilities
	Chapter 4:	Meeting Your Needs and the Needs of Others
	Unit 2:	Understanding Human Needs
	Topics:	Meeting the Needs of Patients/Clients
		Defense Mechanisms
	Chapter 9:	Human Growth and Development
	Unit 1:	Development and Behavior
	Topic:	Development and Behavior
	Unit 2:	Aging and Role Change
	Topic:	Role Changes in the Aging
	Unit 3:	Disabilities and Role Changes
	Topic:	Importance of Independence

9. Basic Restorative Services	Chapter 15:	Nurse Assistant/Patient Caregiver
	Topics:	Positioning and Body Alignment
		Range of Motion
		Incontinent Resident
		Prosthetic Devices
		Special Care Devices
	Chapter 19:	Physical Therapy Aide
	Topics:	Guarding Techniques
		Rehabilitation Equipment

ACKNOWLEDGMENTS

The authors wish to express their sincere thanks to the many people who helped develop this book from the outline to the finished product.

- To our families—a warm and loving thanks for their willingness to support us throughout this revision.

- Richmond Ramsey for advising on the Medical Math.

- Sister Suzanne Sassus, Vice-President of Sponsorship, St. Joseph Health System.

- Phyllis Young-Gallagher, R.N. Neonatal and Maternity Health Specialist for Advising on Neonatal and Obstetrics/Maternal Care.

- Gloria Bizjak for reviewing the First Aid Unit.

- Debby Ferguson, BS, REEG/EPT, RPSGT ASET Board Member & PR Committee Representative for the information and editing she provided for the Electroneurodiagnostic Technologist (END techs for short).

- To the reviewers whose suggestions gave us fresh viewpoints on content and contributed to the overall quality of this book.

Reviewers for the Sixth Edition

Donna L. Albercht, RN, BSN
Instructor
Sollers Point Tech
Baltimore, MD

Patti Biro, B.S., M.Ed
Director of Health Care Programs
Center of Business and Community Education
Del Mar College
Corpus Christi, TX

Marilyn F. Collins, BSN, RN, PHN
Director of Health Occupations
Citrus College
Glendon, CA

Toni Decklever, RN, BSN
Career and Technical Education
Larramie County School District #1
Cheyenne, WY

Patty Fay Dimetres, RN, BSN, M.Ed, CAGS
Department of Health and Medical Sciences
Fairfax County Public Schools
Fairfax County, VA

Patty K. Leary, M.Ed
Instructor
Mecosta Osceola Career Center
Big Rapids, MI

Regina Lohre
Director of the Academy of Science and Health
Washington High School
Milwaukee, WI

Kathy S. Menezes, RN, MS
WMA Career Technical Center
Cadillac, MI

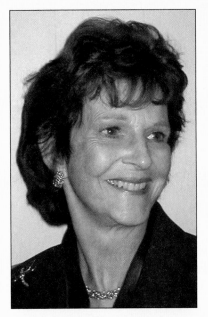

Shirley A. Badasch, M.Ed, RN, is a graduate of California State University at Long Beach. Her career includes acute care nursing, office nursing, industrial nursing, Director of Nursing for a developmentally disabled nursing facility, and Assistant Administrator in Long Term Care. Ms. Badasch's teaching experience includes co-developing the Medical Occupations Program and teaching for nine years in a Regional Occupation Program, and part-time instructor in the Educational Psychology department, California State University at Long Beach. She also taught in the teacher certification program at Cal Poly Pomona and California State University at Sacramento. During her career she worked as a contract consultant to the California State Department of Education, presenting seminars, writing materials, developing programs, and consulting on program development. Ms. Badasch completed her career as the Director of Education for Bristol Park Medical Group. She continues to research and participate in health occupations as a volunteer in her community and as a member of the California Association of Health Career Educators.

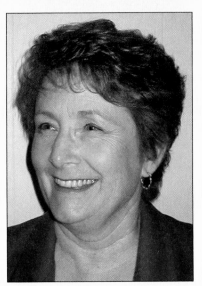

Doreen S. Chesebro, B.Ed, LVN, is a graduate of California State University at Long Beach. Her nursing career includes ambulatory care, long-term care and acute care nursing primarily in intensive care and coronary care units. Mrs. Chesebro's teaching experience includes co-developing and teaching the Medical Occupations Program in a Regional Occupation Program. This program includes long-term care nurse assistant, advanced nurse assistant, home health aide, front and back office medical assistant, and hospital health occupations. She also served as a Program Specialist for the Long Beach Unified School District and has experience as a part-time instructor for teacher certification at California State University at Sacramento and Cal Poly Pomona. As Director of Education in the ambulatory care setting, she was responsible for development, implementation and oversight of

• disease prevention and management classes through patient education
• staff development programs ranging from new employee orientation to management/leadership preparation and mentorship

Mrs. Chesebro is currently the Director of Mission Services for the ambulatory care setting of the St. Joseph Health System in California's Central Orange County Region. In this position, she coordinates and monitors community outreach programs and works closely with medical and business staff to promote the St. Joseph Health System Mission, Core Values and Vision.

THE GRAND PLAN & CAREER LADDER

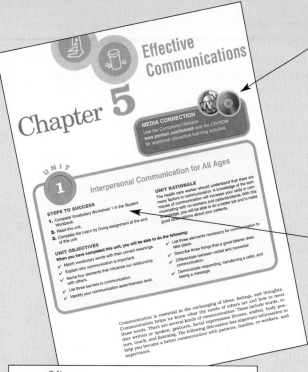

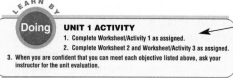

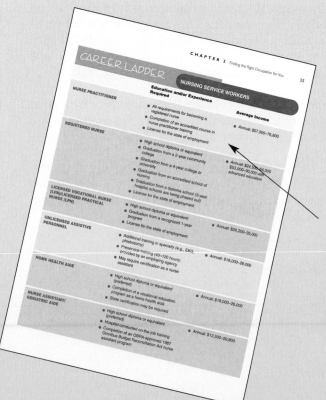

Media Connection

Each chapter begins with an invitation to use the free CD-ROM and Companion Website (www.prenhall.com/badasch) that serve as wonderful study companions to your textbook. Chapter-related audio glossaries, multiple-choice questions, case studies, and other activities help you to preview and to work your way successfully through the chapter. Each chapter ends with a reminder to use the CD-ROM and Companion Website for reviewing, reinforcing, and enriching what you have learned.

Steps to Success

Every unit starts with a plan to help you effectively use your textbook and your workbook to preview and to master the unit skills and concepts.

Learn by Doing

Every unit ends with a plan to help you effectively use your textbook and workbook to review and to reinforce unit skills and concepts.

Career Ladder

What does it take to become a health care professional? Career Ladder helps answer this question with an overview of the education/experience requirements for a variety of health careers from all four National Health Care Skill Standards career clusters. This book also covers more than 230 skills and procedures of 10 representative careers to give you a sense of what health care professionals do in the real world.

PROCEDURES & THE BIG WRAP-UP

Procedures

When performing procedures, it's important to do every step correctly. Brightly colored procedure boxes numbered for easy reference throughout the text clearly outline each procedure, from beginning to end, step by step. When appropriate, procedures are supported with photos and illustrations. Procedure check-off sheets are found on the Companion Website.

Rationale

A short statement of the reason for the procedure. The rationale tells you the "why" for the "what" you will be doing in the procedure.

Charting Examples

Gives a sample way to chart information related to the procedure so that you can become familiar with documentation.

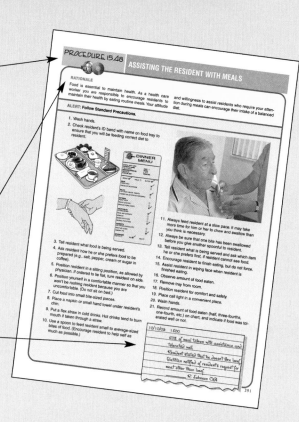

Thinking Critically

These activities will challenge you to do your best thinking and to apply chapter concepts to real life situations in areas such as medical math, computers, law and ethics, patient education, communication, cultural competency, medical terminology, case studies, patient advocacy, patient satisfaction, time management, and safety.

Portfolio Connection

How do you plan and prepare for a career? Portfolio Connection will help you by encouraging you to create a vocational portfolio that shows your job and/or higher education readiness.

Portfolio Tip

Be sure to consider these practical hints on how you create a successful portfolio.

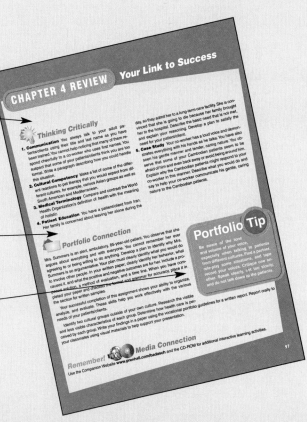

Introduction to
Health Occupations

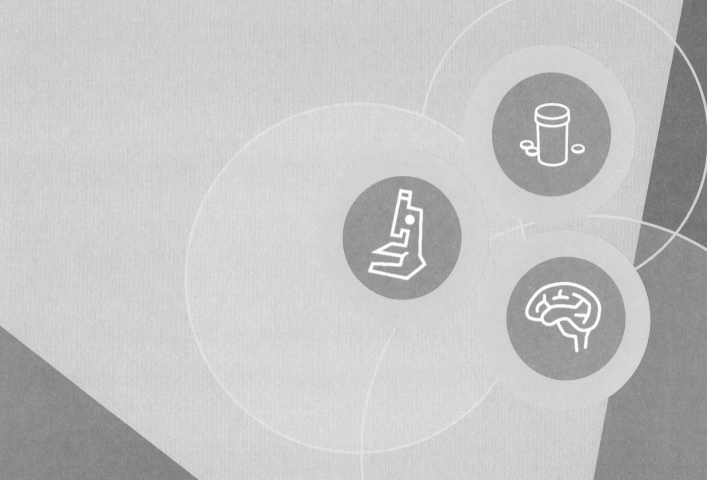

Part 1

Basic Knowledge and Skills

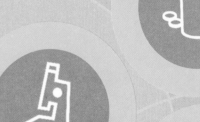

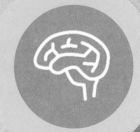

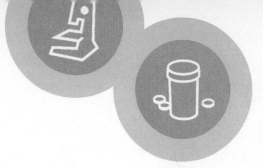

Chapter 1

Introduction to Being a Health Care Worker

MEDIA CONNECTION

Use the Companion Website **www.prenhall.com/badasch** and the CD-ROM for additional interactive learning activities.

UNIT 1

History of Health Care

STEPS TO SUCCESS

1. Complete Vocabulary Worksheet 1 in the Student Workbook.
2. Read this unit.
3. Complete the Learn by Doing assignment at the end of this unit.

UNIT RATIONALE

Health care has developed and changed throughout history. Knowing the history of health care helps you understand current procedures, practices, and philosophies. The experiences and discoveries of the past led to the advances of today. Today's achievements could not have occurred without the trials and errors of the past. When you understand the primitive beginnings of medicine, you appreciate the advances made during the past 5,000 years.

UNIT OBJECTIVES

When you have completed this unit, you will be able to do the following:

✔ Match vocabulary words with their correct meanings.

✔ Identify nine scientists and explain what they contributed to medicine.

✔ Choose one era in the history of health care and write a paper to explain how health care technology changed.

✔ Discuss advances in medicine in the twentieth century.

✔ Research and report on possible advances in medicine for the twenty-first century.

✔ Explain medical ethics and how it affects health care workers and patients/clients.*

✔ Compare health care in the past with health care in the twentieth and twenty-first centuries.

Client is replacing the term *patient* in many health care areas. We will use the terms combined or interchangeably until the transition is complete.

⬤ EARLY BEGINNINGS

Primitive human beings had no electricity, few tools, and poor shelter. Their time was spent protecting themselves against **predators** and finding food. They were **superstitious** and believed that illness and disease were caused by supernatural spirits. In an attempt to heal, tribal doctors performed ceremonies to **exorcise** evil spirits. They used herbs and plants as medicines. Some of the same medicines are still used today. Here are some examples:

■ Digitalis comes from the foxglove plant. Today it is given in pill form, **intravenously,** or by injection. In early times, people chewed the leaves of the foxglove plant to strengthen and slow the heartbeat.

■ Quinine comes from the bark of the cinchona tree. It controls fever, relieves muscle spasms, and helps prevent malaria.

■ Belladonna and atropine are made from the poisonous nightshade plant. They relieve muscle spasm, especially in gastrointestinal (GI) pain.

■ Morphine is made from the opium poppy. It relieves severe pain. It is addicting and is used only when nothing else will help.

predators
Organisms or beings that destroy.

superstitious
Trusting in magic or chance.

exorcise
To force out evil spirits.

intravenously
Directly into a vein.

⬤ MEDICINE IN ANCIENT TIMES

The Egyptians were the earliest people to keep **accurate** health records. They were superstitious and called upon the gods to heal them. They also learned to identify certain diseases. They used medicines to heal disease and learned the art of splinting fractures.

The ancient Greeks were the first to study the causes of disease. They kept records on what they observed and what they thought caused illness. The Greeks understood the importance of searching for new information about disease. This research helped eliminate superstition.

During ancient times, religious custom did not allow bodies to be dissected. The father of medicine, Hippocrates (ca. 469–377 B.C.), based his knowledge of anatomy and physiology on **observation** of the external body. He kept careful notes of the signs and symptoms of many diseases. With these records he found that disease was not caused by supernatural forces. Hippocrates wrote the standard of ethics called the Oath of Hippocrates. This standard is the basis for today's medical ethics. Physicians still take this oath.

The Greeks observed and measured the effects of disease. They found that some disease was caused by lack of sanitation. The Romans learned from the Greeks and developed a sanitation system. They brought clean water into their cities by way of aqueducts (waterways). They built sewers to carry off waste. They also built public baths with filtering systems. This was the beginning of public health and sanitation.

The Romans were the first to organize medical care. They sent medical equipment and physicians with their armies to care for wounded soldiers. Roman physicians kept a room in their houses for the ill. This was the beginning of hospitals (Figure 1.1). Public buildings for the care of the sick were established. Physicians were paid by the Roman government. It is interesting to note that the Roman physician wore a death mask. This mask had a spice-filled beak, which the Romans believed protected them from infection and bad odors.

accurate
Exact, correct, or precise.

observation
Act of watching.

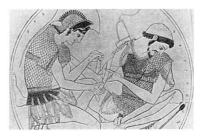

Figure 1.1

Roman physician.

THE DARK AGES (A.D. 400–800) AND THE MIDDLE AGES (A.D. 800–1400)

When the Roman Empire was conquered by the Huns (nomads from the north), the study of medical science stopped. For a period of 1,000 years, medicine was practiced only in **convents** and **monasteries.** Because the Church believed that life and death were in God's hands, the monks and priests had no interest in how the body functioned. Medication consisted of herbal mixtures, and care was **custodial.** Monks collected and translated the writings of the Greek and Roman physicians.

Terrible epidemics caused millions of deaths during this period. Bubonic plague (the black death) alone killed 60 million people. Other uncontrolled diseases included smallpox, diphtheria, syphilis, and tuberculosis. Today, these illnesses are not always life threatening. Scientists have discovered vaccines and medications to control these diseases. It is important to remember that some diseases can become epidemic if people are not vaccinated.

convents
Establishments of nuns.

monasteries
Homes for men following religious standards.

custodial
Marked by watching and protecting rather than seeking to cure.

THE RENAISSANCE (A.D. 1350–1650)

The Renaissance period saw the rebirth of learning. During this period, new scientific progress began. There were many developments during this period:

■ The building of universities and medical schools for research

■ The search for new ideas about disease rather than the unquestioning acceptance of disease as the will of God

■ The acceptance of **dissection** of the body for study

■ The development of the printing press and the publishing of books, allowing greater access to knowledge from research

These changes influenced the future of medical science.

dissection
Act or process of dividing, taking apart.

THE SIXTEENTH AND SEVENTEENTH CENTURIES

The desire for learning that began during the Renaissance continued through the next two centuries. During this time, several outstanding scientists added new knowledge. Here are some examples:

■ Leonardo da Vinci studied and recorded the anatomy of the body (Figure 1.2).

■ William Harvey used this knowledge to understand physiology, and he was able to describe the circulation of blood and the pumping of the heart.

■ Gabriele Fallopius discovered the fallopian tubes of the female anatomy.

■ Bartolommeo Eustachio discovered the tube leading from the ear to the throat (eustachian tube).

■ Antonie van Leeuwenhoek invented the microscope, establishing that there is life smaller than the eye can see. Van Leeuwenhoek scraped his teeth and observed the bacteria that cause tooth decay. Although it was not yet realized, the germs that cause disease were now visible.

Unfortunately **quackery,** mass death from childbed fever, and disease continued. The causes of infection and disease were still not understood.

quackery
Practice of pretending to cure diseases.

Figure 1.2

Human body as depicted by Leonardo da Vinci. (Courtesy of Galleria Dell'Accademia.)

THE EIGHTEENTH CENTURY

Many discoveries were made in the eighteenth century that required a new way of teaching medicine. Students not only attended lectures in the classroom and laboratory, but also observed patients at the bedside. When a patient died, they dissected the body and were able to observe the disease process. This led to a better understanding of the causes of illness and death. The study of physiology continued, and more new discoveries were made:

- René Laënnec invented the **stethoscope.** The first stethoscope was made of wood. It increased the ability to hear the heart and lungs, allowing doctors to determine if disease was present.
- Joseph Priestley discovered the element oxygen. He also observed that plants refresh air that has lost its oxygen, making it usable for respiration.
- Benjamin Franklin's discoveries affect us in many ways. His discoveries include bifocals, and he found that colds could be passed from person to person.
- Edward Jenner discovered a method of vaccination for smallpox. Smallpox killed many people in epidemics. His discovery saved millions of lives. His discovery also led to immunization and to preventive medicine in public health.

stethoscope
Instrument used to hear sound in the body (e.g., heartbeat, lung sounds, bowel sounds).

THE NINETEENTH AND TWENTIETH CENTURIES

Medicine continued to progress rapidly, and the nineteenth century was the beginning of the organized advancement of medical science. Important events during the nineteenth and twentieth centuries include the following:

- Ignaz Semmelweis identified the cause of childbed fever (puerperal fever). Large numbers of women died from this fever after giving birth. Semmelweis noted that the patients of midwives (women who delivered babies but were not physicians) had fewer deaths. One of the differences in the care given by the physicians and the midwives was that the physicians went to the "dead room," where they dissected dead bodies. These physicians did not wash their hands or change their aprons before they delivered babies. Their hands were dirty, and they infected the women. Semmelweis realized what was happening, but other physicians laughed at him. Eventually, his studies were proved correct by others, and handwashing and cleanliness became an accepted practice. Today, handwashing is still one of the most important ways that we control the spread of infection.
- Louis Pasteur discovered that tiny **microorganisms** were everywhere. Through his experiments and studies, he proved that microorganisms cause disease. Before this discovery, doctors thought that microorganisms were *created by* disease. He also discovered that heating milk prevented the growth of bacteria. Pasteurization kills bacteria in milk. We still use this method to treat milk today.
- Joseph Lister learned about Pasteur's discovery that microorganisms cause infection. He used carbolic acid on wounds to kill germs that cause infection. He became the first doctor to use an **antiseptic** during surgery. Using an antiseptic during surgery helped prevent infection in the incision.
- Ernst von Bergmann developed **asepsis.** He knew from Lister's and Pasteur's research that germs caused infections in wounds. He developed a method to keep an area germ-free before and during surgery. This was the beginning of asepsis.

microorganisms
Organisms so small that they can only be seen through a microscope.

antiseptic
Substance that slows or stops the growth of microorganisms.

asepsis
Sterile condition, free from all germs.

■ Robert Koch discovered many disease-causing organisms. He is considered the father of microbiology. He also introduced the importance of cleanliness and sanitation in preventing the spread of disease.

■ Wilhelm Roentgen discovered x-rays in 1895. This discovery allowed doctors to see inside the body and helped them discover what was wrong with the patient.

■ Paul Ehrlich discovered the effect of medicine on disease-causing microorganisms. His treatment was effective against some microorganisms but was not effective in killing other bacteria. His discoveries brought about the use of chemicals to fight disease. In his search to find a chemical to treat syphilis, he completed 606 experiments. On the 606th experiment, he found a treatment that worked.

anesthesia

Loss of feeling or sensation.

Before the nineteenth century, pain was a serious problem. Surgery was performed on patients without **anesthesia.** Early physicians used herbs, hashish, and alcohol to help relieve the pain of surgery. They even choked patients to cause unconsciousness to stop pain. Many patients died from shock and pain. During the nineteenth and twentieth centuries, nitrous oxide (for dental care), ether, and chloroform were discovered. These drugs have the ability to put people into a deep sleep so that they do not experience pain during surgery. The knowledge of asepsis and the ability to prevent pain during surgery are the basis of safe, painless surgery today.

Scientists and physicians learn from the discoveries of the past. They continue to study and research new ways to treat diseases, illness, and injury. Some of the most important discoveries in recent times include the following:

■ Gerhard Domagk discovered sulfonamide compounds. These compounds were the first medications effective in killing bacteria. They changed the practice of medicine by killing deadly diseases.

■ In 1892 in Russia, Dmitri Ivanovski discovered that some diseases are caused by microorganisms that cannot be seen with a microscope. They are called *viruses.* These viruses were not studied until the electron microscope was invented in Germany. These are some of the diseases caused by viruses:

  • Poliomyelitis • Rabies • Measles • Influenza • Chicken pox • German measles • Herpes zoster • Mumps

■ Sigmund Freud (Figure 1.3) discovered the conscious and unconscious parts of the mind. He studied the effects of the unconscious mind on the body. He determined that the mind and body work together. This led to an understanding of psychosomatic illness (physical illness caused by emotional conflict). His studies were the basis of psychology and psychiatry.

■ Alexander Fleming found that penicillin killed life-threatening bacteria. The discovery of penicillin is considered one of the most important discoveries of the twentieth century. Before penicillin was discovered, people died of illnesses that we consider curable today, including pneumonia, gonorrhea, and blood poisoning.

Figure 1.3

Sigmund Freud.

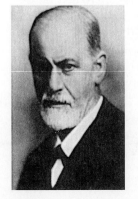

■ Jonas Salk discovered that a dead polio virus would cause immunity to poliomyelitis. This virus paralyzed thousands of adults and children every year. It seemed to attack the most active and athletic people. It was a feared disease, and the discovery of the vaccine saved many people from death or crippling.

■ In contrast to Salk's virus, Albert Sabin used a live polio virus vaccine, which is more effective. This vaccine is used today to immunize babies against this dreaded disease.

The discovery of methods to control whooping cough, diphtheria, measles, tetanus, and smallpox saved many lives. These diseases kill unprotected children and adults. It is important for everyone to be immunized. Immunizations are available from doctors, clinics, hospitals, and public health services.

Our society is discovering new approaches to medical care every year. Patients/clients are being taught more about wellness, and they are learning more about self-care. Family and friends are learning patient care skills, including how to perform detailed procedures. Nurses and technicians are visiting patients/clients at home or caring for them in an ambulatory care setting. Just a few years ago, patients were admitted to the hospital for surgery and recovered in the hospital over a period of several days. Today, many patients enter the hospital, have surgery, and are sent home the same day.

People are living longer and are usually healthier. New inventions and procedures have changed medicine as we once knew it. Here are some examples:

- The possibility of eliminating disabling disease through genetic research
- The ability to transplant organs from a donor to a **recipient**
- The ability to reattach severed body parts
- The use of computers to aid in diagnosis, accurate record keeping, and research
- The ability to use **noninvasive** techniques for diagnosis
- The advancement in caring for the unborn fetus
- The rediscovery and the medical profession's greater acceptance of alternative medicine and complementary medical practice including acupuncture, acupressure, herbal therapy, and healing touch

Every day, science makes new progress. We are living in a time of great advancement and new understanding in medicine. People are living longer, creating a need to better understand **geriatric** medicine. Frontiers in medical science include hope for treatment and eventually cures for: diabetes, cancer, AIDS, multiple sclerosis, arthritis, and muscular dystrophy.

recipient
One who receives.

noninvasive
Not involving penetration of the skin.

geriatric
Pertaining to old age.

⊙ THE ADVANCEMENT OF NURSING

In the nineteenth century, nursing became an important part of medical care. In 1860, Florence Nightingale (1820–1910) attracted well-educated, dedicated women to the Nightingale School of Nursing (Figure 1.4). The graduates from this school raised the standards of nursing, and nursing became a respectable profession. Before this

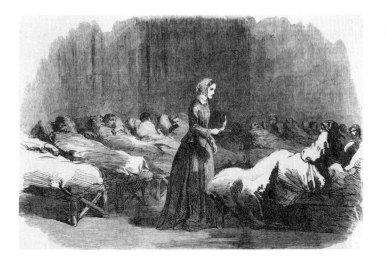

Figure 1.4

Florence Nightingale, founder of modern nursing.

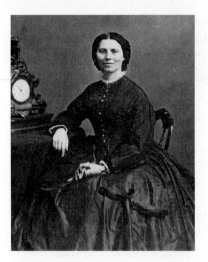

Figure 1.5

Clara Barton, founder of the Red Cross.

time, nursing was considered unsuitable for a respectable lady. The people giving care to patients were among the lowest in society—"too old, too weak, too drunken, too dirty, or too bad to do anything else."

Florence Nightingale came from a cultured, middle-class family who opposed her interest in caring for the ill. However, she convinced her father to give her money to live, and she gained experience by volunteering in hospitals. During the Crimean War, she took a group of 38 women to care for soldiers dying from cholera. More soldiers were dying from cholera than from war injuries. She became a legend while she was there because of her dedication to nursing. After the war she devoted much of her life to preparing reports on the need for better sanitation and construction and management of hospitals. Her primary goal was to gain effective training for nurses. The public established a Nightingale fund to pay for the training, protection, and living costs of nurses. This was established in recognition of her services to the military during the Crimean War. She also designed a hospital ward that improved the environment and care of the patients. Prior to this time, patients were crowded into small areas that were often dirty. The ward that she designed allowed for a limited number of beds, permitted circulation of air, had windows on three sides, and was clean.

During this time, Clara Barton (1821–1912) served as a volunteer nurse in the American Civil War (Figure 1.5). After the war, she established a bureau of records to help search for missing men. She also assisted in the organization of military hospitals in Europe during the Franco-Prussian War. These experiences led her to establish the American Red Cross.

Another step forward in the field of nursing was contributed by Lillian Wald (1867–1940). She was an American public health nurse and social reformer. She established the Henry Street Settlement in New York to bring nursing care into the homes of the poor. This led to the Visiting Nurse Service of New York. Today, visiting nurse services are found in most communities.

● PATIENT CARE TODAY

Nursing care has changed many times throughout the years. Patients have been cared for by teams that included a registered nurse as team leader, a licensed vocational nurse or practical nurse (LVN/LPN) as a medication nurse, and a nursing assistant who provided personal care. In primary care nursing, which followed team nursing, all patient care was provided by a registered nurse. Today, unlicensed assistive caregivers are part of the patient caregiver team. There are many titles and new job descriptions for these positions, including clinical partner, service partner, nurse extender, health care assistant, and patient care assistant. These new positions extend the role of entry-level employees. The nurse assistant performs additional tasks, such as phlebotomy and recording an electrocardiogram (EKG). Employees from departments other than nursing learn patient care skills. Environmental service workers and food service workers may help with serving food and providing some routine patient care. The registered nurse delegates patient care tasks according to the training and expertise of the assistive personnel.

A LOOK BACK AND AN OVERVIEW OF THE FUTURE

In the twentieth century, medicine is making great strides in improving health care. During this century, we experienced many changes, including these:

- Antibiotics for bacterial diseases
- Improved life expectancy
- Organ transplants
- Healthier hearts (reduced smoking, better diets)
- Dentistry without pain
- Childhood immunizations
- Noninvasive diagnosis with computers (CAT, MRI)
- End of smallpox
- Childhood immunizations
- New understanding of DNA and genetics
- Control of diabetes
- Decline in polio

The future of medicine holds many promises for better health. Current and future research will provide us with many new advances, including these:

- Cure for AIDS
- Decrease in the cases of malaria, influenza, leprosy, and African sleeping sickness
- Cure for genetically transferred diseases (e.g., Tay-Sachs, muscular dystrophy, multiple sclerosis, cerebral palsy, Alzheimer's, lupus)
- Improved treatment for arthritis and the common cold
- Isolation of the gene that causes depression
- Use of electronics to allow disabled persons to walk
- Nutritional therapy to decrease the number of cases of schizophrenia

MEDICAL ETHICS

Advancement in medicine creates new problems. How will the recipient of an organ be chosen? Who will be allowed to receive experimental drugs? How will the creation of in vitro embryos be ethically managed? Is it ethical to provide continuing confidentiality about AIDS patients, or should they be required to report their condition? Does a terminally ill patient have the right to assisted death (euthanasia)? There are many questions now, and there will be more questions in the future as health care changes.

SUMMARY

You have learned that the science of health care has grown and developed over the last 5,000 years. These changes increased the average life expectancy. Our standards of living improved with the progress of medical science. The dedication of the many scientists discussed in this unit is responsible for the improvements in health care that we enjoy today. Their research is the foundation of the high technology that is developing in medicine.

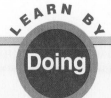

Doing   UNIT 1 ACTIVITY

1. **Complete Worksheets 2 and 3.**
2. **Ask your instructor for directions to complete Worksheets/ Activities 4 through 7.**
3. **When you are confident that you can meet each objective listed above, ask your instructor for the unit evaluation.**

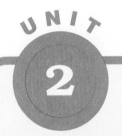

UNIT 2

Health Care Providers

STEPS TO SUCCESS

1. Complete Vocabulary Worksheet 1 before beginning the reading.
2. Read this unit.
3. Complete the Learn by Doing assignment at the end of this unit.

UNIT OBJECTIVES

When you have completed this unit, you will be able to do the following:

✔ Match vocabulary words with their correct meanings.

✔ Write a report on a volunteer agency.

✔ Define *managed care.*

✔ Define *ambulatory care.*

✔ Evaluate how managed care and ambulatory care meet the needs of the changing health care system.

✔ List six types of outpatient care and the type of treatment given.

✔ Define *wellness* and *preventive care.*

UNIT RATIONALE

It is the responsibility of every health care worker to help patients/clients solve their health problems. Since the health care industry has many delivery systems, it is important for future health care workers to be aware of health care agencies and facilities, their delivery systems, their organization, and some of their major services. When you understand how health care facilities and agencies serve the public, you will become a resource person for members of your community.

✔ Contrast the current trends with health care in the twentieth century.

✔ Fill in an organizational chart.

✔ Give two reasons why the organization of health care facilities is important.

✔ Explain a chain of command.

✔ List and define the major services in health care.

✔ Identify two departments in each major service.

facilities

Places designed or built to serve a special function (e.g., hospital, clinic, doctor's office).

 ● **TYPES OF HEALTH CARE PROVIDERS**

There are several **facilities** and agencies that provide medical care. Some are familiar, and others will be new to you. The following descriptions will help you understand the differences among the many providers of medical care (Figure 1.6).

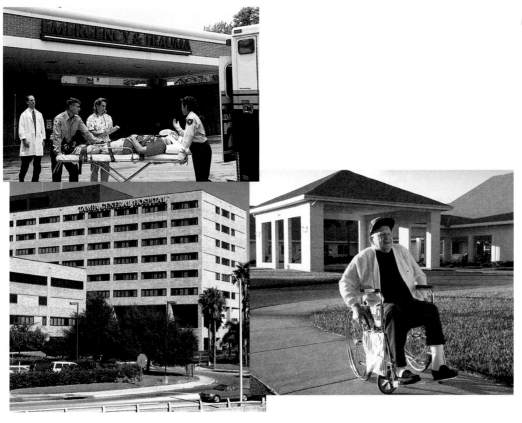

Figure 1.6

Types of providers and the facilities in which they provide care.

General hospitals are facilities where patients are hospitalized for a short time, a few days to a few weeks. They provide a wide range of **diagnostic,** medical, **surgical,** and emergency care services.

Specialty hospitals provide care for specific illnesses, such as **chronic** diseases, **tuberculosis,** and **psychiatric** problems. Patients/clients in these hospitals are generally hospitalized for a long time.

Convalescent care (e.g., nursing home, long-term care) facilities generally care for elderly people needing nursing services and personal care. They also care for physically ill or injured people of all ages who require an extended convalescence for recovery.

Ambulatory care/clinics are facilities where several physicians with different **specialties** combine their practices. This allows the patient/client to have immediate care for many different illnesses.

Physician and dental facilities provide care that promotes wellness and diagnosis of illness. Simple surgery, bone setting, counseling, and administration of drugs also take place here. Physicians and dentists may choose to provide care in an ambulatory care setting.

Rehabilitation centers provide care for patients/clients who require physical therapy, **hydrotherapy,** and other therapies for loss of limb or organ function. They may receive **prosthetics** and learn how to use adaptive devices. Patients may stay in the center or be treated as **outpatients.**

Health maintenance organizations (HMOs) stress wellness (preventive health care). This avoids unnecessary hospitalization and other unnecessary major medical expenses. They provide health services that include hospitalization, basic medical services, **immunizations,** and basic checkups.

Home health care agencies provide care in the home for patients/clients who need health services but not hospitalization. Services include nursing, physical therapy,

diagnostic

Pertaining to the determination of the nature of a disease or injury by examining (e.g., using x-ray and laboratory tests).

surgical

Repairing or removing a body part by cutting.

chronic

Continuing over many years or for a long time (e.g., chronic illness).

tuberculosis

Disease caused by tubercle bacilli; may cause death if untreated.

psychiatric

Pertaining to the mind.

specialties

Fields of study or professional work (e.g., pediatrics, orthopedics, obstetrics).

hydrotherapy

Treatment that uses water therapy for disease or injury.

prosthetics

Artificial parts made for the body (e.g., teeth, feet, legs, arms, hands, eyes, breasts).

outpatients

Patients/clients who do not require hospitalization but are under a physician's care.

immunizations

Substances given to make disease organisms harmless to the patient; may be given orally or by injection (e.g., tetanus, polio).

rehabilitation

Process that helps people who have been disabled by sickness or injury to recover as many of their original abilities for activities of daily living as possible.

communicable

Capable of passing directly or indirectly from one person or thing to another.

maternal

Relating to the mother or from the mother.

licensing

Giving an agency or person permission to carry on certain activities and telling what they may not do as well as what they are authorized to do.

environmental sanitation

Methods used to keep the environment clean and to promote health.

endowments

Gifts of property or money given to a group or organization.

personal care (bathing, dressing, etc.), and homemaking (e.g., housecleaning, food shopping, and cooking). Home health care workers provide care for all ages, from infants to the elderly.

Senior day care provides care for those elderly people who are able to live at home with their families but need care when the family is away. These centers provide a place where the elderly can be cared for during the day. They provide activities, **rehabilitation,** and contact with other people. The elderly are given their medications and are aided in mobility.

The *World Health Organization* is a special agency of the United Nations founded in 1948. It is concerned with world health problems and publishes health information, compiles statistics, and investigates serious health problems worldwide.

Hospices are important in our health care system. They are discussed in this book on page 220.

GOVERNMENT AGENCIES

The federal, state, and local governments provide health services. These services are funded by taxes. They are responsible for giving direct health care, safeguarding our food and water supplies, and promoting health education.

Veterans Administration hospitals are federally supported and provide care for veterans who served in the armed forces.

The *U.S. Public Health Department* is a federal agency that has six major responsibilities:

- Performing research on diseases that kill, handicap, or cripple
- Preventing and treating alcohol and drug abuse
- Preventing and controlling diseases that are transmitted by insects, animals, air, water, and people
- Checking the safety of food and drugs that consumers purchase
- Planning more effective ways to deliver health services
- Making quality care available and affordable by encouraging health personnel to work in underserved areas

State psychiatric hospitals serve the mentally ill.

State university medical centers provide training for health workers, give medical care, and conduct medical research.

State public health services provide health education materials. They are responsible for water and food purity, **communicable** disease control, alcohol and drug abuse control, **maternal** health, and **licensing** of various health agencies.

County hospitals provide care for the ill and injured, especially those patients/clients who require financial help in order to receive care.

Local *public health departments* provide services to local communities—focusing on the reporting of communicable diseases, public health nursing, health education, **environmental sanitation,** and maternal and child health services.

Senior centers have clinics that provide special services for geriatric patients (e.g., podiatry clinic, hypertension clinic, general medical care).

VOLUNTEER AGENCIES

Volunteer organizations receive support from donations, gifts, membership fees, fund-raisers, and **endowments.** They are not supported by the government, and many of the people who work for them are not paid. They raise funds for medical research and for public education about various health problems. Some well-known agencies include these:

- American Cancer Society
- March of Dimes
- American Red Cross
- American Heart Association
- American Diabetes Association
- National Association of Mental Health

All of these agencies and facilities help bring good health to individuals and communities.

MANAGED CARE: QUALITY CARE AND MANAGED COSTS

The managed care provider's goals are to give quality care at reasonable costs. Policies help **ensure** quality care at minimal cost. Some of these policies are discussed here.

Preventive care, such as routine physicals, well-baby care, immunizations, and wellness education, helps keep patients healthy. Wellness education stresses the importance of good nutrition, weight control, exercise, and healthy living practices. Health education programs, wellness centers, weight-control programs, fitness centers, health food distributors, and health care organizations all promote wellness and preventive care. Being healthy helps prevent serious illness and lowers medical costs.

Primary care providers may include family and general practice physicians, internists, nurse practitioners, and physician's assistants. Primary providers care for all routine medical problems. The providers also **refer** patients/clients to specialists.

Specialty care is care given by a provider who is trained in one special area. Specialists usually limit their practice to treating one type of problem. Specializing gives them a broad knowledge of that area. A few specialties are

- Surgery
- Podiatry
- Audiology
- Obstetrics
- Orthopedics
- Chiropractic
- Urology

Emergency care and *urgent care* provide different services. Emergency care is for life-threatening conditions that require hospitalization. Urgent care is for non-emergencies that require prompt treatment. Emergencies requiring hospital care are expensive. Excellent care is available in the urgent care setting, and costs are lower.

The *preadmission authorization requirement for hospitalization* allows necessary hospitalization and prevents unnecessary hospitalization. Good-quality outpatient care is encouraged when possible. Outpatient care is much less expensive, and patients/clients often prefer being in their own homes.

ensure
To make certain.

refer
To send to.

trend

General direction or movement.

familiar

Known.

AMBULATORY CARE

The current **trend** is to develop large managed care organizations that provide good-quality, cost-effective health care. Ambulatory care providers are following managed care concepts. One change keeps patients/clients at home for their care whenever possible. Most patients like to be at home because it is comfortable and **familiar.** It also reduces health care costs. Only the very ill and severely injured are hospitalized. All other patients are cared for in facilities like these:

- Rehabilitation centers
- Outpatient surgery
- Outpatient medical centers/clinics
- Physicians' offices
- Day care

Such facilities provide what is called *ambulatory care.* The patient/client goes to a facility for care and returns home. Some patients also need home health care to help with bathing, range of motion, dressing changes, intravenous therapy, and special treatments.

In ambulatory care there are opportunities for health care workers to use their multidisciplinary skills: For example, a person with an EKG certificate, phlebotomy certificate, or limited radiology certificate is an asset to an ambulatory care organization.

QUALITY HEALTH CARE COSTS AND PAYMENTS

Health Plan Employer Data Information Set

Under the direction of the National Committee for Quality Assurance (NCQA), the Health Plan Employer Data and Information Set (HEDIS) sets guidelines and gives a report card that

- Measures health plan performance
- Helps identify physicians who give high-quality medical care to their patients/ clients
- Helps identify physicians who do not meet the quality care guidelines

Diagnostic-Related Groupings

The federal government passed legislation in 1983 to regulate the price of medical care. This legislation approved the grouping of medical conditions, the reasonable cost for each condition, and its standard treatment. These groupings are known as *diagnostic-related groupings* (DRGs). DRGs help reduce unnecessary procedures and encourage self-care and home care.

Health Insurance: Third-Party Payers

Health care costs, including dental, are so high that most people have some type of insurance plan. These plans are called *third-party payers.* Insurance companies require the subscriber to pay a fee for insurance coverage and in return agree to pay for specific medical and dental care. Each insurance company determines what it will and will not pay for and how much it will pay. The subscriber must pay any fees that the insurance company does not pay.

Health Maintenance Organizations

Health maintenance organizations (HMOs) require members to pay a co-payment, or co-pay, for medical services. The member must get medical care from the physicians, labs, hospitals, and so on that agree to the fee the HMO is willing to pay. If the member gets medical care outside the HMO, he or she will have to pay for the care.

Preferred Provider Organizations

Physician groups and hospitals work together to give comprehensive health care at a reduced cost to various companies. Employees of these companies contract with a preferred provider organization (PPO) and agree to see providers on the PPO list. If they see other providers, they pay a larger fee.

Medicaid

Health insurance is provided by the state and federal government. Benefits and eligibility are different in each state. People who are blind, disabled, or of low income are generally able to get Medicaid insurance.

Medicare

Health insurance is provided to people over the age of 65. Subscribers pay a monthly payment to the Social Security Administration. Some health care providers accept Medicare payments as payment in full for services; others charge more than Medicare pays. To cover the extra costs, many people buy a third-party payer insurance to cover all of their medical costs. There are many programs for Medicare recipients that provide care for a small co-pay.

○ ORGANIZATION

An efficient health care facility must be well organized. An organizational chart shows how each department fits into the system and identifies the line of authority (Figure 1.7). When you look at an organizational chart, you can see who your immediate supervisor is. It tells you the areas of responsibility for all of the employees. The organizational chart also establishes the chain of command.

Chain of Command

The chain of command tells you to whom you take questions, reports, and problems. This is always your immediate supervisor. It is your immediate supervisor's responsibility to resolve any problem that occurs. If your immediate supervisor is unable to find a solution, he or she takes the problem to his or her immediate supervisor. This provides an efficient problem-solving structure. Bypassing a link in the chain causes misunderstanding and is unprofessional.

○ MAJOR SERVICES IN HEALTH CARE

As you can see in Figure 1.7, each service has specialized departments. These departments are determined by the type of service they give:

- *Therapeutic services* provide care over time.
- *Diagnostic services* create a picture of health status.
- *Informational services* document and process information.
- *Environmental services* create a therapeutic and supportive environment.

Services can be organized in several different ways. Your facility's organizational chart is your guideline. To find titles of personnel who are employed in these agencies and facilities, refer to "Overview of Careers" in Chapter 2.

Figure 1.7

Sample organizational chart (relates to the National Health Care Skill Standards, Far West Laboratory).

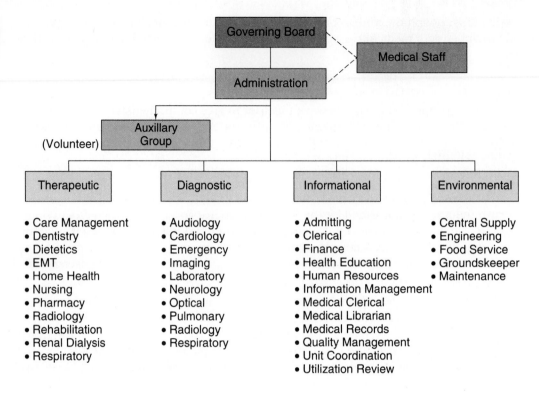

| Governing Board |
| Medical Staff |
| Administration |
| (Volunteer) | Auxillary Group |

Therapeutic
- Care Management
- Dentistry
- Dietetics
- EMT
- Home Health
- Nursing
- Pharmacy
- Radiology
- Rehabilitation
- Renal Dialysis
- Respiratory

Diagnostic
- Audiology
- Cardiology
- Emergency
- Imaging
- Laboratory
- Neurology
- Optical
- Pulmonary
- Radiology
- Respiratory

Informational
- Admitting
- Clerical
- Finance
- Health Education
- Human Resources
- Information Management
- Medical Clerical
- Medical Librarian
- Medical Records
- Quality Management
- Unit Coordination
- Utilization Review

Environmental
- Central Supply
- Engineering
- Food Service
- Groundskeeper
- Maintenance

⊙ SUMMARY

There are many agencies and facilities that help individuals with health problems. They offer a variety of services and are funded in different ways. There are private agencies as well as those funded by federal, state, and local governments. Each agency meets a special need. The current trend in health care is managed care, outpatient care, and ambulatory care. The emphasis is on wellness and preventive care. All facilities and agencies have an organizational chart to help them be more efficient and to establish a chain of command. In health care facilities, there are four services: **therapeutic,** diagnostic, information, and environmental.

therapeutic

Pertaining to the treatment of disease or injury (e.g., physical therapy, radiology, diet, nursing).

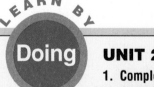

UNIT 2 ACTIVITY

1. **Complete Worksheet 2.**
2. **Ask your instructor for directions to complete Worksheets/ Activities 3 through 5.**
3. **Complete Worksheets 6 and 7.**
4. **When you are confident that you can meet each objective for this unit, ask your instructor for the unit evaluation.**
5. **Prepare responses to each item listed in Chapter Review—Your Link to Success at the end of this chapter.**
6. **Study your worksheets, activities, and unit evaluations in preparation for the chapter evaluation.**

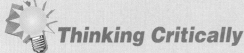

Thinking Critically

1. Legal and Ethical The field of medical ethics is affected by new technology every day. Explain how the legal system is involved in medical matters today. Think about recent medical cases that lawyers have tried.

2. Time Management Make a bar graph plotting a typical day for a nursing assistant in a chosen facility. Work with classmates so that each of you takes a different facility. The bottom line of the graph could represent functions and the vertical line hours. You may draw bars to represent time spent delivering meals, making beds, setting up sitz baths, and so on. Use your graphs to think about how assistants spend their days and what kind of work appeals most to you.

3. Safety Alert Focus on the different service areas of a health care facility: therapeutic, diagnostic, informational, and environmental. In which areas would safety be most important? Think of some examples. Think of the impact these situations have on staff behavior.

4. Case Study A new patient is telling you how upset he is about a change in his insurance. His company changed from private insurance to an HMO. The patient is very agitated and worried because the system is new to him. Why do you think the patient is so agitated? What can you do to reassure him?

Portfolio Connection

Planning and preparing for a career is a process that allows you to look back on your experiences and learn from them. You can evaluate the things in your past that worked for you and those that did not.

You now have an opportunity to create a file that reflects what you learn. This file is called a *vocational portfolio.* Your portfolio will contain documents that show what you have learned during your vocational preparation. Your work will show the abilities and skills you gain throughout your training. You will also create a job search packet that helps you identify ways to share your portfolio with schools or potential employers. Developing your portfolio provides a chance to express the positive results of your learning experiences in a professional manner.

Think about a time when you surprised yourself by accomplishing something that you were not sure you could do. What caused you to try it when you were unsure about it? What went well in that experience? What would you do differently? Explain your answers in a short paper. Your explanation must clearly identify your self-evaluation and show how you would approach uncertain experiences in the future.

This assignment helps you review and evaluate your past experience. Some of the future assignments for your portfolio will require a similar process, with a focus on your vocational training. Turn in this assignment to your instructor. When you create your portfolio in Chapter 2 your teacher will return it to you. Put it in your portfolio in Section Four, "Written Samples."

Portfolio Tip

Remember the wide variety of health care settings in which you could work. Try to collect samples for your portfolio from as many settings as possible (hospital, clinic, doctor's office, home care, etc.) as you continue your studies.

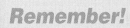

Remember! Media Connection

Use the Companion Website **www.prenhall.com/badasch** and the CD-ROM for additional interactive learning activities.

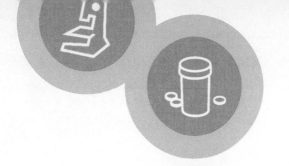

Chapter 2

Finding the Right Occupation for You

MEDIA CONNECTION

Use the Companion Website
www.prenhall.com/badasch and the CD-ROM
for additional interactive learning activities.

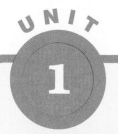

UNIT 1

Career Search

STEPS TO SUCCESS

1. Read this unit.
2. Review the portfolio guidelines and structure on Worksheet 7. Read the Vocational Portfolio packet in the Student Workbook addendum.
3. Complete the Learn by Doing assignment at the end of this unit.

UNIT OBJECTIVES

When you have completed this unit, you will be able to do the following:

✔ Define *interests, values,* and *abilities.*

✔ List five work-related values.

✔ Identify three resources for occupational research.

✔ Research three health careers.

UNIT RATIONALE

When you consider an occupation in the health care field, it is important to focus on your interests, values, and abilities. When you understand yourself, it is easier to select the right occupation. There are many different career opportunities in the health care field. Researching several careers will help you choose the right career for you. Learning how to use the resources for researching occupations will make it easier for you to choose a career.

✔ Explain the importance of a vocational portfolio.

✔ Write a paper titled "What I Learned About Selecting a Career."

INTERESTS

Your interests tell what you like to do and what you do not like to do. Recognizing your interests helps you make a good career choice. For instance, if you like to work alone, a career in direct patient/client care probably is not right for you. Working in one of the computer areas might be better. When you know your interests early in your career search, you can identify careers that use those interests. If you discover that many of the tasks listed in an occupation are not interesting to you, reconsider your choice, and research careers that require your interests.

VALUES

A value is the importance that you place on various elements in your life. Money might be more important to you than leisure time. Working with people might be more important to you than what shift you work. Knowing what values you feel most strongly about helps you avoid **compromising** the things that are most important to you. Recognizing your values also helps you **prioritize** your work-related values, such as job security, leisure time, wages, recognition, creativity, advancement, working environment, home life, responsibility, and management. Ask yourself the following questions.

compromising
Giving up something important.

prioritize
To put in order of importance.

- **Job security.** Is it important that you find a job immediately upon the completion of your training program? How important is job availability?
- **Leisure time.** Is it important for you to have extra time for leisure activities?
- **Wages.** Is an average wage acceptable if you like your work, or is a very high wage necessary?
- **Recognition.** Is it important that the job you choose is respected by the people in your community?
- **Creativity.** Do you like to come up with new ideas to solve problems, or do you prefer a job in which there is exactly one way to do things?
- **Advancement.** Do you want a career that provides opportunities for promotion?
- **Working environment.** Do you prefer to work indoors or outdoors?
- **Home life.** Do you want to work a daytime schedule (9 to 5) with some overtime and with weekends and holidays off, or are you willing to do shift work (all hours, any day of the week)?
- **Responsibility.** Do you want a job that requires you to make a number of decisions?
- **Management.** Do you want to be responsible for supervising the work of other people or for organizing many tasks at once?

All of these factors affect your job choice. Make a list of these work values and put them in order of their importance to you. When you research an occupation, refer to your list so you do not choose a job that conflicts with many of your values.

ABILITIES

An ability is something you do well. You have many abilities. For example, you may work well with your hands, or you may be very good at mathematics. It is much more pleasant to work in an occupation that uses your abilities. If you choose an occupation that is too far below your ability level, you will be bored. If it is too far above your ability level, you will be frustrated. It is important to evaluate your abilities during your career search. List your abilities, and use the list when researching an occupation. Match your abilities to the job description.

RESOURCES FOR OCCUPATIONAL RESEARCH

There are many resources you can use in your research. Two of them are the *Dictionary of Occupational Titles,* which lists job titles, tasks, and duties for 20,000 occupations, and the *Occupational Outlook Handbook,* which discusses the nature of the work, employment outlook, training and qualification requirements, earnings, and working conditions for a variety of occupations. *Work Briefs* by Science Research Associates, the Career Exploratory Kit, the *Encyclopedia of Careers,* and computer programs are also good resources. In addition, check career-related pamphlets, microfilm, and videos. You can find all of these resources in libraries and career centers. Interview individuals who are already working in health care occupations, as well as looking at written materials.

By conducting occupational research, you learn about the tasks performed, the job outlook, the education required, the working environment, and many other things. It requires time and effort to research the occupations that interest you and to prepare for a specific career. However, your efforts allow you to find a job that gives you satisfaction.

◎ HOW TO DO A CAREER SEARCH

1. Choose a health career that interests you. Use the information from the resources listed in this unit and the information in the following unit for your research. Instructions for your research are in the Student Workbook.

2. Interview for information. Interview a worker in the occupation that interests you. Prepare a questionnaire before the interview.

3. Write a paper telling how the occupation you researched matches your interests, abilities, and values.

When you complete your research, you have a guideline to follow that will help you choose an occupation that you enjoy.

◎ DEVELOPING A VOCATIONAL PORTFOLIO

A portfolio is a collection of materials that show the knowledge, abilities, skills, and insights you gain in your search for a career. The purpose in developing a portfolio is to show your mastery of vocational requirements to an employer, a college, or a higher-level training program. You also see your own growth and accomplishments over time. Follow the directions in "Vocational Portfolio" at the back of the Student Workbook to assemble your own portfolio.

Completing this project shows your commitment to a set of values and your ability to plan, organize, and create a product. It provides an opportunity to pursue a specific interest and to meet professionals in health care occupations. This project leads you through planning, evidence of progress, final product, and oral presentations.

◎ SUMMARY

In this unit you learned that it is important to identify and evaluate your work interests, values, and abilities. You learned how to use this information when you choose a career, how to use many resources to research career possibilities, and the importance of developing a vocational portfolio.

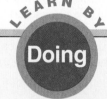

UNIT 1 ACTIVITY

1. **Complete Worksheets/Activities 1 and 2 as assigned.**

2. **Complete Worksheet 3 as assigned.**

3. **Complete Worksheets/Activities 4 through 6 as assigned.**

4. **Read the Vocational Portfolio packet in the addendum of the Student Workbook and complete Worksheet/Activity 7.**

5. **When you are confident that you can meet each objective listed above, ask your instructor for the unit evaluation.**

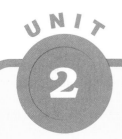

Overview of Careers

STEPS TO SUCCESS

1. Complete Vocabulary Worksheet 1 in the Student Workbook.

2. Read this unit.

3. Complete the Learn by Doing assignment at the end of this unit.

UNIT RATIONALE

There are hundreds of job opportunities in the health care field. The occupations in the four occupational clusters in this unit introduce you to some of the possible health care careers. These occupational clusters follow the National Health Care Skills Standards (see page 16). These standards are a guide to the information you need to be a successful health care worker. Part One of this text provides the health care core foundation skills for all health services that are covered in the national standards. Part Two has entry-level occupations from each cluster in the standards. You can learn the skills from several occupations and become a multidisciplinary/unlicensed assistive personnel health care worker. Finding several areas of interest in the following occupations enhances your education and provides the skills to increase your employability. After carefully researching these careers, you can make an informed decision.

Employment in all of the medical occupations is expected to grow faster than the average for all occupations through the year 2006. Population growth, the increase of middle-aged and elderly people, new medical technology, and the need for more rehabilitation and long-term care make a health care occupation a very good choice for the future.

UNIT OBJECTIVES

When you have completed this unit, you will be able to do the following:

✔ Define the vocabulary words.

✔ Compare and differentiate the services performed by the therapeutic, diagnostic, information, and environmental services.

✔ Define *therapeutic, diagnostic, information,* and *environmental services.*

You learned in Chapter 1 that there are four major health care service areas, each containing many occupations. On the following pages you will study some of the possible occupations in each service and the duties that you might have as an entry-level employee. Remember that the entry-level jobs are the first step in a career ladder or lattice. The career ladder moves upward in your career. The career lattice allows you to use your transferable skills to move into other career areas. Both allow you many choices. The following information is from the *Dictionary of Occupational Titles,* the *Occupational Outlook Handbook,* and *Descriptions and Organizational Analysis for Hospitals and Related Health Services.*

⬤ THERAPEUTIC SERVICES

Therapeutic service workers observe the patient/client, instrumentation, and environment. They report results and assist the treatment team by performing procedures accurately. They also assist in reaching treatment goals.

Respiratory Therapy/Respiratory Care Workers

Every breath is the breath of life, and helping patients/clients with their breathing is a very important part of health care. Patients/clients may live without water for a few days. They may live without food for a few weeks. But without air, they will suffer brain damage within a few minutes and may die after 9 minutes. Respiratory therapy workers and respiratory care practitioners evaluate, treat, and care

Respiratory Technician cleaning and assembling equipment.

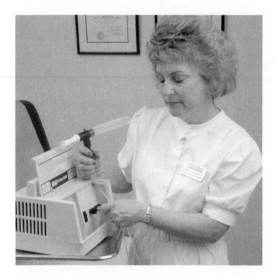

for patients/clients of all ages who have breathing problems. Therapists test lung capacity and check blood for oxygen and carbon dioxide content. They give treatments and teach self-care to patients/clients with chronic respiratory problems. They also give emergency care for drowning, stroke, shock, heart failure, and other emergencies. Other duties may include keeping records and making minor repairs to equipment (Figure 2.1).

Respiratory care workers have many career options (see Career Ladder box) and work in acute hospitals, cardiopulmonary laboratories, ambulatory care units, health maintenance organizations, home health agencies, and nursing homes. They work indoors and may be exposed to flammable gases and body fluids. Their jobs may require shift work and weekend work. They stand for long periods of time and carry or push equipment throughout the facility.

TASKS

- Spend most time taking care of equipment
- Follow tasks under the direction of a respiratory therapist
- Scrub and wash equipment, such as respirators, intermittent positive-pressure breathing machines, pulmonary function machines, and oxygen administration sets
- Inspect equipment for damage, and report problems to supervisor
- Start and test gauges, and notify supervisor of malfunction
- Deliver oxygen tanks and other equipment where needed
- Assist in administration of gas or aerosol therapy as directed
- Record amount of oxygen used by patient/client, and prepare billing forms
- Assist the respiratory technician and therapist as needed

For more information, write
American Association for
Respiratory Care
11030 Ables Lane
Dallas, TX 75229

Pharmacy Workers

Pharmacy workers prepare and dispense medications prescribed by physicians, podiatrists, dentists, and other health care professionals (Figure 2.2). They provide information to health care professionals and to the public about medicines.

Pharmacy worker, preparing medications.

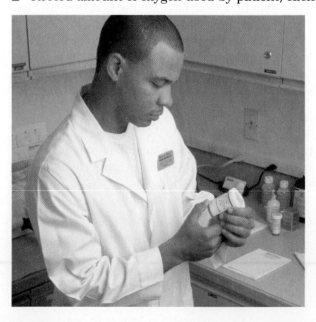

CAREER LADDER   RESPIRATORY THERAPY WORKERS

	Education and/or Experience Required	Average Income
RESPIRATORY THERAPIST (RRT)	• High school diploma or equivalent • Completion of AMA-approved respiratory therapist training program in a community college or a 4-year bachelor's degree program • Registered respiratory therapist (RRT) • Two years of experience in the field following training • Passing grade on a written examination given by the National Board of Respiratory Therapy	• Annual: $32,500–48,000
RESPIRATORY THERAPY TECHNICIAN	• High school diploma or equivalent • Completion of respiratory technician training • Certified respiratory therapy technician (CRTT) • Completion of AMA-approved respiratory therapy technician program • One year of work experience • Passing grade on a written examination given by the National Board of Respiratory Therapy	• Annual: $22,000–28,500

RESPIRATORY THERAPY AIDE	• No educational requirements
	• It is desirable to
	  • Have a high school diploma or the equivalent
	  • Have completed a vocational education program in respiratory therapy
		• Annual: $18,000–21,000

Another important task is to review the medicines that patients/clients are taking. This reduces the chance that the patient/client will have a drug interaction that can cause illness or an allergic reaction. They also help in the strict control of distribution and use of government-controlled products, such as narcotics and barbiturates. Since vaccines and other drugs deteriorate, pharmacy workers are responsible for careful inventory control.

Pharmacy workers have many career options (see Career Ladder box) and work in acute hospitals, community pharmacies, health maintenance organizations, home health agencies, and clinics. A pharmacist may also work for state and local health departments, as well as for pharmaceutical manufacturers. Pharmacy workers work indoors and may be required to work in a restricted environment, such as areas where sterile solutions are prepared. In large hospitals or community pharmacies,

CAREER LADDER   PHARMACY WORKERS

	Education and/or Experience Required	Average Income
PHARMACIST	• Completion of 5 years in an accredited pharmacy program • One year of pharmacy internship • License in state of employment	• Annual: $38,000–80,000
PHARMACY TECHNICIAN	• Two to 12 months of on-the-job training or completion of a 1 to 2-year program in a community college • Some states offer a pharmacy technician certification upon successful completion of an examination	• Annual: $13,500–30,000
PHARMACY CLERK/PHARMACY HELPER	• High school diploma or equivalent • Good typing skills • Two to 3 months of on-the-job training or completion of a pharmacy vocational program	• Annual: $12,500–16,500

they may work in shifts. Their work requires lifting, carrying, pushing items, and climbing ladders in storage areas. They need good vision for close-up work. They stand for long periods of time and must take proper safety precautions when working with products that can be dangerous.

Pharmacy Assistants
TASKS

■ Type labels for medication and records and transactions in the pharmacy log

■ Clip typed labels to medication requests and deliver to the pharmacist

■ Assign prescription numbers

■ List patient's/client's name, physician, and prescription numbers in the log book

■ Copy physician's instructions for use of medication

■ Calculate charges, type billing slips for prescriptions, and enter charges on medication forms

■ Compile periodic reports from log book

■ Mix pharmaceutical preparations using the metric system

■ Label pharmaceutical preparations by using a typewriter, printer, or computer, and maintain records and files

■ Rotate stock to keep dated items current and order supplies

■ Run errands and deliver orders

■ Clean equipment and work areas according to department procedures

- Destroy damaged drugs according to department standards
- Use aseptic techniques, follow procedure for working under purification hood, and wear appropriate clothing and disposable caps

For more information, write
American Association of Colleges
of Pharmacy
1426 Prince Street
Alexandria, VA 22314

Occupational Therapy Workers

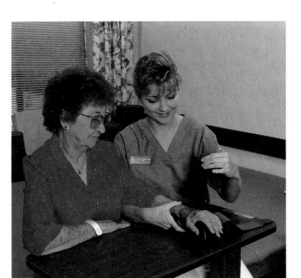

Figure 2.3

Occupational therapy worker applying hand support to prevent contractures.

Occupational therapy workers treat people who are mentally, physically, developmentally, or emotionally disabled (Figure 2.3). They evaluate the self-care, work, and leisure skills of their patients/clients. They plan and develop programs that help restore, develop, and maintain patients' ability to manage the activities of daily living. The goal is to improve clients' quality of life by helping them compensate for their limitations.

Occupational therapy workers have many career options (see Career Ladder box) and work in general hospitals, schools for handicapped children, nursing homes, outpatient clinics, rehabilitation centers, day care centers, mental health agencies, special workshops, health maintenance organizations, and psychiatric hospitals. They work a 40-hour week and may have to work evenings or weekends occasionally. The work environment depends on the type of facility. In a large rehabilitation center, therapists may work in a spacious room equipped with machines, hand tools, and other devices. In a psychiatric hospital, they may work on the ward. They carry and lift equipment and transfer patients from wheelchairs. Their work requires both standing and sitting.

Occupational Therapy Aides/Assistants
TASKS

Occupational Therapy Aides
- Transport patients, assemble equipment, and prepare and maintain work areas
- Perform clerical tasks, restock and order supplies, answer the phone, and schedule appointments

Occupational Therapy Assistants
- Teach work-related skills (e.g., use of power tools)
- Help clients with rehabilitative activities and exercises
- Teach proper method of moving from a wheelchair to bed
- Observe patient activities for progress and make reports to aid in evaluation of patient progress
- Assist in adaptation of equipment, splints, and other self-help devices
- Transport patients
- Store equipment, clean work areas, and help maintain tools and equipment
- Perform other clerical duties (e.g., filing)

CAREER LADDER   OCCUPATIONAL THERAPY WORKERS

	Education and/or Experience Required	Average Income
PHYSIATRIST	● Graduation from an accredited medical school ● License to practice medicine or osteopathy in state of employment ● Residency in physical medicine and rehabilitation	● Annual: $70,000–120,000
OCCUPATIONAL THERAPIST (OT) (OTR REGISTERED)	● Bachelor's degree in occupational therapy (4-year course in an approved program) ● Certification by the Board of Registry of the American Occupational Therapy Association ● Up to 6 months of on-the-job training ● Occupational therapist chief or supervisor	● Annual: $30,500–47,000
CERTIFIED OCCUPATIONAL THERAPY ASSISTANT (COTA)	● High school diploma or equivalent ● Completion of a 2-year program in a community college ● Completion of a certified vocational or technical program ● Supervised fieldwork ● Completion of a 2-year program approved by the American Occupational Therapy Association (AOTA)	● Annual: $13,000–39,000
OCCUPATIONAL THERAPY AIDE	● High school diploma or equivalent ● On-the-job training ● Completion of a vocational education program as an occupational therapy aide	● Annual: $12,000–16,000

For more information, write
American Occupational Therapy Association
Division of Credentialing
4720 Montgomery
PO Box 31220
Bethesda, MD 20824-1220
http://www.aota.org

Physical Therapy Workers

Physical therapy workers (Figure 2.4) help people with injuries or diseases of the muscles, nerves, joints, and bones to overcome their disabilities. The client may be disabled from an accident, a stroke, or a disease. Some of the conditions that require treatment are multiple sclerosis, cerebral palsy, nerve injuries, amputations, fractures, arthritis, and heart disease. Patients vary in age from newborn to aged. Physical therapy workers help the patient regain as close to normal activity as possible.

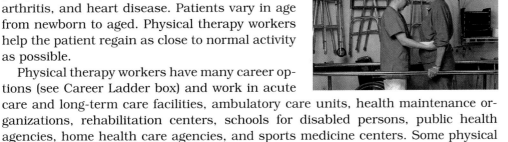

Figure 2.4

One of the many duties of a physical therapy aide is assisting patients/ clients with walking.

Physical therapy workers have many career options (see Career Ladder box) and work in acute care and long-term care facilities, ambulatory care units, health maintenance organizations, rehabilitation centers, schools for disabled persons, public health agencies, home health care agencies, and sports medicine centers. Some physical therapists are in private practice. They contract to work for health care agencies or may have an office where they provide care. They work in specially equipped physical therapy departments, in clinics, and in private homes. Their work requires lifting and carrying up to 50 pounds, stooping, pushing, and pulling patients and equipment. They stand and walk during their shifts.

Physical Therapy Aides/Assistants

TASKS

Physical Therapy Aides

■ Prepare equipment (e.g., hydrotherapy pools, paraffin baths, and hot packs)

■ Assist patients/clients to treatment area using a wheelchair or offering a shoulder to lean on

■ Inform therapist or assistant if patients/clients are having difficulty with their treatment

■ Change linen on beds and tables

CAREER LADDER PHYSICAL THERAPY WORKERS

	Education and/or Experience Required	Average Income
PHYSICAL THERAPIST	● Four-year degree in physical therapy ● Supervised 4-month clinical internship ● Passing grade on a state licensure examination	● Annual: $26,000–73,000
PHYSICAL THERAPY ASSISTANT	● Training requirements are not uniform ● Twenty-four states require graduation from an accredited community college ● Students may be required to pass a written licensure examination	● Annual: $15,600–25,000
PHYSICAL THERAPY AIDE	● High school diploma or equivalent (preferred) ● On-the-job training ● Completion of a vocational education program as a physical therapy aide	● Annual: $13,000–24,000

- Clean equipment and work area
- Inventory materials and supplies
- Assist with clerical tasks

Physical Therapy Assistants

- Apply heat, cold, and ultrasound
- Massage and perform therapeutic exercises

For more information, write
American Physical Therapy Association
1111 North Fairfax Street
Alexandria, VA 22314-1488
http://www.apta.org

Emergency Medical Service Workers

First responders are often the first trained people to treat patients/clients. They provide emergency medical care before emergency medical technicians (EMTs) reach the scene. They may be law enforcement officers, members of the fire service, company employees, or private citizens.

Emergency medical technicians are providers of prehospital medical care in an emergency. A heart attack, unscheduled birth, automobile accident, or near drowning all require immediate attention. The EMT administers basic life support and transports sick and injured people to medical facilities (Figure 2.5).

Emergency medical service workers have many career opportunities (see Career Ladder box) and may work in rescue, police, and fire departments, ski patrols, hospital emergency departments, and private ambulance services. They must usually work shifts and weekends. They work inside and outside in all weather conditions. They may be exposed to body fluids.

Emergency medical service workers must be in good physical condition. For example, they must have good eyesight, hearing, and speech. They must also be able to lift heavy loads, reach, stoop, and climb as the job requires.

First Responders/Emergency Medical Technicians
TASKS

First Responders

- Gain access to patient, assess patient, provide appropriate care, and report assessment and care given
- Lift or move patient to a safe place if necessary

Figure 2.5	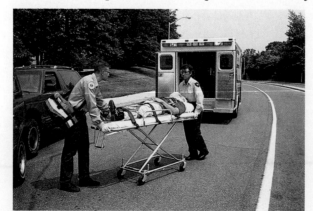
EMTs transporting an injured or sick patient to a medical facility.	

Emergency Medical Technicians/A (Basic)

- Drive an ambulance
- Determine the nature of the victim's illness or injury
- Give appropriate care

• Open and maintain the airway • Restore breathing • Control bleeding • Treat for shock • Immobilize fractures • Bandage wounds • Assist

CAREER LADDER   EMERGENCY MEDICAL SERVICE WORKERS

	Education and/or Experience Required	Average Income

REGISTERED EMT-PARAMEDIC	• Completion of EMT-paramedic training in an approved program offered by one of the following:
	  • Vocational school
	  • State educational facility
	  • Community college
	  • Hospital
	  • Medical school
	  • University
	• Six months of field experience as an EMT-paramedic
	• Passing grade on a written and practical examination given by the National Registry of Emergency Medical Technicians or the state emergency medical systems board
		• Annual: $29,000–40,000

REGISTERED EMT-AMBULANCE/ I (INTERMEDIATE)	• Graduation from an approved EMT Basic program and 35–55 hours of additional instruction • Passing grade on a written and practical examination given by the National Registry of Emergency Medical Technicians or the state emergency medical systems board	• Annual: $29,000–35,000
BASIC EMT-AMBULANCE/ A (BASIC) (EMT)	• At least 18 years of age • High school diploma or equivalent • Valid driver's license • Completion of a minimum 110-hour program offered in vocational programs • Passing grade on a written and practical exam given by the National Registry of Emergency Medical Technicians or the state emergency medical systems board	• Annual: $18,600–23,000

with childbirth • Give initial care to poison and burn victims • Use automated external defibrillators

■ Use correct equipment and techniques to remove trapped victims safely

■ Transport patients to hospital

  • Place patient on stretcher • Constantly watch patient while in transport
  • Notify hospital of arrival

■ Report to the emergency staff observations of and care given to the victim

■ Maintain clean, well-equipped ambulance

■ Ensure ambulance is in good running order

　• Check gas, oil, tire pressure, siren, communication equipment

For more information, write
National Association of Emergency Medical Technicians
408 Monroe
Clinton, MS 39056

National Registry of Emergency Medical Technicians
PO Box 29233
Columbus, OH 43229

Medical Assistants

Medical assistants are responsible for the efficient operation of a physician's office. They also work in clinics, health maintenance organizations, and ambulatory care units. Medical assistants have varied duties. Some specialize in back office procedures (Figure 2.6), while others choose to work in the front office. They work indoors in a clean environment, 40 hours a week, and some weekends. They have varied job opportunities, (see Career Ladder box) and their work requires standing on their feet most of the day (back office), lifting, reaching, and helping patients/clients. They may be exposed to body fluids. The front office worker sits at a desk for long periods.

The current trend toward large medical groups has relocated administrative/front office responsibilities. Billing, insurance verification, medical records, appointment scheduling, and payroll have been relocated to departments that specialize in handling work for the increased number of patients/clients. See "Administrative Support Service Workers" later in this unit for more information.

Medical Assistants

TASKS

Administrative/Front Office Medical Assistants

■ Greet patients/clients

■ Answer phones

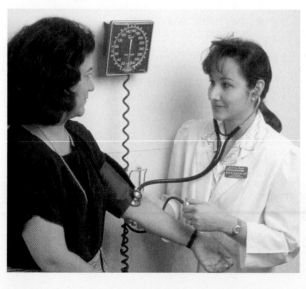

Figure 2.6

A back office medical assistant performing one of many duties—taking a client's blood pressure.

■ Handle mail

■ Make appointments

■ Arrange hospital admissions

■ Arrange for laboratory services

■ Prepare insurance forms (e.g., Medicare, medical insurance, workers' compensation)

■ Type medical reports

■ Maintain patient files

■ May handle billing and receipts

■ Prepare payroll for office staff

CAREER LADDER   MEDICAL ASSISTANTS

	Education and/or Experience Required	Average Income

OFFICE MANAGER	• Completion of administrative and clinical medical assistant program
	  • Workshops
	  • Seminars
	  • Home study courses
		• Annual: $20,000–34,000

CLINICAL/BACK OFFICE MEDICAL ASSISTANT	• High school diploma or equivalent • On-the-job training in a physician's front office • Completion of an administrative medical assistant program • Completion of an examination by the American Association of Medical Assistants, which offers a certified medical assistant (CMA) certificate (optional)	• Annual: $16,500–27,000
ADMINISTRATIVE/FRONT OFFICE MEDICAL ASSISTANT	• High school diploma or equivalent • On-the-job training in a physician's back office • Completion of an administrative medical assistant program	• Annual: $16,500–27,000

Clinical/Back Office Medical Assistants Tasks vary according to state law.

■ Sterilize instruments using an autoclave

■ Prepare clients for examination

■ Assist physician during examination

■ Give injections

■ Take and record temperatures, pulse, respiration, and blood pressure

■ Measure height and weight

■ Perform routine urinalysis

■ Collect blood samples

■ Perform simple blood tests

■ Record electrocardiograms

■ Assist with minor surgery

■ Direct patients in preparation for x-rays and tests

■ Instruct patients about medication and special diets

For more information, write
American Association of Medical Assistants
20 North Wacker Drive, Suite 1575
Chicago, IL 60606-2903

Figure 2.7

A dental assistant performing one of many tasks—assisting the dentist.

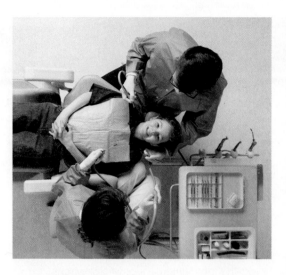

Dental Workers

Dental workers (Figure 2.7) are responsible for maintaining oral health and repairing dental abnormalities. They emphasize treatment and prevention of problems associated with the hard and soft tissues of the mouth.

According to their level of education, dental workers have many different opportunities. They work in private practices, dental schools, hospital dental departments, private clinics, health maintenance organizations, and state and local public health departments (see Career Ladder box). Dental laboratory technicians work in a dental laboratory. Dental workers work indoors in a clean environment. They are subject to respiratory infections due to close contact with patients and may be exposed to body fluid. Their work requires standing most of the day, reaching, and handling dental instruments, equipment, and supplies.

Dental Assistants
TASKS

- Make the patient comfortable in the dental chair
- Prepare the client for treatment
- Hand the dentist proper instruments and materials
- Suction the patient's mouth
- Prepare materials for making impressions and restorations
- Take and process dental x-rays
- Teach oral health (e.g., flossing, brushing, postoperative care)
- Prepare instruments for sterilizing
- Make casts of teeth and mouth from impressions taken by the dentist
- Apply medications to the teeth and oral tissue, remove cement used in the filling process, and place rubber dams on the teeth (in some states)
- May manage the office (e.g., make appointments, keep treatment records, send bills, receive payments, and order supplies and materials)

For more information, write
Commission on Dental Accreditation, American Dental Association
211 East Chicago Avenue, Suite 1814
Chicago, IL 60611
http://www.ada.org

National Association of Health Career Schools
750 First Street NE, Suite 940
Washington, DC 20005
FAX: (202) 842-1565
E-mail: NAHCS@aol.com

American Dental Assistants' Association
203 North Lasalle, Suite 1320
Chicago, IL 60601

CAREER LADDER DENTAL WORKERS

	Education and/or Experience Required	Average Income
DENTIST	• Graduation from a dental school approved by the American Dental Association • Passing grade on written and practical examinations • State licensure by passing written examinations given by the National Board of Examiners	• Annual: $109,000–200,000
DENTAL HYGIENIST	• Graduation from an accredited dental hygienist program in a 2-year community college, a 4-year bachelor's degree program, or a 5-year master's degree program • Passing grade on a written and clinical examination • License in the state of employment (given by the National Board of Dental Examiners)	• Annual: $27,500–57,000
DENTAL LABORATORY TECHNICIAN	• High school diploma or equivalent • Two-year vocational program • On-the-job training (3 to 4 years) • May become certified by passing a written and practical examination given by the National Board for Certification	• Annual: $23,000–50,000
DENTAL ASSISTANT	• High school diploma or equivalent • On-the-job training • Completion of a 1- or 2-year community college or vocational training program • Completion of an examination by the Certifying Board of the Dental Assisting National Board (CDA) (optional)	• Annual: $14,700–24,000

Nursing Service Workers

Nursing service workers provide many varied and essential services (Figure 2.8). They care for patients who are physically ill or disabled and provide preventive care (e.g., immunizations). They work in industries, community health nursing, general hospitals, long-term care facilities, government agencies, schools, educational institutions, visiting nurse associations, clinics, physicians' offices, ambulatory care units, homes, and health maintenance organizations. Nurses work indoors. They may have rotating shifts and work on weekends. Their work requires standing,

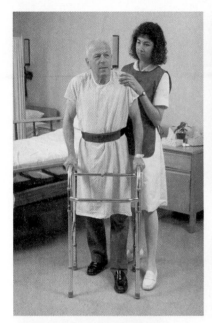 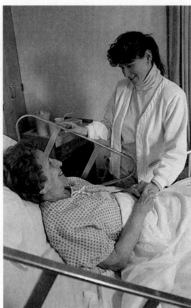 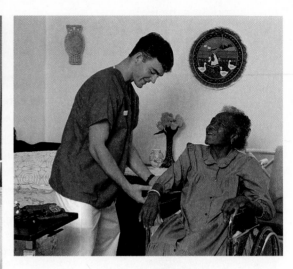

Figure 2.8

Nurse assistants (a and b) and home health aide (c) helping clients.

walking, lifting, and pushing patients, carts, and wheelchairs. They are exposed to unpleasant odors and body fluids.

Nurse Assistants/Home Health Aides

Home health aides care for patients/clients in their homes instead of in a health facility. They care for patients of all ages who need more care than their families can give. Their job requires them to go to different homes. Nurse assistants and home health aides stand, walk, and lift patients and may push wheelchairs. They may be exposed to body fluids. They have many career options (see Career Ladder box) ranging from nurse assistant to director of nursing.

TASKS
Nurse Assistants
- Answer patient/client call lights
- Bathe patients
- Dress and undress clients
- Assist with personal hygiene (e.g., shaving, hair care, oral care, and dental care)
- Serve and collect food trays and feed patients who need help
- Provide between-meal nourishment and fresh drinking water
- Transport patients in wheelchair or stretcher or help patients walk
- Take and record temperature, pulse, and respiration and record blood pressure
- Record food and liquid intake and output
- May apply ice bags or heat packs
- Give back rubs, if appropriate
- Observe and report any unusual conditions

CAREER LADDER NURSING SERVICE WORKERS

	Education and/or Experience Required	Average Income
NURSE PRACTITIONER	• All requirements for becoming a registered nurse • Completion of an accredited course in nurse practitioner training • License for the state of employment	• Annual: $57,000–76,800
REGISTERED NURSE	• High school diploma or equivalent • Graduation from a 2-year community college • Graduation from a 4-year college or university • Graduation from an accredited school of nursing • Graduation from a diploma school (3-year hospital schools are being phased out) • License for the state of employment	• Annual: $24,500–64,000 $53,000–90,000 with advanced education
LICENSED VOCATIONAL NURSE (LVN)/LICENSED PRACTICAL NURSE (LPN)	• High school diploma or equivalent • Graduation from a recognized 1-year program • License for the state of employment	• Annual: $20,200–35,000
UNLICENSED ASSISTIVE PERSONNEL	• Additional training in specialty (e.g., EKG, phlebotomy) • Preservice training (40–120 hours) provided by an employing agency • May require certification as a nurse assistant	• Annual: $18,000–26,000
HOME HEALTH AIDE	• High school diploma or equivalent (preferred) • Completion of a vocational education program as a home health aide • State certification may be required	• Annual: $18,000–26,000
NURSE ASSISTANT/ GERIATRIC AIDE	• High school diploma or equivalent (preferred) • Hospital-conducted on-the-job training • Completion of an OBRA-approved 1987 Omnibus Budget Reconciliation Act nurse assistant program	• Annual: $12,500–20,800

- Tidy clients' rooms, change bed linen, and collect soiled linen
- Write in patients' charts

Home Health Aides

- Transfer patients from place to place and assist with bathing, walking, and pre-scribed exercises
- Assist with medication routines
- Help with braces or artificial limbs
- Check and record pulse, respiration, and blood pressure
- Change nonsterile dressings
- Provide emotional support and take client outside home as a companion
- Change bed linen, clean laundry, and clean clients' living quarters
- Shop for patients' food and prepare meals
- Report findings and observations to supervisors
- Act as a companion on shopping trips, doctor visits, and outdoor activities

For more information, write
National Association of Health Career Schools
750 First Street NE, Suite 940
Washington, DC 20002
FAX: (202) 842-1565
E-mail: NAHCS@aol.com

National Association for Home Care
228 Seventh Street SE
Washington, DC 20003

Veterinary Workers

Veterinary assistant animal caregivers usually care for small animals such as dogs and cats. They provide basic care such as feeding, grooming, cleaning cages, exer-cising animals, providing companionship, and observing animals for behavioral changes that can indicate an illness or injury. Other positions in animal care in-clude working with horses, zoo animals, and laboratory animals used for research.

Animal care workers have many career opportunities (see Career Ladder box). They may work in kennels, animal shelters, veterinary hospitals and clinics, stables, laboratories, aquariums, and zoological parks. Job titles and duties vary by em-ployment setting. In some positions shift work may be required because the animals need 24-hour care. The work environment depends on the type of facility. Some ken-nels have outdoor animal runs; veterinary offices have exam and treatment rooms. Concern for and interest in animals may cause emotional upsets due to witnessing the results of abuse or having to **euthanize** the animal. The work can be physically demanding. You may have to lift large bags of food and the work can involve kneel-ing, bending, crawling, and restraining of animals. There is also a chance of injury due to bites and scratches. Odors can be unpleasant.

TASKS

Animal Caretaker/Assistant

- Keep constant eye on condition of animals in their charge
- Watch animals recover from surgery
- Check dressing

euthanize

To painlessly end the life or permit the death of a hopelessly sick or injured animal or individual for reasons of mercy.

CAREER LADDER VETERINARY WORKERS

	Education and/or Experience Required	Average Income
VETERINARIAN (DVM OR VMD)	• Completion of 3–4 years of preveterinary college • Graduation from an accredited veterinary college and a Doctor of Veterinary Medicine degree • License in state of employment	• Annual: $36,000–128,000
ANIMAL HEALTH TECHNICIAN (ATR REGISTERED)	• Completion of certificate or associate's degree • Registration, certification, or licensure required in many states	• Annual: $14,200–28,700
VETERINARIAN ANIMAL CARETAKER/ASSISTANT	• High school diploma or equivalent • On-the-job training • Home study through American Boarding Kennels Association (ABKA) • Passing grade on oral and written exam to become ABKA Certified Kennel Operator (CKO)	• Annual: $11,200–20,000
GROOMER	• Completion of 6–10 weeks of informal apprenticeship • Four to 18 weeks at a state-licensed grooming school • Completion of National Dog Groomers Association of America written and practical skills exam	• Annual: $11,200–20,000

- Observe animals' overall attitude
- Notify doctor of anything out of the ordinary
- Maintain sanitary conditions

Kennel Staff
- Clean cages and dog runs
- Fill food and water dishes
- Exercise animals

Experienced Attendants
- Provide basic animal health care
- Bathe animals
- Trim nails
- Attend to other grooming needs

■ Sell pet food and supplies

■ Assist in obedience training

■ Help with breeding

■ Prepare animals for snipping

Groomers

■ Do initial brush-out

■ Clip hair with electric clippers, cobs, and grooming shears

■ Cut nails

■ Clean ears

■ Bathe

■ Blow-dry animal

■ Do final clipping and styling

Groomer/Owners

■ Operate own grooming business

■ Answer telephones

■ Schedule appointments

■ Discuss pets' grooming needs

■ Collect information on pets' disposition

■ Collect information on pets' veterinarian

■ Inspect and report medical problems such as skin or ear infection

For more information, write
The Humane Society of the United States
2100 Street NW
Washington, DC 20037-1598
http://www.hsus.org

◉ DIAGNOSTIC SERVICES

Diagnostic service workers help with the diagnosis of illness and disease. Some diagnostic service workers have direct contact with the patient/client, whereas others do not. They plan services and prepare and perform tests accurately. They also understand quality control and report results in a timely manner.

Medical Laboratory Workers

Medical laboratory workers (Figure 2.9) perform many varied tests. Some of these tests are highly technical, whereas others are not as technical. In many cases, tests are performed on computerized equipment. Medical laboratory workers determine changes

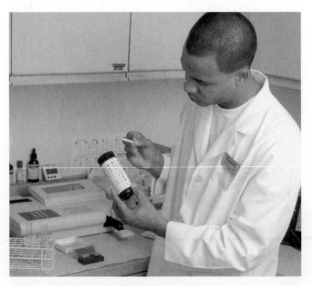

Figure 2.9

One of the many duties of a medical laboratory aide is reading reagent strips.

that have occurred in the blood, urine, lymph, and body tissues. They identify increases or decreases in white or red blood cells, cross-match blood for transfusions, identify microscopic changes in cells, and determine the presence of parasites, viruses, or bacteria in the blood, tissue, or urine. These tests help the physician make an accurate diagnosis and correctly treat the patient.

Medical laboratory workers have many career opportunities (see Career Ladder box). They work for acute care hospitals, private laboratories, physicians' offices, clinics, ambulatory care units, health maintenance organizations, public health agencies, pharmaceutical firms, and research institutions. Their work requires a lot of walking, standing, reaching, stooping, lifting, and carrying of equipment. In addition, they need good eyesight for close work. They work indoors and may be exposed to unpleasant odors and body fluids and have frequent contact with water and cleaning solutions. Their jobs often require them to work shifts and weekends.

CAREER LADDER — MEDICAL LABORATORY WORKERS

	Education and/or Experience Required	Average Income
MEDICAL PATHOLOGIST	● Graduation from a medical school approved by the Council on Medical Education and Hospitals of the American Medical Association ● State license to practice medicine or osteopathy ● Certification by the American Board of Pathology	● Annual: $70,000–120,000

MEDICAL LABORATORY SUPERVISOR, ADMINISTRATOR, OR CHIEF PATHOLOGIST, HISTOLOGIST, CYTOLOGIST	● Several years of experience as a medical technologist
	● Graduate education in one of the following:
	  • Biological sciences
	  • Chemistry
	  • Management
		● Annual: $70,000–120,000

MEDICAL LABORATORY TECHNOLOGIST	● Graduate of 4-year medical technology program in college or university ● Graduate of 4-year medical technology program and certification (CMT) ● Successful completion of a written examination prepared by the Board of Registry of the American Society of Clinical Pathologists, Medical Technologists ● Registered medical technologist (RMT) ● Successful completion of a written examination prepared by the International Society of Clinical Laboratory Technology	● Annual: $32,500–45,000

CAREER LADDER

MEDICAL LABORATORY WORKERS (cont.)

	Education and/or Experience Required	Average Income
MEDICAL LABORATORY TECHNICIAN	• Two years of training in a community college, 4-year college or university, or vocational/technical school • Two years of training in a laboratory technician program • Successful completion of requirements for certification (CLT) established by the National Certification Agency for Medical Laboratory Personnel	• Annual: $23,500–30,00
MEDICAL LABORATORY ASSISTANT BLOOD AND PLASMA	• High school diploma or equivalent • Completion of an approved 12-month medical laboratory technician certificate program in a community college, vocational school, or private program	• Annual: $12,500–24,500
MEDICAL PHLEBOTOMIST	• High school graduate or equivalent • Ten to 20-hour certification program in a hospital, physician's office, or laboratory • Completion of a vocational education program as a phlebotomist	• Annual: $15,500–23,000
MEDICAL LABORATORY AIDE	• High school diploma or equivalent • On-the-job training for at least 2 months • Completion of a vocational education program as a laboratory aide	• Annual: $12,500–15,500

Medical Laboratory Aides/Phlebotomists

TASKS

Medical Laboratory Aides

■ Clean laboratory equipment

■ Prepare cleaning solutions

■ Dry glassware and instruments using a cloth, hot-air dryer, or acetone bath

■ Examine clean equipment for cracks or chips and store equipment properly

■ Operate an autoclave to sterilize equipment

■ Prepare stains, solutions, and culture media following appropriate procedures

Phlebotomists/Venipuncture Technicians

■ Draw blood from patients for testing by the technician or technologist

For more information, write
American Society of Blood Banks
8101 Glenbrook Road
Bethesda, MD 20814-2749

For more information, write
International Society for Clinical Laboratory Technology
917 Locust Street, Suite 1100
St. Louis, MO 63101-1413

Board of Certified Laboratory Assistants
9500 South California Avenue
Evergreen Park, IL 60642

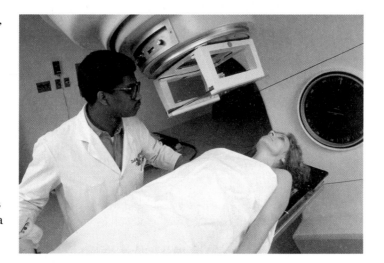

Figure 2.10

A radiologic technologist preparing to take an x-ray of a patient.

Radiology Workers

Radiology workers operate x-ray equipment to take pictures of the internal parts of the body (Figure 2.10). The x-rays provide information for the diagnosis and treatment of patients. For example, x-rays of the chest help detect lung diseases, such as lung cancer and tuberculosis. Some of the diseases or injuries that x-rays help diagnose or treat are ulcers, blood clots, cancer, and fractures. The use of imaging techniques like ultrasound and magnetic resonance imaging (MRI) is growing. The term *diagnostic imaging* includes these procedures as well as x-ray techniques.

Radiology workers have a variety of job opportunities (see Career Ladder box) and may work in general hospitals, physicians' offices, trauma centers, chiropractic offices, private consulting offices, clinics, federal and state agencies, public school systems, health maintenance organizations, and ambulatory care facilities. They work indoors and may be in confined areas. They wear protective gloves, aprons, and film badges because the hazards of radiation are present. Shift work and evening work may be part of their schedule. Their work requires the lifting and positioning of patients, standing during most of the shift, and pushing mobile equipment. They may be exposed to body fluids.

The career ladder in the radiology field does not have an aide or assistant position. The following information is included in this book because radiology is an important career for you to consider. Some facilities use transport aides in radiology. Being a transport aide in a radiology department allows you to learn about the radiology department.

Diagnostic Medical Sonographers

Diagnostic medical sonographers use diagnostic ultrasound under the supervision of a physician. They are also called *ultrasound technologists.* They use equipment to transmit sound waves at high frequencies into the patient's body, resulting in an image viewed on a screen and automatically recorded on a printout strip or video. The use of ultrasound is important in prenatal care and for cardiology.

Sonographers work in acute care hospitals, in clinics, and sometimes with a group of obstetrics specialists. They work five-day weeks and generally have weekends and evenings off.

For more information, write
American Society of Radiologic Technologists
15000 Central Avenue SE
Albuquerque, NM 87123-3917

CAREER LADDER

RADIOLOGY WORKERS

	Education and/or Experience Required	Average Income
RADIOLOGIST	● Graduation from an accredited medical school ● License to practice medicine in the state of employment ● Three years of special training in radiology recognized and approved by the board and by the Council on Medical Education and Hospitals of the American Medical Association	● Annual: $70,000–120,000
RADIOLOGIC TECHNOLOGIST/ SONOGRAPHER/ULTRASOUND RADIOLOGIC TECHNOLOGIST CHIEF	● Graduation from an accredited program ● Bachelor's degree in radiologic technology ● Experience in 2 or more radiologic disciplines (e.g., nuclear medicine, radiation therapy) ● Should be registered as a radiologic technologist through the American Registry of Radiologic Technologies (ARRT)	● Annual: $25,000–50,000
DIAGNOSTIC MEDICAL TECHNOLOGIST	● High school diploma or equivalent ● One-year certificate program ● No experience in health occupation	● Annual: $24,800–34,900

American Registry of Radiologic Technologists
1255 Northland Drive
Mendota, MN 55120

Society of Diagnostic Medical Sonographers
12770 Coit Road, Suite 708
Dallas, TX 75251

Electrocardiography Workers

Electrocardiographic Technicians

Electrocardiography workers operate an EKG machine to record the electrical changes that occur during a heartbeat (Figure 2.11). These recordings help physicians diagnose any irregularities or changes in the patient's heartbeat. These tests are done routinely after a certain age, before surgery, and as a diagnostic tool. EKG technicians also apply Holter monitors. EKG technicians have many job opportunities (see Career Ladder box) and work in acute care hospitals, clinics, private physicians' offices, health maintenance organizations, and ambulatory care facilities. They work indoors and may work shifts, evenings, and weekends. They spend a lot of their time standing and walking.

TASKS

- Escort client to treatment room
- Take portable equipment to patient's room
- Explain the test procedure
- Help client remove necessary clothing
- Paste or attach electrodes to correct areas on patient's chest, arms, legs; connect leads from EKG machine to electrodes; and operate selector switch on EKG machine
- Reposition chest electrodes to record various positions
- Check recording for accuracy (leads placed incorrectly give an incorrect reading)
- Recognize significant deviations from normal heartbeat and report immediately
- Edit and mount final results
- Send copy of graph to the physician
- Maintain EKG records

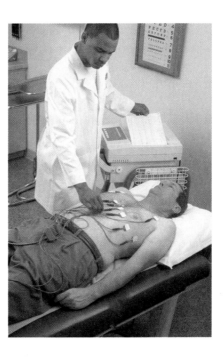

Figure 2.11

An EKG technician performing an electrocardiogram.

CAREER LADDER — ELECTROCARDIOGRAPHY WORKERS

	Education and/or Experience Required	Average Income
CARDIOLOGIST	• Graduation from an accredited school of medicine • One-year internship • One- to 2-year residency in internal medicine • One to 2 years of clinical fellowship in cardiology • Passing grades on examinations for board certification in cardiology	• Annual: $70,000–200,000
CARDIOVASCULAR TECHNOLOGIST	• Completion of a 2-year community college program in cardiovascular technology • Completion of a 4-year college or university program	• Annual: $23,000–40,000
EKG TECHNICIAN	• High school diploma or equivalent • One to 6 months of on-the-job training • Completion of a vocational education program as an EKG technician • One to 2 years of study at a community college	• Annual: $17,000–27,000

- Type physician's diagnosis
- Care for equipment by cleaning electrodes and keeping all equipment well supplied with paper, etc.
- Conduct vectorcardiograms (multidimensional traces), stress testing (exercise tests), and pulse recordings
- Apply Holter monitoring (12- to 24-hour recording of an EKG)

For more information, write
National Society for Cardiovascular Technology
120 Falcon Drive, Suite 3
Fredericksburg, VA 22408

Electroneurodiagnostic Technologists

Electroneurodiagnostic (END) technologists use computers to record electrical impulses transmitted by the brain and the nervous system. They perform several different neurological tests including electroencephalograms (EEGs), evoked potentials (EPs), nerve conduction studies (NCSs), polysomnographs (PSG/sleep studies), and surgical monitoring. EEGs assist in the diagnosis of various brain disorders such as seizures, stroke, head trauma, and brain tumors. EPs are performed on patients with possible multiple sclerosis, brainstem tumors, and spinal cord problems. NCSs evaluate peripheral nervous system problems such as carpal tunnel syndrome. Sleep studies are performed on patients to diagnose sleep disorders such as sleep apnea and narcolepsy. The brain, nerves and/or muscles can be monitored by END technologists during various brain and spinal cord surgeries. END technologists take medical histories, apply electrodes for the procedure being performed, record electrical impulses from the central and peripheral nervous systems, maintain equipment, and interact with patients to reduce anxiety during tests. END technologists have many job opportunities (see Career Ladder box). They work in hospitals, neurologist's and neurosurgeon's offices, sleep centers, and psychiatric facilities. Some positions may require on-call duty, and sleep disorder technologists usually work evenings and nights.

TASKS

- Take medical histories
- Apply electrodes to designated spots
- Record and monitor the patient's waveforms on a computer
- Interact with neurologists and other health care staff

CAREER LADDER — ELECTRONEURODIAGNOSTIC TECHNOLOGIST

	Education and/or Experience Required	Average Income
ELECTRONEURODIAGNOSTIC TECHNOLOGIST	• Graduation from an accredited 2-year associate's degree END program • Experience running END procedures • Registration in one or more of the five END areas by the American Board of Electroencephalographic and Evoked Potential Technologists	• Annual: $26,610–38,500

- Write technical reports (possibly)
- Keep records
- Schedule appointments
- Order supplies
- Maintain equipment

For more information, write
Executive Office, American Society of Electroneurodiagnostic Technologists
204 West Seventh Street
Carroll, IA 51401
http://www.aset.org

Association of Polysomnographic Technology
2025 South Washington, Suite 300
Lansing, MI 48910-0817

Joint Review Committee on Electroneurodiagnostic Technology
Route 1, Box 63A
Genoa, WI 54632

American Board of Registration of Electroencephalographic and Evoked Potential
Technologists
PO Box 916633
Longwood, FL 32791-6633

American Association of Electrodiagnostic Technologists
35 Hallett Lane
Chatham, MA 02633-2408

INFORMATION SERVICES

Information service workers are an important support to all other medical services. These workers analyze, **extract,** and document information using automated systems. They understand the sources, routes, and flow of information within the health care environment.

extract

Identify and take out or emphasize.

Administrative Support Service Workers

Administrative support service workers (medical clerical workers) handle complaints, interpret and explain policies or regulations, prepare payrolls, resolve billing disputes, and collect delinquent accounts. They are responsible for the everyday situations that medical organizations must deal with smoothly and efficiently to maintain business operations and good customer service. The following list of occupations are included in administrative support services. See Chapter 19 for more detailed information on these services.

- Claim representative
- Insurance processor or enrollment clerk
- Billing and account collector
- Clerical worker
- Computer or data processor
- Receptionist
- Appointment scheduler
- Material/supply and distribution clerk or purchasing clerk

- Payroll and timekeeping clerk
- Personnel clerk
- Secretary or word processor
- Telephone operator

Admitting Department Workers

Admitting department workers are responsible for the admitting and discharging of patients. They interview patients/clients for information necessary for accurate record keeping (Figure 2.12). The workers in the admitting department are usually the first hospital employees that the patient sees. Employees in this department help the patient feel confident about the hospital and the care that they will receive.

Admitting workers have a variety of job opportunities (see Career Ladder box) and work in an acute care hospital. They may assist with lifting patients and carrying their belongings. They may also push wheelchairs or stretchers. Their work is in an office environment and requires sitting and reaching. They may work shifts and evenings.

Admitting Clerks
TASKS

- Interview incoming patients/clients and record information required for admission
- Assign rooms
- Prepare identification band
- Explain hospital rules and policies
- Store patients' valuables in hospital safe and arrange escort to room
- Send admitting forms to appropriate departments
- Prepare daily census and preadmission forms and arrange transfers
- May act as cashier and receptionist (depending on the size of the facility)
- Use a computer for records

For more information, write
American Hospital Association
840 North Lake Shore Drive
Chicago, IL 60611

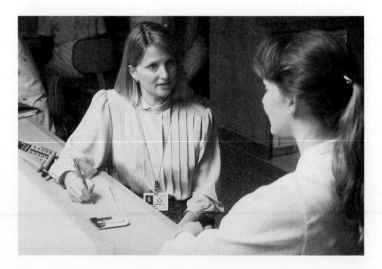

Figure 2.12

One of the many duties of an admitting clerk is interviewing patients/clients.

CAREER LADDER — ADMITTING DEPARTMENT WORKERS

	Education and/or Experience Required	Average Income
ADMITTING OFFICER	• High school diploma or equivalent • Bachelor's degree • Two to three months of on-the-job training • One to 2 years of experience working in a health care facility (may be required)	• Annual: $15,500–27,000
ADMITTING CLERK	• High school diploma or equivalent • Computer skills • One to 2 months of on-the-job training	• Annual: $11,000–21,500

Medical Records/Health Information Management Workers

Medical records/health information management workers keep permanent records that describe the patient's condition and the treatment that he or she receives.

Physicians and allied health personnel use medical records to provide care for the patients. Medical records are also legal documents that can be used in a court of law. Insurance companies use the records to determine what they will pay for the patient's care. Records are used in medical research, as well.

Medical records must be accurate and carefully filed (Figure 2.13). Medical records/ health information management workers have many job opportunities (see Career Ladder box) and are employed by acute care hospitals, long-term care hospitals, public health departments, manufacturers of medical record systems, and insurance companies.

Medical records/health information management specialists may have a private practice as a consultant. Their work requires frequent reaching and stretching for files, long periods of time at a desk, and some lifting of records.

Medical Records/Health Information Management Clerks

TASKS

- File and pull medical records
- Maintain a sign-out system for records
- Update index file of patients and check for prior records of newly admitted clients
- File cards according to established system and file medical records by numerical system
- Answer routine staff requests for information about patients
- Gather statistics for state health department
- Transcribe reports of operations, x-rays, and laboratory examinations

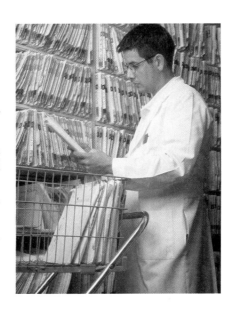

Figure 2.13

One of the many duties of a medical records/health information management file clerk is filing and pulling medical records.

CAREER LADDER
MEDICAL RECORDS/HEALTH INFORMATION MANAGEMENT WORKERS

	Education and/or Experience Required	Average Income
REGISTERED MEDICAL RECORDS ADMINISTRATOR (RRA)	• Bachelor's degree from an accredited college program • Passing grade on the certification examination given by the American Health Information Management Association	• Annual: $30,200–48,000
MEDICAL RECORDS TECHNICIAN (ART REGISTERED)	• Graduation from a program accredited by the American Health Information Management Association (AHIMA) or the AHIMA Independent Study Program and a passing grade on the AHIMA certification exam	• Annual: $21,000–31,200
MEDICAL TRANSCRIPTIONIST	• High school diploma or equivalent • On-the-job training • Completion of a vocational education program in the area of medical transcriptionist • Completion of a correspondence course	• Annual: $14,000–30,000
MEDICAL RECORDS/HEALTH INFORMATION MANAGEMENT CLERK	• High school diploma or equivalent • Typing and filing skills • Knowledge of office methods and medical terminology • Three to 6 months of on-the-job training • Completion of a vocational education program in the area of medical records clerk	• Annual: $10,000–18,000
MEDICAL RECORDS/HEALTH INFORMATION MANAGEMENT FILE CLERK	• High school diploma or equivalent preferred • On-the-job training • Completion of a vocational education program in the area of admitting file clerk	• Annual: $10,000–18,000

For more information, write
American Health Information Management Association
919 North Michigan Avenue, Suite 1400
Chicago, IL 60611-1683
http://www.ahima.org

Unit Secretaries and Health Unit Coordinators

Unit secretaries and health unit coordinators are responsible for clerical, reception, and communication duties in the nursing unit. One of their main duties is to transcribe physicians' orders. Health unit coordinators are essential to the nursing units, as they relieve the nursing staff of many duties. This gives the nurses more time to devote to patient care.

Health unit coordinators have various career options (see Career Ladder box) and may be employed in acute care hospitals, long-term care facilities, and clinics. Their work is indoors in a clean environment. They may work shifts and weekends. Their work requires sitting at a desk for long periods of time, frequent telephoning, and reaching for and handling charts.

Health Unit Coordinators

TASKS

- Transcribe physicians' orders
- Prepare and compile records, including patient's name, address, and names of attending physicians
- Copy information into charts, including patients' temperature, pulse, respiration rate, and blood pressure
- Prepare requisitions for laboratory tests (e.g., special procedures, diagnostic tests, pharmaceutical orders)
- Order necessary supplies for the client
- Answer patients' call lights and send appropriate person for request
- Provide physicians with clients' charts, check charts for new orders, and keep charts up-to-date
- Use a computer if applicable

For more information, write
National Association of Health Unit Clerks/Coordinators
709 West Seldon Lane
Phoenix, AZ 85021

CAREER LADDER — HEALTH UNIT COORDINATORS

	Education and/or Experience Required	Average Income
MANAGER OF HEALTH UNIT COORDINATORS	● High school diploma or equivalent ● Associate's degree from a community college in unit management as a health unit coordinator	● Annual: $14,000–23,000
UNIT SECRETARY/HEALTH UNIT COORDINATOR	● High school diploma or equivalent ● Community college ● Hospital training program ● Completion of a vocational education program in the area of unit secretary or health unit coordinator	● Annual: $10,900–19,000

Figure 2.14

A central supply worker loading an autoclave.

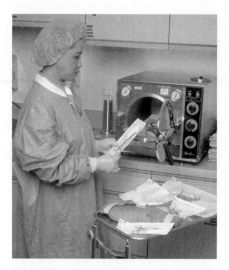

⊙ ENVIRONMENTAL SERVICES

Environmental service workers provide a therapeutic environment for the delivery of care. They repair and maintain medical and general equipment, follow aseptic procedures, and ensure high-quality food.

Central Processing/ Supply Workers

Central processing/supply workers supply various departments with equipment and materials (Figure 2.14). The equipment must be in working condition. Malfunctioning equipment is life threatening. The workers keep an inventory of supplies and equipment. Supplies and equipment are properly packaged, cleaned, and sterilized. The workers in this department are key members of the health care team. Other health care workers cannot give necessary care without proper tools. Central processing/supply workers work in acute care hospitals and large outpatient clinics. The department is often in a basement or at the rear of the building. Lifting and moving articles and equipment are required. The workers stand on their feet for long periods of time and may be exposed to body fluids. See Career Ladder box for career opportunities.

Central Processing/Supply Technicians
TASKS

- Use solutions to scrub and wash surgical instruments, containers, syringes, and equipment
- Sterilize articles (e.g., instruments, equipment, linens) using the steam autoclave, gas autoclave, or antiseptic solution
- Prepare packs of supplies, instruments, dressings, and treatment trays; carefully wrap, label, and seal each pack
- Store and inventory prepared articles, supplies, and equipment

CAREER LADDER — CENTRAL PROCESSING/SUPPLY WORKERS

	Education and/or Experience Required	Average Income
TECHNICIAN	● High school diploma or equivalent ● On-the-job training (3 to 6 months) ● Completion of a vocational education program as a central supply technician	● Annual: $10,500–18,300
CHIEF TECHNICIAN	● On-the-job experience	● Annual: $12,500–22,000

■ Fill requisitions (gathering supplies and equipment as requested) and post charges

■ Check expiration dates on sterilized materials

For more information, write
American Hospital Association
840 North Lake Shore Drive
Chicago, IL 60611

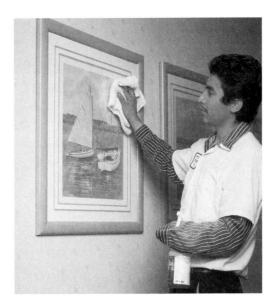

Figure 2.15

A housekeeping attendant cleaning public areas, one of housekeeping's many duties.

Hospital Cleaners (House-keepers)/Environmental Services Technicians

Housekeepers are responsible for the cleanliness of the environment (Figure 2.15). Cleanliness helps prevent the spread of infection and creates a more pleasant environment for patients/clients, staff, and visitors.

Hospital cleaners (housekeepers)/environmental service workers have many job opportunities (see Career Ladder box) and work in long-term care facilities, acute hospitals, and clinics. They have frequent contact with water and cleaning solutions. They walk, stand, and stoop during their shift. They also push and pull equipment, climb on ladders when necessary, and may be exposed to body fluids. Their hours may include shift work and weekend work.

Hospital Cleaners/Housekeeping Attendants
TASKS

■ Load service cart

■ Clean assigned areas (e.g., rooms, offices, laboratories)

■ Dust, vacuum, and clean blinds, floors, furniture, and equipment

■ Polish floors using a buffing machine

■ Wash walls, ceilings, windows

■ Empty ashtrays and trash

■ Scour sinks, tubs, and mirrors

■ Disinfect bedsprings and unit equipment

■ Replenish soap and towels

■ Replace cubicle curtains and soiled draperies

■ Report malfunctioning equipment

■ Move furniture, equipment, and supplies and turn mattresses

For more information, write
Institute of Sanitation Management
1710 Drew Street
Clearwater, FL 33515

National Executive Housekeepers Association
204 Business and Professional Building
Second Avenue
Gallipolis, OH 45631

CAREER LADDER   HOUSEKEEPING WORKERS

	Education and/or Experience Required	Average Income
DIRECTOR OF HOUSEKEEPING SERVICES	● High school diploma or equivalent ● College degree in housekeeping management or completion of courses in housekeeping and institutional management ● Experience in the housekeeping department	● Annual: $18,000–40,000
HOUSEKEEPING CREW LEADER/SUPERVISOR	● High school diploma or equivalent ● Completion of courses in hospital housekeeping and institutional management ● One to 4 months of on-the-job training ● Up to 2 years of experience as a housekeeping attendant ● Completion of a vocational education program	● Annual: $12,000–23,000
HOUSEKEEPING AIDE/ATTENDANT	● One to 3 months on-the-job training ● Completion of a vocational education program	● Annual: $10,900–18,750

Food Service Department Workers

Food service workers are responsible for providing nutritional care to clients. They plan special and balanced diets. They also distribute menus, prepare food trays, and deliver food to the patients throughout the hospital (Figure 2.16).

Food service workers have many career options (see Career Ladder box) and may work in acute care hospitals and in long-term care facilities. They generally work 40 hours a week and may work in shifts. The areas might be very warm, with much activity in a relatively small area. Some lifting, reaching, moving of equipment, and occasional bending are required. They walk and stand most of the shift.

Food Service Workers
TASKS

■ Prepare and deliver food trays to patients/clients

■ Read color-coded menu cards to determine appropriate items to place on trays

■ Measure food servings according to diet list; prepare individual servings of salad, desserts, sandwiches

■ Prepare foods for soft or liquid diets using a blender

■ Check trays for accuracy and completeness, push food tray carts to client floors, and serve trays to patients (according to hospital policy)

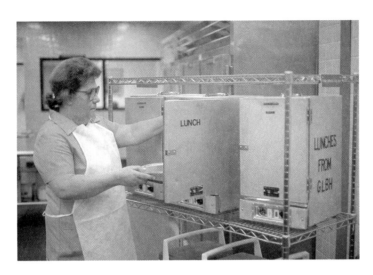

Figure 2.16

One of the many duties of a food service worker is preparing meals.

- Return food tray carts to kitchen
- Clean work area, wrap silverware, and restock condiments for tray line

For more information, write
American Dietetic Association
216 West Jackson Boulevard, Suite 800
Chicago, IL 60606-6995
http://www.eatright.org

CAREER LADDER   FOOD SERVICE DEPARTMENT WORKERS

	Education and/or Experience Required	Average Income
ADMINISTRATIVE DIETITIAN	• Must be a registered dietitian • Graduate study credits in institutional or business administration	• Annual: $40,000–60,000
REGISTERED DIETITIAN	• Bachelor's degree with a major in foods and nutrition or institutional management • Six- to 12-month internship in a dietary department	• Annual: $35,300–45,000
DIETETIC INTERN	• Bachelor's degree with a major in foods and nutrition or institutional management	• Annual: $20,000–31,000
DIETETIC TECHNICIAN	• Completion of a dietetic technician program in a community college	• Annual: $15,000–24,000
FOOD SERVICE WORKER/DIETETIC AIDE	• On-the-job training • Completion of a vocational education program as a food service worker	• Annual: $12,000–16,400

American Home Economics Association
2010 Massachusetts Avenue NW
Washington, DC 20036

ADDITIONAL HEALTH CARE AREAS

There are many other positions in the health care area. You may use the skills that you have learned in Unit 1 to do a career search for other areas that interest you. Here are some suggestions for you to consider in the health-related field:

Dental Occupations

- Dental ceramist

Medical Practitioners

- Chiropractor
- Ophthalmologist
- Optometrist
- Osteopath
- Physician (all specialties)
- Physician's assistant
- Veterinarian

Medical Technologists, Technicians, Assistants, and Aides

- Artificial plastic-eye maker
- Audiometrist
- Cardiopulmonary technician
- Chiropractor
- Contact lens technician
- Cytotechnologist
- Dialysis technician
- Electroencephalographic (EEG) technologist
- Heart-lung machine operator/perfusionist
- Mental health worker
- Mental retardation assistant
- Operating room technician
- Orthopedic technician
- Orthotist
- Physician's assistant
- Prosthetic aide
- Psychiatric aide
- Surgical technician/assistant
- Transporter
- Ultrasound technologist/sonographer

Nursing Occupations

- Licensed psychiatric aide
- Midwife
- Nurse anesthetist
- Nurse practitioner

Therapy and Rehabilitation Occupations

- Alcoholic rehabilitation center attendant
- Audiologist
- Dance therapist
- Kinesiotherapist
- Music therapist
- Recreation therapist
- Speech pathologist

Other Health-Related Occupations

- Clinical engineer and biomedical equipment technician
- Director of volunteer services
- Dispensing optician
- Funeral director
- Grounds maintenance and facilities worker
- Health service administrator
- Insurance clerk
- Medical illustrator
- Medical writer
- Morgue attendant/embalmist
- Nursing home administrator
- Orthodontist
- Prosthetist
- Social service worker
- Speech pathologist
- Transporter

○ SUMMARY

In this unit, you reviewed many health occupations. You learned that each occupation has different tasks and different educational requirements. You also learned that different occupations require different traits in the worker. With this information, you can evaluate an occupation before you research it carefully. Use the information in Unit 1 to research any occupational area.

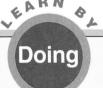

UNIT 2 ACTIVITY

1. Complete Worksheets 2 and 3 as assigned.
2. Complete Worksheet/Activity 4.
3. Prepare responses to each item listed in Chapter Review—Your Link to Success at the end of this chapter.
4. When you are confident that you can meet each objective listed above, ask your instructor for the unit evaluation.

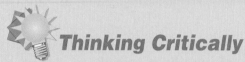

Thinking Critically

1. **Communication** How does your ability to communicate affect those around you? What are you doing to increase your ability to communicate effectively?

2. **Time Management** Many health occupation careers require staff to be willing to work shifts covering 7 days a week, 24 hours a day. Think of your present lifestyle and the life you hope to lead in the future. Plot a chart of when you would be willing to work on a daily and weekly basis, year-round. File this in a private, personal area of your portfolio to look at when you are considering specific careers and jobs. Update this document if your thinking changes.

3. **Legal and Ethical** Give an example of each of the following:
   a. Legal considerations that relate to becoming a health care worker
   b. Ethical dilemmas that a health care worker may face

4. **Cultural Competency** Cultures throughout our communities are very different. In the health care environment, we also experience a variety of cultures. Identify the ser-

vices and departments that require workers to have the ability to interact effectively with people from other cultures. Explain your reasoning.

5. **Computer Tip** If you have access to a computer, consider keeping an electronic portfolio as well as a hard copy version. You may create folders for different topics and save the portfolio to a disk if it is not your personal computer. Doing this will save space and paper and give you important practice in using a computer.

6. **Case Study** Glenda needs to find a good job as soon as she graduates. She is unsure about how to find the right career. She must earn enough to pay for an apartment, a car, living expenses, and leisure activities. She wants a position that is well respected, provides a clean environment, and offers potential for professional growth. She enjoys working with people and feels really good when she is able to help others. List the steps Glenda should take to help her identify the best career options for her.

Portfolio Connection

The following provides a guideline for creating the structure of your portfolio. When you are done you can add and exchange documents as you complete them. Keeping your file current shows your organizational skills and provides you immediate access to materials that reflect the positive results of your learning. To create your portfolio, follow the instructions on Worksheet 7 of your Student Workbook. You must acquire a three-ring notebook, three-ring pocket inserts, and tab dividers. Label each tab with the following:

Portfolio

- Title page
- Table of contents
- Letter of introduction
- Résumé
- Letter(s) of recommendation
- Advanced training or college requirements
- Certificates/licenses
- Skills check-off sheets
- Practical experience evaluation
- Evaluation of paid or unpaid time working in your vocation

Portfolio Tip

File portfolio items as soon as you complete them.

- Written reports and assignments in your vocation area
- Personal tips and reminders
- Final portfolio checklist

Once your portfolio file is organized, it is ready for your work samples. Add work evaluations from current or previous jobs and keep this file in a place that is easy to access.

In the personal section of the portfolio add any advice or insights that will help you in your career. Be sure that this section can be removed before the portfolio is given to a prospective employer.

Ask your instructor to help you seek a job shadowing opportunity in one health occupation of your choice. Complete a job sharing contract (Worksheet/Activity 4) after you are assigned a time, place, and person to shadow.

Write a report as described in the Vocational Portfolio in the addendum of the Student Workbook.

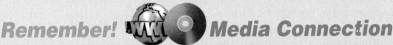

Remember! **Media Connection**

Use the Companion Website **www.prenhall.com/badasch** and the CD-ROM for additional interactive learning activities.

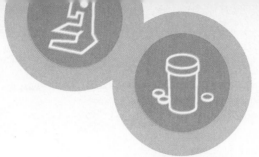

Medical Ethics and Law

Chapter 3

MEDIA CONNECTION

Use the Companion Website
www.prenhall.com/badasch and the CD-ROM
for additional interactive learning activities.

UNIT 1

Ethical Roles and Responsibilities of a Health Care Worker

STEPS TO SUCCESS

1. Complete Vocabulary Worksheet 1 in the Student Workbook.
2. Read this unit.
3. Complete the Learn by Doing assignment at the end of this unit.

UNIT OBJECTIVES

When you have completed this unit, you will be able to do the following:

✔ Match vocabulary words with their correct meanings.

✔ Summarize the code of ethics that every health care worker follows.

✔ Explain why following a code of ethics is important.

✔ Use the value indicators to explain the employee's responsibilities to his or her employer.

UNIT RATIONALE

Members of the health care team must be aware of their ethical roles and responsibilities. This awareness protects them, the patients, their co-workers, and the facility where they work. Ethical behavior ensures quality patient care, positive work relationships, and a well-managed workplace environment.

✔ Explain how each health care worker affects the health care team.

✔ Demonstrate communication objectives that promote patient satisfaction.

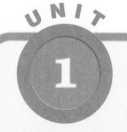 **VALUE INDICATORS**

Quality health care workers show a commitment to certain values. Health care workers are expected to live by values that show others respect. You show respect by treating others with dignity, demonstrating a spirit of service, performing your duties with excellence, and treating others with fairness/justice. Each person determines how values are reflected in his or her day-to-day actions. An employer describes what values are important and how to reflect them while working (Figure 3.1). These de-

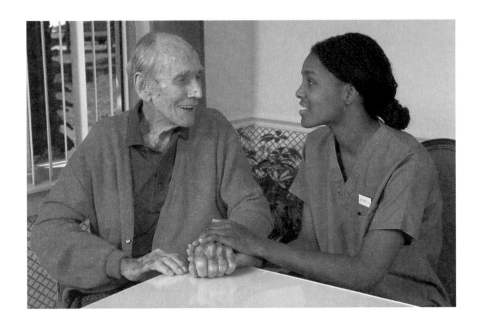

Figure 3.1

Values are reflected in your body language and your verbal responses.

scriptions are usually found in an employee handbook or policy and procedure book. The values below are discussed in many parts of this text. As you read about these values in this book write your thoughts in a diary, describing other attitudes and actions that reflect parts of the four values. To understand your values and to become a values-based health care worker see the *self-reflection exercise* in the Portfolio Connection at the end of this chapter. The following is a brief description of the values we will focus on throughout this book.

■ **Dignity.** You treat people with dignity when you are honest, truthful, trustworthy, sincere and respectful of others. Always do what is needed to the best of your abilities and ask for assistance when tasks are beyond your understanding or ability. Dignity is communicated through listening actively, being positive, showing understanding, and respecting all people.

■ **Service.** Service means responding to patients/clients and co-workers with an understanding of their unique needs. You show kindness and patience. Service also means making comments that are positive, courteous, and helpful.

■ **Excellence.** Performance excellence is taking responsibility for yourself, your team's decisions, and the results. You adapt to changing needs by learning new skills, knowledge, and behaviors that encourage continuous improvement. Accepting and seeking feedback help you improve your performance excellence.

■ **Fairness/Justice.** You treat all people with mutual respect and provide the same dignity, service, and performance excellence regardless of the patient's race, beliefs, ethnic background, or

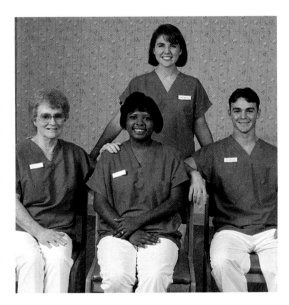

Figure 3.2

Good grooming is important.

Table 3.1 ▪ Code of Ethics

Ethics is a code of conduct representing ideal behavior for a group of people. A health care worker observes the following code of **ethics.**

Dignity	Service	Excellence	Fairness/Justice
Know your limitations. Know what you are trained to do and what you are capable of doing.	*Be a good citizen.* Respond to the needs of others. Demonstrate concern for meeting those needs.	*Be accountable.* Seek out and use feedback from others to learn. Take responsibility for yourself and for your team's actions, decisions, and results.	*Be loyal* to patients/clients, co-workers, and your employer. Always **project** a positive attitude toward the institution where you are employed.
Be sincere. Always be honest and trustworthy in the performance of your duties. Expect your salary in return for your work. Do not solicit gifts or additional money.	*Be caring.* Try to understand the unique needs of others. Respond quickly and effectively to problems that arise while you are working.	*Be informed.* Learn from your experiences. Seek growth and development opportunities for yourself and others.	*Respect the privacy of others.* Always keep privileged information about any personal or private matter **confidential.**
Be well groomed. Always clean your uniform, shoes, hair, nails, skin, teeth, and body to prevent the spread of disease-causing bacteria. Be sure your uniform is free of wrinkles, tears, and runs. All buttons must match. Shoes and laces must be clean and bright. Wear a name tag. This helps people you work with know you and your title. It is required in most states. Do not wear excessive jewelry. It harbors bacteria and can cause you or your patients injury. Wedding rings and watches are acceptable. Never wear perfume or aftershave lotion. They make some people who are ill feel even worse and may trigger an allergic reaction.		*Follow the rules and regulations.* Read the policy manual. Read the procedure manual. Practice Standard Precautions and the Bloodborne Pathogen Rule.	

ethics 🔊
Social values, conduct, description of what is right and wrong.

project 🔊
To show or reflect.

confidential 🔊
Private, personal, restricted, secret.

appropriate
Suitable, correct.

financial resources. You also use supplies and available resources effectively to provide **appropriate** care and a safe environment for everyone.

Health care workers reveal their core values and qualities in everything that they do. Tables 3.1 and 3.2 outline your responsibilities within each of the key value indicators for health care.

● PATIENT OR CUSTOMER SATISFACTION

Patient and customer satisfaction is an essential element in providing effective health care. Demonstrating the values of service and excellence helps patients, their families, and their friends feel satisfied with their care. Satisfaction does not always

Table 3.2 ■ Responsibilities of an Employee

Employees are required to assume certain responsibilities. The responsibilities that are most important to employers include being dependable, honest, and well groomed (Figure 3.1); displaying a good attitude; and following the rules and regulations of the organization.

Dignity	Service	Excellence	Fairness/Justice
Communicate effectively. Express ideas, information, and viewpoints clearly. Use active listening skills, and seek to understand others. Create and maintain positive working relationships. Understand and respect differences in people. Be supportive of others' success when they do well.	*Have a good attitude.* Be willing to help your co-workers. Be aware of your body language and facial expressions, and reflect a positive outlook. Be respectful by changing your behavior when it appears to irritate others. Work effectively under pressure.	*Be dependable.* Be on time. Report in when you arrive. Report to the person taking care of your assignment prior to leaving your area. Do your job to the best of your ability. Call your supervisor ahead of time on those few occasions when you are unable to be at work.	*Be honest.* Never clock in or out for another person. Never take anything from the facility that is not yours. Never say that you have completed a task when you have not. Work with commitment and enthusiasm to improve the care patients/clients receive.

mean that people get what they want, however. It does mean that they receive the very best care available and that the care is given with respect and with a sincere attitude. It also means that each patient/client is fully informed about the service provided by being told:

- What is needed
- Why it's needed
- Who will provide the service
- When it will be provided
- How it will be provided

Health care workers who successfully provide patient/client satisfaction practice the service guidelines outlined in Table 3.3.

Table 3.3 ■ Patient and Customer Satisfaction Guidelines

Communication Objective	Service/Excellence	Behavior
Demonstrate open, honest, and respectful communication. Present ideas, information, and viewpoints clearly, both verbally and in writing. Listen actively and seek to understand others.	Welcome patients, family members, and visitors in a warm, friendly manner.	Introduce yourself to the patient and his or her family. Address the patient by Mr. or Ms. unless directed otherwise. Make eye contact and smile. Explain who you are and what you do. Listen. Wear your name badge. Adhere to the dress code.
	Listen to and communicate with one another and the people you serve.	Listen attentively. Do not interrupt. Make eye contact. Clarify with more questions if necessary. Address the person's needs and take whatever action is necessary.

Table 3.3 ■ (cont.)

Communication Objective	Service/Excellence	Behavior
		Do not argue. Try to eliminate distractions when communicating with patients and families. Communicate clearly and positively. Make sure patients understand their treatment or procedures. Encourage patients to ask questions.
	Have respect for each person's privacy, comfort, and dignity.	Respect patient confidentiality in all settings. Keep noise and conversation levels low. Interview patients in private. Close curtains and doors during exams and procedures. Remember to care for the whole person—body, mind, and spirit.
Anticipate and strive to understand the unique needs of those serving as well as those served. Respond to the needs of those served and demonstrate concern for meeting those needs. Tailor each interaction to the specific needs of the person and/or situation.	Use good elevator manners.	Use the elevator as an opportunity to make a favorable impression. Be friendly. Remember confidentiality—do not discuss patients, their care, or any business on elevators. Once on an elevator, make room for others and push the door open button for them. Stand aside as others enter or exit.
	Provide a safe, clean environment.	Be alert to unsafe conditions. Correct, warn and/or report safety hazards for immediate repair. Pick up and dispose of litter. Keep all areas neat, orderly, and clutter-free.
	Anticipate the wants and needs of those served.	Be aware and sensitive to the different cultures and religious beliefs of patients. Communicate any anticipated delays. Be prepared to address special needs, such as hearing impairments, language barriers, and disabilities. Focus on education, comfort, and privacy needs at all times. Anticipate and provide appropriate comfort measures.
Seek growth and developmental opportunities for yourself and others. Adapt to changing needs by acquiring new skills, knowledge, and behaviors. Learn from your experiences.	Strive to do your best.	Identify better ways to serve patients and their families. Be a role model. Promote cooperation and teamwork. Take opportunities to improve your skills. Seek out and constructively use feedback from others. Show appreciation and thank your co-workers.

THE TEAM CONCEPT

Quality health care depends on every health care worker's doing his or her part. Each member is an important part of the **interdisciplinary** team. Professionals with different backgrounds, different education, and different interests all work together to provide appropriate quality care.

The registered nurse (RN) **delegates** duties to a team of licensed and unlicensed assistive personnel. The RN determines what tasks the members of the interdisciplinary team are assigned. The RN oversees health care workers from various departments and trains them to provide patient care and effectively delegates by using *the five rights of delegation:*

- **Right task.** Identifying an appropriate caregiver-patient relationship.
- **Right circumstances.** Verifying that the correct patient setting and resources are available.
- **Right person.** Identifying a person who is trained and capable of doing the task.
- **Right direction/communication.** Providing a clear, short description of the task and clarifying limitations and the expected result.
- **Right supervision.** Providing appropriate monitoring, assistance, and **feedback.**

All departments are responsible for quality patient care, even if they are not providing hands-on care. For instance, if the medical records department fails to keep correct files of the patient/client chart, the physician will not have the test results and history needed to provide care. If housekeepers do not clean properly and bacteria are present, patients/clients may acquire additional diseases.

Remember: It is the team effort of all health care workers that provides service to the patient/client!

SUMMARY

As a health care worker, you are part of a very important team. You must demonstrate many qualities both in the care of your patients/clients and in your **responsibility** to your employer. Health care workers are expected to conduct themselves in an ethical manner. Ethical behavior protects you, your patients/clients, their families, the staff, and your place of employment. Dignity, service, excellence, and fairness/justice are essential for every health care worker.

interdisciplinary
Involving two or more disciplines.

delegates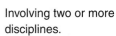
Gives another person responsibility for doing specific tasks.

feedback
Information received as a result of something done or said.

responsibility
One's answerability to an employer in areas such as dependability and honesty.

LEARN BY

Doing **UNIT 1 ACTIVITY**

1. Complete Worksheets 1 and 2.
2. Ask your instructor for directions to complete Worksheet/ Activity 3.
3. Complete Worksheets 4 and 5.
4. When you are confident that you can meet each objective listed, ask your instructor for the unit evaluation.

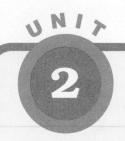

2 Legal Roles and Responsibilities of a Health Care Worker

STEPS TO SUCCESS

1. Complete Vocabulary Worksheet 1 in the Student Workbook.

2. Read this unit.

3. Complete the Learn by Doing assignment at the end of this unit.

UNIT OBJECTIVES

When you have completed this unit, you will be able to do the following:

✔ Match vocabulary words with their correct meanings.

✔ Explain the importance of the Patient's/Client's Bill of Rights.

✔ Explain what natural death guidelines and declarations do.

✔ Describe the purpose of an advance directive and name three forms of advance directives.

✔ Describe the role of an ombudsman in health care.

✔ List three controls on health care workers.

✔ Explain "scope of practice."

✔ Match legal terms with their correct meanings.

✔ Explain why understanding legal responsibilities is important.

✔ Differentiate between policies and procedures.

UNIT RATIONALE

Health care workers must be aware of their legal responsibilities for the protection of the patients/clients, their co-workers, their employers, and themselves. Health care workers may be brought to trial and held liable if they do not perform their duties in a legal manner.

Patient's/Client's Bill of Rights

Document written by the American Hospital Association outlining expected patient/client rights while in a hospital.

⬤ LEGAL RESPONSIBILITIES

It is important for health care workers to remember that patients/clients have rights that represent not only moral and ethical issues, but also rights legislated by both federal and state governments. It is each health care worker's responsibility to recognize the importance of treating patients/clients with dignity. A list of patient/client rights is meaningless unless the person working with the patient understands and follows them. All health care workers must commit to giving the best possible care. The health care worker is legally bound to provide care as it is stated in the **Patient's/Client's Bill of Rights.**

A Patient's/Client's Bill of Rights

A Patient's Bill of Rights was first adopted by the American Hospital Association in 1973.

This revision was approved by the AHA Board of Trustees on October 21, 1992.

Introduction

Effective health care requires collaboration between patients and physicians and other health care professionals. Open and honest communication, respect for personal and professional values, and sensitivity to differences are integral to optimal patient care. As the setting for the provision of health services, hospitals must provide a foundation for understanding and respecting the rights and responsibilities of patients, their families, physicians, and other caregivers. Hospitals must ensure a health care ethic that respects the role of patients in decision making about treatment choices and other aspects of their care. Hospitals must be sensitive to cultural, racial, linguistic, religious, age, gender, and other differences as well as the needs of persons with disabilities.

The American Hospital Association presents A Patient's Bill of Rights with the expectation that it will contribute to more effective patient care and be supported by the hospital on behalf of the institution, its medical staff, employees, and patients. The American Hospital Association encourages health care institutions to tailor this bill of rights to their patient community by translating and/or simplifying the language of this bill of rights as may be necessary to ensure that patients and their families understand their rights and responsibilities.

Bill of Rights

These rights can be exercised on the patient's behalf by a designated surrogate or proxy decision maker if the patient lacks decision-making capacity, is legally incompetent, or is a minor.

1. The patient has the right to considerate and respectful care.

2. The patient has the right to and is encouraged to obtain from physicians and other direct caregivers relevant, current, and understandable information concerning diagnosis, treatment, and prognosis.

   Except in emergencies when the patient lacks decision-making capacity and the need for treatment is urgent, the patient is entitled to the opportunity to discuss and request information related to the specific procedures and/or treatments, the risks involved, the possible length of recuperation, and the medically reasonable alternatives and their accompanying risks and benefits.

   Patients have the right to know the identity of physicians, nurses, and others involved in their care, as well as when those involved are students, residents, or other trainees. The patient also has the right to know the immediate and long-term financial implications of treatment choices, insofar as they are known.

3. The patient has the right to make decisions about the plan of care prior to and during the course of treatment and to refuse a recommended treatment or plan of care to the extent permitted by law and hospital policy and to be informed of the medical consequences of this action. In case of such refusal, the patient is entitled to other appropriate care and services that the hospital provides or transfer to another hospital. The hospital should notify patients of any policy that might affect patient choice within the institution.

4. The patient has the right to have an advance directive (such as a living will, health care proxy, or durable power of attorney for health care) concerning treatment or designating a surrogate decision maker with the expectation that the hospital will honor the intent of that directive to the extent permitted by law and hospital policy.

   Health care institutions must advise patients of their rights under state law and hospital policy to make informed medical choices, ask if the patient has an advance directive, and include that information in patient records. The patient has the right to timely information about hospital policy that may limit its ability to implement fully a legally valid advance directive.

5. The patient has the right to every consideration of privacy. Case discussion, consultation, examination, and treatment should be conducted so as to protect each patient's privacy.

6. The patient has the right to expect that all communications and records pertaining to his/her care will be treated as confidential by the hospital, except in cases such as suspected abuse and public health hazards when reporting is permitted or required by law. The patient has the right to expect that the hospital will emphasize the confidentiality of this information when it releases it to any other parties entitled to review information in these records.

7. The patient has the right to review the records pertaining to his/her medical care and to have the information explained or interpreted as necessary, except when restricted by law.

8. The patient has the right to expect that, within its capacity and policies, a hospital will make reasonable response to the request of a patient for appropriate and medically indicated care and services. The hospital must provide evaluation, service, and/or referral as indicated by the urgency of the case. When medically appropriate and legally permissible, or when a patient has so requested, a patient may be transferred to another facility. The institution to which the patient is to be transferred must first have accepted the patient for transfer. The patient must also have the benefit of complete information and explanation concerning the need for, risks, benefits, and alternatives to such a transfer.

9. The patient has the right to ask and be informed of the existence of business relationships among the hospital, educational institutions, other health care providers, or payers that may influence the patient's treatment and care.

10. The patient has the right to consent to or decline to participate in proposed research studies or human experimentation affecting care and treatment or requiring direct patient involvement, and to have those studies fully explained prior to consent. A patient who declines to participate in research or experimentation is entitled to the most effective care that the hospital can otherwise provide.

11. The patient has the right to expect reasonable continuity of care when appropriate and to be informed by physicians and other caregivers of available and realistic patient care options when hospital care is no longer appropriate.

12. The patient has the right to be informed of hospital policies and practices that relate to patient care, treatment, and responsibilities. The patient has the right to be informed of available resources for resolving disputes, grievances, and conflicts, such as ethics committees, patient representatives, or other mechanisms available in the institution. The patient has the right to be informed of the hospital's charges for services and available payment methods.

The collaborative nature of health care requires that patients, or their families/surrogates, participate in their care. The effectiveness of care and patient satisfaction with the course of treatment depend, in part, on the patient fulfilling certain responsibilities. Patients are responsible for providing information about past illnesses, hospitalizations, medications, and other matters related to health status. To participate effectively in decision making, patients must be encouraged to take responsibility for requesting additional information or clarification about their health status or treatment when they do not fully understand information and instructions. Patients are also responsible for ensuring that the health care institution has a copy of their written advance directive if they have one. Patients are responsible for informing their physicians and other caregivers if they anticipate problems in following prescribed treatment.

Patients should also be aware of the hospital's obligation to be reasonably efficient and equitable in providing care to other patients and the community. The hospital's rules and regulations are designed to help the hospital meet this obligation. Patients and their families are responsible for making reasonable accommodations to the needs of the hospital, other patients, medical staff, and hospital employees. Patients are responsible for providing necessary information for insurance claims and for working with the hospital to make payment arrangements, when necessary.

A person's health depends on much more than health care services. Patients are responsible for recognizing the impact of their life-style on their personal health.

Conclusion

Hospitals have many functions to perform, including the enhancement of health status, health promotion, and the prevention and treatment of injury and disease; the immediate and ongoing care and rehabilitation of patients; the education of health professionals, patients, and the community; and research. All these activities must be conducted with an overriding concern for the values and dignity of patients.

Natural Death Guidelines and Declarations

For many years people were not allowed to make decisions about death with dignity. Today new laws allow individuals to have a say in how they want to live their last days. Each state has adopted natural death guidelines and declarations that give direction to people about how to legally tell others their desire concerning end-of-life issues. These documents ensure the individual the right to accept or refuse medical care. In the United States every person is encouraged to prepare this document called an "advance directive." Advance directives help ensure the right to accept or refuse medical care. Each state has slightly different laws that govern the interpretation of these documents. The advance directive is a written form providing a way for people to express how they want medical decisions made if they are unable to make decisions for themselves. Three common forms of advance directives are a living will, a health care power of attorney, and a durable power of attorney for health care.

- **Living Will:** The living will provides a way for a person to express her or his desire for or against extraordinary measures that could prolong life. A living will takes effect while a person is still alive. Legal assistance may be necessary to ensure that it is interpreted in the way it was intended.

- **Health Care Power of Attorney (HCPOA):** A health care power of attorney allows an authorized person to make health care decisions for an individual if he or she is unable to do so. The HCPOA is more flexible than a living will and can cover any health care decision. A HCPOA can apply in cases of temporary unconsciousness or in case of diseases like Alzheimer's that affect decision making.

- **Durable Power of Attorney for Health Care (DPAHC):** In many states, a durable power of attorney for health care is a signed, dated, and witnessed paper naming an authorized person to make medical decisions for the individual if he or she is unable to make them. This document also includes instruction about treatment to avoid.

It is important to remember that even without a written charge, a patient's wishes stated directly to the doctor generally carry more weight than a living will, health care power of attorney, or durable power of attorney, as long as the patient can decide and communicate his or her wishes.

Ombudsman

An ombudsman is a social worker, nurse, or trained volunteer who makes certain that the patient/client is not abused and that the person's rights are secure.

Controls on Health Care Workers

Licensure, certification, and registration tell what a health care worker may or may not do. They determine the scope of practice for the health care worker. Controls help to improve the quality of care. Although not all health occupations require licensure, certification, or registration, it is important to be aware of these controls.

- *Licensure* is given by a governmental agency when a person meets the qualifications for a particular occupation.

recognition
Acknowledgment as being worthy of approval.

■ *Certification* is given for **recognition.** If specific guidelines must be met, the certification equals licensure.

■ *Registration* is a list of individuals on an official record who meet the qualifications for an occupation (e.g., registered nurse, registered dental assistant).

Legal Terms and Boundaries

Health care workers need to understand how medical-legal problems affect them. Read the following terms. They explain how the health care worker can have a legal problem.

■ *Assault* is a threat or an attempt to injure another person. *Example:* A health care worker threatens to hit a patient/client or co-worker.

resultant
Resulting from an action.

■ *Battery* is the unlawful touching of another person without his or her consent, with or without **resultant** injury. Assault and battery are often charged together because of the successful attempt to injure. *Example:* A health care worker hits a patient/client or co-worker.

■ *Informed consent* is the permission granted by a person in his or her right mind who voluntarily gives consent for treatment. Written consent ensures that patients are informed of all risks and complications of the procedure before signing. *Example:* A patient is asked to sign a consent form for certain procedures in the hospital or physician's office. The procedure must not be done without consent.

omission
Neglect of duty.

■ *Crime* results from performing a forbidden act or from the **omission** of a duty commanded by a public law. This makes the offender liable to punishment by law. *Example:* A health care worker takes a patient/client or co-worker's belongings. Stealing from the workplace is a crime.

defamatory
Statement that causes injury to another's reputation.

■ *Libel* is writing **defamatory** matter about an individual or group to a third party. *Example:* A newspaper writes damaging information about a local health care institution. The newspaper cannot provide proof of the statement. The paper is charged with libel. What you write in a patient record could be libel if you make a statement such as, "Mr. M. is nasty."

misrepresentations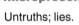
Untruths; lies.

■ *Slander* is a spoken statement of false charges or **misrepresentations** that defame or damage another's reputation. *Example:* A health care worker tells friends that a famous person was treated for a drug overdose when in fact he or she was treated for a serious medical problem.

■ *False imprisonment* is the holding or retaining of a person against his or her will. *Example:* A physician or a health care worker refuses to allow a patient to leave the hospital.

■ *Felony* is a serious crime that carries a penalty of imprisonment for more than 1 year and possibly the death penalty. *Example:* A health care worker withholds treatment for a terminally ill patient, which causes the patient's premature death.

■ *Invasion of privacy* is a civil wrong that unlawfully makes public knowledge of any private or personal information without the consent of the wronged person. *Example:* A health care worker gives personal information to a newspaper about a patient/client or co-worker.

faulty
Defective or imperfect.

dismantles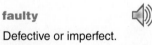
Takes apart.

■ *Malpractice* means "bad practice." It is care that leads to **faulty** practice or neglect. *Example:* A respiratory therapy aide dislikes cleaning equipment, so he **dismantles** each item and places it on the racks as though it were clean. This action leads to a serious infection in a patient/client.

prudent
Careful or cautious.

■ *Negligence* is the failure to perform in a reasonably **prudent** manner. *Example:* A health care worker forgets to lock the brakes on a wheelchair, and the patient/client is injured.

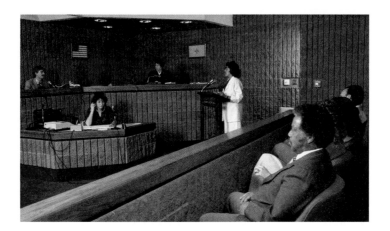

Figure 3.3

Health care worker testifying before a judge and jury.

- *Privileged communication* concerns any personal or private information given by a patient/client to medical personnel that is **relevant** to his or her care. *Example:* A health care worker should consider all information in the chart as privileged communication (Figure 3.3).

- *Reasonable care* is the legal **obligation** of health care workers. They must perform according to the standards of practice expected in their community for comparable workers. *Example:* A laboratory aide draws blood from a patient/client after watching the procedure several times and feeling **competent.** However, she was not taught to do the procedure. Therefore, reasonable care was not exercised.

- *Sexual harassment* is defined by federal regulations as "unwelcome sexual advances, requests for sexual favors, and other verbal and physical contact of a sexual nature." Innocent remarks, inappropriate pictures, and written material can be perceived as sexual. You can guard against harassment accusations by not making personal remarks or sexual gestures and by not participating in sexually explicit discussions around co-workers. *Example:* A co-worker gets really close and frequently touches another person when talking. The closeness and physical touch may be interpreted as sexual harassment, even if it is innocent.

- A *will* is a legal **document** that defines the **disposition** of property and takes effect after death. *Example:* A patient/client legally declares who will inherit his or her personal property.

- *Reportable incidents and conditions.* The health care worker is obligated to file a confidential report to the county health department when child or adult abuse is suspected. Reports are also required when certain diseases are diagnosed. It is important to check your facility's policy and procedures book for a current listing of reportable diseases and the procedure for reporting abuse.

These definitions and examples provide the knowledge you need to avoid medical-legal problems (Figure 3.4).

relevant

Pertaining to, or having to do with, the patient/client.

obligation

Moral responsibility (e.g., to give the best possible patient/client care, to be on time for work).

competent

Capable or able to perform a skill or task.

document

Written record.

disposition

Act of disposing of (e.g., a person desires that his or her monies be given to an organization after his or her death).

⊙ CONFIDENTIALITY

Patient/client information is confidential. *Confidential* means "secret." Health care workers are obligated to protect and keep all patient/client information confidential. A good rule is to discuss a patient/client only when the discussion affects his or her care in some way—for example,

- When you find candy with the belongings of a diabetic
- When you find alcohol or medications with the belongings of a patient/client

Figure 3.4

All information about patients/clients is confidential.

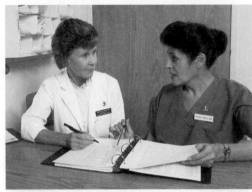

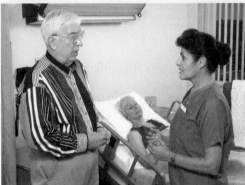

Discuss patient information only with your supervisor. Do *not* discuss patient information with

- Other patients
- Relatives and friends of the patient
- Visitors to the hospital
- Representatives of news media
- Fellow workers, except when in conference
- Your own relatives and friends

■ When patients discuss areas of stress in their personal life, such as financial problems or relationship problems

A medical facility, a physician, or a health care worker can be fined, sued, or lose his or her job for sharing *any* information about patients/clients with others, including family members.

○ POLICIES AND PROCEDURES

manual

Book with guidelines.

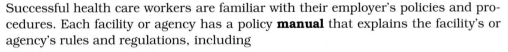

Successful health care workers are familiar with their employer's policies and procedures. Each facility or agency has a policy **manual** that explains the facility's or agency's rules and regulations, including

- Holiday and vacation policy
- Insurance and sick leave benefits
- All other information concerning the operation of that business

A procedure manual explains the step-by-step method of performing tasks, including

- How to take a temperature
- How to fill out forms
- How to package and wrap trays

The facility's policy and procedure manuals are the guidelines that health care workers must follow to do their jobs correctly. Remember your limitations, and do only those procedures that you were taught to do. Always follow your facility's code of ethics. When you follow your facility's policies and procedures, you protect patients, co-workers, your employer, and yourself.

⦾ SUMMARY

In this unit you learned about legal **boundaries** for health care workers. You also learned that confidentiality is an important part of staying within the legal boundaries. When health care workers perform their duties within these boundaries, they help prevent medical-legal problems. Policies are the guidelines that provide information about facility rules and regulations. Procedures tell you how to complete tasks the way your employer wants them done.

boundaries

Legal limits (e.g., you may know how to perform a task, but you may not do it because you are limited by your license, certification, registration, or rules and regulations).

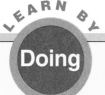

UNIT 2 ACTIVITY

1. Complete Worksheet 2 through 4.
2. When you are confident that you can meet each objective for this unit, ask your instructor for the unit evaluation.
3. Prepare responses to each item listed in Chapter Review—Your Link to Success at the end of this chapter.

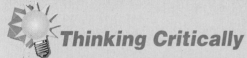

Thinking Critically

1. Communication Being an effective communicator involves active listening, honesty, and assertiveness. Think about the last time you had to tell another person something unpleasant. Were your comments constructive or destructive? Explain in writing how you could change destructive comments into constructive ones. Use the health care value indicators to help you decide what and how to send your message.

2. Legal and Ethical One of your patients tells you he cannot eat because he is worried about having no will. He has no money to pay an attorney. How would you advise this patient? What resources are available in your community for such a person? Use this as a research opportunity. Check with the county court and the local bar association. Let your patient know what resources are available.

3. Cultural Competency One of the members of your care team is having difficulty understanding directions given

by the supervisor. Your co-worker speaks English, but it is her second language, and she frequently misinterprets instructions. How can you treat your co-worker with dignity while helping her understand the instructions?

4. Patient Education A patient/client asks about advance directives. Describe how you will respond.

5. Patient Satisfaction Patient Satisfaction is an important part of the health care worker's role. Go to Table 3.3 and select two communication objectives. Write an explanation of how behavior that reflects these objectives benefits patients and, their families and helps provide appropriate medical services.

6. Computers How can access to the Internet help you with patient care? Set up a table of resources available to you on the Web and keep it updated as you hear of more Web sites. Make the table part of your portfolio for future reference.

Portfolio Connection

Self-Reflection: How you express what you value causes positive or negative responses from others. Your manner encourages open and sincere or closed and guarded responses. Your values and the way you express them affect your success in your occupation. The values discussed in this chapter provide basic guidelines for working closely with others in health care. Think about your most common behaviors. List behaviors you exhibit when you are happy and when you are sad. Compare those behaviors with behaviors that reflect the health care values discussed in this chapter. Write a clear explanation of three behaviors you display. Include

■ At least one behavior that best reflects health care values. Describe why the behavior fits the value.

■ At least one behavior that does not reflect health care values. Describe why the behavior does not fit the values.

Develop and describe a plan to change this behavior into a positive value-based action. Follow these guidelines when preparing your report:

■ Use 8.5-by-11-inch paper.

■ Type, word process, or write neatly in ink.

■ Use correct spelling and grammar.

Portfolio Tip

Before you file your portfolio samples, check that you have followed a step-by-step process in each document. It makes your written or recorded presentations clear and logical.

Include the following in your action plan:

■ Negative behavior, with an explanation about what makes it negative or outside the health care values discussed in this chapter
■ Action that changes the behavior, with an explanation about how it fits the health care values
■ Evaluation plan, including a time line to determine the final outcome of the action plan

When you have completed your plan and checked format and grammar for accuracy, place it in your portfolio in the section for Written Samples.

Patient Advocacy Patient advocacy defends and promotes issues that help ensure appropriate health care. With the many challenges that affect health care today, there is a greater awareness of the need to defend patient rights. The Patient's Bill of Rights is frequently in the news and has been presented to the House of Representatives and the Senate on several occasions. Search the newspapers, public library, and the Internet for the latest information on the struggle to protect patients' rights. Try to identify one way in which you can be an advocate for patient's rights. Write a short report explaining the current status of patient's rights and include your ideas on how you can be a patient advocate.

Remember! **Media Connection**

Use the Companion Website **www.prenhall.com/badasch** and the CD-ROM for additional interactive learning activities.

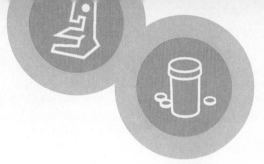

Chapter 4

Meeting Your Needs and the Needs of Others

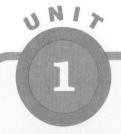

UNIT 1

Holistic Health

STEPS TO SUCCESS

1. Complete Vocabulary Worksheet 1 in the Student Workbook.
2. Read this unit.
3. Complete the Learn by Doing assignment at the end of this unit.

UNIT OBJECTIVES

When you have completed this unit, you will be able to do the following:

✔ Define the vocabulary words.

✔ List three parts of holistic health.

UNIT RATIONALE

Responsible health care promotes lifestyles that encourage wellness. It is important for the health care worker to understand that mind, body, spirit, and social involvement must be balanced. Understanding wellness promotes good health in the health care worker and in the patient/client.

✔ Explain wellness and preventive care.

✔ Compare holistic health to disease-oriented care.

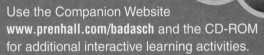 **HEALTH AND WELLNESS**

infirmity
Unsound or unhealthy state of being.

holistic
Pertaining to the whole; considering all factors.

The World Health Organization defines health as follows: "Health is a state of complete physical, mental and social well-being and not merely the absence of disease or **infirmity.**" This definition of health has been expanded with the recent growth and emphasis on **holistic** health. Today we think in terms of the body's working as a unit (mental, physical, spiritual) to maintain and promote optimum wellness through daily actions. The World Health Organization definition of health gives the impression of perfection; wellness implies feeling good regardless of your infirmity or disease.

In health care, *holistic* refers to the well-being of the whole person. It is important to meet physical needs and also mental and spiritual needs when giving care. Holistic health care is a part of the wellness approach, which encourages good health. Understanding these needs helps you care for yourself and for your patients/clients.

⬤ WELLNESS AND PREVENTIVE HEALTH CARE

Wellness and preventive health care emphasize keeping patients well, not waiting until they are ill to provide treatment. Health education is vital to helping clients maintain good health. A holistic approach includes all of the following:

- *Physical fitness* makes us alert and energetic in activities of daily living. It gives us enough energy to enjoy leisure time and to respond when emergencies arise. It can be achieved through
  - Routine physicals • Adequate rest • Good nutrition • Weight control
  - **Elimination** of waste • **Aerobic** exercise • Immunizations • Well-baby checks
  - Avoiding substance abuse, including
  - Drugs • Alcohol • Tobacco • Excessive food intake

- *Mental fitness* allows us to interact effectively with others and to feel balanced. Mentally healthy people
  - Self-direct (being the captain of your own ship) • Have a sense of belonging
  - Trust their own senses and feelings • Accept themselves • Have **self-esteem**
  - Practice stress management

- *Spiritual fitness* allows us to experience meaning and purpose in life. It provides a sense of comfort with others, creating greater acceptance of behaviors, attitudes, and beliefs. (Figure 4.1). It includes
  - Enjoying companionship • Sharing ideas and thoughts • Having a sense of belonging • Showing enthusiasm for life

Holistic health requires health care workers to promote physical, mental, and spiritual well-being. For example, a patient experiencing stomach pain may be referred to a psychologist if the physician suspects that the patient is under a lot of emotional stress. The psychologist may refer him to a biofeedback specialist for stress management. This process continues until the patient's/client's needs are met in all areas.

elimination
Process of getting rid of.

aerobic
Requiring oxygen.

self-esteem
Belief in oneself.

⬤ JOBS AND PROFESSIONS

- Psychologist
- Psychiatrist
- Social worker (rehabilitation worker)
- Biofeedback specialist
- Physician
- Nurse
- Parish nurse specialist
- Acupressurist
- Acupuncturist
- Palliative care specialist

Figure 4.1

Enjoying companionship, sharing ideas, having a sense of belonging, and showing enthusiasm for life are vital to well-being.

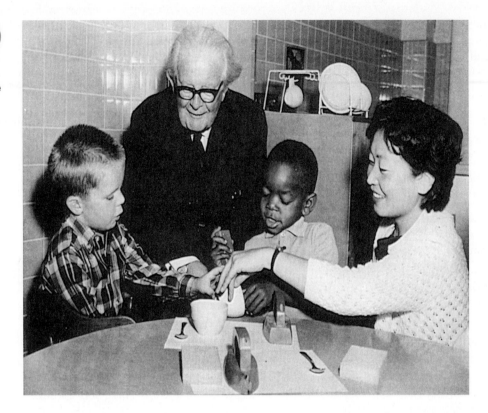

⊙ SUMMARY

You have learned that the holistic approach to health is important because it includes all aspects of a person's well-being. When we are in balance physically, mentally, and spiritually, we experience life in a positive way creating a greater sense of well-being. The trend in health care is toward wellness and preventive care.

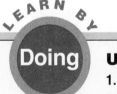

LEARN BY Doing

UNIT 1 ACTIVITY

1. **Complete Worksheets 2 and 3 in the Student Workbook.**

2. **When you are confident that you can meet each objective for this unit, ask your instructor for the unit evaluation.**

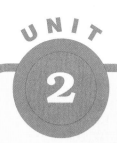

UNIT 2

Understanding Human Needs

STEPS TO SUCCESS

1. Complete Vocabulary Worksheet 1 in the Student Workbook.

2. Read this unit.

3. Complete the Learn by Doing activities at the end of this chapter.

UNIT OBJECTIVES

When you have completed this unit, you will be able to do the following:

✔ Match vocabulary words with their correct meanings.

✔ Name four psychological needs that must be met to maintain stability.

✔ Name four physiological needs that must be met to maintain stability.

UNIT RATIONALE

Understanding a person's physiological and psychological needs is essential for every health care worker. Every person has needs that must be satisfied to maintain stability. Health care workers must be aware of these needs to maintain their own stability and to meet the needs of patients/clients and co-workers.

✔ Explain five benefits of pet-facilitated therapy.

✔ Match five defense mechanisms with the correct descriptions.

✔ Explain how you use defense mechanisms daily.

⬤ MEETING THE NEEDS OF PATIENTS/CLIENTS

Physiological Needs

Physiological needs are divided into 4 categories. Biological needs are listed in Table 4.1a, safety needs in Table 4.1b, sensory needs in Table 4.1c, and motor activity needs in Table 4.1d.

Psychological Needs

Psychological needs are divided into 4 categories. Adequacy and security needs are listed in Table 4.2a, social approval and self-esteem needs in Table 4.2b, order and meaning in life needs in Table 4.2c, and self-growth needs in Table 4.2d.

Understanding people's **physiological** and **psychological** needs helps you be a better health care worker. You are able to recognize the reasons for certain behaviors and respond appropriately to help meet your patients' needs. Always report evidence of all unmet needs to your supervisor. Your supervisor will determine what to include in the next patient care meeting. A plan will be determined concerning how to best meet the patient's/client's need.

physiological
Pertaining to normal body functions.

psychological
Pertaining to the mind.

Table 4.1a ■ Biological Needs—Food, Water, Sleep, and Elimination

Threatened by Illness	Communication Needs	Age-Specific and Communication Needs	Cultural Awareness	Reporting and Recording Observations
• Food and water may be withheld before various procedures or surgery is performed. • Sleep may be interrupted because of the environment, noises, or anxiety. • Elimination is frequently affected by changes in routine, foods, or medication.	• Be committed to reflecting the value of dignity. Use effective communication skills that demonstrate holistic care. Be alert to the biological needs and communicate how they will be met during patient care. • For new patients explain: 　–Physician's orders concerning activity, food, use of the bathroom, and any expected special procedures; 　–Mealtimes; 　–How to request assistance or ask questions. • Always ask patients if they have any special requests or questions. • When sleep must be interrupted, inform the patient before he or she goes to sleep.	• Use words that the patient can understand. Ask a translator to ensure that words and thoughts are fully communicated. • Allow decisions concerning food and sleep to be made by the patient when possible. • Tell patients what to expect. • Reassure children and parents of times they can be together. • Address people by their proper names and titles. • Ask coherent patients if they have any specific fears. Address their fears honestly and with sensitivity, always treating people with dignity. Ask for assistance when necessary. • Remember that comments like "Don't worry" are never helpful.	• Many cultures of the world: 　–Believe that illness is caused by a supernatural power; 　–Use various herbs to treat illness and may request a specific diet; 　–Consider white bad luck. Medical personnel in white may cause an increase in fear; 　–Believe that hot and cold air currents negatively affect health. Be alert to drafts. • See Unit 3 of this chapter for more information.	• Report to your supervisor and record in the medical record: 　–Special requests; 　–Expressed fears; 　–Your instructions about the medical routine; 　–Your observations of how the patient and family received instructions concerning the routine and potential limitations of food, water, interrupted sleep, and expected preparation for procedures that may affect elimination.

Table 4.1b ■ Safety Needs—Need to Feel Secure and to Avoid Bodily Harm and Injury

Threatened by Illness	Communication Needs	Age-Specific and Communication Needs	Cultural Awareness	Reporting and Recording Observations
• Patients needing medical procedures and treatments may feel insecure. They may be facing hospitalization for the first time and are afraid they will be hurt or die. They may be entering a long-term care facility where they will live for the rest of their lives. They may wonder: –What will happen to me? –How will I be treated? –Will I be safe? • Patients may also be worried about pain or accidents that could occur during procedures.	• Be sure that the patient fully understands what you are saying. Use pictures, culturally appropriate gestures, writing and/or a translator to ensure understanding. • Tell patients what they can expect from you and your team. Introduce yourself and your team. Your reassuring presence and warm touch may be enough to help a patient feel safe. • For new hospital patients: –Tell patients how to request assistance or contact you—explain the call system and intercom. • Show your commitment to service and treating others with dignity by always doing what you say you're going to do. This helps create trust and builds a sense of security for patients and their families.	• Think of the patient's age and ability to understand before speaking. Use the patient's words as much as possible. Speak at his or her level. • When caring for pediatric patients, ask the family if special words or objects communicate special things. For example, a child may call a special toy or blanket a "binki." • When possible, allow family or significant others to be present if the patient requests their presence.	• Be alert to body language and other forms of communication that may provide clues to the patient's state of mind. • See Unit 3 of this chapter for more information on various cultural beliefs that may affect the way health care is given.	• Report to your supervisor and record in the medical record: –Special requests; –Expressed fears; –Your instructions about medical routine; –Your observations of how the patient and family received instructions.

Table 4.1c ▪ Sensory Needs—Stimulation of the Five Senses (Hearing, Seeing, Feeling, Smelling, Tasting) as Well as Intellectual Stimulation

Threatened by Illness	Communication Needs	Age-Specific and Communication Needs	Cultural Awareness	Reporting and Recording Observations
• When the senses are not stimulated they diminish. For example, when a patient is not able to eat, intravenous fluids may be used. Because the smell and taste sensors are not stimulated, when the patient begins to eat again it will take time for taste and smell to return to normal. • The senses are less responsive to stimulation as we age. Geriatric patients may have lost one or more of their senses. They may have difficulty hearing or seeing which may increase their fear and cause anxiety.	• Communicating with people who are experiencing a sensory loss takes patience and imagination. Try some of the following to stimulate their senses. —People with hearing loss can experience music by touching a speaker while it plays music. They can feel rhythm vibrate through the speaker. —Patients with touch-impaired senses usually lose feeling in their hands and feet. When it is reasonable, touch their face or arms with things that they want to feel, such as a warm towel. —Visual, smell- and taste-impaired patients appreciate your description of colors, smells, or flavors in their environment. For example, you might say "Remember the smell of turkey roasting and fresh bread baking? That's what it smells like today." • When working with people show your commitment to excellence by being sensitive and remembering to use techniques that help people experience their senses.	• The loss of senses during the aging process also adds to the loss of well-being. As a health care worker you can help restore a sense of well-being by being aware and using techniques that help people experience or remember the feelings of their five senses. • When you are aware of sensory loss, talk to the person and ask what helps him or her experience the lost sense. Try various techniques that will help stimulate the senses, always explaining what you are doing.	• The various cultures of the world relate differently to touch, gestures, and personal space. As a health care worker it is important that you are mindful of the various cultures and the potential barriers relative to the body senses. See Unit 3 of this chapter for details.	• Report to your supervisor and record in the medical record: —Special requests; —Expressed fears; —Your instructions about medical routine; —Your observations of how the patient and family received instructions.

Table 4.1d ■ Motor Activity—Movement or Exercise of the Body

Threatened by Illness	Communication Needs	Age-Specific and Communication Needs	Cultural Awareness	Reporting and Recording Observations
• When muscles are not stimulated they atrophy (shrink) and eventually weaken and can even become frozen. The results of a lack of muscle stimulation may or may not be reversible depending on the length of time the muscle was not stimulated. For example, when a cast is removed from an arm or a leg after a long period the arm or leg is usually much smaller than the one which was not in a cast. The casted limb was not able to stimulate the muscles so they shrank and became weak. Weakened muscles can prevent free and easy movement. People with weakened muscles often feel less able to take care of their basic needs and do the things they want to do.	• Be sure that the patient fully understands what you are saying. Use pictures, culturally appropriate gestures, writing and/or a translator to ensure understanding. • People who experience difficulty moving around must be informed about how to reach you and others at all times. • Inform the person that you are aware of his or her condition and will take precautions to protect any special needs. • Explain the procedures that you will use to ensure the patient's safety as you help him or her move or as you do procedures. • Your commitment to service excellence makes an important difference for patients. Share expected times for changing or moving your patients, and always follow through.	• Remember to ask patients if they follow a certain procedure that best accommodates their limited or painful movement. Caution: Never do anything contradictory to your training or good judgment. • When appropriate, encourage people to do as much as possible on their own to promote self-sufficiency.	• Be alert to your patient's customs concerning personal space. Always tell the patient what you are going to do before you start to move or touch him or her. • Be aware of cultural taboos about touching the head and appropriate versus inappropriate hand gestures. • See Unit 3 of this chapter for details.	• Report to your supervisor and record in the medical record: –Special requests; –Expressed fears; –Your instructions about medical routine; –Your observations of how the patient and family received instructions.

Threatened by Illness	Communication Needs	Age-Specific Communication Needs	Cultural Awareness	Reporting and Recording Observations
• When a condition occurs that requires medical treatment it is easy to feel a loss of control. Medications and various procedures and disease processes can change the way the body feels and what a person is capable of doing. • Loss of a sense of control affects physical and emotional well-being.	• Discuss what must be done to promote good health and to treat specific conditions. Encourage the patient to comment and make decisions as much as possible. • Show your commitment to dignity and justice by providing opportunities for patients to be involved as much as possible in decision making.	• When possible, provide opportunity for patients to make decisions such as what they will eat or wear.	• Be aware of cultural customs that show respect or disrespect. For example, making direct eye contact in some cultures is disrespectful. Adapt your behavior and language to show respect for each person's dignity.	Report to your supervisor and record in the medical record: –Signs of insecurity; –Voiced inadequacies; –Your observations; –Special requests; –Your observations of how the patient and family received instructions.

Threatened by Illness	Communication Needs	Age-Specific Communication Needs	Cultural Awareness	Reporting and Recording Observations
• When illness limits what a person is able to do at work, socially and personally, depression can occur. This in turn can affect the success of treatment. The patient's ability to support his family may be taken away by an illness that causes job loss. This causes extreme stress. (See Figure 4.2.)	• It is important to spend time with patients who feel isolated. Patients in quarantine or who have body changes that others can see may feel different and isolated from their friends and family. Spending time with them and learning about their life can help them feel accepted. • Encourage family and friends to include them in activities and events when possible. • Show your commitment to dignity by practicing active listening skills. Show interest in the patient's concerns and past experiences. • Inform the patient and family of available resources that may be helpful. For example, social services.	• When caring for children use terms they can understand. • Be positive even when you want to say something negative. • As a health care worker you can help restore a sense of well-being by staying alert to your patient's moods, using resources within your facility to encourage and promote socialization with others who may be having similar experiences. • Use age-appropriate vocabulary. Do not use childish gestures or language to talk with an elderly person.	• Use culturally appropriate gestures and words to show respect. Honoring a person's culture is an effective way of reinforcing self-esteem and showing social approval. • Be aware of dietary preferences. • Encourage family and friends to display pictures and articles that may bring warm and comforting memories.	• Report to your supervisor and record in the medical record: –Signs of low self-esteem; –Voiced inadequacies; –Your observations concerning any change in behavior. For example, withdrawal, passive behavior, wanting to give things away, refusing to see people; –Special requests; –Your observation of how the patient and family received instructions.

Table 4.2c ■ Order and Meaning in Life—Understanding of What Is Going on in One's Environment

Threatened by Illness	Communication Needs	Age-Specific Communication Needs	Cultural Awareness	Reporting and Recording Observations
• When illness occurs it is difficult to know what to expect or how to plan for the future. • Meaning and purpose in life are in question if an illness changes the way we do things. • Order that brings a sense of control is lost, leaving a feeling of being out of control and uncertain.	• Tell patients what to expect before, during, and after procedures to help them psychologically prepare for the experience. • Listen to the patient so you will have an understanding of his or her concerns. • Respond with understanding. For example, "We will be starting your physical therapy today and I am bringing you the schedule so you will know when to expect the therapist."	• Use words that the patient can understand. Ask for a translator to ensure that words and thoughts are fully communicated. • Write information and schedules on a paper that the patient and family can refer to. Use pictures for children, like a clock with the hands pointing to a time you will return.	• Use culturally appropriate gestures and words to show respect. Honoring a person's culture is an effective way of reinforcing self-esteem and showing social approval. • Be aware of routine cultural activities that bring meaning to the patient.	• Report to your supervisor and record in the medical record: –Signs of low self-esteem; –Voiced inadequacies; –Your observations concerning any change; –Special requests.

Table 4.2d ■ Self-Growth—Need for Fulfillment Beyond Basic Needs

Threatened by Illness	Communication Needs	Age-Specific Communication Needs	Cultural Awareness	Reporting and Recording Observations
• Illness often consumes our thoughts. Patients who experience a long illness or physical changes that limit their abilities may experience a loss of personal growth.	• Use active listening skills to identify patients' special interests. Allow them to share the details of these interests. When appropriate, discuss possible options with the care team that will allow the patient to experience learning. Your service excellence and commitment to treating others with dignity are a reality when you take action in this way.	• Use words that the patient can understand. Ask for a translator to ensure that words and thoughts are fully communicated. • When caring for children introduce activities at the child's level of understanding. • Be sure enough time is given to teach and not frustrate the patient of any age.	• Seek culturally appropriate learning for the patient. • Some cultures view games as childish; being sensitive to cultural attitudes will help the patient accept new opportunities.	• Report to your supervisor and record in the medical record: –Voiced discouragement or being bored; –Your observations concerning mood changes; –Special requests; –Involvement of any kind that promotes learning.

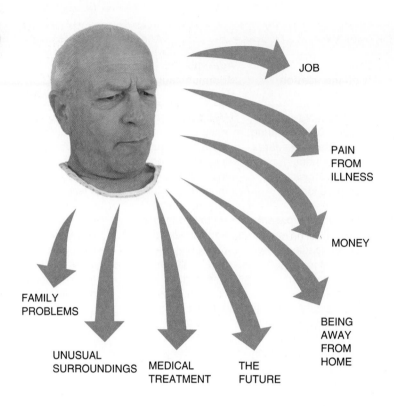

Figure 4.2

Clients worry about many
things when hospitalized.

JOB

PAIN
FROM
ILLNESS

MONEY

BEING
AWAY
FROM
HOME

FAMILY
PROBLEMS

UNUSUAL
SURROUNDINGS   MEDICAL   THE
                TREATMENT   FUTURE

⬤ PET-FACILITATED THERAPY

value

Importance, worth.

There is a great deal of interest focused on the **value** of the human-pet bond. Recent studies show that petting or stroking a pet has an immediate effect on the body. Most people studied showed

- A slowing heartbeat
- Deeper breaths
- Fewer abnormal heartbeats
- Lowered blood pressure
- An increased sense of well-being

Over 50% of American households have pets in the home, primarily for the companionship that they provide. Research shows that even when people do not respond well to other people, they do respond to pets. They talk to their pets. They care for the needs of their pets. When there is a human-animal bond, the patient often finds new meaning in life. They feel less lonely. They feel needed because their pets are totally dependent on them. They have a reason to get out of the house to buy food for their pets. The pet may be just the friend or responsibility they need to help them feel better or to feel good about themselves. Research also shows that fish swimming gracefully in a pleasant aquarium with swaying plants creates a very relaxing environment that reduces stress.

All of this research has alerted the medical community to methods of providing new ways to promote healthier lifestyles through the companionship of pets. People who are experiencing many changes in their lives may find a pet to be the one unchanging element. Other people may be lonely and find that a pet is a good companion. Yet others may just enjoy the pleasure and presence of a pet.

In some places, pet-facilitated therapy is used as a treatment. Animals are taken into convalescent homes and children's hospitals. Some hospitals have arranged to have a pet live on the premises. Other programs have been developed with the Humane Society, and pets are brought in to visit on a regular basis. Hospitals are certainly only one place where pet-facilitated therapy is successful. It is especially effective in the home. An aging person may feel very depressed and alone. A pet brings new meaning to life. Now there is something that really needs him or her and is affectionate and loving. The same kind of therapy is effective for a sick child.

Pet-facilitated therapy has become a form of treatment. It is successful. When working with your patients, be alert to their needs. Perhaps a pet will meet a need that no other care can.

● MEETING THE NEEDS OF CO-WORKERS AND OTHER STAFF

Recognizing human needs in your patients/clients makes you a better health care worker. Recognizing human needs in the staff you work with helps make you a successful member of the health care team.

Physiological Needs

When the *biological needs* of every staff member are not met, **friction** may occur. It is important to eat properly and to get adequate sleep. Many disagreements occur when people are irritable and easily upset because they failed to meet their biological needs.

> **friction**
> Disagreement because of a difference of opinion.

It is important that every member of the staff have their *safety needs* met. They should feel secure and know that bodily harm can be avoided. As a staff member, always follow safety regulations, such as cleaning up spills, reporting damaged equipment, and taking care to protect others. When someone needs help lifting, help the person. This establishes a sense of safety for all the staff and creates a good working environment.

As a fellow staff member, it is important that you realize what the *sensory needs* are. This helps you understand fellow staff members who have sensory impairments. For instance, if a co-worker's hearing or sight is impaired, you need to be aware of this impairment. Your awareness allows you to be patient and to build a good working relationship.

Psychological Needs

Adequacy and *security* are important to all people and help all of us maintain **stability.** Your attitude toward other staff members is either cooperative or disruptive. When staff members work together, they establish a sense of a job well done.

> **stability**
> Ability to maintain a balance, both mentally and physically.

Social approval and *self-esteem* can be met in our relationships with our fellow employees. It is important that you develop **rapport** with other staff members. As you work together to create a healthy environment for the patients/clients and the staff, everyone feels accepted and worthwhile.

> **rapport**
> Harmony; a close relationship with another.

Order and *meaning* needs are met by the day-to-day activities on the job. If every staff member does his or her share and comes to work when scheduled, these needs are met.

The need for *self-growth* is met as you and the other staff members are able to accomplish your jobs and look toward promotion and new learning.

● DEFENSE MECHANISMS

All people use defense mechanisms to help them feel more comfortable with themselves and to make their behavior seem reasonable. Defense mechanisms are mental devices that help people cope with various situations. Health care workers who are aware of defense mechanisms better understand themselves, their co-workers, their supervisors, and their patients' behavior. Following are some key defense mechanisms:

- **Rationalization:** Finding good reasons to replace the real reason for behavior in order to maintain self-esteem. *Example:* Mark did poorly on a test and explained it by saying, "I'd rather be popular than smart."
- **Compensation:** Substituting one goal for another. *Example:* Mary really wanted to be on the track team but wasn't good enough. Instead, she joined the choir and became a soloist.
- **Projection:** Placing the blame for your actions on someone or something else because you cannot accept the responsibility. *Example:* "I didn't get a good grade in my health occupations class because the teacher doesn't like me."
- **Sublimation:** Redirecting feelings toward a constructive objective. *Example:* You enjoy playing tennis and you use the game to work out **aggressiveness** and **hostility** instead of directing those feelings toward others.
- **Identification: Idolizing** someone you would like to be like. *Example:* Margaret especially admired her music teacher. She began to walk and dress like her.

When you are aware that everyone uses defense mechanisms, and when you know what they are, you are able to understand your behavior and the behavior of others. As a health care worker, it is important for you to realize that a defense mechanism may be involved in certain behavior. This allows you to give better care. Your knowledge of defense mechanisms also helps you understand the behavior of the people with whom you work.

aggressiveness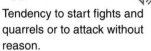

Tendency to start fights and quarrels or to attack without reason.

hostility

Unfriendliness; ill will toward another.

idolizing

Loving to excess.

⬤ SUMMARY

You have learned that human beings have physiological needs, which include biological needs, safety needs, sensory needs, and motor activity needs. They also have psychological needs, which include the need to feel adequate and secure, to have social approval and self-esteem, to have order and meaning in life, and to experience self-growth. These needs must be met at all times. It is important that we are always aware of these needs in our patients/clients, our co-workers, our supervisors, and ourselves. You have also learned that all people use defense mechanisms to help them feel comfortable inside. These include rationalization, compensation, projection, sublimation, and identification.

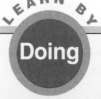

Doing   **UNIT 2 ACTIVITY**

1. **Ask your instructor for direction to complete Worksheet/Activity 2.**
2. **Ask your instructor for directions to complete Worksheet/Activity 3.**
3. **Complete Worksheets 4 and 5.**
4. **Ask your instructor for directions to complete Worksheet/Activity 6.**
5. **When you are confident that you can meet each objective for this unit, ask your instructor for the unit evaluation.**

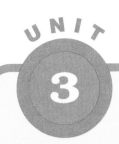

UNIT 3

Cultural Cross-Terms and Principles

STEPS TO SUCCESS

1. Read this unit.
2. Complete the Learn by Doing assignment at the end of this unit.

UNIT RATIONALE

Health care workers interact with people from many cultural backgrounds. It is important to know culturally acceptable and effective gestures, terms, and behaviors. This knowledge allows the health care worker to adapt his or her care and communication techniques. The patient/client receives quality care, and the experience is positive.

UNIT OBJECTIVES

When you have completed this unit, you will be able to do the following:

✔ Explain how culture influences behavior.

✔ Identify culturally acceptable and effective gestures, terms, and behaviors.

✔ Recognize communication techniques that create a positive exchange of information.

✔ Identify common folk medicine practices.

✔ Compare and contrast cultural differences.

✔ Explain how understanding cultural beliefs affects you as a health care worker.

⬤ CULTURE AND BEHAVIOR

When caring for and working with people from different cultures, you must understand their cultural background. Understanding allows you to have positive experiences and to communicate effectively. Our understanding and opinions of other cultures develop through our life experiences. Culture includes a shared background. This means that cultural groups have shared experiences. Among those experiences common to most groups are:

- Language
- Communication style
- Belief system
- Customs
- Attitudes
- Perceptions
- Values

Language and communication styles and some customs are visible to people outside of a specific cultural group. Belief systems, some customs, attitudes, perceptions, and values are less visible. Think of a tree (see Figure 4.3). The trunk, branches, and leaves are all visible—like language, communication styles, and some customs are visible in people. The roots of a tree, however, grow deep underground and nourish it to keep it strong—but they are not visible. So it is with culture: Belief systems, some customs, attitudes, perceptions, and values all come together to create a strong foundation that helps form a person. It is important to remember that there are no rights and wrongs when comparing various cultures. Cultures are only different. Cultural differences do not weaken society, but in fact strengthen society if there is a sense of openness that allows understanding. This does not mean

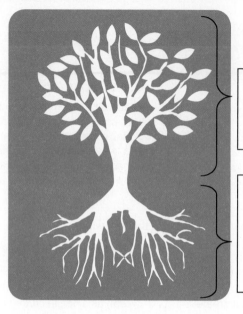

Culture can be compared to a tree because some cultural characteristics are visible like the trunk, branches, and leaves of tree whereas others are less visible like the root system of a tree which is underground.

Visible

ß   Language
ß   Communication style
ß   Some customs

Less Visible

ß   Some customs
ß   Belief systems
ß   Attitudes
ß   Perceptions
ß   Values

changing one culture to adopt another cultural view. It only means that there is understanding and consideration that reflect the value of dignity toward those from different cultures. Taking interest in different cultures broadens your thinking and opens doors to new adventures. Think for a moment about what life would be like if our ancestors were afraid to start a fire or go into the water. How different would your life be today without fire or an appreciation of the ocean? When we refuse to be open and do not try to understand, we can easily **prejudge** and form prejudices. Some prejudices include:

prejudge

To decide or make a decision before having the facts.

- **Age prejudice:** A person is too old or too young.
- **National prejudices:** A person comes from a foreign country.
- **Physical prejudices:** How the person looks different from you.
- **Mental prejudice:** A person judges an individual by how smart a person is, how much a person knows, how well a person thinks.
- **Religious prejudices:** A person's beliefs are different from yours.
- **Racial prejudice:** A person belongs to a different race from you.

You can over come prejudice by learning about others. Here are some suggestions:

- Keep an open mind.
- Look for additional information. Why do people think the way they think? (For example, why does someone think people of another culture are lazy or not smart?)
- Watch documentaries, read books, magazines, and newspapers for information.
- Look at many resources before you form an opinion.
- Evaluate all the information. Ask yourself if it is true or false?

There are some basic points to keep in mind when experiencing aspects of a different culture.

- Values are an important part of every culture. Cultures have values and ideals that they believe are true, yet individual conduct may not always reflect those values. For example, a culture may value and honor their national flag, but not everyone in the cultural group may have a flag or display it.

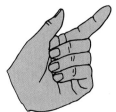

■ Behavior is not only the result of culture. Age, financial status, education, gender, experience, relationships, health, and many other factors influence behavior.

Figure 4.4

Motioning with a finger for someone to come.

■ It helps to look for the common characteristics of different cultures or to seek a common ground. For example, we are all part of the human race so food is common to all of us. We can explore different flavors, which are created by spices, cooking techniques, and so on. We also all have seasons of the year that have special meaning and that are celebrated through traditions.

■ Being open and willing to learn about others includes choosing your words carefully so they express your desire to learn. It is best to avoid saying things like:

- "We're all alike; we're all human"—A statement like this ignores the important differences that bring depth and richness to life. A person's dignity could be diminished causing her to feel that she needs to blend in more. People may change their names to fit in or avoid traditions that may draw attention to the differences.

- "We should stay with our own culture, we are too different"—This statement may cause fear and separation. When fear causes separation, defensive attitudes and behavior often follow. Arguments or fights are often the result of such fear. Learning about other cultures is enriching and broadens our view about life. Understanding other cultures usually brings a more complete understanding of your own culture and helps you communicate better with others.

Now decide what your opinion is.

Our behavior sends a message to others. They receive or understand the message by the way they interpret behavior. When more than one culture is involved, the interpretation of a behavior is often different. For example, to use the motion illustrated in Figure 4.4 to get a person to come is acceptable in the United States. In many other cultures, it is insulting and rude. Learning about communication in other cultures helps the health care worker understand the true meaning of behavior. This information allows you to respond with understanding.

GESTURES AND BODY LANGUAGE
Personal Space and Touching

Personal space and touching are defined in different societies as close contact and more distant contact. Personal space is the space needed to feel comfortable when we are with other people. Figures 4.4 to 4.6 show examples of societies where more distant contact is expected.

People in close-contact societies are comfortable with less space between them. Close-contact societies may be more likely to touch an arm or shoulder of the person they are talking with in the United States. It is important to use caution when touching. A touch can be easily misunderstood.

Some Southeast Asian cultures believe that a person's spirit is on the head. Touching the head is often considered an insult. Table 4.4 explains who is permitted to touch or not touch the head.

Table 4.3 ■ Close-Contact and Distant-Contact Regions		
	Close-Contact Regions	**Distant-Contact Regions**
REGIONS	• Africa • Indonesia • Latin America • Mediterranean • Southern Europe	• Canada • Great Britain • Northern Europe • United States
COMMON BEHAVIOR	• Men hold hands with men and women hold hands with women. • Men and women greet one another by kissing on both cheeks.	People greet one another with a handshake or hand gesture. Close friends or family members may hug each other.

Figure 4.5

Talking intimately.

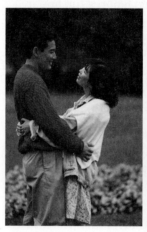
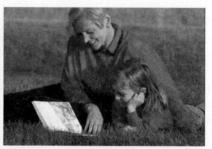
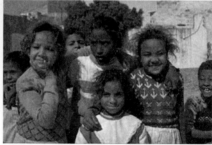

Greetings

Greeting another person is important in all cultures. The way a greeting is given and received often determines how positive or negative the meeting is. Table 4.5 describes greetings in various cultures.

Hand Gestures

Hand gestures help communicate many things. It is very important to use correct gestures so that others are not offended. Figure 4.8 illustrates gestures that are offensive in other cultures.

Eye Contact

In some cultures, eye contact may indicate that a person is listening, sincere, or honest. In other cultures, direct eye contact is considered to be hostile or disrespectful. Table 4.6 explains some cultural views about eye contact.

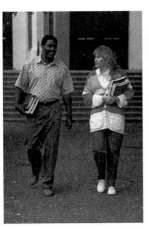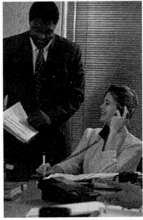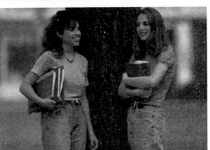

Figure 4.6

Respecting personal distance.

Table 4.4 ■ Guidelines Restricting Touch and Physical Closeness in Southeast Asian Cultures.

Cambodian	Vietnamese	Laotian
• Only a parent can touch the head of a child.	• Only elderly people can touch the head of a child.	• It is necessary to ask permission to move near another person.
• Members of the opposite sex never touch each other in public, not even brothers and sisters.		

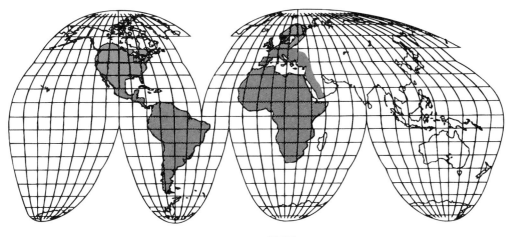

Close-contact cultures   More-distant cultures

Figure 4.7

Regions of the world showing the location of close-contact and more-distant cultures.

Table 4.5 ■ Guidelines for Greeting People

Anglo-American	Latin American	Cambodian, Laotian	Vietnamese	Hmong
Shake hands if desired.	Shake hands or hug.	Do not shake hands. Instead, put hands together at different levels. 1. Equal status—hands must be at chest level. 2. Older person or stranger—hands must be at chin level. 3. Relative or teacher—hands must be at nose level.	Salute by joining both hands and moving them against the chest.	Bow head or shake hands.

Table 4.6 ■ Eye-Contact Guidelines

Anglo-American	African Americans	Navajo	Japanese, Southeast Asian, Hispanic
Eye contact is important; it indicates interest, honesty, and listening.	Eye contact may not be important. Being in the same room indicates attentiveness.	Direct eye contact is avoided. • Peripheral vision is used. • Direct stares are considered hostile or a way to scold children.	Eye contact is avoided as a form of respect.

COMMUNICATING EFFECTIVELY WITH PEOPLE FROM OTHER CULTURES

When speaking with people from other cultures, the tone of your speaking voice is similar in importance to the gestures you use. Speaking tone includes voice quality, volume, and pitch. Voice tones cause positive or negative reactions from others. Clear pronunciations are more easily understood. When speaking to others who are learning English,

■ Speak clearly; do not slur words.

■ Speak so that they can hear you easily.

■ Do not raise your voice or yell.

■ Speak in moderate tones.

SAME GESTURE, SAME MEANING, BUT VERY DIFFERENT CONNOTATIONS

Figure 4.8

Hand gestures.

	American Culture	Asian Cultures
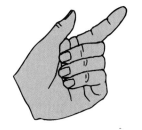	OK for "Come here."	Absolutely *taboo* for calling a person, even a child. It's the way to call an animal (a dog, in particular), especially when accompanied by a whistle. Considered *very insulting.*
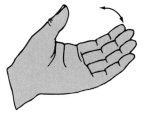	OK for "Come up here."	Never use. Only an inferior person would be summoned this way. Considered *insulting,* even to a child.
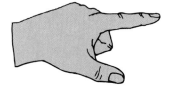	OK to point at someone or something.	OK to point at *something* but not at *someone.* Considered too direct a reference, amounting to confrontation, which the Indo-Chinese avoid by all means.
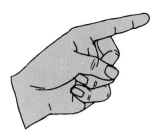	Slight threat (or warning) when making a point to someone.	Relatively strong threat made by a person of superior rank to an inferior (father to son, teacher to student). This is one step ahead of corporal punishment. (A parent would *never* use this gesture to a girl because it is considered too brutal.)

■ Pronounce the entire word; do not draw it out or shorten sounds.

■ Summarize often.

■ Confirm their understanding.

■ Clarify when necessary.

■ Do not assume that they understand.

You gain greater interpersonal effectiveness when you strive to understand and respect people of a different culture and viewpoint. Making every effort to understand and to be understood is one way to treat others with dignity.

traditional

Customary beliefs passed from generation to generation.

⬤ FOLK MEDICINE

Folk medicine is a collection of **traditional** beliefs and customs for treating pain or illness. Many who practice folk medicine believe that natural materials, such as herbs, spices, and tree herbs, and spiritual prayers and rituals keep evil spirits away and allow the body to heal.

It is very important to respect the beliefs of other cultures. If you insult the patient, you will be ineffective in providing care. Some caregivers work with their patients' beliefs to create positive relationships. Then they can introduce other suggestions for care.

Learn about the common practices in your clients' cultures. Read magazines and books about other cultures. Ask questions. Learn about ritual healing, folk medicine, and spiritual healing. Keep informed! Your understanding helps the patient get well faster and feel respected. The experience will be positive for both of you.

The following information is an overview of some common folk medicine practices in various cultures. Some practices that cause painful symptoms are not considered abusive because they are based on a belief of the culture.

Armenians

- Give the mother a party 1 week after a baby is born. The mother is served bread, which she dips into a paste of margarine, sugar, and flour. This is a celebration of the birth of the child.
- **Prohibit** a menstruating woman from attending church, taking a shower, or eating spicy foods.

prohibit

To not allow.

Cambodians

- Use herbs as medicine.
- Use cupping for headaches. Cupping leaves a round mark on the forehead. A cotton ball saturated in alcohol is placed in a glass and set on fire. After burning for a few seconds, the cotton is discarded. The heated glass is placed upside down over the painful area.
- Use coining for pain. Oil or ointment is applied to the skin. Then a large coin is used to rub the painful area in one direction until the blood is raised to just below the surface of the skin. This leaves red areas on the skin.
- Consider the color white to be a sign of bad luck. White indicates mourning and death. Think about a Cambodian's first visit to a caregiver. Is it possible that the white uniform might seem frightening?

Central and South Americans

- Use herbal home remedies.
- Teach a menstruating woman not to get her head wet and to avoid eating cucumbers, oranges, lemons, pork, lard, and deer meat.

Chinese

- Use herbs as medicine.
- Practice acupuncture and use herbs over puncture sites.
- Use cupping with heated bamboo.

Hmong and Mien Tribes

■ Perform spiritual ceremonies to please the spirits that cause illness.

■ Use herbal home remedies, including opium.

Iranians

■ Believe that poor health is predetermined (fatalism).

■ Use herbs, foods, rituals, and magic formulas for healing.

■ Believe the "Evil Eye" (a person or animal that causes injury through a look) causes sudden illness.

■ When of the Islamic faith, require washing of the face and hands before prayer.

■ Require periodic baths for cleansing.

Koreans

■ Practice alchemy, a medieval practice of magic and natural herbal remedies.

■ Use acupuncture.

■ Go to hot springs for bath rituals and massage.

■ Use energy and brain stimulants.

Native Americans

■ Use herbs and spices.

■ Use modern medical practices.

■ Some rely on a shaman (medicine man or woman) to remove pain and evil spirits.

Vietnamese

■ Commonly use herbal medicine.

■ Use cupping for head pain, cough, muscle pain, and motion sickness.

■ Use acupuncture for musculoskeletal problems, visual problems, and other ailments.

Table 4.7 lists typical terms used by non-English-speaking Asian cultures to describe health problems.

Table 4.7 ■ Terms that Describe Health Problems

Terms	Condition
Weak heart	Palpitations, dizziness, faintness, feeling of panic
Weak kidney	Impotence, sexual dysfuntion
Weak nervous system	Headache, malaise, inability to concentrate
Weak stomach or liver	Indigestion
I'm skinny.	Sickliness
Fire, hot	Dark urine, flatulence, constipation
Air/wind, cold	Illness was caused by too much air

○ SUMMARY

Cultural beliefs are very important to all societies. You give quality care when you take the time to understand and respect patients of other cultures. Your caring about them as individuals will help them improve more quickly. If they are not ill, your caring builds mutual respect for future meetings.

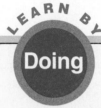

Doing   **UNIT 3 ACTIVITY**

1. Complete Worksheets/Activities 1 and 2 as assigned.

2. Complete Worksheets 3 and 4 as assigned.

3. Complete Worksheets/Activities 5 and 6 as assigned.

4. Prepare responses to each item listed in Chapter Review—Your Link to Success at the end of this chapter.

5. When you are confident that you can meet each objective for this unit, ask your instructor for the unit evaluation.

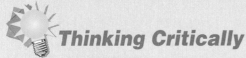

Thinking Critically

1. **Communication** You always talk to your adult patients/clients using their title and last name as you have been trained. You cannot help noticing that many of them respond cheerfully to a co-worker who uses first names. You suspect that some of your patients/clients think you are too formal. Write a paragraph describing how you could handle this situation.

2. **Cultural Competency** Make a list of some of the different reactions to pet therapy that you would expect from different cultures, for example, various Asian groups as well as South American and Mediterranean.

3. **Medical Terminology** Compare and contrast the World Health Organization's definition of *health* with the meaning of *holistic*.

4. **Patient Education** You have a patient/client from Iran. Her family is concerned about leaving her alone during the day, so they admit her to a long-term care facility. She is convinced that she is going to die because her family brought her to the hospital. Describe the basic need that is not met, and explain your reasoning. Develop a plan to satisfy the need for your patient/client.

5. **Case Study** Your co-worker has a loud voice and demonstrates everything with his hands as he talks. You have also seen his gentle manner and tender, caring nature. You observe that some of your Cambodian patients seem to be afraid of him and even back away or avoid being around him. Explain why the Cambodian patients might respond to your co-worker in this manner. Describe what you would do and say to help your co-worker communicate his gentle, caring nature to the Cambodian patients.

Portfolio Connection

Mrs. Summers is an alert, ambulatory, 85-year-old patient. You observe that she argues about everything and with everyone. You cannot remember her ever agreeing to or being willing to do anything. Develop a plan to identify why Mrs. Summers is so argumentative. Your plan must clearly identify what you would do to involve other people. In your written paper, clearly identify her behavior, what causes it, and what the positive and negative outcomes are for her. Include a proposed solution, a method of evaluation, and a time line. When you have completed your paper and checked the format and grammar for accuracy, place it in the section for written samples.

Your successful completion of this assignment shows your ability to organize, analyze, and evaluate. These skills help you work effectively with the various needs of your patients/clients.

Identify two cultural groups outside of your own culture. Research the visible and less visible characteristics of each group. Determine how health care is perceived by each group. Write your findings in a paper using the vocational portfolio guidelines for a written report. Report orally to your classmates using visual materials to help support your presentation.

Portfolio Tip

Be aware of the tone and volume of your voice, especially when talking to patients from different cultures. Find a partner, role-play some situations, and tape record your voices. Critique one another. Speak clearly, not too slowly, and do not talk down to the patients.

Remember! 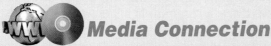 *Media Connection*

Use the Companion Website **www.prenhall.com/badasch** and the CD-ROM for additional interactive learning activities.

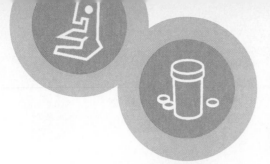

Effective Communications

Chapter 5

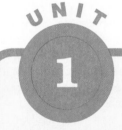

UNIT 1

Interpersonal Communication for All Ages

STEPS TO SUCCESS

1. Complete Vocabulary Worksheet 1 in the Student Workbook.
2. Read this unit.
3. Complete the Learn by Doing assignment at the end of this unit.

UNIT RATIONALE

The health care worker should understand that there are many factors in communication. A knowledge of the techniques of communication will increase your skills in communicating with co-workers and patients/clients. With this knowledge, you will be able to do a better job and to make good observations about your patients.

UNIT OBJECTIVES

When you have completed this unit, you will be able to do the following:

✔ Match vocabulary words with their correct meanings.

✔ Explain why communication is important.

✔ Name four elements that influence our relationship with others.

✔ List three barriers to communication.

✔ Identify your communication assertiveness level.

✔ List three elements necessary for communication to take place.

✔ Describe three things that a good listener does.

✔ Differentiate between verbal and nonverbal communication.

✔ Demonstrate responding, transferring a caller, and taking a message.

Communication is essential in the exchanging of ideas, feelings, and thoughts. Communication helps us know what the needs of others are and how to meet those needs. There are several kinds of communication. These include words, either written or spoken, gestures, facial expressions (frowns, smiles), body posture, touch, and listening. The following discussion has important information to help you become a better communicator with patients, families, co-workers, and supervisors.

○ ELEMENTS THAT INFLUENCE YOUR RELATIONSHIPS WITH OTHERS

Prejudices

All people form opinions or **biases** as they are growing up. These **prejudices** affect how they feel about other people and how they relate to them. You may have very strong feelings about the backgrounds or the values of your patients or co-workers. Your feelings affect how you communicate. For instance, if you believe that certain people are lazy, overly emotional, or **inferior,** you need to think about your prejudices. When you understand your prejudices and feelings, you have an opportunity to overcome them.

Frustrations

When you care for and work with others, you may experience **impatience, annoyance,** and probably anger. Perhaps other people do not understand your directions, or they may move too slowly. You feel irritated. These feelings interfere with your ability to communicate. Take time to understand why you feel frustrated. Evaluate the situation, and then try to correct it. It is your responsibility to control your behavior and to understand that patients, families, and co-workers have problems that are the cause of their behavior.

Attitudes

How you act toward others and how they act toward you affect the quality of **communication.** If you are disinterested or bored, if you are in a bad mood, if you wish you were someplace else—communication breaks down. However, if you show interest and concern for others, you will experience worthwhile communication, your job will become easier, and you will be more effective.

Life Experiences

People have new experiences every day. These help us know what to expect in day-to-day living. They also help us know how to act in certain situations. This understanding gives health care workers a knowledge of their own behavior and helps them communicate more effectively.

○ BARRIERS TO COMMUNICATION

Recognizing barriers to communication allows you to become an understanding health care worker. The following are three major communication barriers:

- **Labeling.** Deciding the other person is mean, lazy, a complainer, or difficult causes a breakdown in communication. You do not pay attention to the message being sent. If you listen, you might find out the reason for the behavior.

- **Sensory impairment.** Deafness or blindness can be a communication barrier. Always evaluate the people you are communicating with to be certain that they do not have a sensory impairment.

- **Talking too fast.** It is especially important when you are working with elderly people to speak slowly. Communication can break down when the message is delivered too rapidly.

Developing skills in communication helps you become a better health care worker. It is important always to be **courteous** and understanding. Take time to evaluate gestures, facial expressions, and tone of voice in order to understand what

biases
Tendencies; prejudices.

prejudices
Judgments or opinions formed before the facts are known.

inferior
Lower (e.g., one product is inferior in quality to another product).

impatience
Unwillingness to tolerate.

annoyance
Irritation (e.g., to feel irritated with a co-worker or patient).

communication
Act of exchanging information.

labeling
Describing a person with a word that limits them (e.g.,lazy, stupid).

courteous
Polite; considerate toward others.

is really being said. You may feel frustrated, angry, or irritated, but as a health care worker, it is up to you to attempt to understand and to listen. Hearing accurately and then responding appropriately are essential. Remember to communicate your messages so that they can be understood easily.

ELEMENTS OF COMMUNICATION

For communication to take place, there are three essential elements:

convey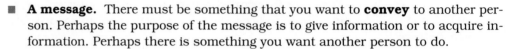

To say, tell, or express.

- **A message.** There must be something that you want to **convey** to another person. Perhaps the purpose of the message is to give information or to acquire information. Perhaps there is something you want another person to do.

- **A sender.** Unless there is someone who wants to send a message, there cannot be communication.

- **A receiver.** Even if there is a message and a sender, there must be a receiver. If there is no one to receive the message, communication is incomplete.

GOOD LISTENING SKILLS

When you think of communication, you may not think of listening. However, listening is a very important element in all communication. If you do not receive the message that is being sent, communication has not taken place. Your understanding of how to be a good listener makes you a better health care worker.

- **Show interest.** It is important for you to show interest in the person who is sending you a message (Figure 5.1). If you follow all of the other rules of being a good listener but tune out the message because you are not interested, communication will not take place.

- **Hear the message.** Health care workers frequently think that they understand what is being said to them when they really do not. It is important to repeat what you believe you heard being said to be certain you heard correctly. It is not necessary to repeat exactly what was said, but check to see if you have understood the general message.

Figure 5.1

Good eye contact, a gentle touch, and your body inflections show that you are interested in what is being said.

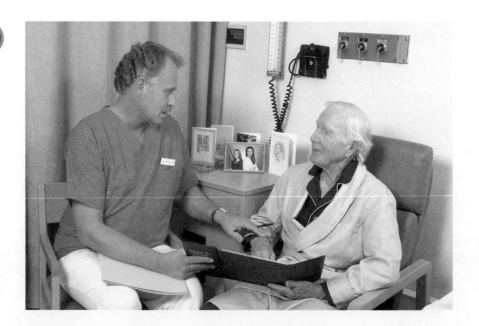

■ **Do not interrupt.** Have you ever tried to send a message and been frustrated by the receiver's interrupting you? Allow the sender to give you the entire message without interruptions. If you need to ask a question to clarify the meaning, be patient and wait until the sender is finished. She or he may give you the information you need without your questions.

Being a good listener takes patience. You need to concentrate on being a good listener until the skills become easy for you. As a health care worker, good listening is an essential skill. Good listening skills also help you follow directions, make good observations of patients, and understand your fellow workers.

ASSERTIVE COMMUNICATION

Communicating assertively is an honest and direct way to say what you feel or think. Being assertive allows you to express your feelings and thoughts. You must believe that you have the right to be heard and believed by others. You recognize that it is OK for you and for others to say no when it is appropriate—for example, when you are asked to do something you are not trained to do. It is OK to ask for something you want or need to accomplish a goal or task. This type of open, honest communication shows that you are a genuine person with self-respect and confidence. Assertiveness says that you have an awareness of and respect for others. To communicate strong health care values effectively, it is important for you to be an assertive communicator.

There are three common styles of communication:

■ *Unassertive, or passive, communication* allows others to control the conversation.

■ *Assertive communication* does not take power or authority away from others. It empowers individuals to speak up and be heard.

■ *Aggressive communication* occurs when power is taken away from others and communication breaks down.

Most people communicate in all three of these styles, depending on their feelings or thoughts at the time. Health care workers are more effective when they use assertive communication skills. You can develop your skills over time. Start by rating your preferred communication style on the assertiveness inventory in the Student Workbook, and follow the portfolio directions at the end of this chapter.

NONVERBAL COMMUNICATION

Communication also takes place in nonverbal ways. It is not necessary to speak in order to send a message. You send messages with your eye contact, facial expressions, **gestures,** and touch.

■ **Eye contact.** Making eye contact with the person with whom you are communicating is important. Eye contact lets others know that you are paying attention. When you do not make eye contact, you send others a message that you are not interested or that you wish to avoid them.

■ **Facial expressions.** A smile sends a different message than a frown does. It is possible to say something very kind and still send a message of anger with your eyes. Try to think of an instance when you knew that what was being said was not what was meant. How did you know? The expression on the sender's face probably sent you a different message.

■ **Gestures.** Shrugging your shoulders, turning your back, and leaving the room while someone is talking to you certainly convey a lack of interest in the sender's message. You need not say "I am not interested" because you have effectively sent that message through your gestures.

gestures

Motions of a part of the body to express feelings or emotions (e.g., nodding the head yes or no).

■ **Touch.** Touch can convey great caring, warmth, concern, and tenderness. It can also convey anger, rejection, and distaste. Touch is a very important part of your communication. It is important that your nonverbal communication be supportive and positive.

⬤ VERBAL COMMUNICATION

Verbal communication includes spoken and written messages.

■ **Spoken messages.** When you speak to someone, you send a message. The tone of your voice, the language you use, and the message you send are interpreted by the receiver. Always speak clearly and concisely. This ensures that your message is understood.

■ **Written messages.** You communicate frequently with the written word. You take messages and orders. You may write notes in the patient's/client's chart, and you may need to leave instructions for fellow workers. It is important to spell correctly, use proper grammar, and write in a clear and concise manner.

Telephone Communication

The telephone is an important communication tool between you and those you serve. All departments in the health care setting require good telephone communication skills. You may be asked to answer the telephone, take a message, or respond to a request. Always follow good communication standards when answering an incoming or placing an outgoing call.

Telephones at workstations are for communication of health care issues pertinent to those you serve. Personal calls and socializing must be done on your break or outside of your assignment or work time. See Table 5.1 for indicators that promote patient/client satisfaction when talking on the telephone and Table 5.2 for telephone guidelines.

Table 5.1 ■ Indicators That Promote Patient/Client Satisfaction When Talking on the Telephone

Communication Objective	Service/Excellence	Behavior	
• Demonstrate open, honest, and respectful communication. • Present ideas, information, and viewpoints clearly both verbally and in writing. • Listen actively and seek to understand others.	Use good telephone manners.	Answer the telephone cheerfully. • Use a pleasant, caring, and sincere tone of voice. • Answer the telephone on the first ring if possible. • Speak clearly and courteously. • Remember to thank the caller when a call is returned. • Identify yourself and give your title (e.g., "This is Monica, nurse assistant."). • Identify your department or doctor's office (e.g., "Dr. Smith's office"). • Thank the caller for calling. • Allow the caller to hang up first to ensure that the caller has said everything he or she wanted to say. • Use appropriate words and phrases:	
		Appropriate	Inappropriate
		• May I have your name, please? • Would you repeat that, please? • How may I assist you? • I'm sorry; I didn't understand.	• What's your name? • What did you say? • What do you want? • Huh?

Table 5.2 ■ Telephone Guidelines

Being Prepared	Placing a Caller on Hold	Transferring a Caller	Writing a Message	Leaving a Message

• Have the necessary materials
  –Pencil
  –Message pad
  –Telephone
  –Facility and public telephone directory
• Before placing a call
  –Prepare questions to ask.
  –Gather information to share with the person you are calling.
  –Determine appropriate action to take.
• Follow the patient/client satisfaction indicators in Table 5.1.
	• Ask the caller if he or she can hold and wait for the response.
	• Check every 30 seconds to see if the caller wants to continue to hold.
	• Ask if you may take a message.
	• Transfer the call as soon as possible.
	• Follow the patient/client satisfaction indicators in Table 5.1.
		• Explain where you are transferring the caller and to whom.
		• Give the caller the number you are transferring to.
		• If possible, stay on the telephone and introduce the caller to the person receiving the call.
		• Follow the patient/client satisfaction indicators in Table 5.1.
			• Record time and date.
			• Write clearly
			  –The caller's name—verify spelling.
			  –The telephone number–read back the number.
			• Summarize information with the caller by repeating the message.
			• Sign or initial the message.
			• Record the action you take to deliver the message.
			• Follow the patient/client satisfaction indicators in Table 5.1.
				• State
				  –Whom you are calling for.
				  –Your name and where you are calling from.
				  –Your message—remembering to follow confidentiality guidelines.
				  –The times that you will be available for a return call.
				• Document date, time, and message left.
				• Follow the patient/client satisfaction indicators in Table 5.1.

⬤ SUMMARY

Communication requires a sender, a receiver, and a message. The message may be verbal or nonverbal, and many factors influence the effectiveness of communication. These factors include prejudices, frustrations, attitudes, and life experiences. Good listening skills are important to ensure successful communication, and an awareness of barriers to good communication is important.

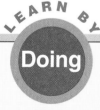

LEARN BY **Doing**

UNIT 1 ACTIVITY

1. Ask your instructor for directions to complete Worksheet/ Activity 2.

2. Complete Worksheet 3.

3. Ask your instructor for directions to complete Worksheet/Activity 4.

4. Complete Worksheets 5 through 7.

5. Ask your instructor for directions to complete Worksheet/Activity 8.

6. When you are confident that you can meet each objective listed, ask your instructor for the unit evaluation.

Charting and Observation

STEPS TO SUCCESS

1. Read this unit.

2. Complete the Learn by Doing assignment at the end of this unit.

UNIT RATIONALE

Observation and documentation of your observations are a key component of health care. Your ability to observe patient/client behavior and symptoms will directly affect their care. Accurate documentation provides information needed to make decisions about their care. It is important that you develop sharp observation, reporting, and documentation skills.

UNIT OBJECTIVES

When you have completed this unit, you will be able to do the following:

✔ Explain the difference between subjective and objective observations.

✔ Explain which type of reporting allows immediate feedback and action.

✔ List information that must be on all health records.

✔ Apply five general charting guidelines.

○ OBSERVATION

Every health care worker is responsible for observing the patient/client. Even if you are not responsible for charting, you must report your observations to your supervisor. You are responsible for making good observations moment by moment. Your observation skills must be fine-tuned so that you are aware of the patient's mental and physical state. This awareness helps you and your co-workers be more effective.

When interacting with patients and their families, use all of your tools to evaluate the situation. Your tools are four of your five senses: sight, hearing, touch, and smell.

- *Look* for all visible signs that may indicate a reason for the client's complaint.

- *Listen* carefully. Don't put thoughts or words into others' minds. Be sure that you understand fully what you are told.

- *Feel* for changes in the skin, body temperature, abnormal structures, and so on.

- *Smell* unusual odors, which are often the first clue to a problem (e.g., fruity breath, foul stools).

There are two types of observations:

- *Subjective observations* cannot be seen. They are ideas, thoughts, or opinions. If you cannot see it, feel it, hear it, or smell it, it is a subjective observation. (The patient complains of pain—you cannot see it, feel it, hear it, or smell it.)

- *Objective observations* can be seen. If you can see it, feel it, hear it, or smell it, it is an objective observation. (The patient has a cut—you can see it.)

The health care worker must report and document all subjective and objective observations. Any unusual event or change in a patient must be reported verbally to the supervisor and then documented on the client's legal record.

REPORTING

Reporting unusual events or any change in behavior or condition is every health care worker's responsibility. Observation of people in a waiting area or a patient care area is important. Verbal reports to a supervisor allow immediate feedback and action when necessary. For example, you must always report changes in blood pressure, breathing, or coloring (e.g., pale, **flushed**) and any indications that a person is in distress. It is also important to report anyone who acts strangely, threateningly, or weakly or appears to be in pain. Do *not* wait for others to report unusual observations. You may prevent a serious situation by reporting your observation in a timely manner.

flushed

Showing reddening of the skin.

DOCUMENTATION

Documentation is required in all health care settings. Documentation is a record of the patient's progress throughout treatment. Many people may be responsible for documenting information on a single patient/client. This record provides the information needed to allow each health care provider to give the care that best benefits the patient.

All records must contain certain information:

- Client's name
- Client's address
- Diagnosis
- Client's age
- Identification number
- Physician's orders

Depending on the department where the record is kept, other information may be required. Each health care worker who cares for the patient makes a notation on the chart. (Your facility policy tells you if you are required to chart. Even if you do not chart, you must always report your observations.) These notations should contain specific information about the client, including

- Care or treatment given
- Time of treatment
- How the patient tolerated the care or treatment
- Any observations that would be helpful to other health care workers
- Information that the patient has given that would affect treatment

This documentation is admissible in a court of law. This means that anything you write is considered to be true. If you do not write down something that you did for the patient, it is assumed that it was not done. As you can see, it is very important to be accurate and careful when you chart.

Everyone must follow these general guidelines for charting:

- Use ink for record keeping. In some facilities, different colors are used for different shifts.
- Entries must be **legible.** If your writing is difficult to read, you should print.
- If you make an error, do not erase it or scratch it out or cover it up. Draw a single line through the error so that it can still be read. Write "error" next to it, and then place your initials next to the correction (e.g., "error/KG Patient tolerated procedure well.")
- Entries should be in short phrases. You do not need to write complete sentences. You do not need to use the patient's name because you are writing in the patient's chart. Your entries should be concise, clear, and meaningful.
- All entries that you make are followed by your signature. You sign with your first initial, your last name, and your title.

legible

Capable of being read easily.

Hospital Chart

The rules listed above apply to all charting. However, additional charting may be required. This is especially true for the nurse assistant. Each facility has its own policy and procedures for charting. Learn what these are. There are some standard types of charting that all nurse assistants are required to do:

■ *Nurses' notes* may be in narrative or check-off form. These notes state

• What personal care was given • What activities the client participated in • The patient's skin condition • General observations about the client • Any unusual occurrences • Any complaints that the client has • What treatments were given • Any information that is important to the patient's well-being

During your career you may be asked to document in many different styles. To avoid confusion in this book, we will use the following style:

Date

Military time

A description of the care or treatment given, complaints and problems, all written as ordinary sentences

Signature (first initial, full last name) and certification.

Many facilities provide flow sheets with charting examples and when employed you will follow those examples.

■ The *graphic chart* is a record of the patient's vital signs. All graphic charts have time blocks and numbers that relate to temperature, pulse, and respiration. On some graphic charts there is also space for blood pressure, intake and output, bowel movements, and weight (Figure 5.2).

Figure 5.2

Graphic chart with intake and output section.

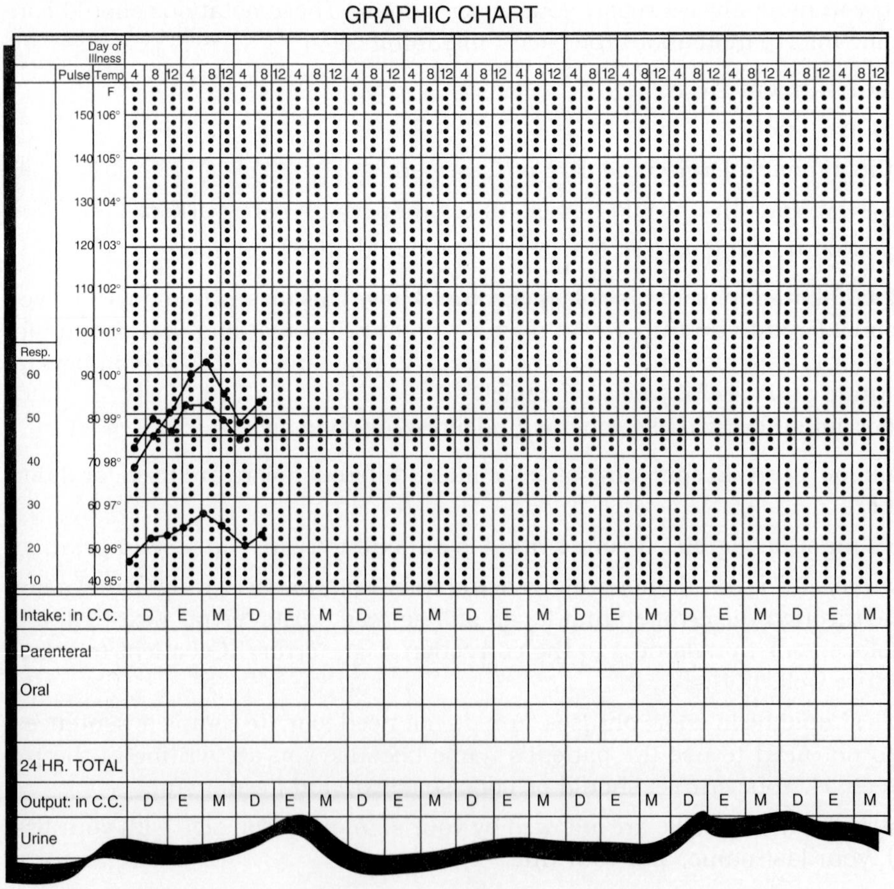

GRAPHIC CHART

Other parts of the chart include

- A front sheet with personal information, such as name, address, marital status, place of employment, and admission diagnosis
- A physical examination and a medical history
- The daily progress report written by the physician
- There may be

   • A discharge plan • A social worker's report • Treatment records from other departments in the hospital or from specialists

Documentation is a very important responsibility. Learn how to write good records, and always be responsible and careful when you chart.

◯ CONFIDENTIALITY

It is important to remember our discussion of confidential information in Chapter 3. When communicating any information concerning the client, remember that it is confidential and is not discussed unless it affects the treatment. The physician and patient will decide if family members or others will share the information.

◯ JOBS AND PROFESSIONS

- PBX operator
- Psychologist
- Social worker
- Psychiatrist
- Receptionist
- Speech pathologist

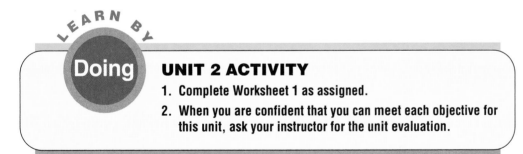

Doing **UNIT 2 ACTIVITY**

1. Complete Worksheet 1 as assigned.
2. When you are confident that you can meet each objective for this unit, ask your instructor for the unit evaluation.

Computers in Health Care

STEPS TO SUCCESS

1. Complete Vocabulary Worksheet 1 in the Student Workbook.

2. Read this unit.

3. Complete the Learn by Doing assignment at the end of this unit.

UNIT OBJECTIVES

When you have completed this unit, you will be able to do the following:

✔ Match vocabulary words with their correct meanings.

✔ List and explain how four computerized diagnostic tests help diagnose disease or illness.

✔ State how environmental services use computers.

✔ Describe ways that information services use computers.

✔ Discuss ethics and confidentiality as they relate to computers.

UNIT RATIONALE

Computers are essential in health care. Health care agencies use computers in most departments to help save time and improve accuracy. They are used for record keeping, diagnostic tests, education, research, and many other tasks. Health care workers must have a basic understanding of how computers work and how they are used in health care in order to be employable.

⬤ COMPUTERS IN GENERAL

During the past 40 years, computer technology has grown at an unbelievable rate. The early computers were made of vacuum tubes and required large, environmentally controlled rooms. They often overheated and became inoperable for many hours. Repairing them was time consuming. Large systems were very expensive, and only the largest organizations were able to afford them. Today's computer technology allows computers to be smaller, more powerful, and less expensive.

⬤ BASIC COMPUTER COMPONENTS

Computers have basic components that you need to learn in order to understand computer terminology. All computers must allow users to input information, must be able to process information, and must have some way to output information.

Inputting

Several devices are used to input information into a computer. The most common are the keyboard and the light pen. The keyboard looks like a typewriter with a few extra keys. One key plays a very important function. This is the Enter key. When you finish putting your information into the computer, you must signal the computer, "I'm done. Now it's your turn." You do this with the Enter key.

The light pen looks like a pencil, but it is designed to sense the writing on the computer screen. The user selects one of the choices displayed on the screen and moves the light pen across the choice. Then the user presses the Enter key.

Other input devices include keypunch cards, floppy diskettes, and magnetic disks or tapes. These devices are used for both inputting and storing records.

Processing

A computer processes the information that is input and returns the information to the person who input it or to someone in another department. The central processing unit (CPU) is the working unit of the computer. The CPU consists of many electronic components and microchips. The CPU can process only the information it receives; if it receives incorrect information, it processes incorrect information. This is where the phrase "Garbage in, garbage out" comes from. You must be accurate when you enter information.

Outputting

Just as there are several devices for inputting information into a computer, there are several devices for outputting it. The two most common are the monitor and the printer. The health care worker uses both of these devices.

Monitor

A monitor or video screen, also called a *cathode ray tube (CRT)*, looks much like a television screen. As you input information, you can see it on the screen of the monitor. When it is processed, you see the results on the screen. You can also recall stored information to the screen.

Printer

A printer is used to print the processed information on paper. Information printed on paper is called *hard copy* and can be filed with the patient's records.

COMPUTERS IN HEALTH CARE

Computers are processors of information. They process large amounts of information at incredible speeds, accurately and consistently. Wherever your career path in the health field takes you, you will do a portion of your work on a computer. Hospitals and medical and dental offices are converting medical records, accounting, and purchasing functions to computers. Some health care agencies have computer diagnostic services where a complete physical examination is analyzed by a computer.

In the hospital, a computer performs many functions. The following are some of the procedures computers assist with:

- Recording physicians' notes and orders
- Charting at bedside
- Ordering or changing diets
- Ordering unit supplies
- Processing charges for nursing care equipment
- Ordering lab work and receiving lab results
- Recording lab results for patient records
- Scheduling x-rays, special tests, and surgeries
- Processing discharges
- Performing Diagnostic testing
- Researching via the Internet

In medical and dental offices, computers can be used to schedule appointments, set up a recall system, bill patients, schedule lab work, dial the telephone, manage the security system, and keep the inventory. Computers are an important part of the search for correct specific patient/client data that meets the **HEDIS** requirements. Electronic medical records are a necessary method of monitoring patient/client progress and quality health care. Electronic records provide data that allows physicians to provide timely disease management.

The key benefit to electronic medical record systems is that they make information available to multiple staff at locations hundreds of miles apart at the same time. This also increases flexibility for medical professionals. Web services also play a role in providing data; for example, laboratory results are immediately sent to a Website,

HEDIS

Health Plan Employer Data and Information Set; an organization that provides quality care guidelines.

allowing physicians or other professionals to access them. Medical professionals can access complete patient/client data that previously was available only in the paper medical record. Not all medical environments have the funds and training available to implement electronic medical data systems; however, the systems will gradually become more affordable and therefore more accessible over time.

Therapeutic Services

If you choose to enter an occupation in the therapeutic services, you will have opportunities to work with a computer each day. In the pharmacy, drugs are inventoried using a computer. A computer also assists the pharmacist in keeping track of medications that a person receives. The computer can alert the pharmacist when one medication acts as an **antagonist** to another medication or contains a substance that causes an allergic reaction. In physical and occupational therapy, a computer assists paralyzed patients to walk. In respiratory therapy, a computer keeps critically ill patients in **homeostasis.** In emergency services and intensive care areas, computers do direct patient/client monitoring and are programmed to warn health care workers when a potentially dangerous condition occurs.

Diagnostic Services

In diagnostic services, highly sophisticated computers are being used. In the past, surgery and other **invasive** procedures were used to reach a diagnosis. Today, computerized diagnostic equipment helps diagnose many illnesses. Using computerized equipment removes the risks of surgery and reduces the pain and discomfort of invasive tests. Computerized tests include the following:

- The *CAT scanner* does computerized axial **tomography.** This test allows an organ to be transversely dissected to help find abnormalities (such as tumors) without surgery. A photograph is taken to provide the radiologist and the physician with a permanent record for future use.

- The *Coulter counter* completes multiple examinations of many blood specimens in seconds.

- The *electrocardiogram computer* creates pictures on a computer screen. It prints out the electrical activity of the heart. This helps the physician diagnose heart disease correctly.

- The *magnetic resonance imaging* (MRI) computer scans the body. The scanner produces a cross-sectional image of the body. This helps the physician find tumors, see the results of medication and treatment, and diagnose the cause of an illness or disease.

- The *positron emission tomography* (PET) computer is also a scanner. It produces a three-dimensional image that shows an organ or bone from all sides.

- The *ultrasound imager* computer produces a picture of internal organs, tumors, aneurysms, and other abnormalities. It also produces pictures of the fetus developing in the uterus to help with fetal monitoring. These pictures can be seen on the monitor or can be processed on a photographic film.

The latest electronic technology scans an organ and provides not only pictures, but also creates a three-dimensional object out of plastic. This object is an exact replica of the organ scanned in the patient's body. It allows the physician to practice difficult or experimental surgical procedures on the plastic replica before performing the procedure on the patient.

Environmental Services

Environmental careers also offer an opportunity to work with computers. Central supply services/central processing services are computerized for reordering inven-

antagonist

Something that works against.

homeostasis

Constant balance within the body. This balance is maintained by the heartbeat, blood-making mechanisms, electrolytes, and hormone secretions.

invasive

Entering the body.

tomography

X-ray technique that produces film of detailed cross sections of tissue.

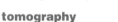

tory and for billing. Supplies are even categorized and identified by bar scanners like those you see in the grocery store.

Information Services

In information services, the computer is used in a variety of ways. Medical records workers manage and process records on computers. With diagnostic-related groupings, the computer is used to help categorize and track patients in the medical system. Health unit coordinators/unit secretaries use the computer to process many of the orders, transmitting requests to other departments.

The growing need to access medical data from patient/client files quickly is forcing health care providers to use computerized information systems. This means that to be employable, every health care worker must know the basics of computer keyboarding.

Contingency Planning

Whenever human beings depend on machines, **contingency** plans need to be made just in case the machine stops functioning. When a computer is not functioning, it is said to be *down*. Downtime can be scheduled to allow a new program to be entered into the computer's memory or to make changes. Downtime can also be unexpected (e.g., due to a power failure or component failure). Hospitals and medical/dental offices have learned that it is important to have an alternative plan if failure occurs. Despite modern technology, you still need to know manual methods of entering orders. The use of computers can make you more efficient in your job. With time, you will learn all of the things the computer can do, and you will learn how to do them. Practice is important in learning how to use the computer to its fullest capability.

contingency
Event that may occur but is not intended or likely to happen.

Ethics and Confidentiality

The health care worker must remember the importance of ethics and confidentiality when using a computer. Computers contain privileged information that must be protected. Keep your identification code or password confidential to protect you and the patient.

⚪ SUMMARY

In this unit you read that computers are an essential part of health care. All health care services have gained a greater ability to treat, diagnose, and care for patients/clients through computerization. Computers do shut down occasionally, making contingency planning important. The responsible use of computers means that all users must keep information learned about patients/clients confidential. Keeping your identification code or password a secret is also your responsibility.

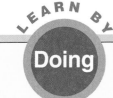

UNIT 3 ACTIVITY

1. **Complete Worksheets 2 and 3 as assigned.**
2. **Prepare responses to each item listed in Chapter Review—Your Link to Success at the end of this chapter.**
3. **When you are confident that you can meet each objective for this unit, ask your instructor for the unit evaluation.**

Thinking Critically

1. Communication Describe a recent event in which you or someone else did not use good listening skills. Explain what you or the person you observed could have done differently to demonstrate good listening skills in that situation.

2. Time Management Have you ever thought of good communication as a time saver? Write down the pluses and minuses of taking time to communicate properly. Describe in writing some problems that are caused by failure to communicate properly. Put this list in the personal section of your portfolio to remind you why you should speak with care.

3. Patient Education Explain how you know when patients/clients understand and can do what you have instructed them to do.

4. Legal How would you explain to a new employee the legal importance of clear and complete documentation? Create a bulleted list of points to be made.

5. Case Study The licensed nurse you are working with has been waiting all morning for a physician to call her back about a patient. Ten minutes after the nurse leaves the facility for a late lunch, you answer the telephone and it is the physician calling her back. Explain in writing what you will say and do.

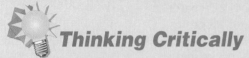 **Portfolio Connection**

The ability to communicate effectively is essential to successful interactions with others. Your decision to develop effective communication skills directly affects your success or failure in the work world. Your experience in a health occupations program is the perfect place to focus on developing assertive communication skills.

There are many easy-to-read books on assertiveness training that are helpful in learning about and practicing assertiveness. Go to your local library or resource center, and select and read a book that teaches assertive communication skills.

Identify your most common and least common communication type (unassertive, assertive, aggressive). Think of three recent experiences that demonstrate your use of unassertive or aggressive communication. What caused you to respond the way you did? What could you have done or said that would have made your responses assertive? What was the outcome of the unassertive or aggressive communication?

Explain your answer for all three experiences by writing a short paper. Your explanation must clearly identify the unassertive or aggressive statements or actions, indicate what you would change to create an assertive, effective communication, and compare the expected results with those of the unassertive or aggressive communication.

This assignment helps you evaluate the effectiveness of your most frequently used communication skill and allows you to express it in writing. Assertive written communication skills reflect your ability to communicate effectively in the health care environment. Your ability to demonstrate this skill in your portfolio presents you as an appropriate candidate for higher education or job opportunities. Place this assignment in Section Four, "Written Samples."

Portfolio Tip

How you deliver your message in both words and body language may be more important than the message itself: it may decide whether your audience is willing to listen. Think before you speak.

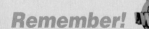 **Remember!** **Media Connection**

Use the Companion Website **www.prenhall.com/badasch** and the CD-ROM for additional interactive learning activities.

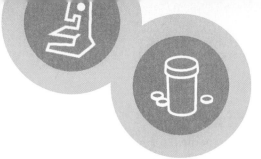

Medical Terminology

Chapter 6

MEDIA CONNECTION
Use the Companion Website
www.prenhall.com/badasch and the CD-ROM
for additional interactive learning activities.

UNIT 1

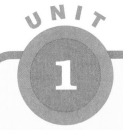

Pronunciation, Word Elements, and Terms

STEPS TO SUCCESS

1. Read this unit.
2. Complete the Learn by Doing assignment at the end of this unit.

UNIT RATIONALE

Health care workers use medical terminology in their work every day. It is the professional language that helps them communicate effectively and quickly. All caregivers use medical terminology to record orders, write instructions, take notes, and to chart. Health care workers are unable to perform their job if they cannot use and understand medical terminology.

UNIT OBJECTIVES

When you have completed this unit, you will be able to do the following:

✔ Define roots, prefixes, and suffixes.

✔ Define the word elements listed.

✔ Match medical terms with their correct meanings.

✔ Divide medical terms into elements.

✔ Combine word elements to form medical terms.

● INTRODUCTION TO MEDICAL TERMINOLOGY

Medical **terminology** can be fun, interesting, and challenging. At first medical terminology may seem hard to learn. However, with practice it becomes easier and easier. You need to learn how to build a medical term, how to pronounce it, and what it means. This unit gives you the tools that you need to learn and understand medical terms.

terminology
Specialized terms used in any occupation.

PRONUNCIATION

If you have never heard medical terms pronounced, they may seem very difficult. To make it easier for you, the following are some hints to help you pronounce the terms correctly:

- **ch** sounds like *k*

    Examples: chyme (kīm), cholecystectomy (kō-lē-sis-tek'-ō-me), chronic (kro-nic), chondroid (kon'-droyd)

- **ps** sounds like *s*

    Examples: psychiatric (sī-kē-a'-trik), pseudomonas (sū-dō-mō'-nas), psychology (sī-kol'-ō-ji), psoriasis (sō-rī'-a-sis)

- **pn** sounds like *n*

    Examples: pneumonia (nū-mō'-ni-a), pneumatic (nū-mat'-ik)

- **c** sounds like a soft *s* when it comes before *e, i,* and *y*

    Examples: cycle (sī-kl), cytoplasm (sī'-tō-plazm), cisternal (sis-ter'-nal), centrifuge (sen' tri-fūj)

- **g** sounds like *j* when it comes before *e, i,* and *y*

    Examples: giant (jī'-ent), gestation (jes-tā'-shun), generic (jen-er'-ik), gyration (jī-rā'-shun)

- **i** sounds like *eye* when added to the end of the word to form a plural

    Examples: glomeruli (glō-mer'-ū-lī), villi (vil'-lī), alveoli (al-vē'-ō-lī), bacilli (ba-sil'-lī)

FORMING MEDICAL TERMS FROM WORD ELEMENTS

Medical terms are words that consist of several parts. All medical terms have a word root. Most medical terms have the root word and a prefix, a combining vowel, and a suffix. In some cases, the word has only a prefix or suffix added to the root. When you add different prefixes and suffixes to the word root, you change the meaning of the medical term. The combining vowel makes the word easier to pronounce. You build a large medical term vocabulary when you learn the meanings of word parts and how to combine them (Figure 6.1).

- The *word root* is the main part of the word and tells what the word is about. For instance, *cardio* is the root word that means "heart." This is the subject of the word you are going to build.

- The *prefix* is a word element added to the beginning of a word root. The prefix is added to the root to change the meaning or to make it more specific. The prefix *electro* means "pertaining to electricity."

- The *suffix* is an element added to the end of the word root that changes or adds to the meaning of the root. The suffix *gram* means "record."

Figure 6.1

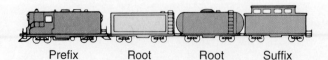

Prefix Root Root Suffix   Prefix   Root   Root   Suffix

■ The *combining vowel* makes it possible to combine several word roots. It also makes the word easier to pronounce (Figure 6.2).

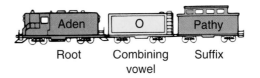

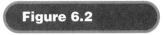

Root Combining vowel Suffix

When all the previous word elements are combined, the word is *electrocardiogram* (electr/o/cardi/o/gram). It means "an electrical record of the heart."

The following are some examples of (common) English words (Figure 6.3):

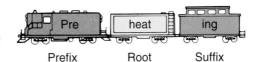

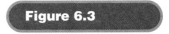

Prefix Root Suffix

Combining Word Elements

Prefix	Root	Suffix	Word
pre	heat	ing	preheating
	gentle	ness	gentleness
	speed	o/meter	speedometer

Rules for Combining Word Elements

Rules help make medical terminology easier to learn. When everyone uses the rules, there are fewer mistakes. A mistake in combining a word can change its meaning and cause confusion.

Combining Vowels

■ The combining vowel is usually an *o*, for example, *oste/o. Oste* means "bone," and the *o* is the combining vowel. The *o* can be added to join a word root with another word root or a suffix. Sometimes an *i, y,* or *u* is used. Combining vowels make it easier to pronounce the term. For example, *osteomyelitis* is easier to pronounce than *ostemyelitis.*

■ When the suffix begins with one of the vowels *(a, e, i, o, u),* the *o* on the root word is not used. Since *oste/o* ends in *o* and the suffix *-itis* begins with a vowel, the *o* is dropped. The word is *osteitis,* which means "inflammation of the bone."

■ The combining vowel is placed between root words, for example, *osteoporosis* (oste/o/por/osis). Pronounce the word with the combining vowel, and you can tell that it is easier to say than *osteporosis.*

The following words are examples of word elements that have been combined to form a medical term:

aden/o/pathy	disease of the glands
hepat/o/rrhagia	hemorrhage of the liver
poly/arthr/itis	inflammation of many joints
hyster/ectomy	surgical removal of the uterus
hyster/o/salping/ectomy	surgical removal of the uterus and fallopian tubes
oste/o/por/osis	condition of pores in the bone

After you learn the roots, prefixes, and suffixes, you can combine many word parts to form medical terminology. There is always at least one root word, and there may be more than one root word. When you add a prefix or a suffix you create a new word.

Changing Words from Singular to Plural

■ Use the rule for changing words from singular to plural that applies to the language the word comes from; for example, the English word *wavelength* adds an -*s* to become *wavelengths*. Since many medical terms come from Greek or Latin, use the following rules for Greek or Latin words.

■ Add an -*e* to a word ending in -*a*—for example, *axilla* to *axillae*.

■ Drop the -*ax* at the end of a word and add -*aces*—for example, *thorax* to *thoraces*.

■ Change the -*x* to -*g* in a word that ends in -*nx* and add -*es*—for example, *phalanx* to *phalanges*.

■ Drop -*ix* or -*ex* at the end of the word and add -*ices*—for example, *appendix* to *appendices*.

■ Drop the -*y* at the end of a word and add -*ies*—for example, *myringotomy* to *myringotomies*.

■ Drop the -*us* at the end of a word and add an -*i*—for example, *alveolus* to *alveoli*.

■ Drop the -*on* at the end of a word and add an -*a*—for example, *ganglion* to *ganglia*.

■ Drop the -*is* at the end of a word and add -*es*—for example, *metastasis* to *metastases*.

■ Drop the -*um* at the end of a word and add -*a*—for example, *ischium* to *ischia*.

■ Drop the -*ma* at the end of the word and add -*mata*—for example, *stoma* to *stomata*.

When you learn the following word elements, you have the tools to combine hundreds of medical terms. Learn which words are prefixes, which are roots, and which are suffixes. When you know the terms, it is easy to learn the specialized language of a health care worker.

Prefix	Meaning	Prefix	Meaning
a, an	without	intra	inside, within
ab	away from	macro	large
ad	toward	mal	bad
ante	before	micro	small
anti	against	mono	one, single
bi	both, two	neo	new
brady	slow	ortho	straight
circum	around	pan	all
con	with	para	beside, beyond
contra	against	peri	around
diplo	double	poly	many
dors	back	post	behind, after
dys	painful, difficult	pre	before, in front of
ecto	outside	pro	forward
endo	inside, within	pseudo	false
epi	upper, above	retro	backward
ex	out from	semi	half
hemi	half	sub	below
hyper	excessive, above, more than	super	above
		supra	above
hypo	deficient, below, less than	tachy	rapid
		trans	across
inter	between		

Root	Meaning	Root	Meaning
acro	extremities	faci	face
aden	gland	fascia	band, fibrous
angio	vessel (blood)	gastro	stomach
ankyl	crooked, looped	gingiva	gum
arterio	artery	gloss	tongue
arthro	joint	gyne	woman
aud, aur	ear, hearing	hemo	blood
blepharo	eyelid	hepat	liver
brachi	arm	hydro	water
bronchi	bronchial	hystero	uterus, womb
bucca	cheek	iri	iris (eye)
carcin	cancer	kerat	cornea, scaly
cardio	heart	labia	lip
caud	tail	lacrim	tear
cephal	head	lacto	milk
cerebro	brain	lapar	abdomen
cervic	neck	laryng	larynx
cheil	lip	leuko	white
chole	bile	lingua	tongue
cholecyst	gallbladder	lip	fat
chondro	cartilage	lith	stone
coccus	round	lymph	fluid
col	colon	mamm, mast	breast
colp	vagina	melan	black
costo	ribs	mening	membrane (pertaining to the covering of the brain or spinal cord)
cranio	skull	meno, mens	menstruate
cut	skin	myelo	bone marrow
cyan	blue	myo	muscle
cysto	bladder, sac	nares	nose, nostrils
cyt, cyte	cell	necr	death
dacry	tear duct	nephro	kidney
dactyl	fingers, toes	neuro	nerve
dent	tooth	ocul	eye
derma	skin	odont	tooth
dextr	right	oophoro	ovary
duoden	duodenum	ophthal	eye
edema	swelling	orchis	testes
electr	electric	osteo	bone
emesis	vomit	oto	ear, hearing
enter	intestine		
erythro	red		
esophag	esophagus		
esthesi	feeling		

Root	Meaning
ovario	ovary
ovi	egg
part	birth, labor
ped, pod	foot
ped	child
phagia	swallow
pharyng	pharynx
phasia	speak
phleb	vein
pleur	pleura of the lung
pneumo	lung
procto	rectum
psycho	mind, soul
pulm	lung
pyelo	pelvis of the kidney
pyo	pus
ren	kidney
rhin	nose
salpingo	tube
semin	seed
soma	body
splen	spleen
spondyl	spine
squam	scaly
stoma	mouth
stric	narrowing
therm	heat
thorac	thorax
thrombo	clot
trachi	trachea
vas	vessel
vesic	bladder, sac
viscera	organ

Suffix	Meaning
a, ac	pertaining to
al	like, similar, pertaining to
algia	pain
cele	hernia
cente	puncture

Suffix	Meaning
crine	secrete
desis	surgical fixation
ectomy	surgical removal
emia	blood
genesis, genic	source, origin
gram, graph	pictures
ia	a disease; an unhealthy state or condition
ic, ical, is	pertaining to
itis	inflammation
lysis	destruction
malacia	softening
megaly	enlarged
oid	like, similar
ology	study of
oma	tumor
orrhagia	hemorrhage
orrhaphy	suture
orrhea	flow
osis	condition of
ostomy	surgical opening
otomy	incision into
pathy	disease
penia	deficiency
pexy	fixation
phobia	fear
plasty	surgical repair
plegia	paralysis
ptosis	drooping down
sarcoma	tumor, cancer
sclerosis	hardening
scope	picture, inspection
spasm	contraction
stasis	stoppage
um	pertaining to
uria	urine
y	the act of or result of an action

How to use Medical Terminology

Medical terminology provides a system for health workers to communicate with each other. When a patient complains to the doctor about a "pain in the stomach," it can mean many different things. Often the patient is referring to pain in the lower abdominal cavity and not the stomach. For instance, the patient may be assuming that "the stomach" is the entire area between the ribs and the pelvis. The doctor must ask exactly where the pain is, how it feels, how long it has been a problem, and other questions. After making a diagnosis the primary case provider must be able to tell the health care workers exactly what the problem is. When the entire health care team understands the problem they can treat the patient in the most effective way.

The patient in the above situation could have any of the following or any number of other problems:

Gastritis	Gastralgia
Hepatitis	Ileitis
Appendicitis	Colitis
Pancreatitis	Diverticulitis

○ SUMMARY

Medical terminology is formed by using three components: prefixes, roots, and suffixes. To make the words easier to pronounce, a combining vowel such as *i, o, y,* or *u* may be used. In this unit, you memorized many word elements to help you be a better prepared health care worker.

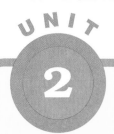

Doing

UNIT 1 ACTIVITY

1. Complete Worksheet/Activity 1 as assigned.
2. Complete Worksheet 2 and Worksheet/Activity 3 as assigned.
3. When you are confident that you can meet each objective listed above, ask your instructor for the unit evaluation.

2

Medical Abbreviations

STEPS TO SUCCESS

1. Read this unit.
2. Complete the Learn by Doing assignment at the end of this unit.

UNIT RATIONALE

Health care workers use abbreviations to convey information about their patients/clients. Abbreviations help save time and save space on medical documents.

UNIT OBJECTIVES

When you have completed this unit, you will be able to do the following:

✔ Recognize and define abbreviations that are commonly used by health care workers.

✔ Replace terms with abbreviations.

abbreviations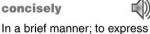

Words that have been shortened.

concisely

In a brief manner; to express in a few words.

● INTRODUCTION TO ABBREVIATIONS

Abbreviations are the shortened form of words. They are an efficient way of communicating quickly and **concisely** with other health care workers. You must be very careful when you use abbreviations. Always use standard abbreviations. Never make up an abbreviation. Doing so is confusing and will be a problem if a record is used in a legal action, because no one will understand what you wrote. Never use an abbreviation if you are unsure about its meaning. It is better to write out the word so that it is easily understood. Be considerate about when you use an abbreviation. Your patients/clients do not know what the abbreviations mean. For instance, *NPO* posted over the bed means "nothing by mouth." You know what it means, but you should always explain it to your patient/client. The following abbreviations are the most common abbreviations that health care workers use.

Abbreviation	Meaning	Abbreviation	Meaning
abd.	abdomen	dc, d/c	discontinue
a.c.	before meals	Del. Rm.	delivery room
ADL	activities of daily living	Dr.	doctor
ad lib	as desired	dx	diagnosis
adm	admission	ECG/EKG	electrocardiogram
am/AM	morning (midnight to noon)	EEG	electroencephalogram
amb	ambulate/walk	EENT	eye, ear, nose, and throat
amt.	amount	ER	emergency room
approx.	approximately	°F	Fahrenheit degree
ax	axillary, armpit	ft	foot
bid/BID	twice a day	fx	fracture
bm/BM	bowel movement	GI	gastrointestinal
B/P	blood pressure	GU	genitourinary
BR, br	bed rest	Gyn	gynecology
BRP	bathroom privileges	H_2O	water, aqua
°C	Celsius degree, centigrade	hr	hour
c̄	with	hs	bedtime, hour of sleep
CA	cancer	ht	height
cath.	catheter	hyper	above, high
CBC	complete blood count	hypo	below, low
cc	cubic centimeters	ICU	intensive care unit
CCU	coronary care unit	I & O	intake and output
c/o	complains of	IV	intravenous
CO_2	carbon dioxide	lab	laboratory
CPR	cardiopulmonary resuscitation	liq.	liquid
CS	central supply	LPN	licensed practical nurse
CVA	cerebrovascular accident/stroke	LVN	licensed vocational nurse
		M.D.	medical doctor

Abbreviation	Meaning	Abbreviation	Meaning
med.	medicine	q̄	every
min.	minute	qd	every day
NA	nurse aide/nursing assistant	q2h	every 2 hours
		q3h	every 3 hours
ng	nasogastric tube	q4h	every 4 hours
noct, noc.	night	qhs	every night at bedtime
NPO	nothing by mouth		
O₂	oxygen	qid, QID	four times a day
Ob	obstetrics	qod/QOD	every other day
OOB/oob	out of bed	qs	quantity sufficient
OPD	outpatient department	r	rectal
		RN	registered nurse
OR	operating room	ROM	range of motion
ord.	orderly	R.R.	recovery room
ORTH	orthopedics	Rx	prescription or treatment ordered by a physician
O.T.	occupational therapy		
pc	after meals	s̄	without
PEDS	pediatrics	sob	short of breath
per	by, through	spec.	specimen
pm/PM	afternoon (noon to midnight)	s̄s̄	one half
		stat	at once, immediately
po	by mouth		
post	after	surg.	surgery
postop, PostOp	postoperative	TID/tid	three times a day
pre	before	TLC	tender loving care
preop, PreOp	before surgery	VS	vital signs
prn	whenever necessary, when required	WBC	white blood count
		w/c	wheelchair
Pt, pt	patient	wt	weight
P.T.	physical therapy		

⦿ SUMMARY

Health care workers use abbreviations to help communicate quickly and effectively. Abbreviations are the shortened form of words and help reduce the time needed to chart important information. You have learned the most commonly used abbreviations; however, in your work experience you may find other abbreviations that are not listed here.

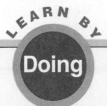

UNIT 2 ACTIVITY

1. Complete Worksheet/Activity 1 as assigned.

2. Complete Worksheets 2 and 3 as assigned.

3. Prepare responses to each item listed in Chapter Review—Your Link to Success at the end of this chapter.

4. When you are confident that you can meet each objective listed above, ask your instructor for the unit evaluation.

Thinking Critically Check Your Understanding

1. **Communication** You have a patient who is complaining of the following symptoms. Write a description of these symptoms using medical terminology so that your supervisor understands what the patient is experiencing. The symptoms include headache, vomiting, stomach pain, and excessive perspiration.

2. **Computers** Be aware that clients may research their diagnosis on the Internet. Make a list of both the helpful and challenging outcomes of this possibility. In general terms, this may save staff time answering questions, but it may also create misunderstandings. Think of some examples of how this could affect a health occupation aide and write them down for your portfolio.

3. **Legal and Ethical** You are in a hurry to finish your charting and cannot remember some of the abbreviations you

have learned. You can think of several ways to shorten words that you are using. Should you use an abbreviation that you make up? Explain your answer.

4. **Cultural Competency** You have several co-workers who have English as their second language. They are having a problem learning and understanding medical terminology. What are some suggestions you can make to help them learn this new language?

5. **Patient Education** Take a medical condition, such as osteoporosis or polyarthritis, and write an explanation of the disease assuming that the client you are helping has a limited understanding of English.

Portfolio Connection

Imagine that you are the instructor of a medical occupation class. You want your students to learn to communicate effectively in the health care environment. Create five assignments for your students to complete. Use the information in the medical terminology and abbreviation units. Look at the objectives in your textbook to guide you in developing what you want your students to accomplish in the assignment. Develop worksheets and evaluations. Provide clear directions for the student. An employer is interested in your ability to use in a meaningful way the new information you have learned. This exercise for your portfolio develops your skills in organizing what you are learning.

Portfolio Tip

Don't forget that your clients are not experts in medical terminology and may not understand the abbreviations that you and your colleagues use. Always use everyday language when talking to clients and get feedback from them. If you are giving an important instruction or explanation, check to be sure they have understood your comments.

Remember! 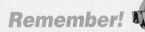 **Media Connection**

Use the Companion Website **www.prenhall.com/badasch** and the CD-ROM for additional interactive learning activities.

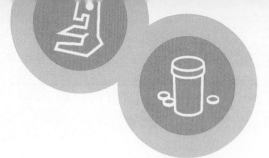

Medical Math

Chapter 7

MEDIA CONNECTION

Use the Companion Website
www.prenhall.com/badasch and the CD-ROM
for additional interactive learning activities.

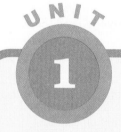

UNIT 1

Math Review

STEPS TO SUCCESS

1. Complete Worksheet 1, Pretest in the Student Workbook.
2. Read "Introduction to the Math Review" and "Numbers," then complete Worksheet 2.
3. Complete the Learn by Doing assignment at the end of this unit.

UNIT OBJECTIVES

When you have completed this unit, you will be able to do the following:

✔ Add and subtract whole numbers, decimals, and percentages.

✔ Multiply and divide whole numbers, fractions, mixed numbers, decimals, and percentages.

UNIT RATIONALE

Health care workers are required to perform simple math calculations when doing various tasks. Knowing basic math concepts and when to apply them is essential for all health care workers. Knowing how to add, subtract, convert standard figures into metric figures, calculate percentages, and manipulate fractions is a part of your responsibility when working in the health care field.

✔ Convert decimals to percentages and percentages to decimals.

INTRODUCTION TO THE MATH REVIEW

Some students have not used math for a long time. This unit review will help you accurately apply basic math concepts and skills necessary to your success as a health care worker. Take the pretest in the Student Workbook. If you pass it with 100 percent, skip this unit. If you do not get 100 percent, read through this unit and complete all workbook assignments.

○ NUMBERS

Numbers are expressed in different forms.

- ■ Whole numbers
- ■ Nonwhole numbers
- ■ Mixed numbers
- ■ Percentages

Numbers with more than one digit are defined by their place value. The number 7777 is given the following values:

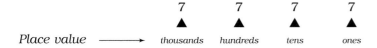

This number is described by saying "seven thousand, seven hundred seventy-seven." Numbers are written with a comma placed to the left of every third digit. The number 7777 is properly written "7,777." The number 22222 is given the following place values:

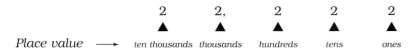

It is written "22,222" and described as "twenty-two thousand, two hundred twenty-two."

Numbers indicating less than a whole number are placed to the right of a decimal. The number 7,777.255 is given the following place values:

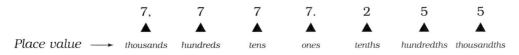

It is written "7,777.255" and described as "seven thousand, seven hundred seventy-seven and two hundred and fifty-five thousandths."

Whole Numbers

Whole numbers are the counting numbers and zero. Whole numbers do not contain decimals or fractions. *Examples:* 1, 2, 3, 10, 15, 18, 0. Ignore zeros before whole numbers. *Example:* 025 → Ø25 and is written 25.

Nonwhole Numbers

Nonwhole numbers are numbers with decimals. *Examples:* 7,777.255, 12.25, 5.9.

Mixed Numbers

Mixed numbers are whole numbers and a fraction. *Examples:* 12¼ or 45¾.

Percentages

The word *percent* means "by the hundred"; 100 percent = the whole or all of something. The symbol for percent is %. (See Figure 7.1.) *Example:* Four turtles = 100% or all of the turtles present. When one turtle is sold, ¼ (one-fourth) or 25% of them are gone and ¾ (three-fourths) or 75% are left.

Figure 7.1

Percentages.

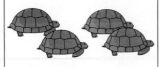
Four turtles = 100%.

One turtle or 25% of the turtles are sold.

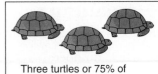
Three turtles or 75% of the turtles are left.

 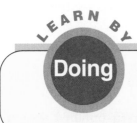

Doing **UNIT 1 ACTIVITY**
1. **Read the following information on addition and subtraction.**
2. **Complete Worksheet 3.**

ADDITION

Adding is the totaling of two or more whole numbers. For example, 2 computers in the reception area + 3 computers in accounting = a total of 5 computers in the office. To add, place numbers in columns. Put a line under the last number in the column. Add all the numbers above the line and write the total or sum of the numbers below the line. *Examples:*

$$
\begin{array}{rr}
& 2 \\
+ & 3 \\
\hline
\text{Total} \quad 5 &
\end{array}
\qquad
\begin{array}{rr}
& 34 \\
+ & 4 \\
\hline
\text{Total} \quad 38 &
\end{array}
$$

When adding more than one column of numbers, always keep the numbers in each column in a line under each other. This helps you add the correct numbers together. Always start adding numbers in the right column first.

Example:

$11 + 234 + 10 + 4$ is written like this:

$$
\begin{array}{r}
11 \\
234 \\
10 \\
+ \quad 4 \\
\hline
\boxed{259}
\end{array}
$$

When figuring numbers that total more than 10 in a column, it is necessary to carry numbers to the left of the column being added. In the next example, the first column of $1 + 4 + 0 + 9 = 14$. In the total, the number to the left of the 4 is 1. Move or carry the 1 to the column at the left and add it to the top number of that column (8), then add the remaining numbers in the column, $1 + 8 + 8 + 1 = 18$. The number to the left of the 8 is 1. Move or carry the 1 to the column at the left and add it to the top number of that column (3), then add the remaining numbers in the column, $1 + 3 = 4$. The total is 484. (See example 1 that follows.)

Example 1:

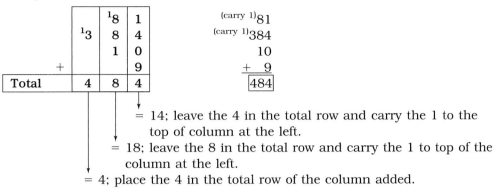

= 14; leave the 4 in the total row and carry the 1 to the top of column at the left.

= 18; leave the 8 in the total row and carry the 1 to top of the column at the left.

= 4; place the 4 in the total row of the column added.

Example 2:

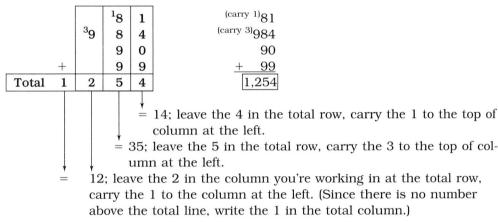

= 14; leave the 4 in the total row, carry the 1 to the top of column at the left.

= 35; leave the 5 in the total row, carry the 3 to the top of column at the left.

= 12; leave the 2 in the column you're working in at the total row, carry the 1 to the column at the left. (Since there is no number above the total line, write the 1 in the total column.)

SUBTRACTION

Subtraction is the opposite of addition. Subtracting numbers means taking a number away from another number. Simple subtraction problems are written in the following way:

$$\begin{array}{r} 84 \\ -23 \\ \hline \boxed{61} \end{array} \quad \text{or} \quad 84 - 23 = \boxed{61} \qquad \begin{array}{r} 136 \\ -12 \\ \hline \boxed{124} \end{array} \quad \text{or} \quad 136 - 12 = \boxed{124}$$

Check your answer by adding the answer to the number subtracted. If your answer is correct, your total will equal the number at the top of your problem. *Examples:*

$$\begin{array}{r} 84 \text{ check} \\ - \boxed{23} \searrow \\ +61 \enspace \boxed{= 84} \end{array} \quad \text{or } 23 + 61 = \boxed{84} \qquad \begin{array}{r} 136 \text{ check} \\ - \boxed{12} \searrow \\ +124 \enspace \boxed{= 136} \end{array} \quad \text{or } 12 + 124 = \boxed{136}$$
Total

Subtracting by Borrowing Numbers

Borrow a number from the column to the left. This allows a larger number, such as 8, to be subtracted from 5. See the following examples to help you understand.

$$2\ \overset{2}{\cancel{3}}{}^{1}5$$ 5 becomes 15 when 1 is borrowed from the 3;

$$\underline{-1\ 8}$$ 3 becomes 2.

$$\boxed{1\ 7}$$

$$1\overset{1}{\cancel{2}}{}^{16}\overset{6}{\cancel{7}}{}^{1}2$$ 2 becomes 12 when 1 is borrowed from the 7;

$$\underline{-1\ 9\ 5}$$ 7 becomes 6 because you borrowed 1; 6 becomes 16

$$\boxed{\cancel{0}\ 7\ 7}$$ when 1 is borrowed from the 2; 2 becomes 1.

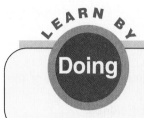

UNIT 1 ACTIVITY

1. **Read the following information on multiplication.**
2. **Complete Worksheet/Activity 4.**

● MULTIPLICATION

Multiplication is a quick, easy way to add. For example, $9 + 9 + 9 = 27$, but an easier process is $3 \times 9 = 27$. Adding large numbers is bulky and takes a lot of time. Multiplication is much easier.

To multiply numbers easily, memorize the multiplication table (Table 7.1). Memorizing this table allows you to calculate numbers quickly and without difficulty. You probably already know most of the multiplication facts. Review the table below and test yourself by completing Worksheet 1, pretest in your Workbook. For instructions on how to read a multiplication table see Worksheet 4 in your Workbook.

The following symbols are used to indicate multiplication: $\times$, ()(), or *. These symbols are used in writing problems. *Examples:*

$$\begin{array}{r} 8 \\ \underline{\times\ 9} \\ 72 \end{array}$$ or $8 \times 9 = 72$ or $8 \cdot 9 = 72$ or $(8)(9) = 72$ or $8 * 9 = 72$

Using calculators is helpful when figuring complicated calculations; however, you are responsible for knowing how to calculate numbers without a calculator. Most

Table 7.1 ▪ **Multiplication Table**									
	1	**2**	**3**	**4**	**5**	**6**	**7**	**8**	**9**	**10**
1	1	2	3	4	5	6	7	8	9	10
2	2	4	6	8	10	12	14	16	18	20
3	3	6	9	12	15	18	21	24	27	30
4	4	8	12	16	20	24	28	32	36	40
5	5	10	15	20	25	30	35	40	45	50
6	6	12	18	24	30	36	42	48	54	60
7	7	14	21	28	35	42	49	56	63	70
8	8	16	24	32	40	48	56	64	72	80
9	9	18	27	36	45	54	63	72	81	90
10	10	20	30	40	50	60	70	80	90	100

of the calculations in your work are simple and easy to figure without the use of a calculator. Do not use a calculator to work through your worksheets. Use your mind, not a calculator.

Long Multiplication

When you are multiplying numbers with more than one digit, it is sometimes necessary to carry and add. See the following examples to review these steps.

The next problem does not require carrying numbers. It does require multiplying and adding.

A.

	5	2	$2 \times 2 = 4$; place 4 in first column, below 2 and 2.
×	3	2	$2 \times 5 = 10$; place 0 in column under the 5 and 3 and place 1 in column at left.
1	0	4	

B.

	5	2	$3 \times 2 = 6$; place 6 in column under the 5, 3, and 0.
×	3	2	$3 \times 5 = 15$; place 5 in column under 1 and place 1 in column at left.
	1	0	4
+1	5	6	

C.

		5	2
	×	3	2
	1	0	4
+1	5	6	
1	6	6	4

} Add together, keeping each number in the correct column.

Answer

This problem requires carrying, adding, and multiplying:

A.

¹8	¹9	8	$2 \times 8 = 16$; place 6 in first column and carry 1 to top of column at left.
× 5	6	2	$2 \times 9 = 18 + 1$ [that was carried] $= 19$; place 9 in column under 9 and 6 and carry
1 7	9	6	1 to top of column at left. $2 \times 8 = 16 + 1$ [that was carried] $= 17$; place 7 in column under 8 and 5 and place 1 in column at left of 7.

B.

⁵8	⁴9	8	$6 \times 8 = 48$; place 8 in column under 9, 6, and 9 and carry 4 to top of column
× 5	6	2	at left. $6 \times 9 = 54 + 4$ [that was carried] $= 58$; place 8 in column under 8, 5, 7
1 7	9	6	and carry 5 to top of column at left. $6 \times 8 = 48 + 5$ [that was carried] $= 53$;
5 3 8	8		place 3 in column under 1 and place 5 in column at left next to 3.

C.

⁴8	⁴9	8	$5 \times 8 = 40$; place 0 in column below 8, 5, 7, and 8 and carry 4 to top of column
× 5	6	2	at left. $5 \times 9 = 45 + 4$ [that was carried] $= 49$; place 9 below 1 and 3. Carry 4 to
1 7	9	6	top of column at left. $5 \times 8 = 40 + 4$ [that was carried] $= 44$; place 4 below 5 and
5 3 8	8		place 4 next to 4 in column at left.
4 4 9 0			

D.

			8	9	8
		×	5	6	2
		¹1	¹7	9	6
	¹5	3	8	8	
+¹4	4	9	0		
5	0	4	6	7	6

} Add together, keeping each number in the correct column.

Answer

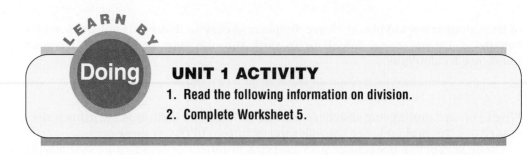

Doing

UNIT 1 ACTIVITY
1. **Read the following information on division.**
2. **Complete Worksheet 5.**

DIVISION

Division is the opposite of multiplication. Knowing the multiplication table is essential when dividing. As a health care worker, you may divide to determine costs per item or to determine the amount of items used daily. Here is a simple example: A medical office budget allows $600 a year for magazines. You are responsible for selecting and ordering the magazines. As you survey appropriate magazine subscriptions, you determine that the average annual cost is $35 per magazine. To determine how many subscriptions you can purchase, you divide $35 into $600. This problem is written as follows:

$600 \div 35$, or $35 \overline{)600}$

$$35 \overline{)600}^{17 \text{ magazine subscriptions}}$$

To understand how 17 magazine subscriptions can be purchased for $600, review the following division skills:

Dividing three-digit numbers by one-digit numbers:

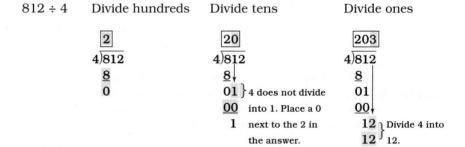

$812 \div 4$ Divide hundreds   Divide tens   Divide ones

Dividing four-digit numbers by one-digit numbers:

$7,216 \div 9$

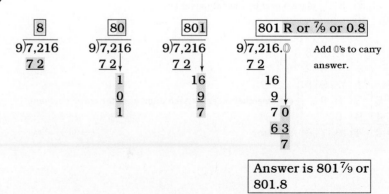

As shown in the example, *R* stands for *remainder.* The remainder is what is left over that is less than a whole. A remainder is usually expressed as a fraction or a decimal.

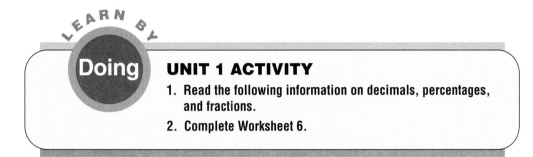

DECIMALS, PERCENTAGES, AND FRACTIONS

Numbers to the left of a decimal are whole numbers. Numbers to the right of a decimal are less than one.

Dividing *decimals* by whole numbers:

$24.5 \div 4 = 4\overline{)24.5}$ Place the decimal point in the answer directly above the decimal point in the dividend.

```
   6.              6.1             6.125
4)24.5          4)24.5          4)24.500
  24              24              24
                   5               5
                   4               4
                   1              10
                                   8
                                  20
                                  20    Add 0's to carry answer.
```

Numbers to the right of a decimal point indicate less than one whole. For example, 1.5 is the same as 1 1/2. *Examples:*

Decimal		Percentage		Fraction(s)
0.10	=	10%	=	$^{10}\!/_{100}$ or $^{1}\!/_{10}$
0.25	=	25%	=	$^{25}\!/_{100}$ or $^{1}\!/_{4}$
6.25	=	625%	=	$6^{25}\!/_{100}$ or $6^{1}\!/_{4}$

Change a decimal number into a percentage by moving the decimal two places to the right. *Examples:*

0.5 = 0.5 0. = 50%

30.0 = 30.0 0. = 3000%

0.04 = .0 4. = 4%

To change a percentage into a decimal number, replace the % sign with a decimal and move the decimal two spaces to the left.

To find the percentage of a number, first change the percentage to a decimal. Then multiply that decimal by the number. *Examples:*

15% of 63 change 15% to 0.15 then multiply 0.15 × 63 = 9.45

9.45 is 15% of 63

20% of 100 change 20% to 0.20 then multiply 0.20 × 100 = 20

20 is 20% of 100

● SUMMARY

In this unit, you reviewed the skills for adding, subtracting, multiplying, and dividing whole numbers, nonwhole numbers, mixed numbers, fractions, and percentages. You also practiced converting percentages, decimals, and fractions.

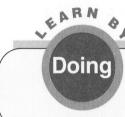

LEARN BY

Doing   **UNIT 1 ACTIVITY**

1. **When you are confident that you can meet each objective for this unit, ask your instructor for the unit evaluation.**

UNIT 2

The Metric System

STEPS TO SUCCESS

1. Read this unit.
2. Complete the Learn by Doing assignment at the end of this unit.

UNIT RATIONALE

The health care worker is expected to measure and calculate weights, heights, and volume in metric units of measure. Understanding how to convert standard and metric units of measure helps you work in a variety of health care settings.

UNIT OBJECTIVES

When you have completed this unit, you will be able to do the following:

✔ Match vocabulary words with their correct meanings.

✔ State the metric unit of measure used to determine length, distance, weight, and volume.

✔ Use metric terms to express 100 and 1,000 units of measure.

✔ Use metric terms to express 0.1, 0.01, and 0.001 units of measure.

✔ List four basic rules to follow when using the metric system.

✔ Identify metric measures of length and volume.

✔ Convert ounces to cubic centimeters/milliliters, pounds to kilograms, and ounces to grams.

◯ USING THE METRIC SYSTEM

The health care industry uses the metric system for measuring. The metric system is used by 90% of the world and is known as the International System of Units. Table 7.2 will help you learn the metric terms, their abbreviations, and what they measure. Each metric unit in this table is a single unit of measure. Table 7.3 explains terms used when *more than one* unit of measure (meter, gram, liter) is being measured. Following are examples of more than one unit:

■ Measures of weight

  • 1 hectogram = 100 grams • 1.5 hectograms = 150 grams • 1 kilogram = 1,000 grams • 1.5 kilograms = 1,500 grams

■ Measures of length

  • 1 hectometer = 100 meters • 1.5 hectometers = 150 meters • 1 kilometer = 1,000 meters • 1.5 kilometers = 1,500 meters

Table 7.4 explains terms used when *less than one* unit of measure is being measured. Following are examples of less than one unit:

■ Measures of length

  • 1 decimeter (dm) = 1/10 or 0.1 of a meter • 1 centimeter (cm) = 1/100 or 0.01 of a meter • 1 millimeter (mm) = 1/1000 or 0.001 of a meter

■ Measures of volume

  • 1 deciliter (dL) = 1/10 or 0.1 of a liter • 1 milliliter (mL) = 1/1000 or 0.001 of a liter

Table 7.2 ■ **Metric Terms, Their Abbreviations, and What They Measure**

Term	Abbreviation	Measures	In Place of
meter	m	length	inch, foot, yard, mile
gram	g	weight	ounce, pound
liter	L*	volume	fluid ounce, cup, pint, quart, gallon

*Capital *L* is commonly used to prevent confusion of lowercase letter *l* and the number 1.

Table 7.3 ■ **Metric Terms, Their Abbreviations, and What They Measure**

Term	Abbreviation	What It Measures
kilo	k	1,000 units
hecto	h	100 units

Table 7.4 ■ **Metric Terms, Their Abbreviations, and What They Measure**

Term	Abbreviation	What It Measures
deci	d	1/10 or 0.1 unit
centi	c	1/100 or 0.01 unit
milli	m	1/1000 or 0.001 unit

There are four basic rules to follow when using the metric system.

decimal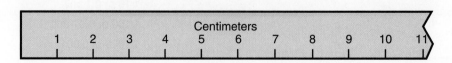

A number containing a decimal point.

- Numbers indicating less than one unit are always written in **decimal** form, *not* as fractions. *Example:* 1/10 = 0.1 or 1/100 = 0.01 or 1/1000 = 0.001.

- When writing decimals, if there is no number before the decimal, it will always be a 0. *Example:* .1 is 0.1, .5 is 0.5, .75 is 0.75.

- Abbreviations for metric terms are never plural; they are always written in singular form. *Examples:* grams is *g*, not *gs*, and liters is *L*, not *Ls*. Always capitalize the abbreviation *L* for *liter* to reduce confusing the lowercase *l* with the number 1.

- Leave a space between the number and the abbreviation, as shown in the following examples: 8 g, 0.1 dm.

○ USING THE METRIC SYSTEM TO MEASURE

Meters, Centimeters, and Millimeters

A meter stick can be used to measure length in the following units:

- centimeters (cm) (Figure 7.2)
- millimeters (mm)
- meters (m)

One meter is slightly more than 3 feet.

Liters, Milliliters, and Cubic Centimeters

- A liter (L) is slightly larger than a quart.
- A milliliter (mL) is 1/1000 of a liter.
- Cubic centimeters (cc) are interchangeable with mL.

Scales can be used to measure weight in grams, hectograms, and kilograms.

Celsius (C) and Centigrade

The metric measure of heat is Celsius or centigrade, which are the same. More information can be found in the unit explaining vital signs (see page 234).

○ CHANGING STANDARD MEASURES TO METRIC MEASURES

It is easy to change liquid or volume measurement by multiplying 30 cc/mL times the number of ounces (Table 7.5).

Health care workers use various types of measuring devices to measure liquid (Figure 7.3).

Figure 7.2

Comparison of standard and metric units of length.

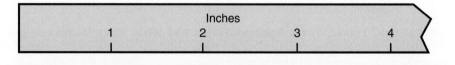

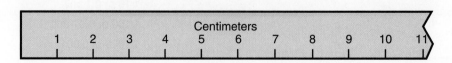

Table 7.5 ▪ Changing Ounces to Milliliters and Cubic Centimeters

1 oz medicine	$1 \times 30 = 30$ mL $= 30$ cc
8 oz water	$8 \times 30 = 240$ mL $= 240$ cc
6 oz soup	$6 \times 30 = 180$ mL $= 180$ cc
4 oz juice	$4 \times 30 = 120$ mL $= 120$ cc
12 oz soda pop	$12 \times 30 = 360$ mL $= 360$ cc

Table 7.6 ▪ Changing Pounds to Kilograms and Kilograms to Pounds

110 lb changed to kilograms: $110 \times 0.45 = 49.5$ kg
200 lb changed to kg: $200 \times 0.45 = 91$ kg
50 kg changed to lb: $50 \times 2.2 = 110$ lb
91 kg changed to lb: $91 \times 2.2 = 200$ lb

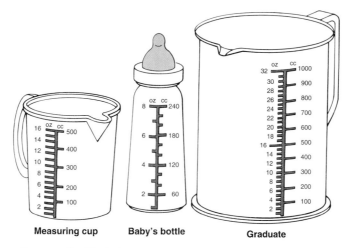

Figure 7.3

Various measuring devices for fluid ounces and cubic centimeters.

Measuring cup   Baby's bottle   Graduate

• They are all calibrated.
• They are made of metal, glass, or plastic.
• They are used for measuring liquids in cubic centimeters (cc).
• They are used for measuring liquids in ounces (oz).
• The measuring cup is used to measure liquids in the home.
• The baby's bottle is used to measure liquids in the home.
• The calibrated graduate is used to measure fluid in the health care institution.

To change measurements of mass or weight, compare pounds with kilograms and grams with ounces. One pound equals 0.45 kilogram; 1 kilogram equals 2.2 lb (Table 7.6).

■ To change pounds to kilograms, multiply the number of pounds by 0.45.

■ To change kilograms to pounds, multiply the number of kilograms by 2.2.

One ounce (oz) equals 30 grams (g). To change ounces to grams, multiply $30 \times$ the number of ounces. To change grams to ounces, divide 30 into the number of grams (see Table 7.7).

There are practice questions in your Student Workbook to help you learn the metric system.

Table 7.7 ■ Changing Ounces to Grams	
1 oz changed to grams: $1 \times 30 = 30$ g	
8 oz changed to grams: $8 \times 30 = 240$ g	

⬤ SUMMARY

We have discussed the basic units of measure in the metric system. These include meters, grams, and liters. When the prefix *kilo* is used before a basic unit of measure, it multiplies the unit 1,000 times. When *hecto* is used, it increases the basic unit by 100 times. We have also discussed how less than one unit is expressed by using prefixes of *deci*, 1/10 of a unit; *centi*, 1/100 of a unit; and *milli*, 1/1000 of a unit. You have learned four basic rules to follow when using the metric system, methods of converting standard units to metric units, and various ways to measure.

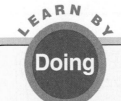

Doing **UNIT 2 ACTIVITY**

1. **Complete Worksheets 1 and 4 and Worksheets/Activities 2, 3 and 5 in the Student Workbook.**

2. **When you are confident that you can meet each objective for this unit, ask your instructor for the unit evaluation.**

The 24-Hour Clock/Military Time

STEPS TO SUCCESS

1. Read this unit.
2. Complete the Learn by Doing assignment at the end of this unit.

UNIT OBJECTIVES

When you have completed this unit, you will be able to do the following:

✔ Recognize time on a 24-hour clock.

✔ Express 24-hour time/military time verbally and in writing.

UNIT RATIONALE

Medical facilities frequently use the 24-hour clock system. The 24-hour clock clearly states time and eliminates confusion when documenting information. A health care worker is required to understand and interpret time in every health care setting.

✔ Convert Greenwich time to 24-hour time.

INTRODUCTION TO THE 24-HOUR CLOCK/MILITARY TIME

In the health care setting, it is important that time be stated in a clear, concise manner. All medical records are legal documents. Time indicates when treatment, medication, and other activities are done and how long procedures or incidents last. A 24-hour clock eliminates the confusion between A.M. (12 midnight to 12 noon) and P.M. (12 noon to 12 midnight) hours. It provides a clear, concise record for recording medical services. The military services were the first to use a 24-hour clock; therefore, the 24-hour system is often referred to as **24-hour time/military time.** Table 7.8 shows you the difference in expressing Greenwich and military time (see also Figure 7.4).

Military time is always expressed in four digits, and no colons are used to separate hours and minutes. Always use a 0 to complete the four-digit number (for example, 0100 instead of 100). When expressing military time, remember to state it in hundreds: for example, zero one hundred hours (0100) is 1:00 A.M.; eleven hundred hours (1100) is 11:00 A.M.; twenty-three hundred hours (2300) is 11:00 P.M.

It is easy to remember that morning hours are 0100 to 1200 hours. The afternoon and nighttime hours can be added to the 1200 hours of noon. For example:

- To determine how 5:00 P.M. is expressed in military time, add 1200 and 0500 (1200 + 0500 = 1700 hours).

- To determine how 12 midnight is expressed in military time, add 1200 and 1200 = 2400 hours.

Table 7.8 will help you understand the relationship between **Greenwich time** and military time.

24-hour time/ military time

Method of telling time by counting each hour consecutively for 24 hours (i.e., . . . 11, 12, 13, . . .).

Greenwich time

Standard time, a 12-hour clock.

Table 7.8 ▪ **Comparison of Greenwich and 24-Hour/Military Time**

Greenwich	Military	Greenwich	Military
1:00 A.M.	0100	1:00 P.M.	1300
2:00 A.M.	0200	2:00 P.M.	1400
3:00 A.M.	0300	3:00 P.M.	1500
4:00 A.M.	0400	4:00 P.M.	1600
5:00 A.M.	0500	5:00 P.M.	1700
6:00 A.M.	0600	6:00 P.M.	1800
7:00 A.M.	0700	7:00 P.M.	1900
8:00 A.M.	0800	8:00 P.M.	2000
9:00 A.M.	0900	9:00 P.M.	2100
10:00 A.M.	1000	10:00 P.M.	2200
11:00 A.M.	1100	11:00 P.M.	2300
12:00 noon	1200	12:00 P.M./ midnight	2400/ 0000

Figure 7.4

24-hour clock: military time.

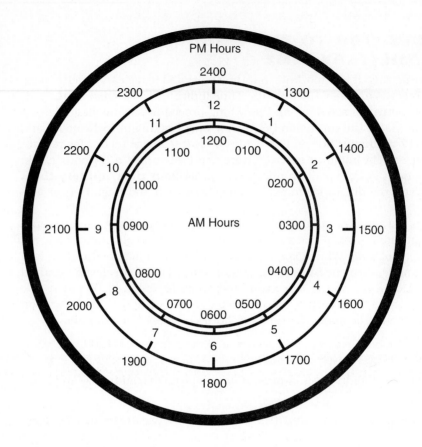

SUMMARY

In this unit, you learned the relationship between Greenwich time and military time and how to determine the time of day using a 24-hour clock. You also learned that the 24-hour clock eliminates confusion between A.M. and P.M. hours.

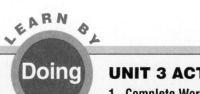

UNIT 3 ACTIVITY

1. Complete Worksheet 1 and Worksheet/Activity 2 in the Student Workbook.
2. When you are confident that you can meet each objective for this unit, ask your instructor for the unit evaluation.
3. Complete Chapter Review—Your Link to Success at the end of this chapter.

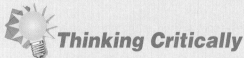

Thinking Critically

1. **Communication** Health care workers are expected to communicate effectively with co-workers, patients, and their families. In the United States, standard units of measure are common, and metric units of measure are less common. Patients or their families may be expected to measure or calculate their medicine, fluid intake, or output. It is essential to explain how to do this in terms a patient will understand. Write instructions to a 75-year-old patient explaining the difference between ounces and cubic centimeters. Your instructions must describe how to measure and calculate the patient's 24-hour fluid intake and output and how to fill in a 24-hour I & O sheet.

2. **Time Management** You have been asked to draw a pie chart to show the percentage of the day a typical worker spends on each of his or her duties. You have been given a list of duties and times, but all are in minutes and fractions. Practice converting the following into percentages: 1 1/4 hours; 3 hours and 20 minutes; 4 hours and 10 minutes; a half-hour.

3. **Safety Alert** Describe two scenarios in which instructions given to patients using a 12-hour clock were confusing and put the patients at risk. Explain how instructions given using a 24-hour clock would have avoided the problems.

4. **Medical Math** The metric system is used in calculating weights and measures appropriately in the medical profession. Describe the equivalents of a meter, gram, and liter, and define *kilo, hecto, deci, centi,* and *milli.*

5. **Patient Satisfaction** A new mother arrives for the baby's first well-baby checkup at 1:00 P.M. You know that she should be taken to an examination room within 5 minutes. Your employer uses military time. Explain how 1:05 P.M. is written in military time. Describe how the receptionist should respond so that the mother knows how much time she will be waiting before seeing the doctor. You call her name and ask her to follow you to the scales. You weigh the baby and find she weighs 6.84 kilograms. What will you tell the mother her baby's weight is in pounds and ounces?

Portfolio Connection

It is time to review your vocational choices once again. This assignment leads you through a cost analysis of schools and associations that can help develop your knowledge and skills.

Review the outcome of your career search from Chapter 2. Write down any new vocational areas of interest you have identified since completing your original career search. Answer the questions in Chapter 2, Unit 1 Worksheets 3 and 4 in your Student Workbook concerning any new areas of vocational interest. Compare your answers to these questions with your values on Worksheet 1 and satisfaction on Worksheet 2 in Chapter 2. Review the vocations that seem best for you at this time.

Research private and public schools for higher education in your vocational choice. Create a spreadsheet that clearly compares costs for each school, using the following criteria:

- Entrance requirements
- Tuition (costs must be compared equally, that is, semester to semester, quarter to quarter, or hours to hours)
- Books (number of books and the cost for new and used books)

Portfolio Tip

Be sure to visit several facilities of the type in which you hope to work. Remember that one facility alone may not be typical. Keep a dated record of each visit with your reactions noted. This will be a private part of your portfolio. This is an important step in your career planning: deciding where you will be happiest working.

- Supplies and materials (list and compare like items)
- Uniforms (identify all required uniform parts, e.g., shoes, name tag)
- Housing
- Transportation (type of transportation, round-trip miles)
- Miscellaneous
- Financial aid resources (eligibility criteria, amount of dollars available, repayment requirements, and interest rates)

This assignment shows your ability to organize data into an easy-to-read, usable document. Use this process to guide future research and cost comparisons. Repeat this assignment as you approach the time for finalizing your decision concerning your professional development.

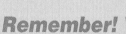 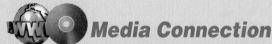

Use the Companion Website **www.prenhall.com/badasch** and the CD-ROM for additional interactive learning activities.

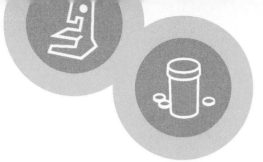

Chapter 8

Your Body and How It Functions

MEDIA CONNECTION
Use the Companion Website
www.prenhall.com/badasch and the CD-ROM
for additional interactive learning activities.

UNIT 1

Overview of the Body

STEPS TO SUCCESS

1. Complete Vocabulary Worksheet 1 in the Student Workbook.
2. Read this unit.
3. Complete the Learn by Doing assignment at the end of this unit.

UNIT OBJECTIVES

When you have completed this unit, you will be able to do the following:

✔ Match vocabulary words with their correct meanings.

✔ List seven cell functions.

✔ Identify three main parts of the cell and explain their functions.

✔ Describe the relationship between cells, tissues, organs, and systems of the body.

✔ Identify terms relating to the body.

✔ Label a diagram of the body cavities.

✔ Explain why health care workers must have a basic knowledge of body structures and how they function.

UNIT RATIONALE

The health care worker assists people who are ill, injured, or seeking a healthy lifestyle. Understanding the body's structure and functions provides the health care worker with the basic knowledge necessary to help each person reach his or her goal. When you understand normal body functions you will recognize disease processes.

○ INTRODUCTION TO THE BODY

The Cell

The **cell** is the building block of the body. Cells are **microscopic.** This means that they are so small they can be seen only with the aid of a microscope. The body is made up of millions of cells. Every cell is programmed to do a specific job that allows the body to **function.** Each cell reproduces, grows, and repairs itself, uses oxygen and **nutrients,** digests food for energy, eliminates waste, produces heat and energy, and is able to move around. The structure of the cell has three main parts (Figure 8.1):

cell
Smallest structural unit in the body that is capable of independent functioning.

microscopic
Too small to be seen by the eye but large enough to be seen through a microscope.

Figure 8.1

Basic cell.

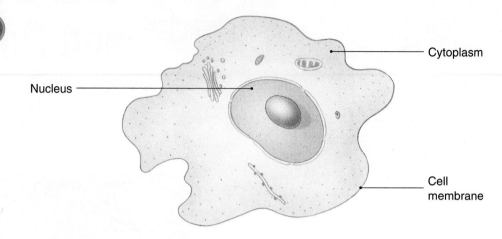

Nucleus

Cytoplasm

Cell membrane

function

Action or work of tissues, organs, or body parts (e.g., the heart's function is to pump blood).

nutrients

Food.

nucleus

The part of a cell that is vital for its growth, metabolism, reproduction, and transmitted characteristics.

reproduction

Process that takes place in animals to create offspring.

cytoplasm

All of the substance of a cell other than the nucleus.

cell membrane

Thin, soft layer of tissue that surrounds the cell and holds it together.

tissues

Group of cells of the same type that act together to perform a specific function.

epithelial

Pertaining to covering of the internal and external organs of the body.

connective tissue

Tissue specialized to bind together and support other tissues.

■ The **nucleus** regulates the activity of the cell and has an important role in the **reproduction** of the cell.

■ The **cytoplasm** is a jellylike liquid where the activities of the cell occur.

■ The **cell membrane** is the outer covering of the cell that keeps the cytoplasm contained. The cell membrane also allows matter to flow in and out of the cell.

Tissues

The body is made up of specialized groups of cells. These groups of cells form tissues. These **tissues** have a specific job. There are five primary kinds of tissue in the body: nerve, **epithelial,** connective, blood, and muscle (Figure 8.2). Table 8.1 describes the locations and functions of each type of tissue.

Organs

Organs are made up of specialized tissues that allow each part of an organ to perform its own specific function. Several different types of tissues make up an entire organ. For example, the heart is an organ made up of **connective tissue,** cardiac tissue, and nerve tissue. These three types of tissue work together in the heart, causing the heart to beat and pump blood throughout the body. The tissues of the body combine to form organs such as the heart, skin, stomach, and all other organs of the body. Figures 8.3a and 8.3b show all the organs of the body and their locations.

Systems

A system is a group of organs working together to perform a certain function. The body is **composed** of several systems. In the next units of this chapter, we discuss the following:

■ Skeletal system

■ Muscular system

■ Circulatory system

■ Lymphatic system

■ Respiratory system

■ Digestive system

■ Urinary system

■ Glandular systems

■ Nervous system

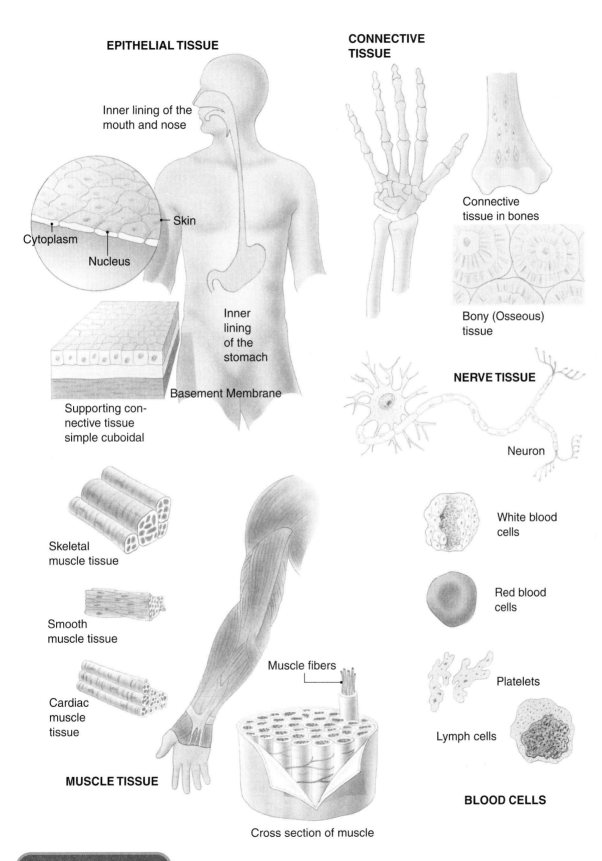

EPITHELIAL TISSUE

Inner lining of the mouth and nose

Cytoplasm

Nucleus

Skin

Inner lining of the stomach

Basement Membrane

Supporting connective tissue simple cuboidal

CONNECTIVE TISSUE

Connective tissue in bones

Bony (Osseous) tissue

NERVE TISSUE

Neuron

Skeletal muscle tissue

Smooth muscle tissue

Cardiac muscle tissue

MUSCLE TISSUE

Muscle fibers

Cross section of muscle

White blood cells

Red blood cells

Platelets

Lymph cells

BLOOD CELLS

Figure 8.2

Types of body tissues.

Type of Tissue	Location in the Body	Function
Nerve tissue	Throughout the body	Sends impulses to/from the central nervous system and to/from the body systems
Epithelial tissue	Forms the outer skin and lines body cavities and passages to the outside of the body	Protects, secretes, absorbs, and receives sensations (e.g., hot, cold, pressure)
Connective tissue	Bones, tendons, fat tissue	Binds, supports, and connects body tissues
Blood and lymph tissue	Moves through the circulatory system	Delivers nourishment, electrolytes, hormones, vitamins, antibodies, heat, and oxygen to all body tissues
Muscle tissue: 1. Cardiac 2. Smooth 3. Striated	1. Heart muscle 2. Internal organs (e.g., stomach, diaphragm) 3. Throughout the body for movement	1. Contracts heart 2. Contracts internal organs 3. Contracts and flexes to allow movement

Table 8.1 ■ Tissues of the Body

composed

Formed by putting many parts together.

structure

Form in which the body is made.

anterior

Located in the front; opposite of posterior (e.g., the abdominal wall is anterior to the back).

distal

Farthest from the point of attachment.

posterior

Behind, to the rear, toward the back (e.g., the heel is posterior to the toes).

sacral region

The area where the sacrum is located; forms the tail end of the spinal column.

- Reproductive system
- Integumentary system

It is important to understand the unique **structure** and functioning of the body. You need to learn that *cells* combine to form tissues, *tissues* combine to form organs, *organs* combine to form systems, and *systems* combine to form the human body (Figure 8.4).

Directions of the Body

To document information about patients, use terms that specify regions or directions of the body; for example, to identify locations of pain or injury, write: 1 cm laceration on the right **anterior** forearm, **distal** to the elbow (Figure 8.5).

The body directions are shown in Figure 8.6. Here are the most common:

- **Cranial:** located near the head.
- **Superior:** above or in a higher position. The head is superior to the torso.
- **Inferior:** below, lower. The knee is inferior to the thigh.
- *Ventral* or *anterior:* located near the surface or in front of the body.
- *Dorsal* or **posterior:** located to the back of the body.
- **Medial:** near the center or midline of the body. Think of the midline as dividing the body in half with a left and a right side.
- **Lateral:** away from the midline.
- **Proximal:** nearest the point of attachment.
- **Distal:** farthest from the point of attachment or the midline.
- **Caudal:** located near the **sacral region.**

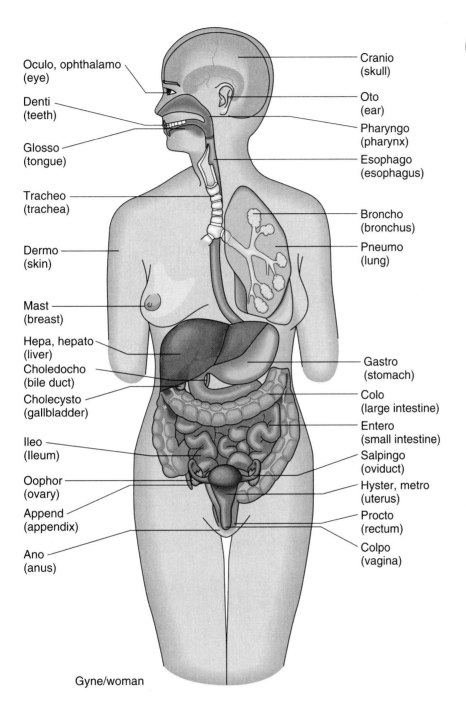

Figure 8.3a

Organs of the body.

Oculo, ophthalamo
(eye)

Denti
(teeth)

Glosso
(tongue)

Tracheo
(trachea)

Dermo
(skin)

Mast
(breast)

Hepa, hepato
(liver)

Choledocho
(bile duct)

Cholecysto
(gallbladder)

Ileo
(Ileum)

Oophor
(ovary)

Append
(appendix)

Ano
(anus)

Gyne/woman

Cranio
(skull)

Oto
(ear)

Pharyngo
(pharynx)

Esophago
(esophagus)

Broncho
(bronchus)

Pneumo
(lung)

Gastro
(stomach)

Colo
(large intestine)

Entero
(small intestine)

Salpingo
(oviduct)

Hyster, metro
(uterus)

Procto
(rectum)

Colpo
(vagina)

Figure 8.3b

Organs of the body.

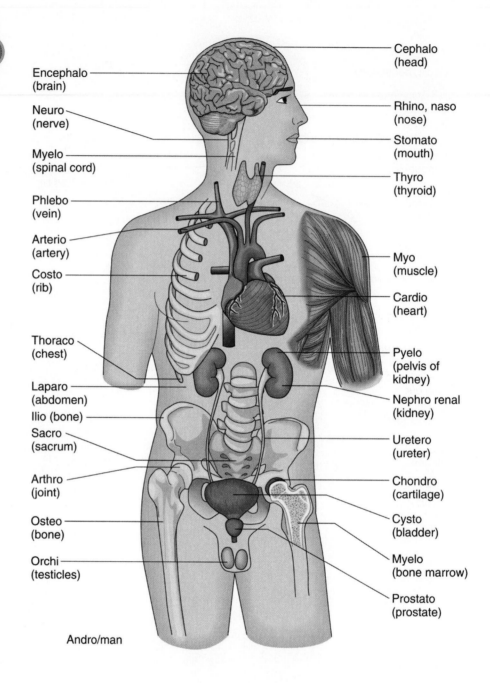

Encephalo
(brain)

Neuro
(nerve)

Myelo
(spinal cord)

Phlebo
(vein)

Arterio
(artery)

Costo
(rib)

Thoraco
(chest)

Laparo
(abdomen)

Ilio (bone)

Sacro
(sacrum)

Arthro
(joint)

Osteo
(bone)

Orchi
(testicles)

Cephalo
(head)

Rhino, naso
(nose)

Stomato
(mouth)

Thyro
(thyroid)

Myo
(muscle)

Cardio
(heart)

Pyelo
(pelvis of
kidney)

Nephro renal
(kidney)

Uretero
(ureter)

Chondro
(cartilage)

Cysto
(bladder)

Myelo
(bone marrow)

Prostato
(prostate)

Andro/man

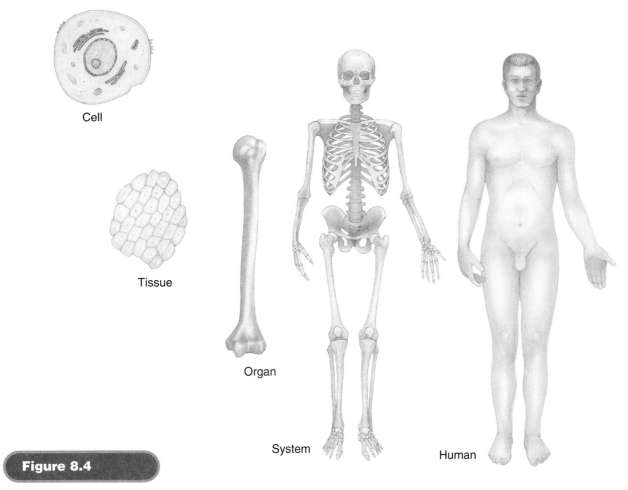

Figure 8.4

Combination of cells, tissues, organs, and systems forms the body.

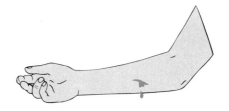

Figure 8.5

To identify the location of this laceration, write: 1 cm laceration on the right anterior forearm, distal to the elbow.

Cavities of the Body

The cavities of the body (Figure 8.7) are another way to identify location of pain or injury (Table 8.2).

Figure 8.6

Directions of the human body.

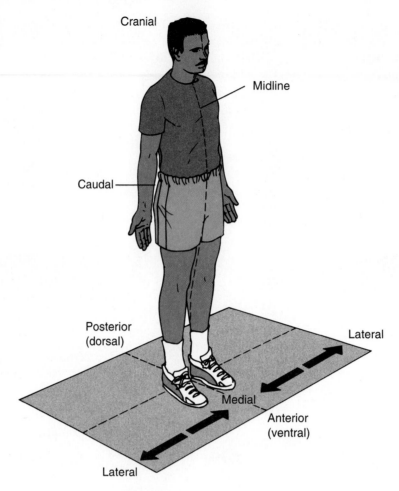

Figure 8.7

Body cavities.

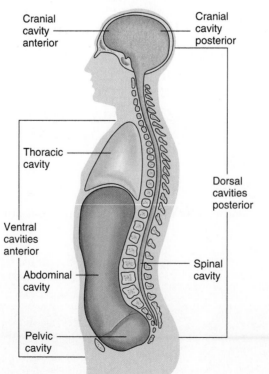

Table 8.2 ■ Cavities of the Body (see Figure 8.7)	
Dorsal Cavities Located to the Back of the Body	**Ventral Cavity Located Toward the Front of the Body**
Cranial cavity—houses the brain	Thoracic cavity—houses the heart, lungs, large blood **vessels**
Spinal cavity—houses the spinal cord	Abdominal cavity—houses the stomach, most of intestines, kidney, liver, gallbladder, pancreas, spleen
	Pelvic Cavity—houses the urinary bladder, part of intestine, rectum, parts of the reproductive system

vessels
Tubes that carry fluid in the body.

MEDICAL TERMINOLOGY

■ aplasia	failure of any part of the body to develop naturally	■ intralobar	within a lobe
■ endogenous	anything occurring within the body	■ necrosis	condition of dead or decaying tissue
■ exogenous	anything occurring outside the body	■ peristalsis	progressive wavelike movement that occurs in some of the tubes of the body (e.g., intestines, esophagus)
■ induration	hardened tissue	■ plasma	liquid part of the blood and lymph
■ infarct	tissue that has lost blood supply and died	■ symptom	any noticeable change in the body or its function
■ interlobar	between lobes	■ visceratonic	lack of normal **tone** in an organ
■ intervisceral	between two organs		

tone   Firmness or tightness.

⬤ JOBS AND PROFESSIONS

- ■ Medical doctor (M.D.)
- ■ Microbiologist
- ■ Pathologist
- ■ Registered nurse (RN)
- ■ Nurse practitioner (NP)
- ■ Licensed vocational nurse (LVN)
- ■ Licensed practical nurse (LPN)
- ■ Nursing assistant (NA)
- ■ Orderly

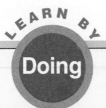

Doing **UNIT 1 ACTIVITY**

1. **Complete Worksheets 2, 4, and 5 and Worksheet/Activity 3 as assigned.**
2. **Ask your instructor for directions to complete Worksheet 6. Study the terms in Unit 1.**
3. **Be prepared to participate in a spelling bee by learning the spellings and definitions of the terminology and the systems in this unit.**

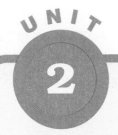

The Skeletal System

STEPS TO SUCCESS

1. Complete Vocabulary Worksheet 1 in the Student Workbook.

2. Read this unit.

3. Complete the Learn by Doing assignment at the end of this unit.

UNIT OBJECTIVES

When you have completed this unit, you will be able to do the following:

✔ Match vocabulary words with their correct meanings.

✔ Label a diagram of major bones in the body.

✔ Select from a list the functions of bones.

✔ Name the long, short, flat, and irregular bones of the body.

✔ Identify immovable, slightly movable, and freely movable joints of the body.

✔ Identify common disorders of the skeletal system.

✔ Label a diagram of four types of bone fractures.

✔ Explain why a health care worker must have a basic knowledge of the skeletal system and how it functions.

⬤ INTRODUCTION TO THE SKELETAL SYSTEM

Structure of the Bone

osseous
Bonelike.

circulation
Continuous one-way movement of blood through the heart and blood vessels to all parts of the body.

components
Parts or elements of a whole; an ingredient.

The skeletal system (Figure 8.8) is made up of bone tissue (**osseous** tissue) (see Figure 8.2). Bones have their own system of blood vessels and nerves which allows **circulation** to occur within the bone.

The **components** of bone change from conception to old age. In the first month after **conception,** an **embryo**'s skeletal framework is made up of **cartilage.** In the second and third months after conception, you can see calcium deposits in the bone. Throughout life, calcium continues to form in the bone structure, causing the bone to become hard. For example, a small child's bone is more **flexible** than the bone of a 30-year-old. The added calcium makes the bones of the 30-year-old harder, less flexible, and more **brittle.** A 60-year-old may lose calcium from the bone. This makes the bone **porous** so that it breaks easily.

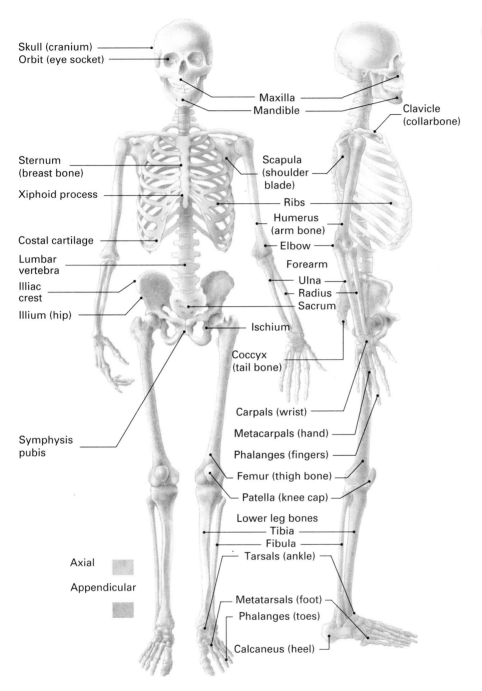

Figure 8.8

The human skeleton is made of bone tissue. There are 206 bones in the body.

Skull (cranium)
Orbit (eye socket)
Maxilla
Mandible
Clavicle (collarbone)
Sternum (breast bone)
Scapula (shoulder blade)
Xiphoid process
Ribs
Humerus (arm bone)
Costal cartilage
Elbow
Lumbar vertebra
Forearm
Ulna
Illiac crest
Radius
Sacrum
Illium (hip)
Ischium
Coccyx (tail bone)
Symphysis pubis
Carpals (wrist)
Metacarpals (hand)
Phalanges (fingers)
Femur (thigh bone)
Patella (knee cap)
Lower leg bones
Tibia
Fibula
Tarsals (ankle)
Axial
Appendicular
Metatarsals (foot)
Phalanges (toes)
Calcaneus (heel)

Functions of the Bone

Bones perform many functions. Some of these are

- To serve as a framework for the body, giving the body structure and support.
- To protect internal structures, such as the brain and spinal cord.
- To act as a storage area for calcium. This calcium is used in the blood if the diet does not provide enough calcium.
- To produce blood cells. The red bone marrow produces most of the red blood cells.
- To allow flexibility when muscles move them.

conception

Occurs when the male sperm fertilizes the female ovum and a new organism begins to develop.

embryo

Living human being during the first 8 weeks of development in the uterus.

cartilage

Tough connective tissue; forms pads at end of bones, is found in the nasal septum and external ear, and forms the major portion of the embryonic skeleton.

flexible

Able to bend easily.

brittle

Fragile, easy to break.

porous

Filled with tiny holes.

Figure 8.9

Types of bones.

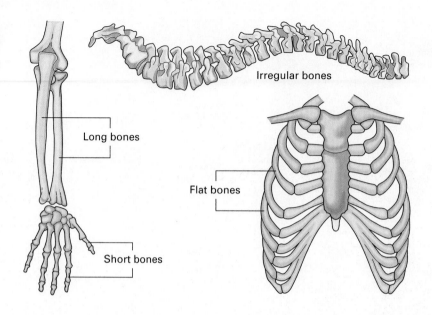

Irregular bones

Long bones

Flat bones

Short bones

Types of Bones

There are four types of bones (see Figure 8.9):

■ *Long bones* (bones that are longer than their width)

  • Humerus • Radius • Ulna • Femur • Tibia • Fibula

■ *Short bones* (length and width are nearly equal)

  • Wrist and hand • Ankle and feet

■ *Flat bones* (two layers of bone divided by a narrow span)

  • Skull • Sternum • Ribs • Shoulder blade

■ *Irregular bones* (bones that do not fit into the shapes of the other three groups)

  • Face • Spine • Hip

Groups of Bones

The human skeleton is divided into two groups of bones. The **axial** skeleton includes 80 bones (see Figure 8.8). These are found in the

■ Skull   ■ Vertebrae   ■ Ribs and sternum

The **appendicular** skeleton includes 126 bones (see Figure 8.8). These bones are found in the

■ Arms   ■ Hands   ■ Legs   ■ Feet   ■ Pelvis

Joints

The point where two bones meet is a joint. Joints are divided into three main groups, depending on the amount of movement permitted (see Figure 8.10). These groups are

■ *Immovable joints*

  • Cranium (suture joints)

■ *Slightly movable joints*

  • Vertebral discs • Symphysis pubis • Sacroiliac joints

axial

Pertaining to the central structures of the body (e.g., vertebrae, skull, ribs, and sternum).

appendicular

Pertaining to any body part added to the axis (e.g., arms and legs are attached to the axis of the body).

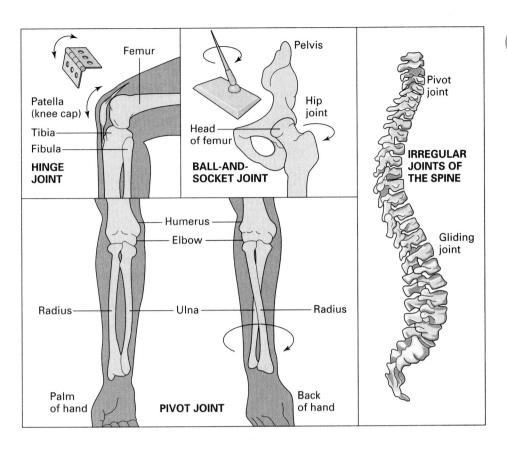

Figure 8.10

Types of joints.

■ *Freely movable joints*

• Shoulder joint • Elbow, wrist, and finger joints • Knee and ankle joints

Ligaments

Ligaments connect to bone and hold bones together. Joints are formed where the bones meet.

⬤ COMMON DISORDERS OF THE SKELETAL SYSTEM

Table 8.3 ■ Common Disorders, Symptoms, and Preventive Measures/Treatment of the Skeletal System

Condition	Disorder	Symptoms	Preventive Measures/ Treatment
Arthritis	Inflammation of the joints. Can be caused when a joint is damaged, causing the edges of bones in the joint to rub against each other and become irritated.	Pain and swelling in the joints. (See Figure 8.11.)	Preventing damaging joints by using good body mechanics and limiting continuous repetitive movements that overuse specific joints.
Degenerative joint diseases— osteoarthritis	Inflammation of the membrane of the joint. Cause unknown, but changes in the structure of joints occur due to the inflammatory process.	Common symptoms include pain, stiffness, tenderness to the touch, deformity of joint regions.	Treating with anti-inflammatory medication. Surgery is sometimes indicated.

Table 8.3 ▪ Continued

Condition	Disorder	Symptoms	Preventive Measures/ Treatment
Fracture • Simple • Compound • Comminuted • Greenstick	Broken bone • The bone is broken, but the skin remains intact. • The bone is broken and **penetrates** the skin. • The bone breaks and there are bone fragments in the tissue. • The bone is bent and splits, causing an incomplete fracture.	Pain, swelling, and abnormal shape. (See Figure 8.12.)	Avoiding falls and situations that may put abnormal stress on bones.
Kyphosis	Abnormal posterior curve of the spine (hunchback). This condition can be caused from a variety of conditions.	Appearance is the main symptom. In advanced conditions pain may occur. Early medical care can identify the cause of this condition and early treatment may prevent progression.	Spine-stretching exercises and sleeping without a pillow. Sleeping on a firm mattress that keeps the back as straight as possible may be helpful.
Osteomyelitis	Infection of the bone that is usually caused by bacteria (often staphylococci) that infects the bone and/or the bone marrow, usually introduced by trauma or surgery.	Persistent, increasing bone pain with tenderness spreading into muscles, along with a fever.	Seeing a physician early for treatment of infections and avoid accidents that may allow the introduction of bacteria into the body.
Osteoporosis	The bone becomes **porous,** causing it to break easily. Occurs more frequently in women after menopause, or in people who are **sedentary** or on steroid therapy for a long time.	Pain, especially in the lower back. Fractures that occur easily or with little trauma associated. Often it is the cause of **spontaneous** fractures in elderly women.	Following a proper diet, doing routine moderate exercise, and employing balanced hormone therapy as aging occurs.
Rickets	The bones do not **calcify** sufficiently, remaining soft.	Bowlegs and knock-knees enlarged. Knoblike enlargement at ends and sides of bones. Muscle pain, enlarged skull, chest deformities, spinal curvature, enlargement of the liver and spleen, increased sweating, and general body tenderness.	Eating a balanced diet, especially foods with calcium, phosphorus, and vitamin D.
Scoliosis	A **lateral** (to the side) curvature of the spine. (See Figure 8.13.)	Congenital malformation of the spine, poliomyelitis, unequal length of legs, and other physical conditions.	Seeking early recognition and treatment may prevent progression of the curvature.

penetrates   Enters or passes through (e.g., a fractured bone passes through the skin).

porous   Filled with tiny openings.

sedentary   Immobilized; do not move around very much.

spontaneous   Occurring naturally without apparent cause.

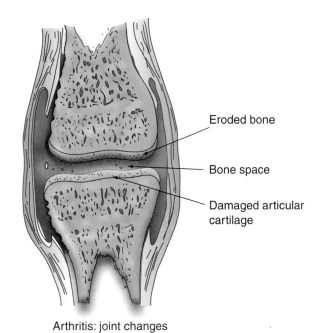

Figure 8.11

Arthritis joint changes.

Eroded bone

Bone space

Damaged articular cartilage

Arthritis: joint changes

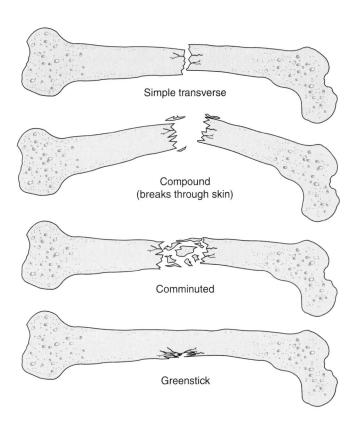

Figure 8.12

Common types of bone fractures.

Simple transverse

Compound
(breaks through skin)

Comminuted

Greenstick

calcify   To harden by forming calcium deposits.

lateral   Relating to the sides or side of.

concave   Curved inward, depressed; dented.

Figure 8.13

Comparison of normal and
scoliosis spines.

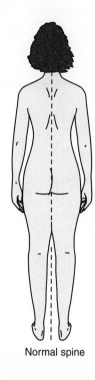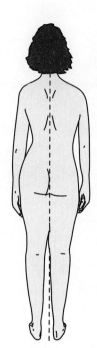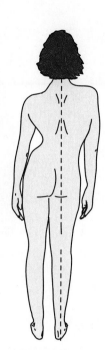

Normal spine   Scoliosis

MEDICAL TERMINOLOGY

■ arthrodesis	surgical **fixation** of a joint	
■ caudocephalad	from tail or coccyx to head	
■ cephalalgia	pain in the head, headache	
■ cephalocentesis	surgical puncture of the head	
■ cerebrotomy	incision into the brain	
■ chondroma	tumor consisting of cartilage	
■ costochondral	pertaining to a rib and its cartilage	
■ craniomalacia	softening of the skull bones	
■ craniosclerosis	thickening of the skull bones	
■ dactyledema	excess fluid in the fingers and toes	
■ dactylology	representing words by signs made with the fingers (sign language)	

■ dactylus	toe or finger
■ ilio	pertaining to the ilium and femur
■ lumbosacral	pertaining to the lumbar vertebrae and the sacrum
■ myelitis	inflammation of the spinal cord
■ osteomalacia	softening of the bone
■ osteoplasty	plastic repair of the bone
■ osteosarcoma	malignant tumor of the bone
■ osteotomy	incision into a bone
■ phalanx	finger or toe bone
■ prosthesis	artificial organ or part of the body

fixation   Repair or fix.

● JOBS AND PROFESSIONS

- Orthopedist
- Orthopedic technician
- Cast technician
- Prosthetist

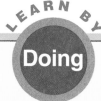

Doing

LEARN BY

UNIT 2 ACTIVITY

1. Complete Worksheets 2 through 4 as assigned.

2. Complete Worksheet 5 after your instructor discusses this unit in class.

3. Ask your instructor for directions to complete Worksheets/Activities 6 and 7.

4. When you are confident that you can meet each objective for this unit, ask your instructor for the unit evaluation.

UNIT

3

The Muscular System

STEPS TO SUCCESS

1. Complete Vocabulary Worksheet 1 in the Student Workbook.

2. Read this unit.

3. Complete the Learn by Doing assignment at the end of this unit.

UNIT OBJECTIVES

When you have completed this unit, you will be able to do the following:

✔ Match vocabulary words with their correct meanings.

✔ Explain the difference between muscle and bone functions.

✔ List three major functions of the muscles.

✔ Match common disorders of the muscular system with their descriptions.

✔ Match basic muscle movements to their correct names.

✔ Label a diagram of the muscular system.

✔ Describe how muscles provide support and movement.

✔ Explain why the health care worker's understanding of the muscular system is important.

digestion

Process of breaking down food mechanically and chemically.

elastic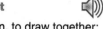

Easily stretched.

contract

To shorten, to draw together; muscles shorten when you flex a body part.

voluntary

Under the control of the person (e.g., you voluntarily raise your arm; it does not rise automatically).

involuntary

Not under control (e.g., muscle twitching).

axis

A center point that can be rotated around.

⬤ INTRODUCTION TO THE MUSCULAR SYSTEM

The muscles of the body make all movement possible. Muscles move body parts, allowing for proper functioning, such as heartbeat, breathing, **digestion** of food, and movement of the body from place to place. The next sections help you understand how muscles work.

Muscle Function

Muscles are made up of **elastic** fibers. These fibers are like a rubber band that lengthens and shortens. The main functions of muscles are to

■ Produce heat ■ Produce movement ■ Maintain posture

Types of Muscle

There are two kinds of muscle:

■ *Voluntary muscles* that you **contract** when you want to move (e.g., skeletal muscles; see Figure 8.14). You control these muscles; the movement is not automatic.

■ *Involuntary muscles,* which contract automatically (e.g., stomach, intestine, and heart). The heart pumps blood automatically. The stomach digests food automatically. You cannot tell the heart or stomach to start or stop.

Tendons

Tendons connect muscles to bones. When the muscle moves, it moves the tendon and bone.

Types of Muscle Tissue

Muscle tissue is classified into three categories:

■ *Skeletal muscles* or *striated muscles* are **voluntary** muscles (see Figure 8.2). These muscles provide movement of the body.

■ *Visceral muscles* or *smooth muscles* form the walls of the internal organs of the body (e.g., digestive tract, respiratory passage, and walls of blood vessels). They are **involuntary** muscles (see Figure 8.2).

■ *Cardiac muscle* forms the wall of the heart. This muscle circulates the blood (see Figure 8.2).

Basic Movements of the Skeletal Muscle

There are six basic movements of skeletal muscles:

■ **Adduct:** moving a body part toward the midline (Figure 8.15a)
■ **Abduct:** moving a body part away from the midline (Figure 8.15b)
■ **Extend:** straightening a body part by moving it away from the body (Figure 8.16)
■ **Flex:** bending a body part toward the body (Figure 8.16)
■ **Rotate:** turning a body part on its **axis**
■ **Open and close openings:** like the anus; called sphincters

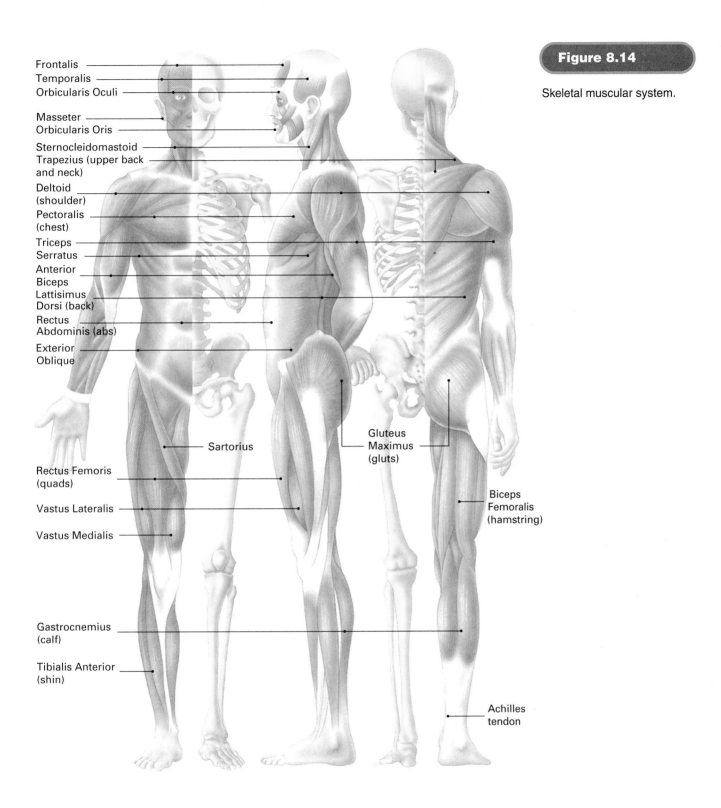

Figure 8.14

Skeletal muscular system.

Frontalis

Temporalis

Orbicularis Oculi

Masseter

Orbicularis Oris

Sternocleidomastoid

Trapezius (upper back and neck)

Deltoid (shoulder)

Pectoralis (chest)

Triceps

Serratus

Anterior

Biceps

Lattisimus Dorsi (back)

Rectus Abdominis (abs)

Exterior Oblique

Sartorius

Rectus Femoris (quads)

Vastus Lateralis

Vastus Medialis

Gluteus Maximus (gluts)

Biceps Femoralis (hamstring)

Gastrocnemius (calf)

Tibialis Anterior (shin)

Achilles tendon

Figure 8.15

(a) Adduction; (b) abduction.

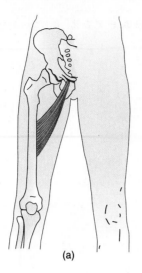
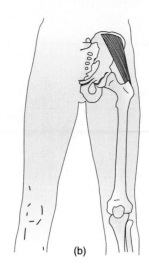

(a)   (b)

Figure 8.16

Extension and flexion.

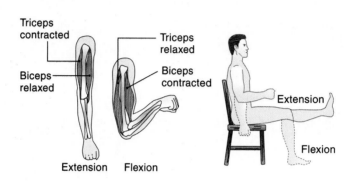

Triceps contracted

Triceps relaxed

Biceps relaxed

Biceps contracted

Extension

Flexion

Extension   Flexion

COMMON DISORDERS OF THE MUSCULAR SYSTEM

Table 8.4 ■ Common Disorders, Symptoms, and Preventive Measures/Treatment of the Muscular System

Condition	Disorder	Symptoms	Preventive Measures/Treatment
Fibromyalgia	Inflammation of the muscle tissues and the fibrous connective tissues.	A chronic stiffness and joint or muscle pain in 8 or more specific muscle sites.	Using rest, heat, massage, and medication to relieve inflammation and swelling.
Muscle strain	A **trauma** to the muscle, usually caused by a violent contraction.	Pain, swelling, warmth, and muscle weakness at the site.	Warming up muscles prior to exercise or strenuous activity. Not overextending muscles by trying to lift or pull objects that are beyond your capacity.
Muscular dystrophy	A group of genetically transmitted diseases that progressively **deteriorate** muscle tissue.	Loss of strength with increased disability and deformity.	Using supportive treatment such as physical therapy and orthopedic procedures to minimize deformity.
Myalgia	Muscle pain.	Muscle pain and malaise; occurs in many infectious diseases.	Resting, taking medication, and identifying the original cause.
Torn muscle	A tear of the muscle tissue, usually caused by extreme trauma to the muscle.	Pain, swelling, warmth, and muscle weakness at the site.	Avoiding strenuous muscle action.

trauma   Damage to the body caused by an injury, wound, or shock; mental trauma occurs from emotional shock.

deteriorate   Break down.

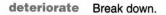

MEDICAL TERMINOLOGY

■ myasthenia	muscle weakness	■ myoma	tumor containing muscle tissue
■ myocardium	heart muscle or cardiac muscle	■ myomelanosis	abnormal darkening of muscle tissue
■ myocele	muscular protrusion (bulging or sticking out) through a muscle	■ myoparesis	weakness or partial paralysis of a muscle
■ myocelialgia	pain of the abdominal muscle	■ myosclerosis	hardening of a muscle
■ myogenic	beginning in the muscle	■ myothermic	pertaining to a rise in muscle temperature
■ myography	record of muscle contractions	■ tenorrhaphy	suturing of a tendon
■ myoid	resembling muscle	■ tenositis	inflammation of a tendon

● JOBS AND PROFESSIONS

- ■ Myologist
- ■ Physical therapist
- ■ Sports medicine assistant
- ■ Tenotomist

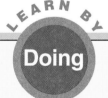

Doing   UNIT 3 ACTIVITY

1. **Complete Worksheets 2 through 5 as assigned.**
2. **When you are confident that you can meet each objective for this unit, ask your instructor for the unit evaluation.**

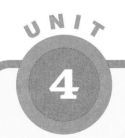

4   The Circulatory System

STEPS TO SUCCESS

1. Complete Vocabulary Worksheet 1 in the Student Workbook.

2. Read this unit.

3. Complete the Learn by Doing assignment at the end of this unit.

oxygen

Element in the atmosphere that is essential for maintaining life.

waste products

Elements that are unfit for the body's use and are eliminated from the body.

adequate

Enough, sufficient.

oxygenated

Containing oxygen.

unoxygenated

Lacking oxygen.

carbon dioxide

A gas, heavier than air; a waste product from the body.

primarily

For the most part; chiefly.

INTRODUCTION TO THE CIRCULATORY SYSTEM

Circulation is the continuous one-way movement of blood throughout the body. All of the systems and organs depend on the circulatory system. Arteries carry blood with **oxygen** and nutrients to each cell, and veins carry away the cell's **waste products.** If the circulation is not **adequate,** cells die. When the cells die, tissues begin to die, and the organs stop working properly. This may cause an entire system to stop functioning.

Kinds of Blood Vessels

■ *Arteries* carry blood from the lower chambers of the heart (ventricles) to all parts of the body. Arteries carry **oxygenated** blood, with the exception of the pulmonary artery. The *pulmonary artery* carries **unoxygenated** blood.

■ *Arterioles* are small arteries that connect arteries with capillaries.

■ *Capillaries* have very thin walls that allow nutrients, oxygen, and **carbon dioxide** to move in and out of the blood (see Figure 8.17).

■ *Venules* are small veins that connect veins with capillaries.

■ *Veins* carry blood from all the different parts of the body and return it to the heart. Veins carry unoxygenated blood, with the exception of the pulmonary vein. The pulmonary vein carries oxygenated blood. Veins have valves that aid in returning blood to the heart.

The Heart

The heart is the pump that forces blood throughout the body (see Table 8.5). The outside of the heart is made **primarily** of muscle, and the inside is divided into four

Figure 8.17

Blood vessels and capillary bed of the body.

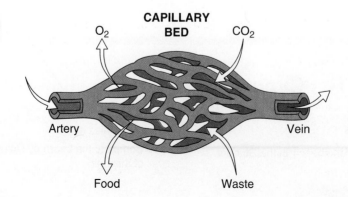

162

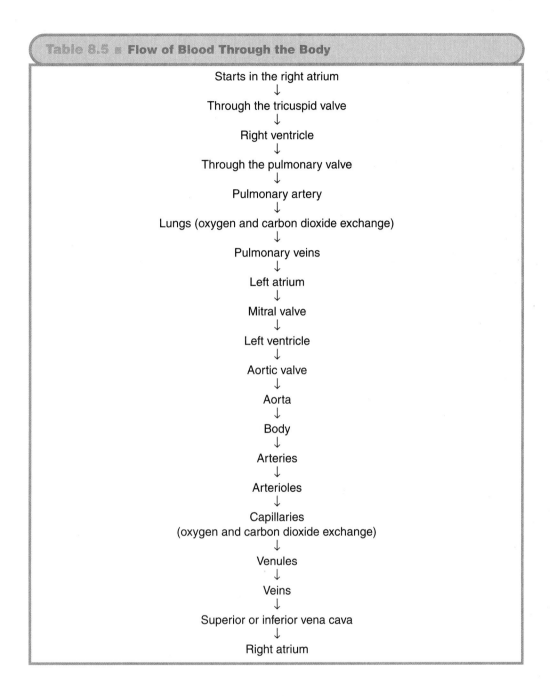

Table 8.5 ▪ Flow of Blood Through the Body

Starts in the right atrium
↓
Through the tricuspid valve
↓
Right ventricle
↓
Through the pulmonary valve
↓
Pulmonary artery
↓
Lungs (oxygen and carbon dioxide exchange)
↓
Pulmonary veins
↓
Left atrium
↓
Mitral valve
↓
Left ventricle
↓
Aortic valve
↓
Aorta
↓
Body
↓
Arteries
↓
Arterioles
↓
Capillaries
(oxygen and carbon dioxide exchange)
↓
Venules
↓
Veins
↓
Superior or inferior vena cava
↓
Right atrium

hollow chambers (see Figure 8.18). The heart wall is made of three different layers of tissue.

■ *Endocardium* is the smooth inside lining of the heart.

■ *Myocardium* is the thickest layer and is made up of muscle.

■ *Pericardium* is a double membrane that lines the outside of the heart.

The inside of the heart is divided into four parts or chambers:

■ The *right atrium* receives unoxygenated blood from the veins.

■ The *right ventricle* receives blood from the right atrium and pumps it to the lungs through the pulmonary artery.

Figure 8.18

Cross section of the heart.

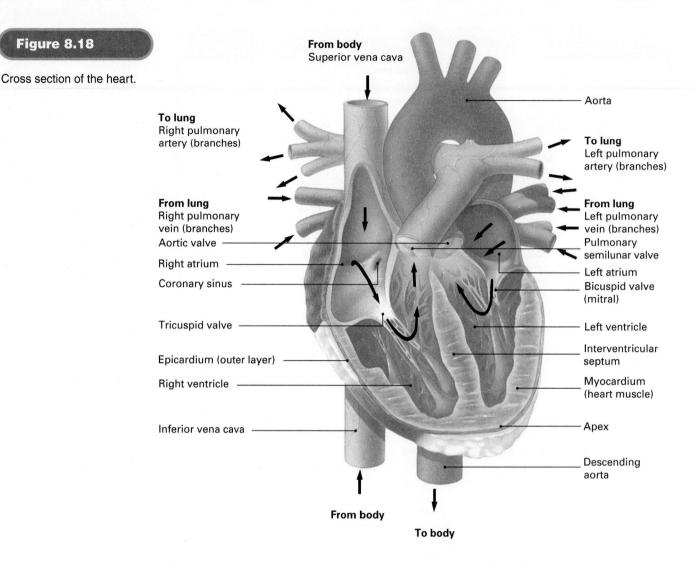

From body
Superior vena cava

To lung
Right pulmonary
artery (branches)

From lung
Right pulmonary
vein (branches)

Aortic valve

Right atrium

Coronary sinus

Tricuspid valve

Epicardium (outer layer)

Right ventricle

Inferior vena cava

Aorta

To lung
Left pulmonary
artery (branches)

From lung
Left pulmonary
vein (branches)

Pulmonary
semilunar valve

Left atrium

Bicuspid valve
(mitral)

Left ventricle

Interventricular
septum

Myocardium
(heart muscle)

Apex

Descending
aorta

From body

To body

- The *left atrium* receives oxygenated blood from the lungs and pumps it into the left ventricle.

- The *left ventricle* pumps blood into the aorta, which is the largest artery in the body. The aorta delivers the blood throughout the body.

Valves separate the chambers in the heart from the vessels leaving the heart.

- The *tricuspid* valve is between the right atrium and right ventricle. It closes when the right ventricle pumps blood out of the heart. This keeps the blood from flowing back into the right atrium.

- The *pulmonary semilunar* valve lies between the right ventricle and the pulmonary artery. It closes after all the blood from the right ventricle has been pushed into the pulmonary artery. When the valve closes, it stops blood from flowing back into the ventricle.

- The *mitral* (bicuspid) valve is found between the left atrium and the left ventricle. It closes to prevent blood from flowing back into the left atrium when the left ventricle contracts.

- The *aortic semilunar* valve is located between the left ventricle and the aorta. It stops blood from returning to the left ventricle after it has been forced into the aorta.

COMMON DISORDERS OF THE CIRCULATORY SYSTEM

Table 8.6 ■ **Common Disorders, Symptoms, and Preventive Measures/Treatment of the Circulatory System**

Condition	Disorder	Symptoms	Preventive Measures/ Treatment
Aneurysm	An aneurysm is present when the wall of a blood vessel is weakened. Aneurysms may be found in any part of the circulatory system. Among the most serious are those that occur in the head, heart, and aorta. An aortic aneurysm that ruptures usually causes immediate death. A ruptured cerebral aneurysm can cause paralysis, speech and vision disturbances, and death.	Pulsating swelling that produces a blowing sound through a stethoscope. Pain may or may not be present.	Maintaining healthy living can be helpful in keeping blood pressure within normal range. Exercise and diet may also be a factor, but will not ensure the prevention of aneurysms.
Arteriosclerosis	Arteriosclerosis is present when the walls of the arteries become thick and harden, causing vessels to be less elastic. Less blood is able to flow through the arteries because the arterles are narrowed.	This is common in geriatric patients. Typical signs include changes in skin temperature and color, changes in peripheral pulses, headache, dizziness, and memory changes.	Continuing activity throughout aging, getting adequate rest, and avoiding stress.
Endocarditis	An inflammation of the inside lining of the heart that may affect the heart valves. This condition can be caused by a variety of diseases. Survival rate is 65 to 85%.	Chest pain, shortness of breath, and elevated body temperature.	Maintaining good health habits may help resist this condition. Early diagnosis helps promote successful treatment.
Heart murmur	The valve does not close completely, allowing blood to flow back into the chamber it just left. It is most often present in the tricuspid and mitral valves.	Heart sounds that create a blowing sound between heartbeats, which indicate faulty heart valves.	Maintaining a healthy lifestyle may be helpful in preventing murmurs in later life. Some murmurs are present at birth.
Hypertension	A blood pressure greater than 140/90 places increased strain on the entire circulatory system. Risk of hypertension is increased with obesity and can also be caused by many conditions.	Anxiety, heart palpitations, profuse sweating, pallor, nausea, and in some cases the lungs collect fluid. May also experience headaches and blurred vision.	Maintaining good health habits may help resist this condition. Early diagnosis helps promote successful treatment.
Myocardial infarction (MI) or heart attack	Occurs when the coronary arteries are blocked. This blockage can be due to arteriosclerosis, or a blood clot, which is called coronary thrombosis.	Crushing chest pain that may radiate to the left arm, neck, or stomach. The patient may complain of severe heartburn or a gallbladder attack. The patient may look ashen in color and skin may feel clammy. May experience shortness of breath, may feel faint and anxious, and may fear that they are going to die.	Not smoking, maintaining a healthy body weight, eating a balanced diet low in saturated fats, and exercising regularly. Controlling stress is also helpful.

Table 8.6 ■ Continued

Condition	Disorder	Symptoms	Preventive Measures/ Treatment
Myocarditis	An inflammation of the heart muscle caused by viral, bacterial, or fungal infection, serum sickness, rheumatic fever, chemical agents, or complications from a collagen disease.	Chest pain, shortness of breath, and elevated body temperature.	Maintaining good health habits may help resist this condition. Early diagnosis helps promote successful treatment.
Pericarditis	An inflammation of the outer lining of the heart caused by trauma, malignancy, infection, uremia, myocardial infarction, collagen disease, and other nonspecific conditions.	Chest pain, shortness of breath, nonproductive cough, and rapid pulse. A friction rub can be heard over the heart with a stethoscope.	Maintaining good health habits may help resist this condition. Early diagnosis helps promote successful treatment.
Varicose veins	Enlarged veins that are not efficient in returning blood to the heart. They can occur anywhere in the body but are most often found in the lower **extremities.**	Pain and muscle cramps with a feeling of fullness and heaviness in the legs. Some veins near the skin may look enlarged. May be caused by congenital defects of the veins or by congestion and increased pressure.	Minimizing prolonged times of standing and maintaining good posture can reduce the risk of varicose veins in people without congential defects.

extremities   Arms, legs, hands, and feet.

MEDICAL TERMINOLOGY

■ angiocele	hernia of a blood vessel		■ embolus	blood clot in the circulatory system
■ bradycardia	abnormally slow heart rate		■ endocarditis	inflammation of the inside of the heart
■ cardiogenic	beginning within the heart		■ erythrocytosis	disease of red blood cells
■ cardiopulmonary	pertaining to the heart and lungs		■ hemostasis	stoppage of blood flow
■ cardioscope	instrument used to examine the inside of the heart		■ hyperemia	excess of blood in any part of the body
■ cardiovascular	pertaining to the heart and blood vessels		■ hypertension	high blood pressure
■ carditis	inflammation of the heart muscle		■ intravenous	IV, within a vein
■ cyanosis	bluish discoloration of the skin		■ leukocyte	white blood cell
■ ecchymosis	bruised condition		■ leukopenia	deficiency of white blood cells
■ ectopic	pertaining to an abnormal position		■ thrombus	blood clot that obstructs circulation
■ electrocardiogram	ECG/EKG, a tracing of heart activity			

JOBS AND PROFESSIONS

- Internist
- Cardiologist
- Cardiopulmonary technician
- ECG/EKG technician
- Echocardiogram technician

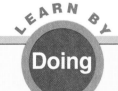

Doing

UNIT 4 ACTIVITY
1. **Complete Worksheets 2 through 5.**
2. **When you are confident that you can meet each objective for this unit, ask your instructor for the unit evaluation.**

The Lymphatic System

STEPS TO SUCCESS

1. Complete Vocabulary Worksheet 1 in the Student Workbook.

2. Read this unit.

3. Complete the Learn by Doing assignment at the end of this unit.

UNIT OBJECTIVES

When you have completed this unit, you will be able to do the following:

✔ Match vocabulary words with their correct meanings.

✔ Describe the general functions of the lymphatic system.

✔ Describe what lymph is.

✔ Match lymph vessels and organs to their function.

✔ Explain the difference between an antigen and an antibody.

✔ Identify common disorders of the lymphatic system.

✔ Describe how the lymphatic system helps provide immunity.

INTRODUCTION TO THE LYMPHATIC SYSTEM

The lymphatic system is an important part of the body's defense against disease. It filters out organisms that cause disease, produces white blood cells, and makes antibodies. It also drains excess fluids and protein so that tissues do not swell up. The lymphatic system and the circulatory system have structures that are joined together by a capillary system. The lymphatic system is made up of the lymph capillaries, lymph vessels, lymph nodes, spleen, tonsils, thymus, lacteals, thoracic duct, right lymphatic duct, and the cisterna chyli.

Kinds of Lymphatic System Vessels and Organs

interstitial

Space between tissues.

- *Lymph capillaries* are tubes that reach into the **interstitial** spaces of most body tissues. The capillaries have very thin walls that allow tissue fluids to move into them. When the fluid moves into the capillary, it is called lymph. The lymph contains waste products and foreign bodies from the cells. The lymph passes from the capillaries to the lymph vessels.

plasma

Watery, colorless fluid containing leukocytes, erythrocytes, and platelets.

- *Lymph vessels* are similar to veins. Muscle contractions help move the lymph from the tissues to the lymphatic trunks. Valves prevent backflow of the lymph. The lymphatic trunks receive the lymph from the body. The lymph from the lymphatic trunks empties into the veins and becomes part of the blood **plasma.**

lymphocytes

Type of white cell.

- *Lymph nodes* lie along the lymph vessels. They are located in the neck, armpit, chest, abdomen, elbows, groin, and knees (see Figure 8.19). They filter out bacteria and other waste products from the lymph as it moves toward the lymphatic trunks. They also produce **lymphocytes,** which help the body defend itself against microorganisms.

- *Tonsils* are masses of lymph tissue that are exposed to the outside. They filter tissue fluid, not lymph. They may filter so many bacteria that the pathogens overwhelm the tonsil. The tonsils then become infected.

monocytes

Large single-nucleus white cells.

- The *spleen* is behind the stomach. It filters microorganisms and waste products from the blood. The spleen makes lymphocytes and **monocytes** to help the body defend itself against microorganisms. The spleen also stores red blood cells and destroys worn-out red blood cells.

- The *thymus* is in front of the aorta and behind the upper part of the sternum. It is lymphatic tissue that stores lymphocytes that work with the lymphatic system to defend the body.

- The *lacteals* pick up digested fats from the small intestine.

- The *cisterna chyli* stores purified lymph before it empties into the bloodstream.

Figure 8.19

Lymph nodes in torso.

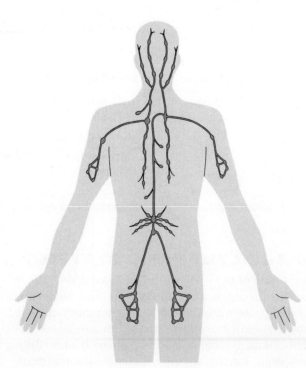

- *Thoracic duct* is the common trunk of all lymphatic vessels in the body except those on the right side.

- *Right lymphatic* duct is the vessel that carries lymph from the right side of the head, neck, thorax, lung, upper right limb, right side of the heart, and the diaphragmatic surface of the liver.

The Lymphatic System and Immunity

The lymphatic system helps the body remove substances that are harmful. These substances may be microorganisms or other foreign bodies. The foreign body is called an **antigen.** Examples of antigens

antigen

Foreign matter that causes the body to produce antibodies.

are poisons, splinters, and microorganisms. When these enter the body, the body responds by producing **antibodies.** The antibodies attack the antigen. This process is called the *immune response.*

Immune Response

The immune system has many specialized cells. Two types of white blood cells are lymphocytes and **phagocytes.** Phagocytes circulate through the body and eat diseased and dead cells. Other types of white cells surround foreign bodies and destroy them. All of the white blood cells are important in protecting the body. Some things that tell you that the immune system is working are fever, inflammation, and pus. When these are present, you know that the immune system is responding to protect the body.

antibodies

Substances made by the body to produce immunity to an antigen.

phagocytes

Cells that surround, eat, and digest microorganisms and cellular waste.

⬤ COMMON DISORDERS OF THE LYMPHATIC SYSTEM

Table 8.7 ▪ Common Disorders, Symptoms, and Preventive Measures/Treatment of the Lymphatic System

Condition	Disorder	Symptoms	Preventive Measures/Treatment
Addison's Disease	Life-threatening condition caused by partial or complete failure of the adrenal glands.	Fatigue, muscular weakness, low blood pressure, nerve impairment, and abnormal **pigmented** skin on the face and hands.	Replacing the chemicals not being produced by the adrenal glands, ensuring adequate fluid intake, maintaining sodium and potassium balance, and eating a diet high in carbohydrate and protein.
Elephantiasis	The worm blocks the lymphatic vessels and causes edema and swelling.	Caused by a **parasitic** thread-like worm, common in tropical and subtropical regions of the world. The worm enters the body from a bite from a host, which is usually a mosquito or other type of insect.	Employing mosquito control is the most effective prevention. Treat following infection with medication.
Hodgkin's Disease	A malignant disorder characterized by painless, progressive enlargement of lymph nodes. It is most common in young men.	Enlarged lymph nodes, weight loss, low-grade fever, night sweats, anemia, leukocytosis, and skin irritation.	Employing radiation and drug therapy treatments. Cause unknown.
Lymphadenitis	Inflammation of the lymph nodes, which may be caused from a variety sources.	Lymph nodes become enlarged, hard, smooth or irregular, red, and may feel hot to the touch.	Using drug therapy treatment.
Tonsillitis	Infection of the tonsils, frequently caused by streptococcus.	Severe sore throat, fever, headache, malaise, difficulty in swallowing, earache, and enlarged, tender lymph nodes in the neck.	Treating with antibiotics and surgery if infections frequently reoccur.

pigmented   Gives color to the skin.

parasitic   Pertaining to an organism that lives in or on another organism, taking nourishment from it.

MEDICAL TERMINOLOGY

■ asplenia	absence of a spleen	■ splenectomy	surgical removal of the spleen
■ lymphadenectomy	surgical removal of the lymph nodes	■ splenitis	inflammation of the spleen
■ lymphadenopathy	enlargement of the lymph nodes	■ splenomegaly	abnormal enlargement of the spleen
■ lymphocytopenia	an abnormally low number of lymphocytes in the blood	■ splenorrhexis	rupture of the spleen
■ lymphocytosis	abnormally high number of lymphocytes in the blood	■ splenotomy	incision into the spleen
■ lymphoma	tumor made up of lymphatic tissue	■ thymectomy	surgical removal of the thymus gland
■ lymphosarcoma	cancer in the lymphatic tissue	■ thymitis	inflammation of the thymus gland

● JOBS AND PROFESSIONS

■ Immunologist

■ Immunology technologist

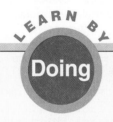

LEARN BY Doing

UNIT 5 ACTIVITY

1. **Complete Worksheets 2 and 3.**
2. **When you are confident that you can meet each objective for this unit, ask your instructor for the unit evaluation.**

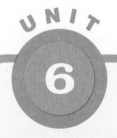

UNIT 6

The Respiratory System

STEPS TO SUCCESS

1. Complete Vocabulary Worksheet 1 in the Student Workbook.

2. Read this unit.

3. Complete the Learn by Doing assignment at the end of this unit.

UNIT OBJECTIVES

When you have completed this unit, you will be able to do the following:

✔ Match vocabulary words with their correct meanings.

✔ Label major organs of the respiratory system on a diagram.

✔ Describe the flow of oxygen through the body.

✔ Identify common disorders of the respiratory system.

✔ Describe how the respiratory system supports life.

✔ Explain why the health care worker's understanding of the respiratory system is important.

⬤ INTRODUCTION TO THE RESPIRATORY SYSTEM

Respiration is breathing. Breathing is necessary to supply life-giving oxygen to each cell in the body and to remove the waste products of each cell. The cell's gaseous waste product is called *carbon dioxide.*

Oxygen enters the body when air is pulled in through the mouth and nose. This process is called **inspiration/inhalation. Expiration/exhalation** occurs when the body forces air out of the lungs. This is the body's way of eliminating the cells' gaseous waste (carbon dioxide).

Structure of the Respiratory System

See Figure 8.20 and Table 8.8.

- The *nasal cavity* (nose) is where air enters the body. The nasal cavity is the preferred passage for air to enter the body. The nasal lining helps stop dust particles and pathogens. If dust and pathogens enter the lungs, the chance for infection is increased.

- The *oral cavity* (mouth) is where air enters the body when the nasal passage is blocked or when a person breathes through the mouth.

- The *pharynx* (throat) is the passageway that air enters after leaving the nose and mouth.

- The *epiglottis* is a flap that closes when food or water is swallowed. When it closes, it covers the opening of the trachea that leads to the lungs. This prevents food and water from entering the lungs.

- The *larynx* (voice box) is located just below the epiglottis. It is a **pouch** containing a cordlike framework that creates voice sounds.

- The *trachea* (windpipe) is the passageway between the pharynx and the lungs.

- The *bronchi* are air passageways that connect to the trachea. The trachea divides into two main branches, the bronchial tubes, that lead into the right and left lungs. The bronchial tubes are lined with hairlike objects called **cilia.** The cilia help move mucus, which catches dust and pathogens, up and out of the lungs.

- The *bronchioles* are the smallest subdivisions of the bronchi.

inspiration/ inhalation
Process of breathing in air during respiration.

expiration/ exhalation
Process of forcing air out of the body during respiration.

pouch
Small bag or sac.

cilia
Hairlike projections that move rhythmically.

Figure 8.20

Respiratory system.

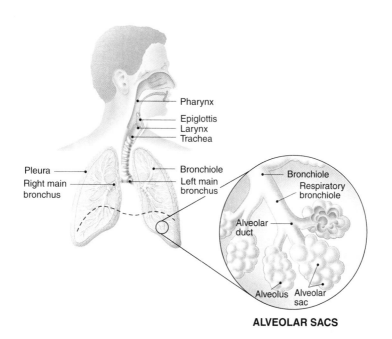

ALVEOLAR SACS

Table 8.8 ■ Flow of Oxygen Through the Body

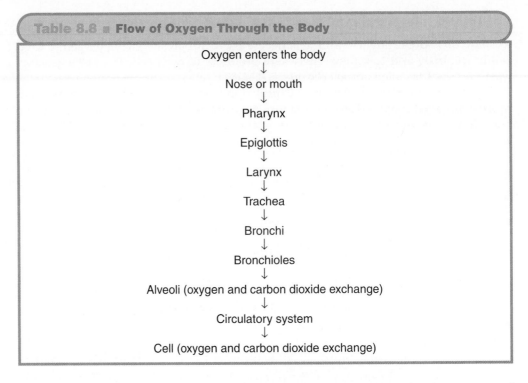

Oxygen enters the body
↓
Nose or mouth
↓
Pharynx
↓
Epiglottis
↓
Larynx
↓
Trachea
↓
Bronchi
↓
Bronchioles
↓
Alveoli (oxygen and carbon dioxide exchange)
↓
Circulatory system
↓
Cell (oxygen and carbon dioxide exchange)

■ The *alveoli* (air sacs) are at the end of each bronchiole. The alveoli are covered with capillaries that absorb oxygen into the blood. Carbon dioxide is forced out of the blood into the alveoli (carbon dioxide and oxygen exchange). Once the carbon dioxide has been released into the alveoli, it can be exhaled from the body.

■ The *diaphragm* is the muscular wall that divides the chest cavity from the abdominal cavity. To begin inspiration, the diaphragm moves down, creating a vacuum that pulls air into the lungs. When the diaphragm relaxes and moves upward again, air is exhaled (forced out) from the lungs.

COMMON DISORDERS OF THE RESPIRATORY SYSTEM

Table 8.9 ■ Common Disorders, Symptoms, and Preventive Measures/Treatment of the Respiratory System

Condition	Disorder	Symptoms	Preventive Measures/ Treatment
Asthma	The bronchial tube walls spasm, narrowing the passageways. With the passageways narrowed, it is difficult to exhale.	A suffocating feeling, breathing is difficult, anxiety can easily occur.	Treating with medication helps reduce the swelling in the bronchical tubes and allows air to move easily through the respiratory system. People with asthma should carry their medication with them at all times.
Emphysema	Leading cause of death. The alveoli become stretched out and are not able to push the carbon dioxide and other **pollutants** out of the lungs. Can be caused from smoking, frequent, untreated respiratory infections, asthma, or abnormal stress on the lungs.	Anxiety, shortness of breath, difficulty breathing, cough, cyanosis, unequal chest expansion, rapid heartbeat, and elevated body temperature.	Achieving a balanced lifestyle that includes adequate rest, a balanced diet, and not smoking helps keep the lungs clean and able to function normally.

Table 8.9 ■ Continued

Condition	Disorder	Symptoms	Preventive Measures/ Treatment
Hay fever	A reaction to trees, grass, or weed pollens.	Runny nose and teary eyes that may feel like a cold.	Removing the specific pollen, tree, or grass from the environment if possible. Medication can also be helpful.
Lung cancer	**Malignant** tissue in the lungs that destroy tissue. Approximately 75% of cases are due to smoking.	Persistent cough, difficulty breathing, purulent or blood-streaked sputum, chest pain, frequent bronchitis and/or pneumonia.	Treating with radiation and chemical therapy. Surgery may also be an option.
Pneumonia	Inflammation of the lungs, usually caused by bacteria, viruses, or an irritation by chemicals.	Chills and fever, headache, cough, and chest pain.	Treating with antibiotic and respiratory therapies.
Tuberculosis	Infectious disease caused by the tubercle bacillus. This bacillus is difficult to destroy. The tubercle bacillus can be carried on air currents and dust particles for a long time. When they are inhaled into the respiratory system, the bacillus may become active and destroy tissue.	Listlessness, vague chest pain, decreased appetite, fever, and weight loss are early symptoms. Tubercle bacillus most often infects the lungs, but it can also infect other organs of the body.	Treating the bacillus to become inactive keeps it from multiplying and from doing more damage to tissue. It is important for people with tuberculosis to always take their medication. If they stop taking it the bacillus may become active again. A major health risk today is a resistant strain of tuberculosis that does not become inactive with current treatments.
Upper respiratory infection (URI)	Infection of the trachea, larynx, throat, or nose.	Sore throat, congestion of the sinuses, nose, and eye with a fever and tiredness.	Getting adequate rest and eating a balanced diet help prevent infections. Infections caused by a virus usually improve after 10–12 days. Bacterial infections may require antibiotics.

pollutants   Things that contaminate the air (e.g., smoke, smog).

malignant   Cancerous.

● JOBS AND PROFESSIONS

- ■ Pulmonologist
- ■ Respiratory therapist
- ■ Thoracic surgeon
- ■ Otologist
- ■ Pulmonary technician
- ■ Oxygen technician
- ■ Otorhinolaryngologist

MEDICAL TERMINOLOGY

▪	apnea	absence of breathing	▪ pneumonolysis	breakdown of lung tissue
▪	bronchiectasis	dilation of the bronchi	▪ pneumothoracic	pertaining to the lungs and chest
▪	bronchitis	inflammation of the bronchial tubes	▪ pulmonary edema	fluid, swelling of the lungs
▪	dyspnea	difficult or painful breathing	▪ rales	rattling or bubbling sounds in the chest
▪	EENT	abbreviation for "eyes, ears, nose, throat"	▪ rhinoplasty	plastic repair of the nose
▪	epistaxis	nosebleed	▪ rhinorrhea	running nose
▪	hypoxia	lack of oxygen	▪ sublingual	beneath the tongue
▪	intercostal	between the ribs	▪ tachypnea	rapid breathing
▪	laryngitis	inflammation of the larynx	▪ thoracotomy	incision into the chest
▪	nares	nostrils	▪ trachelosis	any condition of the neck
▪	pharyngospasm	spasmodic contraction of the pharynx	▪ tracheostomy	opening into the trachea
▪	pleurocentesis	surgical puncture of the pleura	▪ URI	abbreviation for upper respiratory infection

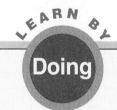

LEARN BY Doing

UNIT 6 ACTIVITY

1. Complete Worksheets 2 through 4.
2. When you are confident that you can meet each objective for this unit, ask your instructor for the unit evaluation.

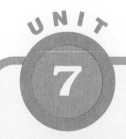

U N I T

7

The Digestive System

STEPS TO SUCCESS

1. Complete Vocabulary Worksheet 1 in the Student Workbook.

2. Read this unit.

3. Complete the Learn by Doing assignment at the end of this unit.

UNIT OBJECTIVES

When you have completed this unit, you will be able to do the following:

- ✔ Match vocabulary words with their correct meanings.
- ✔ Label a diagram of the digestive system and its accessory organs.
- ✔ Explain the functions of the digestive system.
- ✔ Recognize the function of organs associated with the digestive system.

- ✔ Match common disorders of the digestive system with their descriptions.
- ✔ Describe how the digestive system absorbs nutrients.
- ✔ Explain why the health care worker's understanding of the digestive system is important.

⦿ INTRODUCTION TO THE DIGESTIVE SYSTEM

In this unit, we discuss the body's processing of food. This process prepares nutrients so that they can be used by each cell. Body cells cannot absorb nutrients from food. Food must be changed into a substance that the body cells can use. This process of changing food into a usable substance is known as *digestion*. Once digestion occurs, nutrients move into the bloodstream. This transfer of nutrients into the blood is called **absorption.** Digestion and absorption are the two main functions of the digestive system.

Digestive Organs

The digestive system is a very long muscular tube that begins at the mouth and ends at the **anus.** This tube, called the **alimentary canal,** is made up of many parts (Figure 8.21).

- The *mouth* (oral cavity) is where food enters the body. The digestive process begins with the mechanical breakdown (the chewing, mashing, and grinding of food by the teeth).

- The *salivary glands* are located under the tongue, near the jawbone, and at the back of the throat. The purpose of the salivary glands is to produce a **secretion** that dissolves food and coats food with a mucus that allows it to pass through the esophagus more easily.

- The *pharynx* (throat) is located at the back of the oral cavity and is a passageway for food.

- The *epiglottis* is a flap that covers the trachea when food or water is swallowed. By covering the trachea, the epiglottis keeps food and water out of the lungs.

- The *esophagus* receives food and water from the pharynx. Food is moved through the esophagus by a rhythmic wavelike motion called **peristalsis.**

- The *cardiac* **sphincter** is a ring of muscle fibers located where the esophagus and stomach join. This muscle keeps stomach contents from moving up into the esophagus.

- The *stomach* is an enlarged part of the alimentary canal that receives food and water from the esophagus. The stomach holds food until digestive juices have chemically broken down the food particles into **chyme.** Chyme is a creamy semifluid mixture of food and digestive juices.

- The *pyloric sphincter* is a ringlike muscle found at the far end of the stomach. Its main purpose is to keep food in the stomach long enough to become chyme.

absorption

Passage of a substance through a body surface into body fluids and tissues (e.g., nutrients from digested food pass through the wall of the small intestine into the blood).

anus

Outlet from which the body expels solid waste.

alimentary canal

Long muscular tube beginning at the mouth and ending at the anus.

secretion

Producing and expelling a special substance (e.g., sebaceous glands secrete oil; salivary glands secrete saliva).

peristalsis

Progressive, wavelike motion that occurs involuntarily in hollow tubes of the body.

sphincter

Circular muscle that allows the opening and closing of a body part (e.g., anus, pylorus).

chyme

Creamy semifluid mixture of food and digestive juices.

Figure 8.21

The digestive system is also called the alimentary canal.

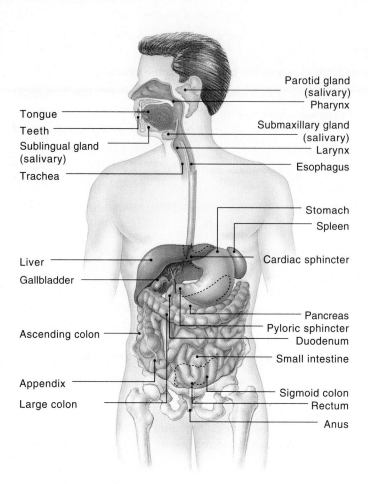

Tongue
Teeth
Sublingual gland (salivary)
Trachea

Parotid gland (salivary)
Pharynx
Submaxillary gland (salivary)
Larynx
Esophagus

Stomach
Spleen
Cardiac sphincter

Liver
Gallbladder

Pancreas
Pyloric sphincter
Duodenum

Ascending colon

Small intestine

Appendix
Large colon

Sigmoid colon
Rectum
Anus

minute

Exceptionally small.

villi

Tiny projections.

The *small intestine* is attached to the stomach at the pyloric sphincter. The small intestine is about 20 feet long. The first 10 to 12 inches of the small intestine are called the *duodenum.* The duodenum receives juices from the pancreas, liver, and gallbladder, which aid in further chemical breakdown of the chyme. This final chemical breakdown is the completion of digestion. The small intestine is the portion of the alimentary canal where most absorption takes place. The lining of the small intestine contains many **minute** projections called **villi.** Each villus contains capillaries that absorb nutrients from the food we eat (Figure 8.22). Those food substances that are not absorbed are moved through the 20 feet of the small intestine by peristalsis to the large intestine.

Figure 8.22

Villi in the lining of the small intestine.

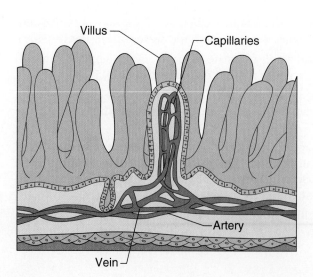

Villus
Capillaries
Artery
Vein

The *large intestine* is attached to the small intestine and receives food substances that are of little value to the body. The large intestine absorbs water, mineral salts, and vitamins. It secretes (discharges) mucus to aid in the movement of **feces** through the intestine.

feces

Solid waste that is evacuated from the body through the anus.

■ The *rectum* is the last 6 to 8 inches of the alimentary canal. It serves as a storage area for feces.

■ The *anus* is the end of the alimentary canal. It is where fecal material is **evacuated** from the body.

evacuated
Emptied out.

Table 8.10 shows common disorders, symptoms, and preventive measures/treatment of the digestive system and accessory structures.

Table 8.10 ■ Common Disorders, Symptoms, and Preventive Measures/Treatment of the Digestive System and Accessory Structures

Condition	Disorder	Symptoms	Preventive Measures/ Treatment
Cholelithiasis (*Accessory Structure*)	Stones in the gallbladder.	Abdominal pain that may radiate toward the back, and heartburn especially after eating.	Eating a low-fat diet. Surgical removal of stones and/or the gallbladder may be necessary.
Cirrhosis (*Accessory Structure*)	Liver cells become damaged, and scarring prevents the liver and other systems from functioning.	Nausea, **flatulence,** decreased appetite, weight loss, light-colored stools, weakness, and abdominal pain.	Eating a balanced diet rich in protein and vitamins (especially folic acid), getting plenty of rest, and abstaining from alcohol. The liver does have the capacity to regenerate given time and the proper diet.
Constipation (*Digestive System*)	Infrequent, difficult **defecation** of fecal material.	Abdominal pain and cramping, inability to defecate.	Eating a balanced diet with adequate amounts of fruits and vegetables, exercising regularly, and drinking adequate amounts of water help to keep elimination of waste regular. When constipation occurs, medication and/or enemas may be necessary.
Diabetes (*Accessory Structure*)	A partial or complete lack of insulin availability preventing **metabolism.**	Excessive thirst, decreased energy.	Diet and exercise. Frequent blood tests to determine the need for medication. Medication may be necessary. Daily inspection of skin for reddened areas or sores, especially the feet. May require shoes with a deep toe box to prevent irritation.
Diarrhea (*Digestive System*)	Abnormal frequent watery stool, usually the symptom of some underlying disorders.	Abdominal cramping that forces frequent defecation and generalized weakness.	Using medication and identifying the condition. It is important to carefully monitor people with diarrhea so they don't become dehydrated which may cause other serious conditions.
Enteritis	Inflammation of the intestines.	Abdominal cramping and **diarrhea.**	See treatment under diarrhea.
Gastric ulcer (*Digestive System*)	Open sore in the stomach.	Pain and sometimes internal bleeding.	Eating a soft bland diet, reducing stress, using medication. When symptoms are not relieved, surgery may be necessary.
Gastritis (*Digestive System*)	Inflammation of the stomach lining. If untreated, it could develop a gastric ulcer.	**Epigastric** pain, indigestion, and burning in the stomach area.	See treatment under gastric ulcer.
Gastroenteritis (*Digestive System*)	Inflammation of the stomach lining and intestines.	Vomiting, abdominal cramping, and diarrhea.	Taking lots of fluids (may be necessary to start an IV to administer fluids if vomiting is excessive) and medication.

Table 8.10 ■ Continued

Condition	Disorder	Symptoms	Preventive Measures/ Treatment
Hepatitis (*Accessory Structure*)	Inflammation of the liver caused by a virus or a poison.	**Jaundice,** enlarged liver, decreased appetite, abdominal and gastric pain, clay-colored stools, and dark-colored urine.	Eating a balanced diet rich in protein and vitamins (especially folic acid), getting plenty of rest, and abstaining from alcohol. The liver does have the capacity to regenerate given time and the proper diet.
Pancreatitis (*Accessory Structure*)	Inflammation of the pancreas caused by an overproduction of its own pancreatic juices.	Severe abdominal pain radiating to the back, fever, loss of appetite, nausea, and vomiting.	Removing any stimulation of the pancreas by removing all stomach contents, IV medication and fluids. Surgery may be necessary.

flatulence   Excessive gas in the stomach and intestines that causes discomfort.

defecation   The pushing of solid material from the bowel.

metabolism   Chemical interactions in the body that provide energy.

diarrhea   Passage of watery stool at frequent intervals.

epigastric   Pertaining to the area over the pit of the stomach.

jaundice   Yellowing of the whites of the eyes, skin, and mucous membranes.

○ THE ACCESSORY STRUCTURES

The accessory structures of the digestive system assist in the process of digestion. These structures are the liver, the gallbladder, and the pancreas (see Table 8.10).

■ The *liver,* the largest gland in the body, has many functions. Some of these functions are

• Production of bile • Removal of poisons that have been absorbed in the small intestines • Storage of vitamins • Production of heparin, which prevents blood from clotting • Production of antibodies, which act against infection and foreign matter

■ The *gallbladder,* a muscular sac, stores the bile that the liver produces. When chyme reaches the duodenum, the gallbladder squeezes bile into the duodenum to aid in chemical breakdown of the chyme.

■ The *pancreas* produces pancreatic juices that also aid in the chemical breakdown of food. It also manufactures **insulin,** which regulates the amount of sugar used by the tissues.

insulin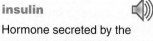
Hormone secreted by the pancreas; essential for maintaining the correct blood sugar level.

○ JOBS AND PROFESSIONS

■ Dietary aide

■ Gastroenterologist

■ Dietitian

■ Hepatologist

MEDICAL TERMINOLOGY

■	anorexia	lack of appetite	■	enterocele	hernia involving the intestine
■	antacid	without acid	■	enterocyst	cyst of the intestinal wall
■	buccolingual	pertaining to the cheek and tongue	■	enterohepatic	pertaining to the intestines and the liver
■	cholecyst	gallbladder	■	gastrointestinal	GI, pertaining to the stomach and intestines
■	cholelithotomy	incision for the removal of a gallstone	■	gastrophrenic	pertaining to the stomach and diaphragm
■	colitis	inflammation of the colon	■	gastrosis	condition affecting the stomach
■	colostomy	opening into the colon	■	hepatopathy	any disease of the liver
■	dysphagia	difficult or painful swallowing	■	hepatoptosis	liver dropping downward
■	emesis	vomiting	■	metabolism	process by which food is changed into energy for the body's use
■	emetic	substance that induces vomiting	■	splenomegaly	enlargement of the spleen

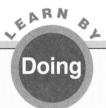

LEARN BY Doing

UNIT 7 ACTIVITY

1. Complete Worksheets 2 through 5.
2. When you are confident that you can meet each objective for this unit, ask your instructor for the unit evaluation.

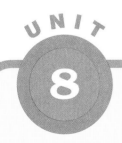

UNIT 8

The Urinary System

STEPS TO SUCCESS

1. Complete Vocabulary Worksheet 1 in the Student Workbook.

2. Read this unit.

3. Complete the Learn by Doing assignment at the end of this unit.

UNIT OBJECTIVES

When you have completed this unit, you will be able to do the following:

✔ Match vocabulary words with their correct meanings.

✔ Label a diagram of the urinary system.

✔ Identify the function of organs in the urinary system.

✔ Match common disorders of the urinary system with their descriptions.

✔ Describe how the urinary system removes liquid waste and eliminates it from the body.

✔ Explain why the health care worker's understanding of the urinary system is important.

⬤ INTRODUCTION TO THE URINARY SYSTEM

The urinary system rids the body of liquid waste and assists in the regulation of water and chemical balance. Its functions include

- The excretion of urine, a liquid waste produced in the body
- The maintenance of water balance; water balance occurs when the intake of water equals the output of water
- Regulation of the chemical balance or acid-base balance of the body; the body must maintain a balance of acids and bases in order to function properly

These functions are accomplished by the organs of the urinary system (Figure 8.23).

Structure of the Urinary System

Two kidneys are located at the back of the upper abdomen. Their primary function is to filter (remove) waste products from the blood. Each kidney has the following structure (see Figure 8.24).

- The *capsule* is the sac surrounding the kidney.
- The *cortex* is the outer part of the kidney.

Figure 8.23

The urinary system removes liquid waste from the body.

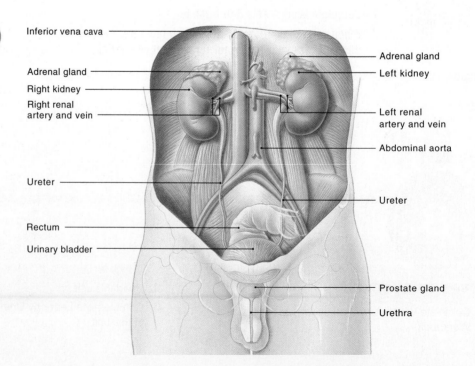

Inferior vena cava

Adrenal gland

Adrenal gland

Left kidney

Right kidney

Right renal artery and vein

Left renal artery and vein

Abdominal aorta

Ureter

Ureter

Rectum

Urinary bladder

Prostate gland

Urethra

- The *medulla* is the inner part of the kidney.

- The **nephron** is the chief filtering **mechanism** of the kidney. Part of the nephron is in the cortex, and part of it is in the medulla. The nephron is made up of

  - A tiny twisted tube called the *convoluted tubule* • A cuplike capsule called *Bowman's capsule* • A cluster of capillaries in Bowman's capsule called the *glomerulus*

- The *ureters* are tubes that carry urine (liquid waste) from the kidneys to the urinary bladder.

- The *urinary bladder* is a muscular sac that expands to hold urine received from the kidneys.

- The *urethra* is a tube extending from the urinary bladder to the outside of the body. This allows for the excretion of urine.

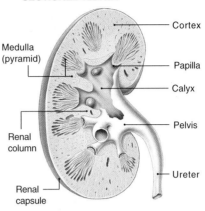

SECTIONED KIDNEY

Cortex
Medulla (pyramid)
Papilla
Calyx
Pelvis
Renal column
Ureter
Renal capsule

Figure 8.24

Cross section of a kidney.

nephron

Functional part of the kidney that filters liquid waste.

mechanism

Process or a series of steps that achieve a result.

COMMON DISORDERS OF THE URINARY SYSTEM

Table 8.11 ▪ **Common Disorders, Symptoms, and Preventive Measures/Treatment of the Urinary System**

Condition	Disorder	Symptoms	Preventive Measures/ Treatment
Cystitis	Inflammation of the urinary bladder due to infection. The bladder is susceptible to infection because bacteria can easily travel up the urethra to infect the bladder.	Frequent, painful urination, possible blood in urine, fever and chills.	Depending on the diagnosis, treating with antibiotics, increased fluid intake, bed rest, medication to control bladder wall spasms, and when necessary, surgery.
Hydronephrosis	Expanded renal pelvis. Normally caused by an **obstruction** (kidney stone or tumor) that keeps urine from flowing down the ureter.	May experience fever and pain on the side (flank), and in some cases urine may contain blood and/or pus.	Removing the obstruction surgically if it does not pass through the ureter and urethra normally.
Kidney or renal failure	Nephron of the kidney is unable to filter liquid waste from the blood.	Early signs include fatigue and mental dullness. Later signs include absences of urination, convulsions, GI bleeding, malnutrition, and (jaundiced) skin that yellowed may be covered with a frostlikesubstance (uremic frost).	Treating with a renal diet and **dialysis,** which is a way to filter waste products from the blood. There are two methods of dialysis: —Hemodialysis, which circulates the body's blood through a machine, that filters out the waste and returns the clean blood to the body. —Peritoneal dialysis, which **infuses** sterile fluids into the **peritoneal cavity** and then drains the fluid from the cavity. While the fluid is in the abdomen, waste products are chemically drawn out of tissues and into the fluid. When the fluid drains from the abdomen, the waste is also removed.

Table 8.11 ▪ Continued

Condition	Disorder	Symptoms	Preventive Measures/ Treatment
Nephritis	Inflammation of the kidney due to infection or arteriosclerosis.	**Edema,** a collection of fluid in the tissues that causes swelling.	Treating with medication or surgery to remove a kidney may be indicated, depending on the cause.
Renal calculi	Kidney stones that develop when the liquid waste from the blood becomes solid.	Sharp, severe pain in the lower back over the kidney, radiating into the groin.	Surgically removing the stones if they do not pass through the ureter and urethra normally.
Uremia	An accumulation of urine substances in the blood occurs when the nephron is unable to completely filter out waste from the blood.	Nausea, vomiting, headache, dizziness, coma or convulsions, breath and perspiration may smell like urine.	Early diagnosis of kidney dysfunction. Treatment is dialysis.

obstruction   Blockage or clogging.

dialysis   Process of removing waste from body fluids.

infuses   Flows into the body by gravity (e.g., IV drips through a tube into the body).

peritoneal cavity

Area of the body containing the liver, stomach, intestines, kidneys, urinary bladder, and reproductive organs.

edema

Swelling; abnormal or excessive collection of fluid in the tissues. Usually, the swelling is in the hands, ankles, legs, or abdomen.

MEDICAL TERMINOLOGY

▪ calculi	stones	▪ nephrorrhagia	renal hemorrhage
▪ cystitis	inflammation of the bladder	▪ nephrostomy	an artificial opening into the kidney
▪ cystoscopy	inspection of the bladder	▪ pyelectasis	dilation of the renal pelvis
▪ diuresis	passage of abnormally large amounts of urine	▪ pyelitis	inflammation of the pelvis of the kidney
▪ glycouria	sugar in the urine	▪ pyelolithotomy	removal of kidney stone
▪ hematuria	blood in the urine	▪ pyelometry	measurement of the kidney's pelvis
▪ nephralgia	renal pain	▪ renal	pertaining to the kidney
▪ nephric	pertaining to the kidney	▪ renal colic	severe pain in the kidney
▪ nephroid	resembling a kidney	▪ uremia	condition in which blood contains toxins usually excreted from the kidneys
▪ nephrolithotripsy	crushing of kidney stones	▪ ureteropyelitis	inflammation of the kidney pelvis and the ureter
▪ nephropexy	surgical attachment of a floating kidney	▪ urethrism	irritability or spasm of the urethra

JOBS AND PROFESSIONS

- Urologist
- Nephrologist
- Dialysis technician

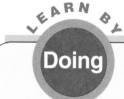

Doing

UNIT 8 ACTIVITY

1. **Complete Worksheets 2 through 4.**
2. **When you are confident that you can meet each objective for this unit, ask your instructor for the unit evaluation.**

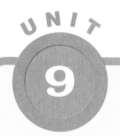

9

The Glandular Systems

STEPS TO SUCCESS

1. Complete Vocabulary Worksheet 1 in the Student Workbook.

2. Read this unit.

3. Complete the Learn by Doing assignment at the end of this unit.

UNIT OBJECTIVES

When you have completed this unit, you will be able to do the following:

✔ Match vocabulary words with their correct meanings.

✔ Label endocrine glands on a diagram.

✔ Identify functions of the endocrine glands.

✔ Identify common disorders of the endocrine glands.

✔ Explain the difference between the endocrine and exocrine glands.

✔ Describe the effects of the endocrine glands on the body.

✔ Explain why the health care worker's understanding of the glandular systems is important.

INTRODUCTION TO THE GLANDULAR SYSTEMS

The glands of the body (Figure 8.25) make substances that help regulate the body processes of growth, **metabolism,** muscle contraction, and many other processes. Glands are divided into two categories. These are the exocrine and endocrine glands.

- *Exocrine glands* have ducts that carry substances to organs, body parts, or the outside of the body. The substance made by the gland is **excreted** and is deposited in the organ or body part. *Examples:*

  • Digestive juices from the salivary glands, pancreas, and gallbladder • Milk from the female mammary glands • Moisture from the sweat glands • Sebum (oil) from the **sebaceous** glands • Tears from the **lacrimal** glands

metabolism
The body's process of using food to make energy and use nutrients.

excreted
Thrown off or eliminated as waste material.

sebaceous
Pertaining to fatty secretions.

Figure 8.25

The glandular systems provide substances that help regulate body processes.

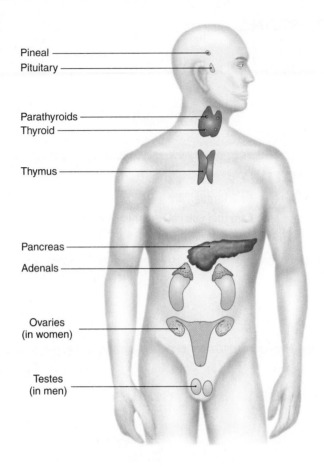

Pineal
Pituitary

Parathyroids
Thyroid

Thymus

Pancreas

Adenals

Ovaries
(in women)

Testes
(in men)

lacrimal

Pertaining to tears.

hormones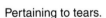

Protein substances secreted by an endocrine gland directly into the blood.

■ *Endocrine glands* are glands without ducts. They secrete **hormones** directly into the bloodstream. The secretions from these glands are separated into two main groups:

• *External secretions* (excretions) are fluids that are carried to a nearby organ or to the outside of the body. • *Internal secretions* are hormones that are carried to all parts of the body through the blood and lymph systems. The endocrine glands that secrete hormones are included in Table 8.12.

Table 8.12 ■ Endocrine Glands, Hormones, and Their Functions

Gland	Hormone	Function
Pituitary	TSH (thyrotropic hormone), ACTH (adreno-corticotrophic hormone), FSH (follicle-stimulating hormone), LH (luteinizing hormone), oxytocin, prolactin, and somatotropic hormone	Controls other glands; stimulates growth
Thyroid	Thyroxin	Controls rate of metabolism
Parathyroid	Parathyroid hormone	Regulates calcium and phosphorus metabolism
Pancreas	Insulin from islands of Langerhans	Enables utilization of glucose
Ovaries	Estrogen and progesterone	Develop and maintain female reproductive organs
Testes	Testosterone	Develop and maintain male reproductive organs
Adrenal medulla	Adrenalin	Prepares the body for fight or flight
Adrenal cortex	Corticoids	Aids body in coping with stress or infection

COMMON DISORDERS OF THE GLANDULAR SYSTEMS

■ Hypothyroidism decreased production of the thyroid secretion.

■ Hyperthyroidism increased production of the thyroid secretion.

Table 8.13 ■ Common Disorders, Symptoms, and Preventive Measures/Treatment of the Glandular System

Condition	Disorder	Symptoms	Preventive Measures/ Treatment
Addison's disease	A life-threatening insufficient amount of hormones from the adrenal glands.	Weakness, decreased endurance, increased pigmentation of the skin and mucous membranes, anorexia, dehydration, weight loss, GI disturbances, anxiety, depression, and decreased tolerance to cold.	Treating with medication, maintaining an adequate intake of fluids, eating a diet high in carbohydrates and protein and low in sodium and potassium.
Diabetes mellitus	Too much sugar (glucose) in the blood, usually the result of the pancreas failing to produce insulin. There are the following types of diabetes: • IDDM—insulin-dependent diabetes mellitus. • NIDDM—noninsulin-dependent diabetes mellitus. • GDM—gestational diabetes mellitus (during pregnancy). • Types of diabetes usually associated with pancreatic disease, hormonal changes, adverse effects of drugs, or genetic abnormalities. • IGT—impaired glucose tolerance.	Increased thirst (polydipsia) and urination (polyuria), and weight loss. Periods of excessive hunger (polyphagia), and low blood sugar levels (hypoglycemia). The eyes, kidneys, nervous system, skin, and circulatory system may be affected, and infections are common. Atherosclerosis often develops.	Maintaining insulin and glucose levels within normal values through diet, exercise, and medication.
Hypoglycemia	Too little sugar in the blood, usually caused by the excessive production of insulin in the pancreas.	Weakness, headache, hunger, visual disturbances, ataxia, anxiety, personality changes, and, if untreated, delirium, coma, and death.	Taking glucose in orange juice by mouth if the person is conscious or administering intravenously if the person is unconscious.

JOBS AND PROFESSIONS

■ Endocrinologist

MEDICAL TERMINOLOGY

■ acromegaly	enlargement of bones of the extremities		■ hyperthyroidism	increased production of the thyroid secretion
■ adenectomy	removal of any gland		■ hypothyroidism	decreased production of the thyroid secretion
■ adenoidectomy	removal of the adenoids		■ lymphocytopenia	deficiency of lymph cells
■ adrenogenic	originating in the adrenals		■ pancreatolysis	breakdown of the pancreas
■ dwarfism	condition of being abnormally small		■ parathyrotoxicosis	poisonous condition of the parathyroid
■ endocrine	ductless; to secrete within		■ pinealoma	tumor of the pineal gland
■ endocrinotherapy	treatment with endocrine preparation		■ pituitarigenic	originating in the pituitary
■ exocrine	to secrete through a duct		■ pituitarism	any disorder of the pituitary gland
■ goiter	enlarged thyroid gland		■ thyroadenitis	inflammation of the thyroid gland
■ goitrogen	any substance that causes a goiter			

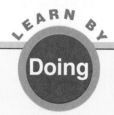

Doing **UNIT 9 ACTIVITY**

1. **Complete Worksheets 2 through 4.**

2. **When you are confident that you can meet each objective for this unit, ask your instructor for the unit evaluation.**

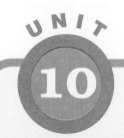

The Nervous System

STEPS TO SUCCESS

1. Complete Vocabulary Worksheet 1 in the Student Workbook.

2. Read this unit.

3. Complete the Learn by Doing assignment at the end of this unit.

UNIT OBJECTIVES

When you have completed this unit, you will be able to do the following:

✔ Match vocabulary words with their correct meanings.

✔ Match and select the functions of various parts of the nervous system.

✔ Label diagrams of the eye and ear.

✔ Match common disorders of the nervous system with their correct names.

✔ Describe the influence of the nervous system on the body.

✔ Explain why the health care worker's understanding of the nervous system is important.

⬤ INTRODUCTION TO THE NERVOUS SYSTEM

The nervous system is a delicate system of nerve cells (Figure 8.26) linked together to receive **stimuli** and to respond to stimuli.

◼ Stimuli are anything that cause a reaction or response (e.g., when your hand touches a hot object or when something flies into your eye).

◼ Response is the reaction to the stimuli (e.g., moving your hand when it touches something hot or tears in the eye when something flies into it).

The nervous system is divided into two parts: the central nervous system and the **peripheral** nervous system.

stimuli

Elements in the external or internal environment that are strong enough to set up a nervous impulse.

peripheral

Situated away from a central structure.

Figure 8.26

Central and peripheral nervous systems; neuron (nerve cell).

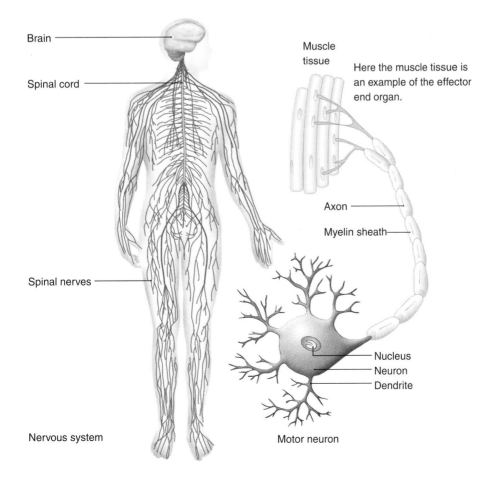

Brain

Spinal cord

Spinal nerves

Nervous system

Muscle tissue

Here the muscle tissue is an example of the effector end organ.

Axon

Myelin sheath

Nucleus
Neuron
Dendrite

Motor neuron

The *central nervous system (CNS)* includes the brain and the spinal cord (see Figure 8.26). Nerves of the spinal cord carry messages to and from the brain. The brain has three main parts:

- The *cerebrum* processes thought having to do with memory and learning. It controls voluntary movements and sense interpretation.
- The *cerebellum* coordinates muscle activity and balance so that muscles function smoothly.
- The *medulla* controls breathing, heartbeat, circulatory action, and digestive movements.

The *peripheral nervous system* includes the nerves and **ganglia** outside the brain and spinal cord. There are

- Twelve pairs of cranial nerves
- Thirty-one pairs of spinal nerves
- Various nerve branches in body organs

All parts of the central and peripheral nervous systems work together to relay messages to the brain. Each message is carried to the correct area of the brain by its specialized **neuron** or nerve cell (see Figure 8.26).

Each specialized neuron leads into a passage that delivers the message or stimuli to the brain or the spinal cord. The areas in the spinal cord that can receive messages cause an action or response to stimuli that does not require interpretation. The stimuli that are received by the brain are interpreted and cause a response. This response can occur anyplace in the body but is most easily recognized in the sense organs. For example, sound waves are received by the ears; light rays are received by the eyes; the nose and tongue respond to smell and taste; and the nerve endings throughout the body respond to pressure, heat, cold, pain, and touch.

The following are the sensory organs of the body.

The Eye

The eye provides vision (Figure 8.27). It is a ball-shaped organ located in the eye orbit of the skull.

ganglia

Mass of nerve tissue composed of nerve cell bodies. Ganglia lie outside the brain and spinal cord.

neuron

Nerve; includes the cell and the long fiber coming from the cell.

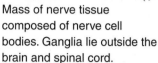
Figure 8.27

Cross section of the eye and external eye.

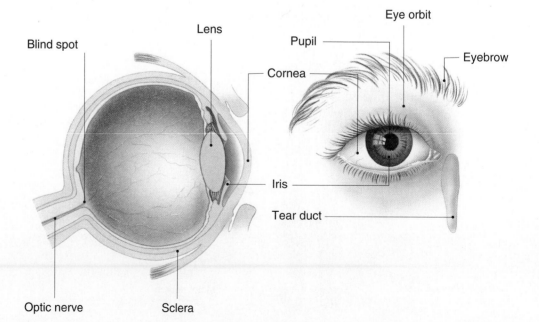

Protection for the Eye

- The lids and eyelashes aid in protecting the eye.
- Tears from the lacrimal **duct** help wash away foreign matter.

Coats of the Eye

- The *sclera*, or the white of the eye, is the outer lining. The front portion of the sclera is clear and is called the *cornea*.
- The *choroid*, the second coating, is heavily **pigmented** to keep light rays from **scattering.**
- The *retina*, the innermost coating of the eye, houses the mechanisms that sense vision.
- The *optic nerve*, located at the back of the eye, receives a picture and sends it to the brain for interpretation.

The Ear

The ear provides hearing and **equilibrium** (Figure 8.28). The ear can be divided into three main parts:

- The *external ear* includes the following:

  • *Auricle*, or outside projection • *External auditory canal* • *Tympanic membrane* or eardrum, which separates the external and middle ear

duct
Narrow, round tube that carries secretions from a gland.

pigmented
Colored; relating to various parts of the body (e.g., iris of the eye, lips, moles, freckles).

scattering
Spreading in many directions, dispersing.

equilibrium
State of balance.

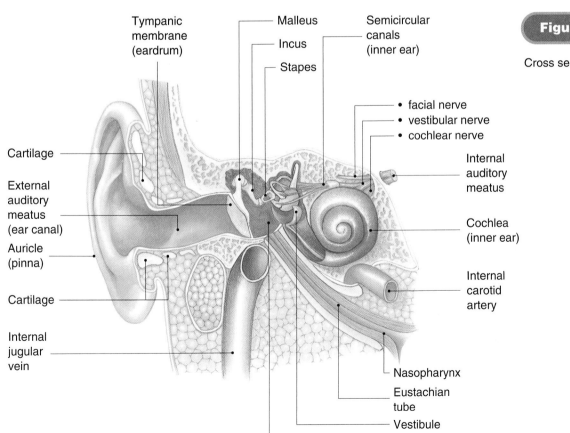

Figure 8.28

Cross section of the ear.

Tympanic membrane (eardrum)
Malleus
Incus
Stapes
Semicircular canals (inner ear)
• facial nerve
• vestibular nerve
• cochlear nerve
Internal auditory meatus
Cochlea (inner ear)
Internal carotid artery
Cartilage
External auditory meatus (ear canal)
Auricle (pinna)
Cartilage
Internal jugular vein
Cavity of middle ear
Nasopharynx
Eustachian tube
Vestibule

ossicles

Three small bones in the middle ear: incus, stapes, and malleus.

amplify

To increase or elevate a sound (e.g., the ossicles of the ear amplify sound waves).

translate

To make understandable.

receptors

Nerves that respond to stimuli.

- The *middle ear* is an air space that contains three bones or **ossicles.** These bones **amplify** sound waves received by the tympanic membrane.
- The *inner ear* contains the semicircular canals, which transmit sound waves received from the middle ear to the nerves that allow us to **translate** sound.

Organs of Taste and Smell

Sense of Taste

Taste is sensed by **receptors** in the tongue called *taste buds.* The taste buds sense four main tastes:

- Sweet
- Sour
- Salty
- Bitter

Sense of Smell

Receptors that receive smells are located high in the upper part of the nasal cavity called the *olfactory epithelium.* The *olfactory nerve* sends the smell to the brain for interpretation.

General Senses

General senses are found throughout the body. These general senses are different from the special senses of sight, hearing, taste, and smell; they are not limited to specific areas of the body (Figure 8.29).

Pressure Sense

subcutaneous

Beneath the skin.

Pressure is sensed by the pressure receptors in the **subcutaneous** tissue layer beneath the skin.

Temperature Sense

Heat and cold are sensed by receptors that respond only to heat or cold and send messages through nerves to the brain.

Sense of Touch

Touch is sensed by receptors called *tactile corpuscles.* These receptors are found in the dermis layer of skin. They are very close together in the fingertips and the toes and also in the tip of the tongue.

Figure 8.29

General senses: heat, cold, touch, pressure, pain.

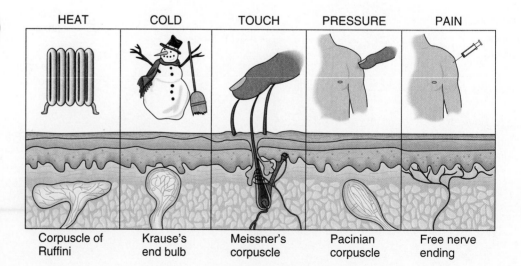

HEAT — COLD — TOUCH — PRESSURE — PAIN

Corpuscle of Ruffini — Krause's end bulb — Meissner's corpuscle — Pacinian corpuscle — Free nerve ending

Sense of Pain

Pain is the most important protective sense because it tells us that something is wrong in the body. Pain receptors are found in the

■ Skin   ■ Muscles   ■ Joints   ■ Internal organs

These receptors are nerve fibers that send messages of pain to the brain when parts of the body are injured.

⚪ COMMON DISORDERS OF THE NERVOUS SYSTEM

Table 8.14 ■ Common Disorders, Symptoms, and Preventive Measures/Treatment of the Nervous System

Condition	Disorder	Symptoms	Preventive Measures/Treatment
Cataract	Formation occurs when the lens of the eye loses its transparency. Light is less able to reach the inner eye. Cataracts are the most common cause of blindness and a very common ailment in the geriatric patient.	At first vision is blurred, then distortion and double vision may develop. If not treated, blindness can occur.	For cataracts that have developed through the aging process, treating with removal of the lens and then prescribing contacts or glasses.
Conjunctivitis	Inflammation of the eyelid lining caused from bacteria or irritation from dirt in the eye.	Red eyes, thick discharge, sticky eyelids in the morning, usually occurring without pain.	Wearing goggles to protect eyes from dirt and debris when possible. For example, when mowing the lawn, sawing wood, etc. Treatment for infected eyes is usually with antibiotics.
Glaucoma	Occurs when there is high pressure within the eye, causing the optic nerve to deteriorate. Glaucoma appears frequently as a person ages.	*Acute glaucoma*—extreme pain, blurred vision, a red eye and dilated pupil. Nausea and vomiting may also occur. *Chronic glaucoma*—there may be no symptoms except a gradual loss of peripheral vision over time and perhaps a dull pain.	Treating with eye drops; surgery may also be helpful.
Neuritis	Inflammation of a nerve caused by injury, malnutrition, alcoholism, or toxic poison.	Pain, numbness, muscle atrophy, change in reflexes.	Eliminating the cause of irritation if possible. Treatment may consist of pain medication, nerve block procedure, and physical therapy to maintain muscle.
Otosclerosis	Hereditary condition in which the bones in the ear change and sounds are not transmitted properly.	Tinnitus (ringing in the ear), then loss of hearing.	No known prevention; treating surgically may be helpful.
Shingles or herpes zoster	Caused by a virus that can affect any sensory nerve but tends to invade nerves in the chest and head near the temple most often.	Many blisters appear on the skin over nerve routes and cause a great deal of pain. The blisters usually disappear in about a week, but the pain may recur for years afterward.	Treating with soothing creams to relieve itching, topical medications, and pain medications when necessary.

MEDICAL TERMINOLOGY

■	audiometer	instrument to measure hearing	■	iridoplegia	paralysis of the iris of the eye
■	blepharitis	inflammation of the eyelid	■	lacrimal	pertaining to tear ducts
■	blepharorrhaphy	suturing the eyelid	■	ophthalmologist	specialist in the study of the eye
■	cerebrocular	pertaining to the brain and eyes	■	otitismedia	inflammation of the middle ear
■	dacryadenitis	inflammation of a tear duct	■	otoneurology	study of the ear and neural disorders
■	gustation	sense of taste	■	otoplasty	plastic repair of cartilage of the ear
■	iridocele	hernia of the iris of the eye	■	otorrhea	purulent discharge from the ear

● JOBS AND PROFESSIONS

- ■ Neurologist
- ■ Ophthalmologist
- ■ Otologist
- ■ Otorhinolaryngologist

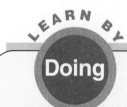

Doing   **UNIT 10 ACTIVITY**

1. **Complete Worksheets 2 through 6.**
2. **When you are confident that you can meet each objective for this unit, ask your instructor for the unit evaluation.**

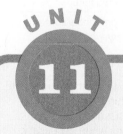

The Reproductive System

STEPS TO SUCCESS

1. Complete Vocabulary Worksheet 1 in the Student Workbook.

2. Read this unit.

3. Complete the Learn by Doing assignment at the end of this unit.

INTRODUCTION TO THE REPRODUCTIVE SYSTEM

Reproduction occurs in all species. Tiny one-celled organisms divide or separate by themselves to reproduce. Most animals require a male and female, each with their own special cells that unite to reproduce. The male and female reproductive systems have several characteristics in common. They are gonads, tubes that carry secretions, and exocrine glands.

- *Gonads* (endocrine glands) or sex glands in the male are called *testes*, and they produce sperm. In the female they are called *ovaries*, and they produce ova.
- The *tubes* form passageways for the **sex cells**, sperm and ova.
- *Exocrine glands* aid in the reproductive process.

The Female Reproductive System

The main function of the female reproductive system is to produce the ovum for fertilization and to house a developing **fetus.** Reproduction occurs when the male and female sex cells unite within the female. After the union of these cells, they grow for 9 months or 40 weeks and develop into a new individual. Look at Figure 8.30 to identify parts of the female reproductive system.

- *Female gonads*, the ovaries, are small oval-shaped structures that produce the female sex cells or *ova* and the hormone called **estrogen.** Approximately every 28 days an ovum **matures** and is forced from the ovary and received by the fallopian tube.
- *Fallopian tubes* are muscular tubes about 5 inches long. The tubes do not connect to the ovaries. When the **ovum** is forced from the ovary into the peritoneal cavity, it floats in the peritoneal fluid. At the end of each fallopian tube, finger-like projections called fimbriae create a current that sweeps the ovum into the tube. Once inside the tube, the ovum is swept forward by small cilia and by peristalsis. The ovum takes about 5 days to move through the fallopian tube and is then deposited into the uterus.
- The *uterus*, a pear-shaped organ, is attached to the fallopian tubes. While the ovum is maturing, the uterus begins to build an interlining called the **endometrium.** If the ovum is not fertilized in the fallopian tube, it deteriorates shortly after entering the uterus. The endometrium then deteriorates, causing bleeding or **menstruation.** The main function of the uterus is to house and nourish the fertilized ovum until delivery of a fully developed fetus.

sex cells
Cells that allow reproduction to occur.

fetus
Infant developing in the uterus after the first 3 months until birth.

estrogen
Female hormone.

matures
Becomes fully developed.

ovum
Female reproductive cell that when fertilized by the male develops into a new organism.

endometrium
Interlining of the uterus.

menstruation
Cyclic deterioration of the endometrium.

Figure 8.30

Cross section of the female reproductive system.

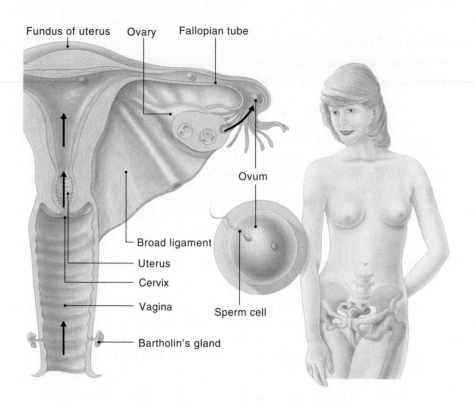

The *vagina* is a muscular tube that houses the neck of the uterus or *cervix.* This tube extends approximately 3 inches to the outside of the body. The vagina is known as the birth canal.

The Male Reproductive System

- *Male gonads* or *testes* are found outside the body, between the legs, in a sac called the *scrotum.* The testes produce the male sex cell or **spermatozoa** (or *sperm*) and the hormone **testosterone.** The *penis* is the primary male sex organ. It lies anterior to the testes (Figure 8.31).

- The *epididymis* is a 20-foot-long tube that is coiled inside the scrotal sac. Sperm are stored here until they mature and are able to move by themselves. As the epididymis extends upward, it becomes the vas deferens.

- The *vas deferens,* the spermatic cord, extends through the abdominal wall and curves over and behind the urinary bladder. It functions as a passageway for sperm.

- *Seminal vesicles* are outpouchings at the end of the vas deferens. They produce a thick yellow secretion that adds to the volume of **semen** and nourishes the sperm.

- The *prostate gland,* located just below the urinary bladder, produces a secretion that maintains mobility of sperm. The *ejaculatory duct* carries sperm from the junction of the vas deferens and the seminal vesicles through the prostate gland and connects to the urethra.

- The *urethra* is a small passage for urine and sperm, and leads from the urinary bladder through the prostate gland and the penis to the outside of the body.

spermatozoa

Male sex cells.

testosterone

Male hormone.

semen

Fluid from the testes, seminal vesicles, prostate gland, and bulbourethral glands. Contains water, mucin, proteins, salts, and sperm.

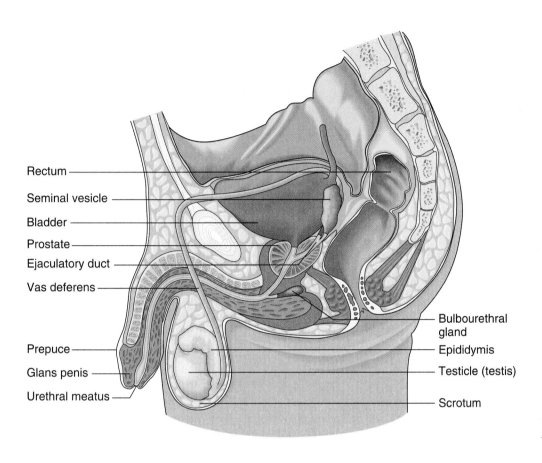

Figure 8.31

Cross section of the male reproductive system.

Rectum

Seminal vesicle

Bladder

Prostate

Ejaculatory duct

Vas deferens

Prepuce

Glans penis

Urethral meatus

Bulbourethral gland

Epididymis

Testicle (testis)

Scrotum

COMMON DISORDERS OF THE REPRODUCTIVE SYSTEM

Table 8.15 ■ Common Disorders, Symptoms, and Preventive Measures/Treatment of the Reproductive System

Condition	Disorder	Symptoms	Preventive Measures/ Treatment
Cryptorchidism	Means "hidden testes." Also called undescended testes.	One or both testes fail to descend into the scrotum.	Administering hormone injections if the testicle does not descend into the scrotum by the age of 1 year. If this treatment is unsuccessful by the age of 5 years, surgery is performed to locate the testicle and place it in the scrotum or remove it.
Fibroid tumors	Common in women over the age of 50. They are usually benign.	There may be breakthrough bleeding between menstrual cycles and pressure from the tumor may cause frequent urination. There are often no symptoms.	Physician will monitor size and growth and determine if surgical removal is necessary.

Table 8.15 ■ Continued

Condition	Disorder	Symptoms	Preventive Measures/ Treatment
Sexually transmitted diseases (STDs)	Affect both male and female. The most common sexually transmitted diseases are:	Symptoms vary as noted below:	For prevention, insisting on sterile needles when receiving medication and maintaining **monogamous** relationships with uninfected partners. Some treatment options are listed below:
–Acquired immune deficiency syndrome (AIDS)	• Acquired immune deficiency syndrome (AIDS) is most commonly transmitted by sexual contact or contaminated needles. It is a contagious disease that causes severe illness and often results in death. The AIDS virus enters the blood of a person from the blood or body fluids of a carrier.	• Symptoms include swollen lymph glands, diarrhea, abnormal or unusual bleeding, fungal infection of the mouth and throat, loss of memory, fatigue, extreme weight loss, and constant cough. All or some of these symptoms may be present.	• Although research is making great strides toward finding a cure, there is no successful treatment that cures AIDS. There are some medications and lifestyle changes that help individuals maintain a fairly healthy state for long periods.
–Chlamydia	• A contagious microorganism that lives in the conjunctiva of the eye and in the urethra and cervix of the uterus.	• Purulent discharge from the urethra in the male or the vagina in the female.	• Treating with antibiotics.
–Gonorrhea	• A contagious organism that affects the genitourinary tract and occasionally the pharynx, conjunctiva, or rectum.	Urethritis, dysuria, purulent greenish-yellow urethral or vaginal discharge, red or swollen urethral meatus, itching, burning, or pain around the vaginal or urethral opening.	• Treating with antibiotics.
–Syphilis	• Caused by a spirochete transmitted through sexual contact. It can affect any organ or system of the body. The spirochete is able to pass through the human placenta causing congenital syphilis in a newborn infant.	*First stage*—small, painless red pustule on the skin or mucous membrane (is contagious). *Second stage*—approximately 2 months later, generalized malaise, anorexia, nausea, fever, headache, loss of hair, bone and joint pain, skin rash that does not itch, sores in the mouth (remains contagious). *Third stage*—may not develop for many years. Appearance of soft, rubbery tumors that may cause a deep burrowing pain. Tumors may appear in any organ or system in the body.	• Treating with antibiotics.

monogamous   Having a sexual relationship with only one partner during a period of time.

MEDICAL TERMINOLOGY

■ amenorrhea	scant or no menstruation	■ mastalgia	pain in the breast
■ cervicitis	inflammation of the cervix	■ menorrhagia	excessive menstrual flow
■ colpectasis	dilation of the vagina	■ metrorrhexis	rupture of the uterus
■ colpoplasty	plastic surgery on the vagina	■ oophorocystectomy	removal of an ovarian cyst
■ dysmenorrhea	painful or difficult menstruation	■ orchiopexy	fixation of the testes in the scrotum
■ ectopic pregnancy	pregnancy outside the uterus	■ orchioplasty	plastic surgery of the testes
■ gonorrhea	flow from the genitals caused by infection	■ orchitis	inflammation of the testes
■ gynecomastia	abnormal enlargement of one or both breasts in men	■ phimosis	refers to a tightness of the foreskin over the end of the penis.
■ hysterectomy	removal of uterus	■ prenatal	occurring before birth
■ hystersalpingo-oophorectomy	removal of the uterus, fallopian tubes, and ovaries	■ postnatal	occurring after birth
■ insemination	injection of semen into the female reproductive system	■ sterile	unable to produce young
■ lactation	secretion of milk from the breast	■ tubal ligation	procedure in which fallopian tubes are blocked
■ leukorrhea	whitish vaginal discharge	■ vasectomy	procedure for male sterilization
■ mammectomy	surgical removal of breast tissue		

○ JOBS AND PROFESSIONS

- ■ Embryologist
- ■ Gynecologist
- ■ Midwife
- ■ Obstetrician

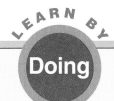

LEARN BY
Doing

UNIT 11 ACTIVITY

1. **Complete Worksheets 2 through 5.**
2. **When you are confident that you can meet each objective for this unit, ask your instructor for the unit evaluation.**

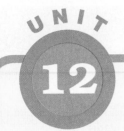

The Integumentary System

STEPS TO SUCCESS

1. Read this unit.

2. Complete the Learn by Doing assignment at the end of this unit.

UNIT OBJECTIVES

When you have completed this unit, you will be able to do the following:

✔ Match vocabulary words with their correct meanings.

✔ Label a diagram of a cross section of skin.

✔ List the five main functions of skin.

✔ Identify three main layers of the skin.

✔ Match common disorders of the integumentary system with their descriptions.

✔ Describe how the integumentary system protects the body.

✔ Explain why the health care worker's understanding of the integumentary system is important.

◯ INTRODUCTION TO THE INTEGUMENTARY SYSTEM

The skin is the body's largest organ and is the body's first line of defense against infection. It contains several kinds of tissue, including epithelial, connective, and nerve tissues. It also contains sweat and oil glands. The combination of these tissues and glands works together as the integumentary system (Figure 8.32). The main functions of the skin are to

■ Protect the underlying body parts from injury and the invasion of pathogens

■ Regulate body temperature by controlling the loss of body heat

■ Eliminate wastes through perspiration

■ Store energy in the form of fat and vitamins

■ Sense touch, heat, cold, pain, and pressure through receptors

Structure of the Skin

Skin is made up of three main layers of tissue.

epidermis

Outer layer of skin.

sloughed

Discarded; separated from (e.g., to shed dead cells, as from the outer skin).

■ The **epidermis** is the outermost layer and has no blood vessels. These cells are constantly **sloughed** off.

■ The *dermis* is just beneath the epidermis and contains many blood vessels. New cells are continually forming to replace those lost from the epidermis.

■ *Subcutaneous* means "under the skin," and this layer connects the skin to muscle.

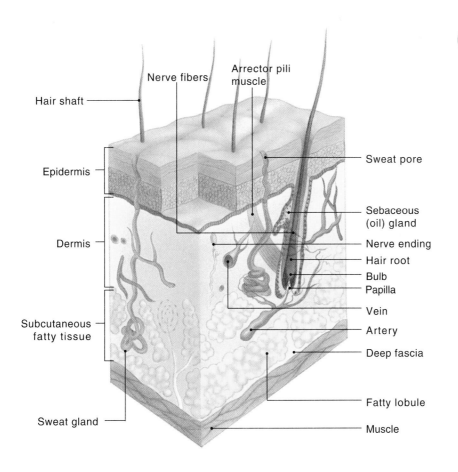

Figure 8.32

Cross section of the
integumentary system (skin).

COMMON DISORDERS OF THE INTEGUMENTARY SYSTEM

Table 8.16 ■ **Common Disorders, Symptoms, and Preventive Measures/Treatment of the Integumentary System**

Condition	Disorder	Symptoms	Preventive Measures/Treatment
Athlete's foot (tinea pedis)	Caused by a fungus. It usually involves the toes and the soles of the feet but is occasionally found on the hands.	Itching, scaling, and sometimes painful lesions.	For prevention, wearing shoes that do not constrict feet and allow good air circulation. Dry feet well after bathing and lightly apply powder between toes. Treating with medication may also be effective.
Atopic dermatitis or Eczema	Reddened areas on the surface of the skin.	• Early stage—areas on the skin may be red, swollen, and weeping purulent fluid. • Later stage is usually reddened, scaly, itchy areas on the skin.	Avoiding allergens. Topical applications and medication may be helpful as a treatment.
Boils (furuncle)	Skin abscess caused when bacteria enters the hair follicles or sebaceous glands.	Pain, redness, and swelling.	To prevent spreading of infection, it is important to avoid irritating or squeezing the lesion. Treatment may include antibiotics and local moist heat. Incision and drainage may be necessary.

Table 8.16 ■ Continued

Condition	Disorder	Symptoms	Preventive Measures/Treatment
Skin cancer	Rapid growth of cells on the skin that can invade blood vessels, lymph glands, and connecting ducts.	• Raised, hard, reddish lesions with a pearly surface. • Slightly elevated cells, tumors that may become sores that don't heal.	For prevention, applying sunscreen and avoiding excessive exposure to the sun. Skin cancers can be cured if treated early. Treatment may include medicated cream, localized laser treatments and radiation. If skin cancer is left untreated, it may cause death.

MEDICAL TERMINOLOGY

■ acne	inflammation of the sebaceous gland	■ keratoderma	scaly skin
■ alopecia	baldness	■ keratogenesis	formation of scaly skin
■ ceraceous	waxlike in appearance	■ pustule	elevation of skin filled with pus
■ ceroma	tumor of waxy appearance	■ scleroderma	hardened, thickened skin
■ debridement	removal of dead tissue	■ sebaceous	pertaining to oily, fatty matter from the sebaceous gland
■ dermatitis	inflammation of the skin	■ sebolith	stone in a sebaceous gland
■ desquamation	shedding skin in scales, sheets	■ seborrhea	excessive discharge of sebum
■ erythema	redness of the skin	■ squamous	platelike, scaly
■ keloid	excessive scarring, resembling a tumor	■ urticaria	itching wheals on the derma, hives

◉ JOBS AND PROFESSIONS

■ Dermatologist

◉ SUMMARY

You have learned that the cell is the building block of the body. Cells form tissues, which form organs. The organs of the body form the systems. All of these components must work together to keep the body in homeostasis (balance). You have also learned about some of the disorders that affect the body. This knowledge helps you take better care of your health and better care of your patients.

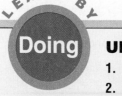

UNIT 12 ACTIVITY

1. Complete Worksheets 1 and 2.
2. When you are confident that you can meet each objective for this unit, ask your instructor for the unit evaluation.

Thinking Critically

1. **Communication** Explain how you think that your understanding of the body systems helps you communicate with patients/clients and co-workers. Your patient/client asks you to explain how the muscles in her upper arm cause the forearm to move. Write how you can communicate this information to a child under 6, an adult over 80, and a teenager.

2. **Medical Terminology** Ms. Wilson looks confused after her doctor has confirmed and explained her diagnosis of diabetes. You know from talking with her family that they usually call diabetes "sugar." How could you help Ms. Wilson better understand her condition? Brainstorm with classmates to think of other words people use for medical conditions or bodily functions that could cause confusion.

3. **Legal and Ethical** A patient's doctor just told him that he has a serious problem in the gastrointestinal system. The doctor thinks that it is probably a malignant tumor. The patient asks you what you know about his condition. What is your responsibility in this case?

4. **Computers** Computers offer many opportunities for learning and for accessing information. They are also used to diagnose disorders of the various body systems. Identify as many computerized tests as you can. Create a list by writing the full name of each test and the name of the computerized equipment used to perform the test.

5. **Patient Satisfaction** As a health care worker your alertness to symptoms and complications associated with the body systems is important for the well-being of your patients. Select and research a chronic disease and write an explanation of potential symptoms and complications.

6. **Patient Education** Many patients have little knowledge of anatomy and may know few correct terms for body parts. Work with classmates to research policy in area facilities on allowing staff to provide patients with illustrated brochures or illustrations taken from the Internet.

Portfolio Connection

Employers look for health care workers who have knowledge of the body and body systems. Assistive personnel work in many different departments and must be able to recognize problems and report them correctly to a supervisor. Complete the following exercise and put it in your portfolio for review in the future: Identify one body system disorder. Research the objective and subjective symptoms that result from this disorder. Explain your findings in a typed or neatly written paper.

Portfolio Tip

Keep in mind that many cultures find it offensive to directly mention body parts: you may need to prompt your patients/clients as to where they feel discomfort.

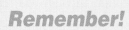 **Remember!** **Media Connection**

Use the Companion Website **www.prenhall.com/badasch** and the CD-ROM for additional interactive learning activities.

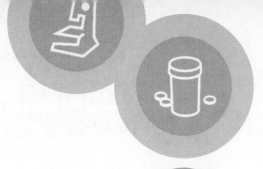

Chapter 9

Human Growth and Development

MEDIA CONNECTION
Use the Companion Website **www.prenhall.com/badasch** and the CD-ROM for additional interactive learning activities.

UNIT 1

Development and Behavior

STEPS TO SUCCESS

1. Complete Vocabulary Worksheet 1 in the Student Workbook.
2. Read this unit.
3. Complete the Learn by Doing assignment at the end of this unit.

UNIT OBJECTIVES

When you have completed this unit, you will be able to do the following:

✔ Match vocabulary words with their correct meanings.

✔ Identify three stages of development between conception and birth.

✔ List four common developments of growth in the first year of life and the age at which they usually occur.

✔ Define and describe characteristics of adolescent development.

UNIT RATIONALE

Health care workers provide care for all age groups. It is important to understand the emotional and physical stages of the life continuum. This knowledge assists you in recognizing normal and abnormal development and behavior. This awareness of life's stages allows you to be an effective health care worker.

✔ Interview a person between the ages of 50 and 80.

✔ Compare your life experiences to each stage described in this chapter.

✔ Design a bulletin board representing one stage of growth and development, including age-specific communication requirements.

---

continuum

Progression from start (birth) to finish (death).

zygote

Any cell formed by the coming together of two reproductive (sex) cells.

⬤ DEVELOPMENT AND BEHAVIOR

People experience many physical and emotional changes over a lifetime. These changes are part of the normal growth and development process. In this unit, we discuss the stages of development and behavior from conception through the life **continuum**.

Conception or fertilization occurs when a male sperm and a female ovum combine. This combination causes the single-cell ovum to divide into many cells. This stage of development is called a **zygote.** Within five weeks, the rapidly multiplying cells duplicate into an embryo.

■ Five weeks after conception, the embryo is about the size of a grain of rice.

■ Six weeks after conception, the nervous system, eyes, and ears are visible.

Fetal and Infant Stage

At 12 weeks or 3 months after conception, the embryo has grown to about 2½ inches (6 cm) long. It is now called a fetus. Babies are born 38 to 40 weeks after conception. See Table 9.1 for stages of average development, behavior, and age-specific communication techniques.

Table 9.1 ■ Infant Through Early Elementary School Age Stages of Average Development, Behavior, and Age-Specific Communication Techniques

Age	Behavior	Age-Specific Communication Techniques	Effective Communication Techniques During Medical Care
6 Weeks	Baby first begins to smile.	Hold, cuddle, and softly speak frequently to infant.	When possible hold, cuddle, and softly speak frequently to infant.
10 weeks	Infant has the ability to roll from a **prone** to a **supine** position.	Hold, cuddle, and softly speak frequently to infant.	Comfort infants by speaking in a soothing tone and touch them gently to communicate your presence and reassurance.
4 to 6 months	Infant raises head and shoulders while in a supine position.	Talking to infants helps them recognize sounds and make associations. It is helpful to talk slowly and clearly when holding, feeding, or bathing infants at this age. Sudden, strange noise may cause fear.	Comfort infants by speaking in a soothing tone and touch them gently to communicate your presence and reassurance.
6 to 8 months	Infant sits without being supported; when placed on abdomen infant may scoot before mastering a crawl; eye color may change.	Distract or move infants when they are headed for trouble.	When possible perform procedures quickly and efficiently to minimize time the infant is exposed to discomfort. Following procedures that cause discomfort or emotional tension take time to comfort infants by speaking in a soothing tone and touch them gently to communicate your presence and reassurance. Allow mom or other family members to be present when possible.
8 to 12 months	Attempts to feed self and begins to crawl, stand, and take steps. As infant becomes toddler, expect frequent falls while learning to walk. Provide a safe environment free of sharp edges and, if possible, keep infant on carpeting instead of cement or tile flooring.	Use simple terms to warn them as they head toward trouble: "Hot!", "Hurt," or "Tastes bad." Always praise good behavior.	When possible perform procedures quickly and efficiently to minimize time the infant is exposed to discomfort. Following procedures that cause discomfort or emotional tension take time to comfort infants by speaking in a soothing tone and touch them gently to communicate your presence and reassurance. Allow mom or other family members to be present when possible.

prone　　Lying on the stomach.　　🔊　　　　**supine**　　Lying on the back.　　🔊

Table 9.1 ▪ Continued

Age	Behavior	Age-Specific Communication Techniques	Effective Communication Techniques During Medical Care
1 year	Learning and experimenting absorbs most of infant's waking hours. Understands simple conversation or commands. Most toddlers at this age can say four or five words clearly.	Speak clearly and slowly, using simple words. Children who are spoken to with clear word pronunciation (not baby talk) develop clearer speech. Resist saying "No," constantly and be patient.	Speak in a calming voice tone. Allow mom or family to be available when possible.
18 months	Walks alone, feeds itself, and stacks objects. "Mine" becomes a favorite expression.	Communicate clear limits about acceptable and unacceptable behavior. Reinforce good behavior. Playing easy games and reading simple stories help develop vocabulary. Time spent in this way provides opportunity to share in positive, nurturing experiences.	*The following is appropriate for children 18 months through 8 years of age.* Refer to the child by his or her favorite name (name, nickname, or special term the family uses). Use the same words the family uses for toileting. Do not blame or scold if toileting accidents occur. Explain in simple terms what is happening to and around the child. Answer their questions honestly and in terms the child will understand. When possible spend time with the child, talking and playing simple games appropriate to their age. Taking time to communicate and enjoy activities with each child is important in creating a positive sense of well-being during medical care. When possible perform procedures quickly and efficiently to minimize time the child is exposed to discomfort. Following procedures that cause discomfort or emotional tension take time to comfort infants by speaking in a soothing tone and touch them gently to communicate your presence and reassurance.
20 to 24 months.	Begins bowel and bladder control. Experiences exploration and a feeling of security. Vocabulary increases rapidly at this age. Pronunciation may take time to develop.	Your patience allows normal speech development to occur. Resist trying to correct pronunciation too frequently. Listen carefully and confirm your understanding of the child's words.	
3 to 4 years	Talks in simple, complete sentences. Experiences a span of emotional growth.	Continue following techniques described above.	
4 to 5 years	Dresses and undresses with little assistance. Experiences a span of emotional growth.	*The following is appropriate for children 4 through 8 years of age.* Children at these ages require frequent reassurance and truthful, caring conversation. Keep discussions short and easy to understand, allowing time for the children to say everything they want to say. Positive acceptance of what the child says is important, and positive reflection back to them helps the child overcome shyness and withdrawal.	
5 to 6 years	Eye and body **coordination** improves. The child is able to hop, skip, and draw figures. Awareness of the ability to choose one action over another is present. Child begins to feel guilt and shame.		**coordination** 🔊 State of harmonized action, such as eye and hand coordination.
6 to 8 years	Physical skills continue to improve. Children start school. They begin to look for reasons that explain why they believe certain things. They also compare themselves with others. At about age 7, they experience emotional withdrawal or shyness.		

Preteen Years or Preadolescent Years

Table 9.2 ■ Preteen Years Through Young Adult Stages of Development, Behavior, and Age-Specific Communication Techniques			
Age	Behavior	Age-Specific Communication Techniques	Effective Communication Techniques During Medical Care
9 to 12 years (preteen or preadolescent years)	Physical growth rate increases, and adult sexual characteristics become noticeable. Girls begin menstruation. Boys develop more hair on their faces and bodies, and voices deepen. Preteens look to their friends for acceptance and approval rather than to their parents. Children ages 8 to 12 experience emotional security; 13-year-olds feel insecure and shy.	Children 9 to 12 years old do best when you listen to them and give them a chance to express themselves. Use positive responses to indicate that you hear what they are saying. It is also important to explain clearly the differences between acceptable and unacceptable behavior. Acknowledge positive actions and discuss why other behaviors are not appropriate. Thirteen-year-olds often require increased words of reassurance and encouragement to overcome feelings of insecurity, shyness and fear.	When appropriate and possible, prior to a medical procedure offer to show them what will be done during procedures. Tell children what to expect concerning how they will physically feel and what they will see and hear. Reassure them by explaining how to get assistance if needed. Explain the importance of asking questions when they are unsure about the way they feel, or what they see or hear.
13 to 18 years (adolescent or teenage years)	The teenage years are the years between childhood and adulthood. Teenagers strive for independence. They also experience puberty, a dramatic sexual development caused by increased hormone production of certain glands. (Girls may start puberty by 11 years; boys usually start at 13 years.) Puberty is a time of both physical and emotional adjustment.	*The following is appropriate for 13 through 20 years of age.* **Adolescents** need others to listen and reflect their words back to them. This type of communication allows teenagers to hear what they are thinking and gain increased understanding of themselves. Respect their privacy. Question personal behavior and habits only when it is pertinent to their health and well-being.	*The following is appropriate for 13 through 20 years of age.* When appropriate and possible, prior to a medical procedure offer to show them what will be done during procedures. Tell teenagers what to expect concerning how they will physically feel and what they will see and hear. Reassure them by explaining how to get assistance if needed.
18 to 20 years (young adulthood)	People become more independent. As they mature, they begin to seek ways of contributing to society.		

adolescent   Pertaining to the period of life between childhood and maturity.

Adulthood

Table 9.3 ■ Adulthood Ages 20 Through 70+ Years Stages of Development, Behavior, and Age-Specific Communication Techniques

Age	Behavior	Communication Techniques With All Adults	Communication During Medical Care
20 to 30 years	This is the beginning of adulthood, when people attempt to build a firm, safe foundation for the future. There is a strong desire to do the right thing. Patterns of living are set during this **decade,** such as: helper patterns (rescuing others), leadership patterns (taking charge, organizing), passive patterns (acting without influence, not taking an active part in things). These are just a few patterns people may fall into; there are many others.	*The following is generally appropriate for ages 20 through the 60s.* Show positive interest in adults' conversation, and interpret and respond to their body language. Use words that are understandable and meaningful to each individual's level. Express your desire to protect privacy; resist questioning personal behaviors and habits unless they are pertinent to the person's health and well-being.	*The following is generally appropriate for ages 20 through the 60s.* Be aware of the impact medical care is having on each person. Be sensitive to fears; honestly explain procedures and expected outcomes. When speaking about a patient, always go to areas away from the patient's view and hearing. Your behavior must communicate respect for others—be aware of your body language and verbal tone. Thoughtfully communicate by being aware of, when words are helpful and when silence is preferred.
30 to 40 years	In this decade, people often feel confined by the guidelines that they established for themselves in their 20s. This confined feeling often leads to restructuring of work, family, and social habits. Through this change, people develop more freedom and a new view of self.		
40 to 50 years	People often evaluate the first part of their life. They make decisions about future directions. Many find themselves adjusting basic values and their emphasis toward life. This time of adjustment is often referred to as "midlife crisis" or the "deadline decade." Women develop assertiveness. Men become more tender and make stronger commitments to ethical issues.		
50 to 60 years	These are the years when people experience a sense of comfort, an acceptance of life, and a new warmth and mellowing. Privacy becomes important, and friends become more cherished. Truth and sincerity become more valued. Renewal of earlier hobbies and interests often sparks new energy and enthusiasm.		

decade   Period of 10 years.

Table 9.3 ▪ Continued

Age	Behavior	Communication Techniques With All Adults	Communication During Medical Care
60 to 70 years	These are the years in which people look forward to retirement. For some people there is a gradual change in their work lives. Others prefer full retirement. The additional hours away from work can now be filled with interests or hobbies. This newfound time often allows people to complete lifelong projects or desires. Sharing of oneself with others aids in maintaining a sense of self-worth.	*The following is appropriate for 60 and older.* Listening and sharing interest in stories and experiences is a way for younger people to learn and to show gratitude for the mentorship of people of this age. When with a hearing impaired person use communication techniques that help promote their understanding. For example: go to a quiet area or eliminate unnecessary sounds, always look at the person when talking and speak clearly.	*The following is appropriate for 60 and older.* When appropriate and possible, prior to a medical procedure offer to show them what will be done during procedures. Tell what to expect concerning how they will physically feel and what they will see and hear. Reassure them by explaining how to get assistance if needed. When possible and if the patient requests, allow a significant other to stay with them.
70 and older	After the 70s, people continue their daily life in the same adult patterns. The effect of aging on the body is discussed in Unit 2 of this chapter. If the body loses its resilience and functions become impaired, the individual's lifestyle may change. It is important to note that of the increasing geriatric population, only 5% require in-patient health care. The remaining 95% are **viable,** active seniors		

viable   Capable of living.

○ SUMMARY

In this unit, you have learned about development from conception throughout the life continuum. You have also become aware of emotional and behavioral experiences and communication issues related to each decade of life.

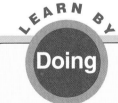

UNIT 1 ACTIVITY

1. Complete Worksheets 1 and 2.
2. Follow your instructor's directions to complete Worksheets/ Activities 3 through 6.
3. When you are confident that you can meet each objective, ask your instructor for the unit evaluation.

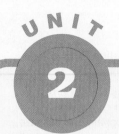

UNIT 2

Aging and Role Change

STEPS TO SUCCESS

1. Complete Vocabulary Worksheet 1 in the Student Workbook.

2. Read this unit.

3. Complete the Learn by Doing assignment at the end of this unit.

UNIT RATIONALE

The population of people over the age of 65 is expanding. Most people over 65 are active, and they adapt well to change. They continue to enjoy physical activities such as tennis, biking, and skiing. Only 5% are in long-term care. To care adequately for senior citizens with health problems, health care workers must be aware of the emotional and physical changes that occur during the aging process. Understanding these changes allows the health care worker to assist the aging person in adapting more easily to new roles and ability levels.

UNIT OBJECTIVES

When you have completed this unit, you will be able to do the following:

✔ Match vocabulary words with their correct meanings.

✔ Identify six body systems and the common physical changes that occur with aging.

✔ Identify basic human needs that are met through work, environment, socialization, and family relationships.

✔ Write an "action plan" to assist another person cope with changes caused by aging.

● PHYSICAL CHANGES OF AGING

The process of aging begins in every person at the moment of birth. Aging is a very natural process, and the health care worker needs to be aware of the physical changes that take place. Understanding these changes helps you be patient and less frustrated with others.

Nervous System

■ The *brain* experiences changes in a number of nerve cells and in the brain mass. Elderly people frequently suffer from arteriosclerosis, which causes a decrease in blood flow and oxygen to the brain. This often results in confusion, which is misunderstood and may be very annoying to the health care worker.

■ *Vision* begins to change with aging:

• Small print, small items, and things at a distance are more difficult to see.
• More light is needed to see things clearly. • Night driving may become difficult. • **Adaptation** to light is more difficult. The eyes take longer to adjust to changes from dark to light and from light to dark. • Diseases may occur:

• *Cataract:* clouding of the normally transparent lenses of the eye

• *Glaucoma:* intraocular pressure causes damage to the optic disks and hardening of the eyeball

■ *Hearing* changes become noticeable in the 60s:

• High-frequency sounds such as a telephone or doorbell may not be heard.
• Loss of understanding of consonants and vowel sounds may result in a person complaining that others mumble or speak too softly.

adaptation

Changing to work better.

◼ *Taste, smell,* and *touch* senses decline with age:

  • Elderly people may not smell gases, spoiled food, or body odor. • Taste buds decline 50%, and food enjoyment is reduced. • Elderly people may request extra salt and sugar because they cannot taste well. • Touch and **reflexes** change. The ability to respond to stimuli is decreased. Elderly people may burn themselves or hold an ice tray too long and damage tissue or take longer to respond to the directions you give.

reflexes
Result when a nerve is stimulated and an involuntary action occurs (e.g., touch a hot stove, and the muscles react involuntarily to move the fingers away).

Musculoskeletal System

◼ Osteoarthritis is an inflammation of the joints and causes pain and slowing down of movement.

◼ Osteoporosis is caused by a loss of calcium in the bone. This is found more in women after menopause, when the bones may become very brittle. They may fracture with very little stress.

◼ With reduced **stamina,** elderly people are often less active, which results in the muscles becoming smaller. They generally slow down, which may cause the health care worker to feel impatient.

stamina
Body's strength or energy.

Respiratory and Circulatory System

◼ The lungs become less elastic, and the **alveolar-capillary** membrane thickens. This makes oxygen exchange more difficult.

◼ The rib cage does not expand as much.

◼ The heart becomes less efficient, and the arteries may become narrowed and clogged. The systolic pressure may rise and result in high blood pressure.

◼ The heart also becomes a less efficient pump. Heart disease is the number one cause of death in older people. Among these diseases are

  • Congestive heart failure • Cardiac arrhythmias • Ischemic heart disease
  • Hypertensive heart disease

alveolar-capillary
Pertaining to air sacs in the lungs.

Gastrointestinal System

◼ Many elderly patients/clients experience **constipation.**

◼ Loss of teeth may interfere with chewing.

◼ The liver is important in metabolism. With age, the liver loses up to 20% of its weight. This is not serious, because the liver can be effective at 50% capacity. However, the liver becomes less effective in metabolizing drugs. Older people must be monitored carefully and be alert to drug side effects.

constipation
Infrequent or difficult emptying of the bowel.

Urinary System

◼ The bladder holds less urine as a person ages. This may cause an urgent and frequent need to urinate.

◼ Bladder infections may occur from **retention** of urine in the bladder. This results in urinary urgency and urinary discomfort.

Your awareness of these changes helps you be patient and understanding. These physical changes often cause frustration in your patient and in you. Remember that these changes occur because the body is aging. Listen and reflect understanding. Explain procedures in understandable terms.

retention
Keeping elements within the body that are normally eliminated (e.g., waste products such as urine and feces).

⬤ ROLE CHANGES IN PEOPLE WHO ARE AGING

Because aging persons are experiencing physical and emotional changes, they need understanding and patience. They want to continue as a part of society, and they need to feel human dignity.

All people have basic needs that are met through the roles they have throughout their life span.

- ■ **Work role.** The work a person does gives a sense of independence, security, and self-esteem. When occupational identity is lost through retirement or physical disability, these needs must be met in some other way.

- ■ **Family relationships.** Being a member of a family meets our needs for emotional warmth, intimacy, and identity. When members of the family begin to leave or die, the person may be left without a means of filling these basic needs. To adapt to these losses, people need help in directing their interests and energies in other areas. Some of these may include social activities, volunteer work, or membership in organizations.

- ■ **Social roles.** Social contacts fill a person's need for interaction with others. Through social contacts, the person feels respected and admired. As the years pass, friends move away or die, and personal relationships change. These losses may cause people to feel that they are no longer socially important. It is very important that the aging person take part in developing new social contacts. Senior centers, churches, and other organizations are available to help meet this need. Becoming involved helps fill the need for interaction with other human beings.

- ■ **Environment.** The home a person lives in is a place where he or she can be in control, where he or she has a feeling of belonging. As aging occurs, it may become necessary to change environments. The home may become a financial burden, or it may be physically impossible to remain there. The older person may move into his or her children's home, a nursing home, or a room of his or her own. This change may be very frightening, and the need for control in their environment is threatened.

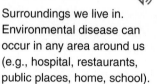

environment

Surroundings we live in. Environmental disease can occur in any area around us (e.g., hospital, restaurants, public places, home, school).

As a health care worker, your understanding of these changes helps you develop the necessary skills to work with older clients. Human beings have a great ability to adjust to changes in their life roles. Acceptance of their needs allows you to be patient and understanding as you care for them.

● SUMMARY

As people age, physical changes occur in the body. These changes affect many body systems. When these changes occur, older patients experience frustration with their conditions. The health care worker has an important role in helping the older patient understand and accept changes.

There are many role changes that occur in aging persons. They may no longer have the identity that their work gave them. They may lose a spouse or other important family members, leaving them lonely. Often, their social role changes as they are less involved in activities. They may find it difficult to develop new friendships. They may have to leave the home where they have their roots and move to a strange place. Awareness of these changes helps the health care worker work effectively with older patients.

LEARN BY Doing

UNIT 2 ACTIVITY

1. **Complete Worksheet 2 as assigned.**

2. **Complete Worksheets 3 through 5 as assigned.**

3. **When you are confident that you can meet each objective, ask your instructor for the unit evaluation.**

Disabilities and Role Changes

STEPS TO SUCCESS

1. Complete Vocabulary Worksheet 1 in the Student Workbook.
2. Read this unit.
3. Complete the Learn by Doing assignment at the end of this unit.

UNIT RATIONALE

Physical disabilities can affect any age group. When a disability, injury, or illness changes a person's lifestyle, he or she must adapt to these changes. This is often difficult and causes frustration and depression. As a health care worker, you need to understand these changes. When you understand such changes, you are more effective, and you can be a positive influence as these patients/clients begin to adapt.

UNIT OBJECTIVES

When you have completed this unit, you will be able to do the following:

✔ Match vocabulary words with their correct meanings.

✔ Define *health.*

✔ List three examples of activities of daily living (ADL).

✔ Define assistive/adaptive devices.

✔ Identify ways to encourage independence.

✔ List eight birth defects.

✔ List ten debilitating illnesses.

✔ Identify seven common changes that occur following the loss of body functions.

✔ State the goal of rehabilitation.

✔ Select a disability and summarize your feelings and expectations concerning

   ✔ What you think it would be like to live with that disability

   ✔ The type of care you would expect

   ✔ The way others respond to the disability

○ DEFINITION OF HEALTH

The World Health Organization defines health as "a state of complete physical, mental, and social well-being and not merely the absence of disease or infirmity." As a health care worker, you strive to help patients/clients reach their highest potential.

○ IMPORTANCE OF INDEPENDENCE

When a person is ill or injured, they often have limitations. These limitations usually affect their activities of daily living. The activities include

■ Bathing

■ Combing hair

■ Going to the bathroom

■ Dressing

■ Eating

■ Brushing teeth

■ Communicating effectively

adapt

To change, to become
suitable, to adjust.

Some patients/clients can do these activities with little or no help. Others need a lot of help to **adapt**. The goal is to allow each person to be as independent as he or she possibly can be. Always encourage a patient to try an activity. (For example, the person may be able to put toothpaste on the brush but needs your help to brush the teeth.) You can encourage the client by being patient and positive and by letting him or her make choices. This helps the patient/client feel more independent and increases feelings of well-being and self-respect. There are many assistive/adaptive devices available (Figure 9.1). Computers are effective assistive/adaptive devices for children and adults with physical disabilities. People who cannot hold a pencil or speak can use computers with special enhancements to communicate. Individualized computer programs are created to guide learning. Computers with e-mail and Internet capabilities provide opportunities for people with disabilities to interact with the outside world. The computer enables people with certain disabilities to communicate their needs, thoughts, desires, and intelligence to their parents and caregivers. These devices help the patient be more independent and self-sufficient. They help clients

- Eat
- Reach objects
- Complete personal care
- Dress and button clothing
- Communicate

⬤ PHYSICAL DISABILITIES

Physical disabilities may be caused by a birth defect, a debilitating illness, or an injury. Understanding these disabilities helps you give better care to your patients.

Birth Defect

syndrome

A number of symptoms
occurring together.

birth defects

Defects present at birth.

debilitating

Causing weakness or
impairment.

Babies who are born with a physical defect, inherited **syndrome,** or other problems have a **birth defect.** As a health care worker, you need to recognize these defects in order to give good care and be supportive to family members. Common birth defects are explained in Table 9.4.

Debilitating Illness

Debilitating illness may occur at any age. Depending on the severity of the disease, physical changes may be minimal or very extensive. Common debilitating illnesses are explained in Table 9.5.

Injury

coma

Deep sleep; unconscious
state for a long period of time.

amputation

Removal of a body part.

Injuries may occur at any age and cause many different disabilities. Some of the most common are

- Spinal cord injuries, which may cause paralysis
- Stroke, which may cause paralysis, brain dysfunction, speech impairments, and/or loss of memory
- Head injuries, which may cause **coma,** loss of memory, and/or paralysis
- **Amputation** of a limb

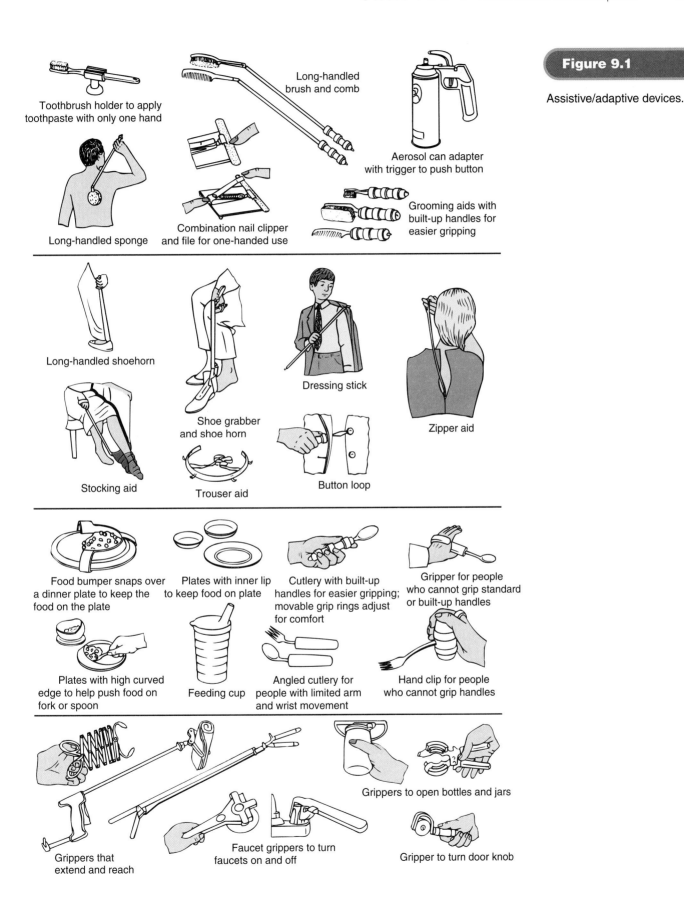

Figure 9.1

Assistive/adaptive devices.

Toothbrush holder to apply toothpaste with only one hand

Long-handled brush and comb

Long-handled sponge

Combination nail clipper and file for one-handed use

Aerosol can adapter with trigger to push button

Grooming aids with built-up handles for easier gripping

Long-handled shoehorn

Shoe grabber and shoe horn

Dressing stick

Zipper aid

Stocking aid

Trouser aid

Button loop

Food bumper snaps over a dinner plate to keep the food on the plate

Plates with inner lip to keep food on plate

Cutlery with built-up handles for easier gripping; movable grip rings adjust for comfort

Gripper for people who cannot grip standard or built-up handles

Plates with high curved edge to help push food on fork or spoon

Feeding cup

Angled cutlery for people with limited arm and wrist movement

Hand clip for people who cannot grip handles

Grippers that extend and reach

Faucet grippers to turn faucets on and off

Grippers to open bottles and jars

Gripper to turn door knob

Table 9.4 ▪ Birth Defects

Condition at Birth	Defect	Identifying Characteristics
Cerebral palsy	A motor function disorder that is caused by a brain defect or lesion present at birth or shortly after.	Spastic hemiplegia; seizures; some degree of mental retardation in some people; impaired vision, speech, and hearing; and stiff, awkward movements.
Cleft lip and/or cleft palate	Fusion of the palate and/or lip does not take place during **embryonic** development.	The cleft is often easily seen, but some display an inability to suck or nurse, crying when the child tries to nurse, with fluid coming out of the nose.
Down syndrome		Varying degrees of mental retardation and multiple defects; slanted eyes; depressed nasal bridge; low-set ears; large, protruding tongue; short, broad hands with a simian crease and stubby fingers; broad, stubby feet with wide spaces between the first and second toes; prone to respiratory infections, visual problems, and abnormalities in tooth development.
Epilepsy	**Neurological** disorders that may be birth defects but can occur later in life due to cerebral trauma, intracranial infection, brain tumor, **intoxication,** or chemical imbalance.	Recurrent **episodes** of convulsive seizures, sensory disturbances, abnormal behavior, loss of consciousness.
Hydrocephaly	Overproduction or underabsorption of cerebro-spinal fluid. May or may not cause increased pressure in the brain.	Globe-shaped head, flat nose bridge, eyes pushed downward and out, becoming widely spread; mild to severe retardation.
Sickle-cell anemia	A **hereditary** disease that is most common among African-American people. The red blood cell is crescent shaped (sickle shaped) and carries an abnormal **hemoglobin.**	Severe joint pain, thrombosis, fever, chronic anemia.
Spinal bifida cystica	A developmental defect. A **hernial** sac containing the **meninges,** spinal cord, or both protrudes at the end of the vertebral column. This sac is easily ruptured, causing the characteristics at the right.	Leakage of spinal fluid, risk of meningeal infection, severe neurological **dysfunction,** paralysis, muscle weakness, retardation.
Tay-Sachs syndrome	An inherited disease caused by an **enzyme deficiency.** It occurs primarily in families of Eastern European Jewish origin.	Difficult breathing and decreased exhange of oxygen and carbon dioxide.

embryonic   Pertaining to the embryo.

neurological   Pertaining to the nervous system.

intoxication   State of poisoning or becoming poisoned.

episodes   Events in a series.

hereditary   Passed from parent to child.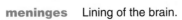

hemoglobin

An iron-containing protein in red blood cells that combines reversibly with oxygen and transports it from the lungs to body tissues.

hernial

Pertaining to projection through an abnormal opening in the wall of a body cavity.

meninges   Lining of the brain.

dysfunction   Impaired or abnormal functioning.

enzyme

Substance that causes a change to occur in other substances.

deficiency

Shortage (e.g., a deficient diet causes the body to function poorly because it is missing an important element).

Table 9.5 ■ Common Debilitating Illnesses		
Debilitating Illness	**Condition**	**Identifying Characteristics/Symptoms**
Acquired immune deficiency syndrome (AIDS)	Caused by a virus that reduces the immune system's ability to respond to **opportunistic infections.**	Common opportunistic infections that result from AIDS include pneumocystis pneumonia, candidiasis, cryptococcus, and herpes. Cancers that may develop are Kaposi's sarcoma and lymphomas.
Alzheimer's disease	A degenerative disorder that affects the brain generally in later, middle life.	Confusion, memory failure, **disorientation,** restlessness, speech disturbances, inability to carry out purposeful movements, and hallucinations.
Arteriosclerosis	Hardening of the arteries, which reduces the elasticity of the arterial walls.	Elevated blood pressure.
Atherosclerosis	**Lipid**-containing material collects on the inside surfaces of the blood vessels causing thickening of the vessel walls and narrowing of the space that blood flows through, thus inhibiting blood flow. Associated with obesity, hypertension, and diabetes.	Angina pectoris, myocardial infarction (MI), coronary heart disease.
Cancer	Uncontrolled growth of immature cells that invade normal tissue and travel to other tissues. More than 80% of cancers are caused by cigarette smoking, carcinogenic chemicals, radiation, and overexposure to the sun.	Signs of cancer vary, but it is wise to see a physician when the following occurs: change in bowel or bladder habits, a nonhealing sore, unusual bleeding or discharge, a thickening or lump anywhere, indigestion or trouble swallowing, an obvious change in a wart or mole, or a nagging cough or persistent hoarseness.
Cardiovascular disease	Any abnormal heart and/or circulatory condition. Cardiovascular disease remains a leading cause of death in the United States.	Dysfunction of the heart and blood vessels commonly causing angina, shortness of breath, weakness, and general fatigue.
Cystic fibrosis	Inherited disorder of the exocrine glands that causes an excessive amount of thick mucus. Most affected are the pancreas, respiratory system, and sweat glands.	Usually diagnosed during infancy or in young children of Caucasian origin. Chronic cough, frequent foul-smelling stools, and persistent upper respiratory infections.
Emphysema	The alveoli in the lungs are overextended and loose their elasticity. The lungs become less and less able to exchange oxygen and carbon dioxide.	Shortness of breath, cough, cyanosis, unequal chest expansion, rapid respiratory rate, elevated temperature. They may also experience, anxiety, restlessness, confusion, and weakness.
Leukemia	Rapid and abnormal growth of leukocytes in the blood-forming organs (bone marrow, spleen, and lymph nodes).	Males are affected twice as often as females. Symptoms include fatigue, pallor, weight loss, easy bruising, extreme weakness, bone or joint pain, repeated infections.

opportunistic infections

Infections that occur when the immune system is weakened. Common organisms that the body normally resists cause infection.

disorientation

State of being confused about time, place, and identity of persons and objects.

arteriosclerosis   Condition of hardening of the arteries.

lipid   Fat.

Table 9.5 ▪ Continued		
Debilitating Illness	**Condition**	**Identifying Characteristics/Symptoms**
Multiple sclerosis	**Progressive** disease that affects the nerve fibers of the brain and spinal cord. It generally begins in young adulthood and continues throughout life.	Muscle weakness, visual disturbances, and dizziness. It affects the whole body, including emotional stability.
Parkinson's disease	Slowly progressive, degenerative, neurological disorder.	Tremors, shuffling gait, masklike face, forward flexion of the trunk, muscle rigidity, and weakness.

progressive   Moving forward, following steps toward an end product.

● ROLE CHANGES IN PEOPLE WHO ARE PHYSICALLY OR MENTALLY CHALLENGED

When people experience a lengthy disability, they require understanding and patience. Disabled people need to remain a productive part of society and to maintain a sense of well-being. The health care worker can be a positive influence on patients/clients during the period of adjustment and rehabilitation.

People who lose a body part or a part of their body functions experience the same stages of loss as do people with a terminal illness. These are denial, rage and anger, bargaining, depression, and acceptance. Many people who suddenly find themselves disabled are dependent on others for many of their daily needs. Being dependent often leads to feelings of not being in control. Physical losses can cause various body functions to be impaired.

Loss of body function often means that changes may occur in the following:

- Communication skills
- Sensory awareness
- Ability to think and comprehend
- Ability to move
- Elimination of waste products
- Eating
- Sexual activity

Loss of physical functions may cause emotional stability to change. The areas of emotional insecurity usually focus around the following:

- Self-esteem   ▪ Self-confidence   ▪ Self-image

Physical impairments that lead to emotional changes may also create a sense of loss concerning the following:

- Ability to develop relationships with others   ▪ Ability to earn a living
- Ability to be a useful member of society

The health care worker helps patients/clients reach their goals by being understanding and knowledgeable about the process involved in acceptance of a disability and rehabilitation.

Rehabilitation

When physical changes occur, the goal of rehabilitation is to help the patient/client return to the highest level of functioning possible. Rehabilitation promotes a healthy return to a productive lifestyle. There are many rehabilitation areas involved in this process. The most common are as follows:

- Physical therapy restores the body to normal functioning when possible.
- Occupational therapy restores the ability to be involved in purposeful activity.
- Speech therapy restores the ability to communicate effectively.
- Psychotherapy changes inappropriate behavior patterns, improves interpersonal relationships, and resolves inner conflicts.

There are several groups available to aid the client and family during the recovery and rehabilitation period. These groups, called *support groups*, are organized to help patients and family members cope with changes during this period. Examples of groups are

- Breast cancer support group
- Ostomy support group
- Vital Options—a support group for young adults with cancer

You can locate groups in your area by contacting the social services department at hospitals, community centers, and organizations oriented to health care.

⬤ SUMMARY

Physical disabilities, injury, and debilitating illness can occur from birth to old age. There are many different types of disabilities. Some of these are caused by accident, heredity, injury, or illness. When any of these are present, the patient may be frustrated or depressed. As a health care worker, you are responsible for the care and support of these patients. It is important to understand their illness and to be familiar with assistive/adaptive devices and support organizations that are available to help patients and their families.

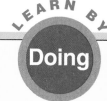

UNIT 3 ACTIVITY

1. Follow your instructor's directions to complete Worksheet/Activity 2.
2. Complete Worksheets 3 and 4 as assigned.
3. When you are confident that you can meet each objective, ask your instructor for the unit evaluation.

End of Life Issues

STEPS TO SUCCESS

1. Complete Vocabulary Worksheet 1 in the Student Workbook.

2. Read this unit.

3. Complete the Learn by Doing assignment at the end of this unit.

UNIT OBJECTIVES

When you have completed this unit, you will be able to do the following:

✔ Match vocabulary words with their correct meanings.

✔ Match the psychological stages of a long terminal illness with their names.

UNIT RATIONALE

As a health care worker, you come in contact with clients who are nearing the end of their life. Your knowledge of the psychological stages experienced by those at the end of life gives you an understanding of their behavior.

✔ Identify and discuss your feelings about terminal illness.

✔ Explain the philosophy of hospice care.

⚪ TERMINAL ILLNESS

Patients/clients who have an illness that cannot be cured are terminally ill. They are expected to die. When the patients learn of their illness, they usually pass through five different psychological stages (Figure 9.2).

isolated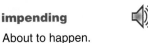

Limited in contact with others.

impending

About to happen.

- **Stage one: Shock and denial.** People find it very difficult to believe that they are really going to die. "No, not me!" During this stage they feel very lonely and **isolated.** *Communication:* If they can discuss these feelings and talk about their **impending** death, they are able to move into the next stage. You may be the only health care worker available to listen to their feelings.

- **Stage two: Rage and anger.** No matter how much kindness you have shown, your client may become very insulting; there might be many complaints about everything you do. You may be tempted to leave them to their anger. *Communication:* If you realize it is not a personal attack, you will be able to listen and to understand that the anger is not directed at you. It is directed at the injustice of the situation. Be a good listener. When patients have exhausted their anger, they will move out of the anger stage.

- **Stage three: Bargaining.** Although they now admit to themselves that they are dying, the clients try to prolong their life with bargaining. For example, they might say, "Just let me live until my children are independent." *Communication:* Listen and reflect what is said, express your understanding, and be aware of your voice tone and body language. Be aware of times when your presence in silence is helpful and when words are not helpful.

- **Stage four: Depression.** Your patients may refuse to talk to you or even look at you. They are experiencing great sadness, for they are losing everyone and everything. *Communication:* Although they may not want to be bothered with friends or visitors, your touch is very important. Your understanding of their feelings of loss enables them to move into the last stage.

- **Stage five: Acceptance.** At last your clients can accept their death. This is a time when your presence lets them know you will not desert them. *Communication:* They may want to discuss their death. Your willingness to be available will help your patients in a very difficult time.

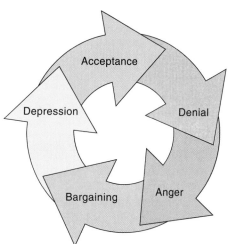

Figure 9.2

Stages of dying.

Friends and family often experience the same stages when someone they love and care about is terminally ill. As a health care worker, you need to be understanding. Family and friends may experience the following stages:

- **Shock and denial.** They may continue to make plans for the future that include the dying person.
- **Rage and anger.** They may be irritable and angry and say unkind things occasionally.
- **Bargaining.** They may ask the physician to keep the patient/client alive for a special occasion.
- **Depression.** They feel extreme sadness and even despair.
- **Acceptance.** They finally accept that death is going to occur. They may ask you to recommend someone for them to talk to.

Decision Making at the End of Life

Decision making related to end of life issues must consider all aspects of care. It involves the patient's perception of death, psychological aspects of culture and spirituality, and all components of treatment and its expected outcome. The patient and family's decision making must be supported in an ethical framework of respect for independence and dignity. Without the support of an individual's right to decision making, there is the risk that the patient will be treated as an object rather than as a person.

Health care decision making is built upon a relationship between patient and health care provider that requires mutual respect, trust, honesty, and confidentiality. Manipulation or intimidation must not hinder the resulting free exchange of information. Patients need to know and be informed of the following:

- Their condition
- The proposed treatment
- Expected results
- Alternative treatment options
- Potential risks, complications, and anticipated benefits

Pain Management

When the terminally ill patient decides jointly with health care providers and the family that prolonging life with therapy is no longer possible, then comfort and pain relief becomes the treatment goal. Most patients with a terminal illness fear physical pain much more than they fear death itself. Pain that is undertreated can have an extreme effect on the patient. It is important to work as a team with your coworkers to address the emotional, physical, spiritual, and psychological effects of pain and relieve discomfort as much as possible. Relieving pain includes maintaining the patient's personal hygiene and body alignment, and speaking gently and clearly to the patient even if he or she is not able to respond to you. Reporting restlessness, excessive sweating, and rapid respirations to the charge nurse will provide information needed to determine if medication is appropriate.

HOSPICE CARE

philosophy

Theory; a general principle used for a specific purpose.

In many communities, hospice care is available for terminally ill people. The hospice **philosophy** is to help patients/clients nearing the end of life live each day to the fullest. This care is provided in the home or in a hospice facility. Patients are kept comfortable and free from pain. When the time for death comes, they are allowed to die peacefully. An important service of hospice is family involvement. Families are counseled and helped to accept the impending death of a loved one. Following the death, the family has continuing support for at least a year. This support helps make the grieving period more tolerable.

You are an important member of the health care team. Your insight into the patient/client and his or her family and friends provides valuable information to decision makers concerning the care process. This knowledge of what your patients/clients may experience helps you meet their needs.

JOBS AND PROFESSIONS

- Gerontologist
- Hospice worker
- Nurse assistant/orderly in long-term care facility
- Ambulatory care clinics
- Assistive personnel

SUMMARY

Most health care workers come in contact with terminally ill patients/clients and are involved in the care of a dying person. The terminally ill patient usually experiences five psychological stages: denial, anger, bargaining, depression, and acceptance. Patients who are terminally ill have an opportunity to choose a hospice for the final days of their illness.

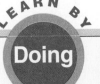

LEARN BY

Doing

UNIT 4 ACTIVITY

1. **Complete Worksheet 2.**
2. **Follow your instructor's directions to complete Worksheet/ Activity 3.**
3. **Prepare responses to each item listed in Chapter Review—your Link to Success at the end of this chapter.**
4. **When you are confident that you can meet each objective, ask your instructor for the unit evaluation.**

Thinking Critically

1. **Communication** Following the medical plan, you are helping Mr. Green learn to use a walker after his stroke. The greatest challenge is that his wife and family tell him that he does not have to bother with learning to get around himself. Now that he is retired due to disability, they tell him that he can just sit in bed and watch television. How would you talk to Mr. Green and his family about the importance of staying mobile?

2. **Legal and Ethical** An elderly husband and wife decide to live in a long-term care facility so that their family won't worry about them. Upon admission, the wife is placed in room 125, and the husband is placed next door in room 126. They ask to share the same room, but the admitting clerk explains that the facility policy doesn't allow men and women to stay in the same room. Describe your remarks to the family and how you would respond to the admitting clerk or your supervisor.

3. **Cultural Competency** Working in the pediatric ward, your team is proud of the progress made with a frightened, withdrawn five-year-old girl. But during visiting hours, her father becomes very angry, telling you that the hospital staff has made his daughter a bad girl because she is noisy and talkative. How would you handle this situation?

4. **Patient Education** A 55-year-old male patient is recovering from a stroke. He is a high school principal and has always been able to take care of himself. His right hand and leg are paralyzed. Each day he is increasingly frustrated because he is unable to bathe or dress himself. Describe devices that could help reduce his frustration. Explain what you would say and do to educate him in the use of assistive/adaptive devices.

5. **Case Study** A 30-year-old woman suffered a head injury, which left her unable to speak. Her daily care provides a bath, clean clothes, and food. People around her rarely speak to her. She stays in her room and looks out the window most of the time. Compare and differentiate between her day and yours. Make specific recommendations that could assist in moving this person toward health as described by the World Health Organization. Explain how your recommendations would change this client's health status.

6. **Patient Satisfaction** Community resources provide people in transition with valuable information and assistance. As a health care worker you have the opportunity to share information about available community resources with your patients and their families. Create a card file of community resources with the following basic information about each: services provided, name of the organization, address, telephone number, e-mail address, and all other pertinent information.

7. **Computers** Patients/clients with disabilities are using computers to communicate and be productive citizens as they live with their disability. Do research on ways computers can be adapted to meet the needs of disabled individuals and write a report explaining what you have learned. Look for *assistive technology, alternative input mechanisms, alternative output mechanisms,* and *computer use with handicapped or disabled children.*

Portfolio Connection

Working with people who are ill causes unfamiliar feelings and experiences. Your ability to identify your feelings and understand how you react to those feelings helps you carry on and continue to care for others. Select a disability described in this chapter. Imagine that you are diagnosed with this disability. Identify your fears, feelings, and expectations. Explain what each day would be like, what type of care you would need, how others would respond to you, and how you would respond to others.

Portfolio Tip

Remember that aging means different things in different cultures.

Your explanation must clearly identify your self-evaluation and new insights about disabilities and behaviors, and must show how you would approach others with disabilities. This assignment helps you investigate your feelings and identify possible behaviors of patients who live with disabilities. Including this assignment in your portfolio gives you easy access to it for review during your training. Comparing assignments throughout your training shows how your experiences have brought about change in your thinking.

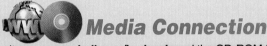

Remember! Media Connection

Use the Companion Website **www.prenhall.com/badasch** and the CD-ROM for additional interactive learning activities.

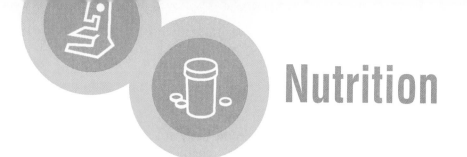

Nutrition

Chapter 10

MEDIA CONNECTION
Use the Companion Website
www.prenhall.com/badasch and the CD-ROM
for additional interactive learning activities.

UNIT 1

Basic Nutrition

STEPS TO SUCCESS

1. Complete Vocabulary Worksheet 1 in the Student Workbook.
2. Read this unit.
3. Complete the Learn by Doing assignment at the end of this unit.

UNIT RATIONALE

Health care workers must maintain good health in order to be efficient in their work. When you eat the proper foods, you have the energy and vitality to function effectively. Patients must have a healthy diet to maintain or to restore good health. Your knowledge of a balanced diet helps you understand how good nutrition maintains good health for yourself and your patients/clients.

UNIT OBJECTIVES

When you have completed this unit, you will be able to do the following:

✔ Match vocabulary words with their correct meanings.

✔ Name the four functions of food.

✔ Name the five basic nutrients and explain how they maintain body function.

✔ Explain the USDA food pyramid.

✔ Compare your diet with the recommendations in the USDA food pyramid.

⬤ INTRODUCTION TO BASIC NUTRITION

Good nutrition promotes a healthier body and mind. It also aids in **resistance** to illness. When we eat a healthy diet, our energy and **vitality** are increased. The right foods speed the healing process and help a person feel better and sleep better.

    Your patients/clients are all from different cultural and religious backgrounds. Each culture and religion has dietary differences. Appetites, food budgets, cultural food preferences, and religious restrictions influence some of these differences. You and your patients need the same basic nutrients provided by a balanced, healthy diet. The health care worker must understand about foods and their effect on the body in order to assess his or her own diet and the patient's diet.

resistance
Ability of the body to protect itself from disease.

vitality
Ability of an organism to go on living.

The Function of Food

When food is taken into the body, it is used in many different ways. The right combination of nutrients work together in the body to

- Provide heat
- Promote growth
- Repair tissue
- **Regulate** body processes

regulate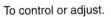

To control or adjust.

Basic Nutrients

Nutrients are chemical compounds found in food. When the food we eat enters the digestive tract, it is changed into a simple form and absorbed into the blood. The blood carries these nutrients to body cells, where they are used to maintain body functions. Table 10.1 lists the basic nutrients.

Water is essential to the body. It carries nutrients to the body cells and carries waste products away from the body cells. It also lubricates the joints and helps regulate body temperature and body processes.

Fiber

Fiber adds bulk to the diet and helps prevent bowel and colon diseases. Fiber also helps prevent constipation. The diet many people eat is high in protein, fats, and carbohydrates but very low in fiber. To keep the bowel healthy, a person should eat several servings of fiber each day. Fiber is found in greens, kale, cabbage, celery, vegetable salads, raw and cooked fruits, whole-grain food, and cereals.

Good nutrition enhances your appearance and increases your stamina. It is important to plan meals and snacks that include all of the basic nutrients each day.

Calories

calories

Units of measurement of the fuel value of food.

proteins

Complex compound found in plant and animal tissues, essential for heat, energy, and growth.

minerals

Inorganic elements that occur in nature; essential to every cell.

vitamins

Group of substances necessary for normal functioning and maintenance of health.

essential

Necessary (e.g., certain food elements are necessary for the body's functions).

Food is the source of energy for our bodies. The body metabolizes food nutrients to create energy. As the body creates energy, it produces heat. Energy is required to ensure that all of the body systems function. The amount of energy created by the food we eat is measured in **calories.** Calorie needs vary from person to person. A large, active man needs more calories than a smaller, inactive man does. The number of calories we eat and the amount of exercise we do balance weight. If we eat

Table 10.1 ■ Basic Nutrients		
Proteins	Build and renew body tissues Provide heat energy	
Carbohydrates	Provide the basic source of energy for body heat and body activities	
Fats	Provide fatty acids for normal growth and development Provides energy Carry vitamins A and D to the cells	
Minerals	Regulate the activity of the heart, nerves, and muscles Build and renew teeth, bones, and other tissues	See Figure10.1
Vitamins	Are **essential** for normal metabolism, growth, and body development	See Figure10.2

Calcium

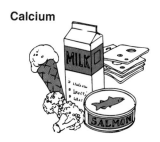

Milk and milk products, except butter; most dark green vegetables; canned salmon.

Iron

Eggs, meat, especially liver and kidney; deep yellow and dark green vegetables; potatoes, dried fruits, whole-grain products; enriched flour, bread, and breakfast cereals.

Iodine

Fish (obtained from the sea), some plant foods grown in soils containing iodine; table salt fortified with iodine (iodized).

Figure 10.1

Minerals are calcium, iron, and iodine.

A

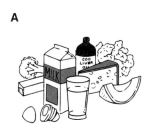

One form of vitamin A is yellow and one form is colorless. Apricots, cantaloupe, milk, cheese, eggs, meat organs (especially liver and kidney), fortified margarine, butter, fish-liver oils, dark green and deep yellow vegetables.

Figure 10.2

Vitamins include A, B complex, B1, B2, B12, C, D, and niacin.

B Complex
B₁ (Thiamine)

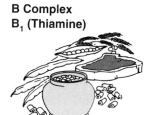

Whole-grain and enriched grain products; meats (especially pork, liver, and kidney); dry beans and peas.

B₂ (Riboflavin)

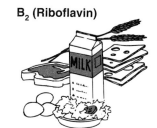

Milk, cheese, eggs, meat (especially liver and kidney), whole-grain and enriched grain products, dark green vegetables.

B₁₂

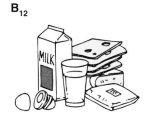

Liver, other organ meats, cheese, eggs, milk.

C (Ascorbic Acid)

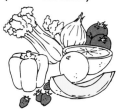

Fresh, raw citrus fruits and vegetables—oranges, grapefruit, cantaloupe, strawberries, tomatoes, raw onions, cabbage, green and sweet red peppers, dark green vegetables.

D

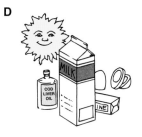

Provided by vitamin D fortification of certain foods, such as milk and margarine. Also fish-liver oils and eggs. Sunshine is also a source of vitamin D.

Niacin

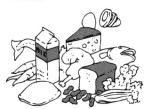

Liver, meat, fish, poultry, eggs, peanuts; dark green vegetables, whole-grain and enriched cereal products.

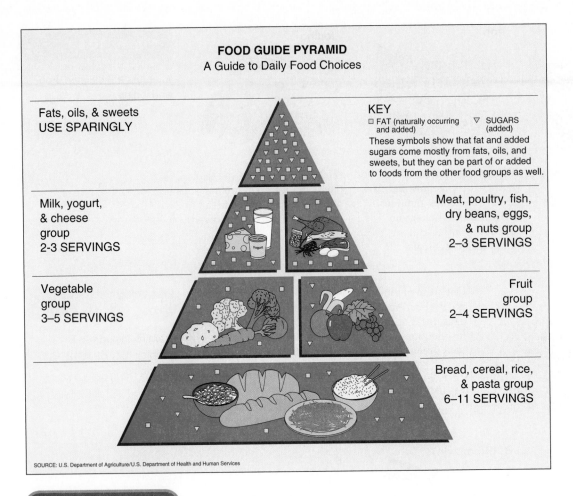

FOOD GUIDE PYRAMID
A Guide to Daily Food Choices

Fats, oils, & sweets
USE SPARINGLY

KEY
□ FAT (naturally occurring   ▽ SUGARS
    and added)   (added)
These symbols show that fat and added
sugars come mostly from fats, oils, and
sweets, but they can be part of or added
to foods from the other food groups as well.

Milk, yogurt,
& cheese
group
2-3 SERVINGS

Meat, poultry, fish,
dry beans, eggs,
& nuts group
2–3 SERVINGS

Vegetable
group
3–5 SERVINGS

Fruit
group
2–4 SERVINGS

Bread, cereal, rice,
& pasta group
6–11 SERVINGS

SOURCE: U.S. Department of Agriculture/U.S. Department of Health and Human Services

Figure 10.3

The "eating right" pyramid.

more calories than we burn, we gain weight. If we burn more calories than we eat, we lose weight. When a patient is inactive and feels ill, she may not want to eat. It is your responsibility to encourage her to take in enough calories to produce the energy needed to heal the body.

The Food Pyramid

Good nutrition and a healthy diet help maintain good health. The U.S. Department of Agriculture (USDA) has provided the food pyramid (Figure 10.3) as a guideline. The "eating right" pyramid focuses on low-fat foods, such as grains, pasta, vegetables, fruits, nonfat dairy products, and lean meats. The pyramid illustrates the recommended daily portions of each food group. Follow these guidelines for yourself and your patients/clients. The food choices of all cultures fit into these guidelines when you plan carefully.

How Poor Nutrition Affects the Body

When we do not supply our bodies with the proper nutrients, many things can go wrong. We lose stamina and vitality. An unhealthy diet often results in illness and disease. The following are a few of the problems that poor nutrition can cause.

■ *Anemia,* a decreased number of red blood cells or a decreased amount of **hemoglobin,** results in

- Fatigue • Dyspnea (shortness of breath) on exertion • Headache • Insomnia (inability to sleep) • Paleness • Indigestion • Rapid heartbeat

■ *Anorexia nervosa* occurs when a person refuses to eat or drastically reduces his or her intake of food. This is related to an emotional disturbance about image (e.g., a person who is very underweight sees herself or himself as overweight). Anorexia nervosa is seen primarily in teenage girls. It results in

- Amenorrhea • Skeletonlike appearance

■ *Bulimia* occurs when a person experiences intervals of food craving and **bingeing** and then **purging.** The side effects are the same as those of anorexia and result in depression.

■ *Constipation* is the infrequent, difficult defecation of fecal material. It is commonly caused by lack of activity and by not eating enough vegetables, fruit, or water.

■ *Dull hair and eyes* are symptoms of poor diet.

■ *Mental slowdown* can occur when nutrition is poor.

■ **Obesity** occurs when a person takes in more calories than the body uses. This results in increasing amounts of fatty tissue.

■ *Osteoporosis* occurs when bones become porous, causing them to break easily. This is caused by inadequate calcium intake or absorption.

■ *Poor skin condition* results from poor nutrition.

hemoglobin
Complex chemical in the blood; carries oxygen and carbon dioxide.

bingeing
Eating excessively.

purging
Causing oneself to vomit.

obesity
Extreme fatness; abnormal amount of fat on the body.

◯ SUMMARY

A balanced, healthy diet is essential for maintaining health and stamina. Everyone needs certain basic nutrients in his or her diet. When you plan your daily meals using the guidelines in the "eating right" pyramid, you meet your body's nutritional needs and help maintain good health. All individuals must eat a healthy diet that provides balanced nutrients and meets cultural and religious needs.

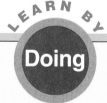

UNIT 1 ACTIVITY

1. Complete Worksheet/Activity 2 as assigned.
2. Complete Worksheets 3 through 5 after your instructor discusses this chapter in class.
3. Complete Worksheets/Activities 6 and 7.
4. When you are confident that you can meet each objective, ask your instructor for the unit evaluation.

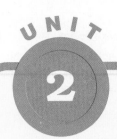

Therapeutic Diets

STEPS TO SUCCESS

1. Complete Vocabulary Worksheet 1 in the Student Workbook.
2. Read this unit.
3. Complete the Learn by Doing assignment at the end of this unit.

UNIT RATIONALE

Some patients/clients have illnesses that require special diets. Therapeutic diets are diets that modify a patient's normal diet in order to treat an illness. Understanding why the diet has been changed helps you encourage clients to eat the food prepared for them. When you are knowledgeable about their diet, you are able to explain how important it is to their recovery.

UNIT OBJECTIVES

When you have completed this unit, you will be able to do the following:

✔ Match vocabulary words with their correct meaning.

✔ List three factors that influence food habits.

✔ Select a correct therapeutic diet for physical disorders.

◯ INTRODUCTION TO THERAPEUTIC DIETS

It is especially important to remember the factors that influence food habits for patients who are on a therapeutic diet. Always respect the patient's personal attitudes and preferences, nationality, race, and religious needs. A therapeutic diet is often very different from the foods the patient normally eats. Your understanding of the reason for the diet and your patients' special needs helps ease their concerns. The dietitian will talk with the patient and try to adapt a therapeutic diet to meet a patient's nutritional and personal needs. An example of a special or personal need is religious restrictions.

Many religions of the world follow specific dietary laws. These guidelines are very important to clients. The stress caused by breaking the law when clients are on a therapeutic diet may cause added worry. Always be respectful of the dietary requests that your clients make, and report their requests to your supervisor. Ask your clients what diet they normally follow. If there is a problem with the diet, report it to your supervisor, who will talk with the dietitian. Table 10.2 lists a few of the restrictions that you may observe.

Purposes of Therapeutic Diets

Therapeutic diets are given to

metabolic

Pertaining to the total of all the physical and chemical changes that take place in living organisms and cells.

- Regulate the amount of food in **metabolic** disorders
- Prevent or restrict edema by restricting sodium intake
- Assist body organs to regain and/or maintain normal function
- Aid in digestion by avoiding foods that irritate the digestive tract
- Increase or decrease body weight by adding or eliminating calories

Table 10.2 ■ Religious Dietary Restrictions

Christian Science Church of Latter-Day Saints (Mormons) Conservative Protestants	Avoid alcohol, coffee, tea.
Greek Orthodox	No meat or dairy products on fast days.
Muslim (Moslem)	No alcohol, pork, or pork products.
Orthodox Jewish	No shellfish, pork, or nonkosher meats. No serving milk and milk products with meat. No eating leavened bread during Passover. Abstain from eating on specific fast days.
Roman Catholic	No food one hour before communion and no meat on Ash Wednesday, Good Friday, and all the Fridays during Lent.
Buddhist	Generally vegetarian.
Hindu	Generally vegetarian.

Types of Therapeutic Diets

Table 10.3 describes the various types of therapeutic diets and their purposes.

The physician may order other diets. Always check the diet that has been ordered for the patient/client. If you have any question about it, ask the person in charge. Correct diets are essential in maintaining good health, and only those foods allowed should be served.

Table 10.3 ■ Some Therapeutic Diets and Their Purposes

Type of Diet	Purpose of Diet	Description
Clear liquid Nutritionally inadequate	Replaces fluids lost from vomiting, diarrhea, surgery	Plain gelatin, ginger ale, tea, coffee (no cream), fruit or apple juice (no pulp), fat-free broth
Full liquid May be **deficient** in iron	Trouble chewing or swallowing, **gastrointestinal** disturbances	All clear liquids, fruit or vegetable juices, strained soup, custard, ice cream, sherbet, milk, cream, eggs, buttermilk, carbonated beverages, eggs, cocoa, eggnog
Soft Nutritionally inadequate	For patients who have trouble chewing, postsurgically	Foods that are soft in consistency, such as fish, ground beef, broth, pureed vegetables, strained cream soup, tender cooked vegetables, fruit juices, cooked fruit, refined cereals, pasta, sherbet, ices, ice cream, custard, plain cookies, angel food cake, tea, coffee, cocoa, carbonated beverages, cheese, cottage cheese

deficient

Lacking something (e.g., a deficient diet causes the body to function poorly because it is missing an important element).

gastrointestinal   Pertaining to the stomach and intestine.

Table 10.3 ▪ Continued

Type of Diet	Purpose of Diet	Description
Bland Nutritionally adequate	Soothes gastrointestinal tract, avoids irritation in ulcers, **colitis**	Foods low in fiber and connective tissue that are mild flavored and easy to digest, such as pear (tender, broiled, boiled), prune juice, applesauce, custard, pudding, ice cream, plain cookies, sponge cake, decaffeinated coffee, milk, cheese, yogurt
Restricted residue Nutritionally adequate	Reduces normal work of the intestine, in cases of rectal diseases, colitis, **ileitis**	Foods low in fiber and low in bulk, such as milk, buttermilk, cottage cheese, butter, margarine, eggs (not fried), tender poultry, fish, lamb, ground beef (broiled, boiled, baked), broth, refined bread, cereals, pasta, gelatin, angel food or sponge cake, mild-flavored cooked vegetables, lettuce, vegetable and fruit juice, applesauce, canned fruit, citrus fruit without membranes
Low carbohydrate (diabetic) Nutritionally adequate	Matches food intake with insulin uptake and nutritional requirements, used for patients with hyperinsulism and **diabetes mellitus**	Foods that supply enough protein, fat, and carbohydrate to maintain health and activities; requires a balance of carbohydrates, protein, and fat to meet the individual need of the patient; restricts sugar, cookies, pies, candies, etc.
Low fat Deficient in fat-**soluble** vitamins	For patients with gallbladder and liver disease, obesity, and heart conditions	Foods high in carbohydrates and proteins; all fats are limited; skim milk, buttermilk, cottage cheese, lean fish, poultry, meats, fat-free soup broths, cooked vegetables, lettuce, fruit juice, bananas, citrus fruits, gelatin, angel food cake, coffee, tea, carbonated beverages, jelly, honey as desired
Low cholesterol Nutritionally adequate	Regulates amount of cholesterol in the blood for patients with coronary disease and **atherosclerosis**	Foods low in fat, such as lean muscle meat, fish, poultry without skin or fat, skim milk, vegetables, fruits
Low calorie (800–2,000 cal) Nutritionally adequate	Reduces number of calories for overweight patients and for clients with arthritis or cardiac conditions	Foods low in fats and calories: skim milk, buttermilk, lean meats, clear soup, vegetables, fresh fruit, coffee, tea, herbs, onions, garlic
High calorie (2,000 cal+) Nutritionally adequate	For persons 10% or more below desired weight; for patients with **anorexia nervosa** and hyperthyroidism	All foods with nutritionally balanced proteins, carbohydrates, fats, vitamins, minerals

colitis   Inflammation of the colon.

ileitis   Inflammation of the ileum (the lower three-fifths of the small intestine).

diabetes mellitus

Condition that develops when the body cannot change sugar into energy; there is an insufficient amount of insulin, leading to an increased amount of sugar in the blood.

soluble   Able to break down or dissolve in liquid.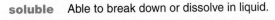

atherosclerosis

Condition of hardening of the arteries due to fat deposits that narrow the space blood flows through.

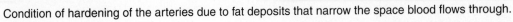

anorexia nervosa

Loss of appetite with serious weight loss; considered a mental disorder.

Table 10.3 ■ Continued		
Type of Diet	**Purpose of Diet**	**Description**
Low sodium Nutritionally adequate	Reduces salt intake for patients with kidney disease, cardiovascular disorders, edema, and **hypertension**	Natural foods prepared without salt, such as fresh fruits, fresh vegetables, foods without salt added
High protein Nutritionally adequate	For children and adolescents needing additional protein for growth; during pregnancy, **lactation;** postsurgically; during illnesses resulting from protein loss	Foods high in protein, such as milk, cheese, eggs, lean meats, fish, and poultry; fruit, cereals, vegetables

hypertension   High blood pressure.

lactation   Body's process of producing milk to feed newborns.

⬤ SUMMARY

There are many factors that influence food habits. Some of these factors are personal attitudes, nationality, race, and religious restrictions. A health care worker must be aware of these factors in order to help the patient/client adapt to therapeutic diets.

The therapeutic diet is prescribed for various ailments. It is important to understand why the diet was prescribed and how it helps in regaining a healthier state. The health care worker should be aware of the foods allowed and not allowed in therapeutic diets and serve only proper foods to his or her patients.

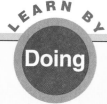

UNIT 2 ACTIVITY

1. **Complete Worksheet 2.**
   Ask your instructor for directions to complete activities.

2. **Complete Worksheet/Activity 3.**

3. **Prepare responses to each item listed in Chapter Review—Your Link to Success at the end of this chapter.**

4. **When you are confident that you can meet each objective, ask your instructor for the unit evaluation.**

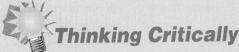

Thinking Critically

1. **Communication** As you are distributing meal trays you notice that one of your patients is tossing all empty food packaging, such as milk cartons and sugar containers, on the floor. Instead of raising your voice and asking, "What do you think you are doing?," how would you speak to the patient about the problem to encourage cooperation and better habits at future meals?

2. **Cultural Competency** The American culture encourages independence regardless of age or gender. In many cultures, however, older people can expect to be waited on by younger family members. How could this affect mealtimes in a facility? Make notes on how you would talk with a patient who appears to be having difficulties opening the packaged foods on the meal tray and coping independently with mealtimes.

3. **Medical Math** Your patient/client is on a therapeutic diet. It is your responsibility to keep a record of all of her intake and output. At the end of the day, she has taken in 1,200 ounces of fluid, and her output is 925 ounces of fluid. How many cc has she taken in? How many cc has she put out?

4. **Case Study** Mrs. Cohen, an Orthodox Jew, has been in St. Andrews Nursing Home for several years. This evening the staff in the kitchen sent her a dinner with mashed potatoes, pork roast, green beans, and custard. She is very upset and is crying: She is hungry, but does not want to eat because of her dietary restrictions. You know that the staff in the kitchen is new. What steps can you take to remedy this problem?

5. **Patient Satisfaction** Your patient, who is on a low-fat diet, is feeling disgruntled and is complaining about everything on his tray. How can you help your patient understand the reason for the diet?

Portfolio Connection

When you care for patients, it is important to know if they are eating a healthy diet. Therapeutic diets do not always meet the standards of a healthy diet.

Choose an illness that requires a therapeutic diet. Write a paragraph about the illness. Explain the symptoms, how the body is affected, and the treatment. Use the food pyramid as a guide to evaluating the therapeutic diet required. Describe in what ways the diet is nutritionally healthy or deficient.

Place this exercise in your portfolio to help you review the food pyramid, healthy diets, and therapeutic diets.

Portfolio Tip

Food preferences and diet can be more of a source of distress and conflict for patients than the actual illness. Make a large photocopy of the food pyramid and keep it in your portfolio.

Write notes for yourself demonstrating how you would explain to patients the importance of a varied diet.

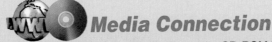

Remember! Media Connection

Use the Companion Website **www.prenhall.com/badasch** and the CD-ROM for additional interactive learning activities.

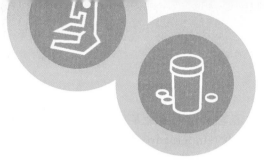

Chapter 11
Measuring Vital Signs

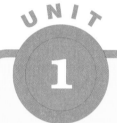

UNIT 1

Temperature, Pulse, and Respiration

STEPS TO SUCCESS

1. Complete Vocabulary Worksheet 1 in the Student Workbook.

2. Read this unit.

3. Complete the Learn by Doing assignment at the end of this unit.

UNIT RATIONALE

Important indicators of your patient's/client's health status are known as *vital signs*. Vital signs give you information about breathing, body temperature, and the heart. They are a good indication of how well the body systems are functioning. As a health care worker, you need to observe patients whenever you are near them. Your knowledge of vital signs and how to measure them helps you know when to report that a patient is having problems.

UNIT OBJECTIVES

When you have completed this unit, you will be able to do the following:

✔ Match vocabulary words with their correct meanings.

✔ Define *vital signs*.

✔ List fourteen factors that influence body temperature.

✔ Name the most common site at which to measure a temperature.

✔ Match the normal temperature to the site where it is measured.

✔ Measure temperature with a glass thermometer.

✔ Demonstrate how to measure oral, rectal, and axillary temperature.

✔ Define *pulse*.

✔ Explain pulse oximetry.

✔ Identify sites where pulse may be counted.

✔ Identify a normal adult pulse rate and a common method for counting a pulse.

✔ List six factors that influence the pulse rate.

✔ Demonstrate counting and recording a radial pulse accurately.

✔ Recognize two parts of a respiration.

✔ Relate types of abnormal respirations to their correct name.

✔ Select eight factors that affect respiration.

✔ Explain the importance of not being obvious when counting respirations.

✔ Demonstrate how to count and record respirations accurately.

✔ Explain the importance of each vital sign.

blood pressure

Highest and lowest pressure against the walls of blood vessels.

TPR

Stands for "temperature, pulse, respiration."

oxidation

The mixing together of oxygen and another element.

excretion

Process of eliminating waste material.

calibration

Standard measure (e.g., each line on a thermometer or a ruler is a calibration).

INTRODUCTION TO VITAL SIGNS

Vital signs include body temperature, pulse, respiration rates, and **blood pressure.** Vital signs are the indicators that tell you how the body is functioning. Pulse oximetry is another important indicator of body functioning. When vital signs are within normal limits, the body is considered to be in homeostasis. When the vital signs are not within normal limits, it is an indication that something is wrong. It is important to be accurate when you measure vital signs and to record the results very carefully and accurately. Other health care workers depend on this information when making decisions about the patient's treatment. In this unit, you learn how to measure body temperature and count the pulse rate and respiratory rate. Together these measurements are referred to as **TPR.** Unit 2 teaches you to measure blood pressure.

TEMPERATURE

Temperature is the measure of body heat. Heat is produced in the body by the muscles and glands and by the **oxidation** of food. Heat is lost from the body by respiration, perspiration, and **excretion.** The balance between the heat produced and the heat lost is the body temperature. Table 11.1 shows the factors that influence temperature.

Thermometers

The thermometer is the instrument used to measure temperature. There are several types of thermometers: glass thermometers, aural thermometers, chemically treated paper or plastic thermometers, and electronic/digital thermometers.

Glass Thermometers (Clinical/Mercury)

A glass thermometer is a hollow glass tube with **calibration** lines on it. At one end of the thermometer is a bulb that is filled with mercury. The mercury is heat sensitive and rises up the hollow tube when exposed to heat. This enables you to read the patient's/client's temperature. There are two types of tips or bulbs on glass thermometers (Figure 11.1).

Aural Thermometers

A tympanic membrane sensor measures body temperature. It is accurate, easy to use, and safe. It is especially effective for babies and children.

Table 11.1 ■ Factors That Influence Temperature	
Increase Temperature	**Decrease Temperature**
Exercise	Sleep
Digestion of food	Fasting
Increased environmental temperature	Exposure to cold
Illness	Certain illnesses
Infection	Decreased muscle activity
Excitement	Mouth breathing
Anxiety	Depression

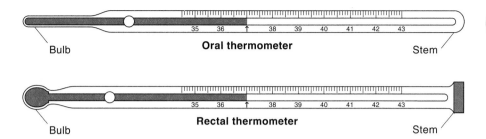

Bulb   **Oral thermometer**   Stem

Bulb   **Rectal thermometer**   Stem

Figure 11.1

Figure 11.1

There are two types of glass thermometers. The rectal thermometer has a rounded bulb that helps prevent perforation of tissue.

Chemically Treated Paper or Plastic Thermometers

This type of thermometer is read by noting the color it changes to. It is disposed of after one use.

Electronic/Digital Thermometers

This thermometer has a probe that you cover with a protective, disposable shield (Figure 11.2). The temperature is measured and registered on a screen. Electronic thermometers are quick and easy to use. There are various types of electronic equipment available. Always follow the manufacturer's instructions.

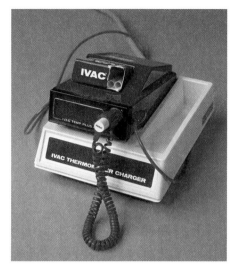

Figure 11.2

Electronic/digital thermometers.

How to Read a Glass Thermometer

1. Hold the thermometer at eye level. Rotate the thermometer until you can see the column of mercury.

2. Look at the lines on the scale at the upper side of the column of mercury. Each long line represents a whole degree. There are four short lines between each of the long lines. The short lines represent ²⁄₁₀ (0.2) of a degree. Only even numbers are shown on a Fahrenheit clinical thermometer (see Figure 11.3) (e.g., 96°, 98°, 100°).

3. If the mercury ends at one of the short lines, look to see which long line is just before it. This tells you the degree of temperature. Then add ²⁄₁₀ for each short line.

4. Read a Celsius thermometer the same way. Each long line represents a degree. Each short line represents ¹⁄₁₀ (0.1) of a degree (see Figure 11.3).

You may be asked to change a temperature from **Celsius** to **Fahrenheit** or from Fahrenheit to centigrade. If you need to make these changes, use the information in Table 11.2.

Sites to Take Body Temperature

Oral

The simplest and most common, convenient, and comfortable site to take a temperature is the **oral** cavity, unless you use the aural thermometer. The average normal oral temperature is 98.6° F or 37° C. Use the oral or aural cavity whenever possible and when the patient has

■ Diarrhea   ■ Rectal surgery   ■ Fecal impaction

Celsius

Measure of heat; in medicine a Celsius thermometer is sometimes used to measure body heat. Also called centigrade.

Fahrenheit

Measure of heat; in medicine a Fahrenheit thermometer is often used to measure body heat.

oral

Referring to the mouth.

PROCEDURE 11.1

USING AN ELECTRONIC THERMOMETER

RATIONALE

As a health care worker it is important to monitor the patient's physical status. One way to determine this status is by measuring the patient's body temperature. There are many different kinds of thermometers. This procedure explains how to use an electronic thermometer to measure body temperature.

ALERT: Follow Standard Precautions.

1. Wash hands.
2. Assemble equipment.*
   a. Plastic thermometer covers
   b. Electronic thermometer with appropriate probe (blue for oral, red for rectal)
3. Identify patient/client.
4. Explain procedure to patient.
5. Place plastic thermometer cover over probe.
6. Insert probe in proper position to measure body temperature (blue-tipped probe under tongue or in axilla, red-tipped probe in rectum).
7. Hold probe in place for 15 seconds.
8. Buzzer will ring when body temperature is displayed on electronic thermometer.

9. Remove plastic sheath and discard.
10. Record temperature. (Report elevated temperature to a supervisor.)
11. Position client for comfort.
12. Wash hands.
13. Return electronic thermometer to its storage place.
14. Report any unusual observation immediately.

*Wear gloves for measuring rectal temperatures. Follow facility policy for measuring oral temperature.

> 12/15/03   1900
>   T-97.4°F Ⓡ
> _____ S. Jones CNA

Figure 11.3

Average normal temperatures shown on Fahrenheit and Celsius thermometers.

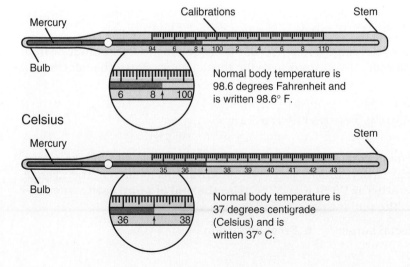

Fahrenheit

Calibrations   Stem

Mercury

Bulb

94 6 8 100 2 4 6 8 110

6 8 100

Normal body temperature is 98.6 degrees Fahrenheit and is written 98.6° F.

Celsius

Mercury

Bulb

35 36 37 38 39 40 41 42 43

36 38

Normal body temperature is 37 degrees centigrade (Celsius) and is written 37° C.

Stem

Table 11.2 ■ Fahrenheit and Celsius Comparison	
Fahrenheit	**Celsius/Centigrade**
32	0
95	35
96	35.5
96.8	36
97.8	36.5
98.6	37
99.6	37.5
100.4	38
101.2	38.4
102.2	39
103	39.4
104	40
105	40.5
105.8	41
106.8	41.5

Rectal

The most accurate temperature reading is taken in the rectum. The normal rectal temperature is 99.6° F or 37.5° C. **Rectal** temperature is taken when patients/clients

- Are under 6 years old
- Have difficulty breathing
- Are extremely weak
- Are confused, unconscious, or senile
- Are being given oxygen
- Experience partial paralysis of the face caused by a stroke or accident

rectal
Referring to the far end of the large intestine just above the anus.

Aural

The aural temperature is also accurate, easy to use, and appropriate for the patients listed above. To measure an aural temperature, a probe is positioned in the aural canal of the ear. A normal aural temperature is 98.6° F or 37° C.

Axillary

The least accurate temperature is taken in the armpit. The normal temperature for this site is 97.6° F or 36.4° C. Use this **axillary** technique only when the temperature cannot be taken orally, aurally, or rectally. Always report a temperature that is above normal to your supervisor.

axillary
Referring to the armpit.

PROCEDURE 11.2

MEASURING AN ORAL TEMPERATURE

RATIONALE

As a health care worker it is important to monitor the patient's physical status. One way to determine this status is by measuring the patient's temperature. This procedure explains how to measure this temperature with an oral thermometer.

ALERT: Follow Standard Precautions.

1. Wash hands.
2. Assemble equipment.*
   a. Clean oral thermometer
   b. Alcohol wipes
   c. Watch with second hand
   d. Disposable thermometer cover
3. Identify patient/client.
4. Explain what you are going to do.
5. Remove thermometer from container and apply disposable cover.
6. Check reading—94° F or 35° C.
7. Ask patient if he or she has been smoking, eating, or drinking. If yes, wait 10 minutes before taking temperature.
8. Place thermometer under tongue.
9. Instruct client to hold with closed lips.
10. Leave in mouth for 5 minutes.
11. Remove from mouth.
12. Remove and discard disposable cover and wipe thermometer from stem to tip.
13. Read thermometer correctly.
14. Wash thermometer in cool water.
15. Put away thermometer.
16. Wash hands.

*Follow facility policy for wearing gloves.

17. Record temperature correctly on pad.
18. Report any unusual observation immediately.

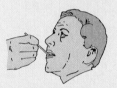

A Insert the thermometer gently into the client's mouth under the tongue.

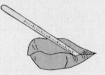

B Position the thermometer to the side of the mouth.

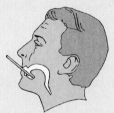

C Instruct the client to keep the thermometer under the tongue by gently closing the lips around the thermometer.

```
12/03/04    1600
        T-99.6°F Ⓡ
_____ S. Jones CNA
```

MEDICAL TERMINOLOGY

■ afebrile	temperature is within normal range		■ pyrexia	above-normal temperature
■ febrile	temperature is elevated		■ pyrogenic	any substance that produces fever
■ hypothermia	temperature is below normal			

PROCEDURE 11.3

MEASURING A RECTAL TEMPERATURE

RATIONALE

As a health care worker it is important to monitor the patient's physical status. One way to determine this status is by measuring the patient's temperature. This procedure explains how to measure this temperature rectally using a rectal thermometer.

ALERT: Follow Standard Precautions.

1. Wash hands.
2. Assemble equipment.
   a. Clean rectal thermometer
   b. Alcohol wipes
   c. Watch with second hand
   d. Lubricant
   e. Disposable nonsterile gloves
   f. Disposable thermometer cover
3. Identify patient/client.
4. Explain what you are going to do.
5. Put on gloves.
6. Remove thermometer from container and apply disposable cover.
7. Check reading—94° F or 35° C.
8. Screen patient.
9. Lower backrest on bed.
10. Put lubricant on tissue and apply to bulb end of thermometer.
11. Separate buttocks.
12. Insert thermometer 1½ inches into rectum.
13. Hold in place 3 to 5 minutes.
14. Remove thermometer.
15. Remove and discard disposable cover and wipe thermometer from stem to tip.
16. Read thermometer correctly.
17. Wash thermometer in cool water.
18. Put away thermometer.
19. Remove and discard gloves.
20. Wash hands.

21. Record temperature correctly on pad.
22. Report any unusual observation immediately.

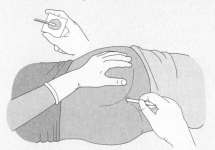

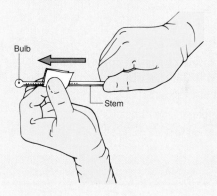

2/14/04   1500
    T-99.2° ℞
        S. Gonzalez CNA

PROCEDURE 11.4 — MEASURING AN AXILLARY TEMPERATURE

RATIONALE

As a health care worker it is important to monitor the patient's physical status. One way to determine this status is by measuring the patient's temperature. This procedure explains how to measure this temperature at the axilla (under the arm).

ALERT: Follow Standard Precautions.

1. Wash hands.
2. Assemble equipment.
    a. Clean thermometer
    b. Alcohol wipes
    c. Watch with second hand
    d. Disposable thermometer cover
3. Identify patient/client.
4. Explain what you are going to do.
5. Remove thermometer from container and apply disposable cover.
6. Check reading—94° F or 35° C.
7. Place thermometer in axilla.
8. Leave in place for 10 minutes.
9. Remove thermometer.
10. Remove and discard disposable cover and wipe thermometer from stem to tip.
11. Read thermometer correctly.
12. Wash thermometer in cool water.
13. Put away thermometer.
14. Wash hands.
15. Record temperature correctly on pad.
16. Report any unusual observation immediately.

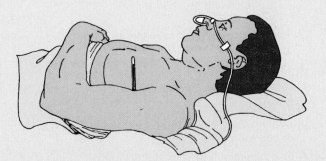

6/14/04   0400
T–97°F AX
_____ H. Ferguson RMA

⬤ PULSE

The pulse rate indicates the number of times the heart beats in 1 minute. It is an important vital sign because it indicates how well the blood is circulating through the body. When you feel the pulse, you are feeling the pressure of the blood against the wall of the artery as the heart contracts and relaxes (Figure 11.4).

Location of Pulse Points

When you count the pulse, place your fingers over an artery and squeeze gently against the bone. Figure 11.5 shows the location on the arteries where the pulse may be taken. The pulse rate should be the same at all pulse sites. Table 11.3 shows the factors that affect pulse rate.

Pulse Characteristics

Just counting the beats is not enough. You must also note the

- **Rate.** Number of pulse beats per minute.
- **Rhythm.** Is the pulse regular? Steady? Or does it skip beats?
- **Arrhythmia.** Does the pulse have uneven intervals between pulses or heartbeats?
- **Force of the beat (volume).** Is it weak, **thready,** or **bounding?** Always report a heartbeat below 60 or over 100.

Pulse Rate

Pulse rate is generally increased with exercise, age, emotional excitement, **hemorrhage,** or elevated temperature. Drugs can increase or decrease the heart rate. When the rate is over 100 beats per minute, it is called *tachycardia.* When the rate is below 60 beats per minute, it is called *bradycardia.* When the rate is irregular, it is called *arrhythmia.* When you record the pulse rate, always report to your supervisor anything that is abnormal. This includes rate (see Table 11.4), rhythm, and force.

Radial Pulse

The radial pulse is the most common site for counting the pulse rate. Always count the pulse for 1 full minute. This prevents missing any abnormalities.

Apical Pulse

You may be asked to count an apical pulse. This is the pulse counted at the **apex** of the heart. Count an apical pulse rate when the heart is too weak to transmit a pulse that you can feel along the arteries. Count the apical heartbeat by placing the stethoscope 2 to 3 inches to the left of the sternum, just below the nipple on the chest.

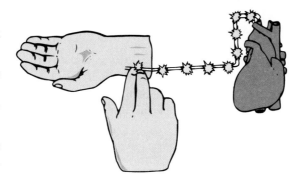

Figure 11.4

The pulse measures the rate of the heartbeat.

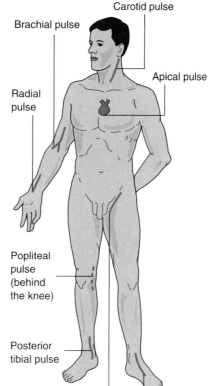

Carotid pulse
Brachial pulse
Apical pulse
Radial pulse
Popliteal pulse (behind the knee)
Posterior tibial pulse
Femoral pulse
Dorsalis pedis pulse

Figure 11.5

Pulse points of the body.

thready

Weak, barely-felt pulse; thin, like a thread.

bounding

Leaping, strong, or forceful (e.g., a very strong pulse is a bounding pulse).

hemorrhage

Large amount of bleeding.

apex

Pointed end of something (e.g., the pointed end of the heart is called the apex of the heart).

Table 11.3 ■ Factors That Affect Pulse Rate

Increase Pulse Rate	Decrease Pulse Rate
Exercise	High level of aerobic fitness
Illness	Depression
Anxiety	Medication
Medication	
Shock	

Table 11.4 ■ Normal Pulse Rates	
Age	**Rate**
Before birth	140–150
At birth	90–160
First year of life	115–130
Childhood years	80–115
Adult	60–80

PROCEDURE 11.5

COUNTING A RADIAL PULSE

RATIONALE

As a health care worker it is important to monitor the patient's physical status. One way to determine this status is by counting the patient's pulse rate. This procedure explains how to count a radial pulse.

1. Wash hands.
2. Assemble equipment.
   a. Watch with second hand
   b. Pad and pencil
3. Identify patient/client.
4. Explain what you are going to do.
5. Place fingers on radial artery—do not use thumb.
6. Count pulse (number of pulsations) for 1 minute.
7. Record pulse rate on pad immediately.
8. Wash hands.
9. Record pulse rate on chart.
10. Report any unusual observation immediately.

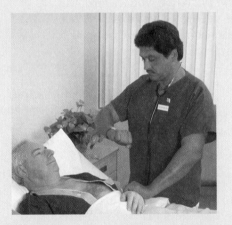

2/14/04   1300
Pulse = 72
Regular and strong
_____ T. Morales CNA

PROCEDURE 11.6

COUNTING AN APICAL PULSE

RATIONALE

As a health care worker it is important to monitor the patient's physical status. One way to determine this status is by counting the patient's pulse rate. This procedure explains how to count an apical pulse.

1. Assemble equipment—stethoscope.
2. Wash hands.
3. Tell patient/client what you are going to do.
4. Uncover left side of patient's chest.
5. Locate apex of heart by placing fingertips on client's chest below left nipple at about the fifth intercostal space.
6. Place stethoscope over apical region and listen for heart sounds.
7. Count the beats for 1 minute; note rate, rhythm, and strength of beat.
8. Record pulse rate on pad.
9. Wash hands.
10. Record apical pulse rate on chart.
11. Report any unusual observation immediately.

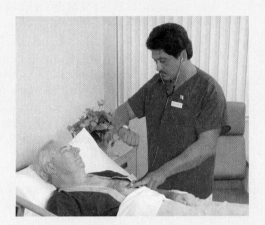

12/14/04 1000
82/78 AP
Pulse deficit = 4
Quality of beat strong
———— S. Padleswki RMA

⊙ PULSE OXIMETRY

The pulse oximeter is an electronic device that determines oxygen (O_2) concentration in the hemoglobin of the arterial blood. When the O_2 concentration in the hemoglobin falls below 90%, the tissues do not have enough oxygen to function. Measuring with the oximeter allows monitoring of cardiac and respiratory patients whose blood O_2 content is an important indicator of their condition. The oximeter has light beams that pass through the tissues. The O_2 content and pulse rate are read and displayed on a monitor. Low concentrations of O_2 or a slow or rapid pulse rate cause an alarm to sound. The sensor is attached to a finger or earlobe, the forehead, the nose, or a toe. The sensor is sensitive to movement, light, and dark nail polish. Do not place a sensor over a break in the skin, a swollen area, or an area where the circulation is poor. To chart the O_2 measurement correctly, use the abbreviation SpO_2. This indicates saturation (S), pulse (p), and oxygen (O_2).

MEDICAL TERMINOLOGY

- **arrhythmia**   absence of rhythm
- **bradycardia**   abnormally slow heartbeat
- **pulsation**   rhythmic beat
- **tachycardia**   abnormally fast heartbeat

⬤ RESPIRATION

Respiration is the process of taking oxygen (O_2) into the body and expelling carbon dioxide (CO_2) from the body. One inspiration (breathing in) and one expiration (breathing out) are considered as one *respiration* (Figure 11.6). When you count a patient's respiration, you do not want the patient to be aware of what you are doing. If the patient realizes that you are counting respirations, he may not breathe normally. Count the pulse rate and respirations while you are taking the temperature. When you finish counting the pulse, count the respiration rate. Table 11.5 shows the factors that affect respiration.

Respiratory Characteristics

Age influences respiration. The rate of newborns may be 40 respirations per minute. The normal adult rate is 14 to 18 respirations per minute. Always note the following:

- **Rate.**   What is the number of respirations per minute?
- **Rhythm.**   Are the respirations regular or irregular?

Figure 11.6

Breathing in once (inspiration) and breathing out once (expiration) make up one respiration.

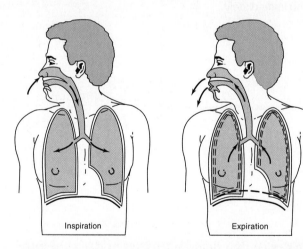

Inspiration   Expiration

Table 11.5 ▪ Factors That Affect Respiration

Increase Respiration	Decrease Respiration
Exercise	Relaxation
Anxiety	Depression
Respiratory disease	Head injury
Medication	Medication
Pain	
Heart disease (e.g., congestive heart failure)	

PROCEDURE 11.7

COUNTING RESPIRATIONS

RATIONALE

As a health care worker it is important to monitor the patient's physical status. One way to determine this status is by count-ing the patient's respiratory rate. This procedure explains how to count the number of times a patient breathes in a minute.

1. Wash hands.
2. Assemble equipment.
   a. Watch with second hand
   b. Pad and pencil
3. Identify patient/client.
4. Do not explain what you are going to do.
5. Relax fingers on pulse point.
6. Observe rise and fall of chest.
7. Count respirations for 1 minute.
8. Note regularity and depth.
9. Wash hands.
10. Record respiratory rate accurately.
11. Report any unusual observation immediately.

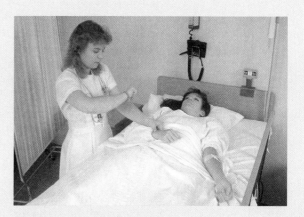

5/22/05   0930
Resp. 20 and regular
_____ M. Taylor CNA

- **Dyspnea.** Is breathing difficult?
- **Apnea.** Has breathing stopped?
- **Cheyne-Stokes.** Are there periods of labored respirations followed by apnea?
- **Rales.** Can you hear bubbling or rattling sounds caused by mucus in the air passages?

Always report any unusual or abnormal respirations to your supervisor.

MEDICAL TERMINOLOGY

- apnea   not breathing
- tachypnea   abnormally fast respirations

RECORDING VITAL SIGNS

Always write the temperature, pulse, and respiration in the same order:

T   P   R

98.6   72   16

Since all health care workers write vital signs in the same way, you do not need to put *T P R* above the figures. Write 98.6/72/16 for an oral temperature. Put an ® next to a rectal temperature (e.g., 99.6®) and an *AX* next to an axillary temperature (e.g., 97.6AX). Some facilities may have a policy and procedure requiring a *T* next to the aural temperature (e.g., 98.6T). These symbols tell other health care workers where you measured the temperature and ensure accuracy. *Always report abnormal or unusual vital signs to your supervisor.*

Taking vital signs may seem routine, but the information is important to the well-being of the patient. Careful recording of vital signs is essential for the protection of the patient.

SUMMARY

You have learned that vital signs are important indicators of the body's condition. Three of these vital signs are temperature, pulse, and respiration. There are many factors that influence TPR in the body, and it is important to be aware of them. You have learned the steps for taking temperature, pulse, and respiration, and you know how to recognize a normal TPR and an abnormal TPR. You may also be responsible for accurate measurement of O_2 in the blood. This information is essential in giving good client care and in recognizing problems with your personal health.

LEARN BY Doing

UNIT 1 ACTIVITY

1. Complete Worksheets 2 through 4 as assigned.
2. Complete Worksheet/Activity 5.
3. Practice the procedures.
4. When you are confident that you can meet each objective listed, ask your instructor for the unit evaluation.

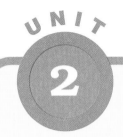

Blood Pressure

STEPS TO SUCCESS

1. Complete Vocabulary Worksheet 1 in the Student Workbook.
2. Read this unit.
3. Complete the Learn by Doing assignment at the end of this unit.

UNIT RATIONALE

You have learned that temperature, pulse, and respiration are signs that indicate whether or not the body is functioning within normal limits. Blood pressure is the fourth vital sign. Measuring the patient's blood pressure gives you a complete picture of his or her vital signs. A complete record of all vital signs helps in the diagnosis and treatment of the patient.

UNIT OBJECTIVES

When you have completed this unit, you will be able to do the following:

✔ Match vocabulary words with their correct meanings.

✔ Define *blood pressure*.

✔ Match descriptions of systolic and diastolic blood pressure.

✔ List four factors that increase blood pressure.

✔ List four factors that can reduce blood pressure.

✔ State the normal range of blood pressure.

✔ Demonstrate how to measure and record a blood pressure accurately.

✔ Explain how vital signs provide information about the patient's health.

⊙ BLOOD PRESSURE

Blood pressure is the force of the blood pushing against the walls of the blood vessels. The *systolic* pressure is the greatest force exerted on the walls of the arteries by the heart. This pressure is exerted when the heart is contracting. You hear the first beat when contraction occurs. The *diastolic* pressure is the least force exerted on the walls of the arteries by the heart. This pressure occurs as the heart relaxes between contractions. When the heart relaxes, there is no sound (beat). Blood pressure depends on the volume of blood in the circulating system, the force of the heartbeat, and the condition of the arteries. When arteries lose their elasticity, they give more resistance, and the blood pressure increases. Table 11.6 shows the factors that affect blood pressure.

Table 11.6 ■ Factors That Affect Blood Pressure

Increase Blood Pressure	Decrease Blood Pressure
Loss of elasticity in the arteries	Hemorrhage
Exercise	Inactivity
Eating	Fasting
Stimulants (e.g., medication, coffee)	Suppressants (e.g., medications that cause blood pressure to lower)
Anxiety	Depression

millimeters

Measure of length.

systolic pressure

Highest pressure against blood vessels. Represented by first heart sound or beat heard when taking a blood pressure.

diastolic pressure

Lowest pressure against the blood vessels of the body. It is measured between contractions.

asymptomatic

Without visible symptoms.

hypotension

Low blood pressure.

apparatus

Equipment needed to perform a task (e.g., blood pressure apparatus includes a blood pressure cuff and a stethoscope).

Normal Blood Pressure

The normal blood pressure range is between 90 and 140 **millimeters** (mm) mercury for the **systolic pressure.** For the **diastolic pressure,** it is between 60 and 90 millimeters (mm) of mercury. When you record a blood pressure, it is written

$$120/80 = \frac{120 \text{ systolic}}{80 \text{ diastolic}}$$

When the blood pressure is above the normal range, it is called hypertension, or high blood pressure. Hypertension is called the silent killer. It is a disease that is **asymptomatic** in most cases. This condition is discovered only when the patient/client has his blood pressure measured. Heredity plays a major role in patients who develop hypertension. Some of the effects are stroke, kidney problems, changes in the retina, and heart disease. When the blood pressure is below the normal range, it is called **hypotension.**

Blood Pressure Apparatus

Blood pressure is measured with an instrument called a **sphygmomanometer.** In the word *sphygmomanometer,*

- **Sphygmo:** refers to pulse
- **Mano:** refers to pressure
- **Meter:** refers to measure

Most health care workers refer to the sphygmomanometer as a BP cuff or blood pressure cuff. There are different kinds of blood pressure apparatus:

- Mercury (This type is not seen often. In many places it is **obsolete.**) (Figure 11.7a)
- Aneroid (Figure 11.7b)
- Electronic/digital (Figure 11.8)

Figure 11.7a

Mercury sphygmomanometer.

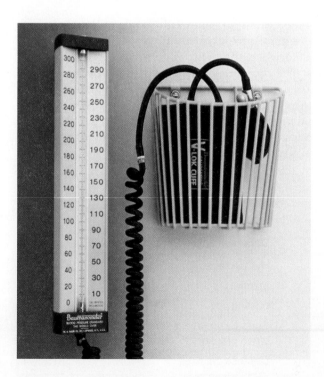

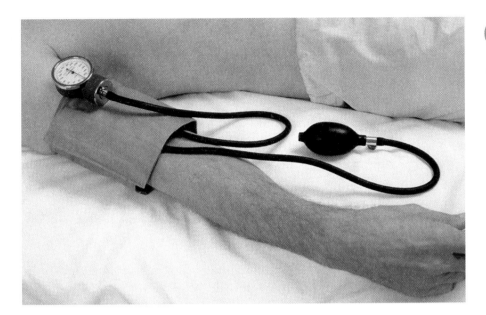

Figure 11.7b

Aneroid sphygmomanometer.

**sphygmo-
manometer**

Measuring device used to
measure the pressure against
the arteries of the body.

obsolete

Out of date.

The mercury and aneroid apparatuses have a **gauge.** The gauge is marked with a series of long and short lines. The long lines are at 10-mm (millimeter) intervals. The short lines are between the long lines. These lines indicate 2 mm (millimeters) each. When you measure a blood pressure, you must do two things at one time. You listen to the heartbeat as it pulses through the artery. You also watch the gauge in order to take a reading.

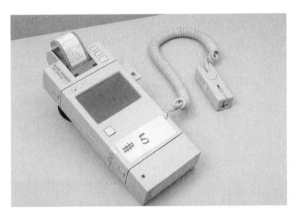

Figure 11.8

Digital sphygmomanometer
and pulse monitor. Place
index finger into finger cuff
and follow directions to
acquire pulse rate and blood
pressure.

The blood pressure cuff is a cloth-covered rubber bladder that fills with air as the bulb is squeezed. When the cuff is **inflated** around the arm, it stops the flow of blood. As the pressure is relieved, the flow returns and you hear a beat. This is the systolic pressure. As the cuff continues to deflate, you hear last a beat and then silence. The last beat you hear is the diastolic pressure.

Stethoscope

When you listen to pulse sounds, you use a stethoscope (see Figure 11.9). A stethoscope picks up sound when it is placed against the body. The stethoscope has earpieces, a spring to help keep the earpieces in the ears, flexible rubber tubing that carries sound, and a bell or diaphragm that magnifies sound.

Ear pieces

Diaphragm

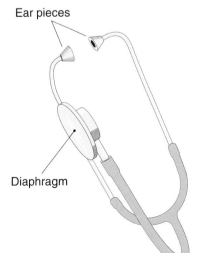

Figure 11.9

Stethoscope.

·gauge

Standard scale for
measurement.

inflated

To swell or fill up with air.

● PALPATING BLOOD PRESSURE

You may be asked to take a blood pressure by first palpating (feeling) the radial pulse. This allows you to determine the correct inflation pressure when inflating the cuff.

PROCEDURE 11.8

MEASURING BLOOD PRESSURE

RATIONALE

As a health care worker it is important to monitor the patient's physical status. One way to determine this status is by measuring the patient's blood pressure. This procedure explains how to determine the patient's systolic (the highest pressure) and diastolic (the lowest pressure) blood pressure.

1. Wash hands.
2. Assemble equipment.
   a. Alcohol wipes
   b. Sphygmomanometer
   c. Stethoscope
   d. Pad and pencil
3. Identify patient/client.
4. Explain what you are going to do.
5. Support patient's arm on firm surface.
6. Apply cuff correctly. (Refer to steps 4 and 5 in procedure "Palpating a Blood Pressure" on page 243.)
7. Clean earpieces on stethoscope.
8. Place earpieces in ears.
9. Locate brachial artery.
10. Tighten thumbscrew on valve.
11. Hold stethoscope in place.
12. Inflate cuff to 170 mm.
13. Open valve; if systolic sound is heard immediately, reinflate cuff to 30 mm mercury above systolic sound.
14. Note systolic at first beat.
15. Note diastolic.
16. Open valve and release air.
17. Record time and blood pressure reading correctly on pad.
18. Wash hands.
19. Wash earpieces on stethoscope.
20. Put away equipment.

21. Record blood pressure in chart.
22. Report any unusual observation immediately.

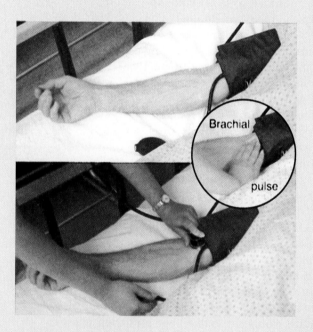

7/29/05   0900
          B/P 134/88
      left arm, sitting
               R. Martin CNA

PROCEDURE 11.9

PALPATING A BLOOD PRESSURE

RATIONALE

As a health care worker it is important to monitor the patient's physical status. One way to determine this status is by measuring the patient's blood pressure. This procedure explains how to palpate a blood pressure so you will know how high to inflate the blood pressure cuff.

1. Wash hands.
2. Tell patient/client what you are going to do.
3. Support patient's arm palm side up on a firm surface.
4. Roll up patient's sleeve above elbow, being careful that it is not too tight.
5. Wrap wide part of cuff around client's arm directly over brachial artery. Lower edge of cuff should be 1 or 2 inches above bend of elbow.
6. Find radial pulse with your fingertips.
7. Inflate cuff until you can no longer feel radial pulse, and continue to inflate another 30 mm of mercury.
8. Open valve and slowly deflate cuff until you feel first beat of radial pulse again.
9. Observe mercury or dial reading. This is the palpatory systolic pressure. It is recorded, for example, as B/P 130 (P).
10. Deflate cuff rapidly and squeeze out all the air.
11. Using your first and second fingers, locate brachial artery. You will feel it pulsating. Place bell or diaphragm of stethoscope directly over artery. You will not hear the pulsation.
12. Tighten thumbscrew of valve to close it.
13. Hold stethoscope in place and inflate cuff until the dial points to about 20 mm above the palpated B/P.
14. Open valve counterclockwise. Let air out slowly until you hear first beat.
15. At this first sound, note reading on sphygmomanometer. This is the systolic pressure.
16. Continue to release air slowly. Note number on the indicator at which you hear last beat or the sound changes to a dull beat. This is the diastolic pressure.
17. Open valve and release all the air.
18. Remove cuff.
19. Record time and blood pressure.
20. Report any unusual observation immediately.

MEDICAL TERMINOLOGY

■ diastolic	least force of pressure exerted against the walls of the arteries		■ stethoscope	instrument used to amplify sound
■ hypertension	high blood pressure		■ systolic	greatest force of pressure exerted against the walls of the arteries
■ hypotension	low blood pressure			

○ SUMMARY

Blood pressure is the fourth vital sign. Many factors influence blood pressure, and an abnormal blood pressure may indicate a serious condition. It is important to be accurate in following the step-by-step instructions for taking a blood pressure, to record the blood pressure of your patient, and to report any abnormalities immediately.

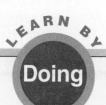

UNIT 2 ACTIVITY

1. Complete Worksheets 2 through 3 as assigned.
2. Practice the procedures.
3. Prepare responses to each item listed in Chapter Review—Your Link to Success at the end of this chapter.
4. When you are confident that you can meet each objective, ask your instructor for the unit evaluation.

Thinking Critically

1. **Communication** You are assigned a patient and you need to take vital signs. Mr. Marks is an elderly man and seems very agitated and upset. You know that his agitation affects his vital signs. What verbal and nonverbal communication skills can you use to help reduce his being upset? Write a brief description of how to help Mr. Marks relax so that you can take accurate vital signs.

2. **Medical Terminology** Define the following medical terms and explain why they are important when taking vital signs: arrhythmia, atypical, aural, axially, centigrade (Celsius), diastole, dyspnea, Fahrenheit, homeostasis, hypertension, hypoxia, hypothalamus, pyrexia, systole, rales, rhonchi, thready, and tympanic membrane.

3. **Safety Alert** Never forget the safety aspects of procedures. For example, when using a glass thermometer, cau-

tion the client not to bite down. Brainstorm with classmates on other safety alerts you should give.

4. **Patient Education** Write a short script for what you would say to a patient as you begin a blood pressure reading. Remember that many patients are frightened of the mounting pressure on their arm.

5. **Case Study** Mr. Ames is on oxygen and cannot breathe comfortably when you remove his oxygen mask. It is time to take his vital signs. He has a severe infection and an accurate temperature is extremely important. What is the correct location for taking his temperature? Explain why. What information is appropriate to give Mr. Ames before you take his temperature?

Portfolio Connection

As a health care worker you are expected to observe clients for their state of health. You are obligated to report any unusual or abnormal signs or symptoms. Write the following in report form. This report demonstrates your evaluating, observing, and reporting skills. Your patient has an elevated blood pressure of 210/140. Does this blood pressure cause concern? What is the medical term for this blood pressure? What are the possible causes of an elevated blood pressure? What can you observe about the patient that is important in your report to your supervisor? Should you report this blood pressure immediately or wait until you report at the end of your day? What are the key things that you must report? Place the report in your portfolio notebook behind the tab marked "Written Reports and Assignments" in the vocational area.

Portfolio Tip

Taking a temperature is a vital procedure, but to many patients it seems a nuisance. Try to explain to the patient as you start the process what a change in temperature will tell the health care staff and how checking it will keep recovery on track.

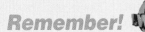

Remember! **Media Connection**

Use the Companion Website **www.prenhall.com/badasch** and the CD-ROM for additional interactive learning activities.

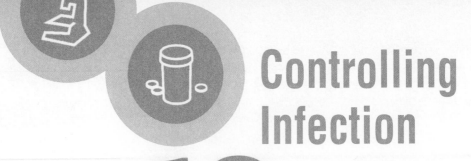

Controlling Infection

Chapter 12

UNIT 1

The Nature of Microorganisms

STEPS TO SUCCESS

1. Complete Vocabulary Worksheet 1 in the Student Workbook.
2. Read this unit.
3. Complete the Learn by Doing assignment at the end of this unit.

UNIT OBJECTIVES

When you have completed this unit, you will be able to do the following:

✔ Match vocabulary words with their correct meanings.

✔ Define *pathogenic* and *nonpathogenic*.

✔ List conditions affecting the growth of bacteria.

✔ List ways that microorganisms cause illness.

✔ List ways that microorganisms spread.

UNIT RATIONALE

Microorganisms are all around us, but we cannot see them. There are both good and bad microorganisms. To help prevent the spread of infection and disease, you must be aware of microorganisms and how they are spread.

✔ List five ways to prevent the spread of microorganisms.

✔ Explain generalized and localized infection.

✔ Explain the difference in signs and symptoms of generalized and localized infections.

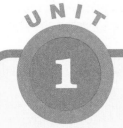

microorganisms

A tiny organism such as a virus, protozoan, or bacterium that can only be seen under a microscope.

anaerobic

Able to grow and function without oxygen.

○ INTRODUCTION TO MICROORGANISMS

We are surrounded by tiny **microorganisms.** They are in the air we breathe, on our skin, in our food, and on everything we touch. You cannot see the organisms without a microscope because they are so small (Figure 12.1). Some of these organisms cause illness, infection, or disease and are called pathogenic. Others are good organisms that help keep a balance in the environment and in the body and are called nonpathogenic.

For microorganisms to live, they must have certain elements in their environment. Some organisms require oxygen in order to survive. These are called *aerobic.* Others live in an environment without oxygen. These are called **anaerobic.** Most microorganisms that cause illness like warm temperatures—about the temperature of the body. All organisms need moisture, and most prefer a dark area to grow in (Figure 12.2). Microorganisms also need food to survive. Some organisms that live on dead matter or tissues are called **saprophytes.** Other organisms that live on living matter or tissues are called **parasites** (Figure 12.2).

Nonpathogenic Organisms

There are many microorganisms that are not **pathogenic.** These organisms, called **nonpathogenic,** are "good" organisms that are used in different ways such as: to make buttermilk, to ferment grain for producing alcoholic beverages, to make bread rise, and so on. Nonpathogenic organisms also **decompose** organic materials in nature. In the body, they work in the digestive system to break down food elements that the body cannot use and eventually eliminates in the form of feces. Nonpathogenic microorganisms also help control the growth of pathogenic organisms.

Pathogenic Organisms

When organisms leave their normal environment in the body and move into other areas, they become pathogens. Some common examples are:

- **Escherichia coli or E. coli** E. coli infections may cause food poisoning and even death. The organism may occur during the butchering process of meat. Organisms from the colon can come in contact with other parts of the beef, thus contaminating the meat. E. coli can be prevented by cooking meat until it reaches a temperature of about 160° F (71.1° C). Poor personal hygiene can allow E. coli to spread from the human colon to the urethra causing urinary tract infections known as **urethritis** and **cystitis.** Health care workers with dirty hands—especially hands that are not washed after toileting—can spread the same E. coli organism to patients' food or onto equipment used to provide care.

- **Salmonella** Salmonella infections may also cause food poisoning or death. Salmonella can occur from eating chicken that is undercooked or from eating foods containing raw eggs. Salmonella can also be spread to food when food service workers do not wash their hands or when cooking utensils or surfaces are not cleaned properly after preparing chicken or egg dishes in particular.

    Health care workers must be aware of the different kinds of pathogenic organisms that cause disease. There are several kinds of disease-causing microorganisms: bacteria, viruses, protozoa, fungi, and **rickettsiae.**

- **Bacteria** Bacteria are responsible for many diseases. For example, strep throat is caused by streptococci, staph infection is caused by staphylococci, and syphilis is caused by **spirochetes.** These are only a few of the diseases that bacteria cause.

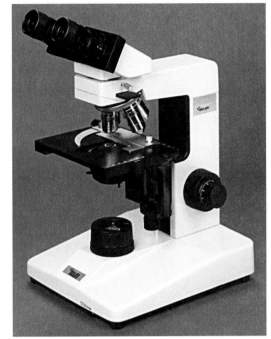

Figure 12.2

Conditions affecting the growth of bacteria.

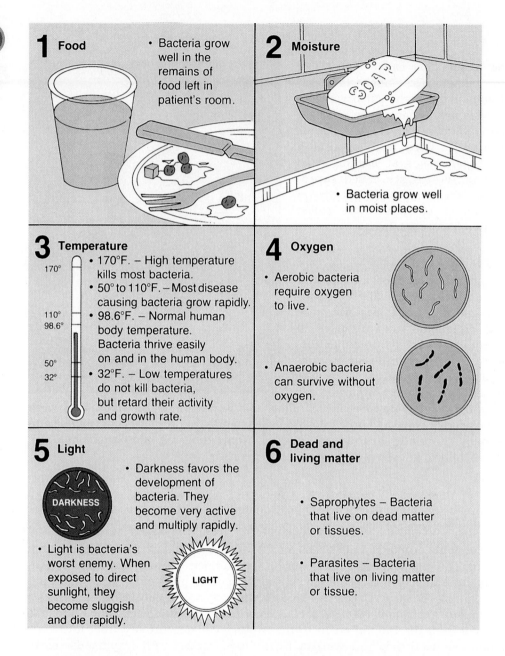

1 Food
- Bacteria grow well in the remains of food left in patient's room.

2 Moisture
- Bacteria grow well in moist places.

3 Temperature
- 170°F. – High temperature kills most bacteria.
- 50° to 110°F. – Most disease causing bacteria grow rapidly.
- 98.6°F. – Normal human body temperature. Bacteria thrive easily on and in the human body.
- 32°F. – Low temperatures do not kill bacteria, but retard their activity and growth rate.

170°
110°
98.6°
50°
32°

4 Oxygen
- Aerobic bacteria require oxygen to live.
- Anaerobic bacteria can survive without oxygen.

5 Light
DARKNESS
- Darkness favors the development of bacteria. They become very active and multiply rapidly.
- Light is bacteria's worst enemy. When exposed to direct sunlight, they become sluggish and die rapidly.

LIGHT

6 Dead and living matter
- Saprophytes – Bacteria that live on dead matter or tissues.
- Parasites – Bacteria that live on living matter or tissue.

Staphylococcus and streptococcus are organisms that are always present in health care environments. Staphylococcus (staph) infections can have a serious impact on patients, staff, and families. An uncontrolled or untreated staph infection in a newborn nursery, for example, can cause infants to die. People who have a stressed immune system have trouble fighting a staph infection and may die. Hospital stays are prolonged because of staph infections. Staph is usually the cause of pimples or boils found on the skin. All drainage from a pimple or boil should be handled according to Standard Precautions to prevent the spread of infection. Patients with staph infections are always treated with Standard Precautions.

■ **Viruses** Viruses are even smaller than bacteria. They cannot grow until they have taken over a living cell. Viruses cause the common cold and many upper respiratory infections. They also cause smallpox, chickenpox, measles, mumps, influenza, and fever blisters. One of the most serious viruses is acquired immunodeficiency syndrome (AIDS). These are only a few of the illnesses caused by viruses.

■ **Protozoa** Protozoa are larger than viruses but also grow within a **host** cell. They cause trichomoniasis, amebic dysentery, and malaria.

■ **Fungi** Fungi are a very low form of plant life. Fungi include molds and yeasts. They can cause athlete's foot, thrush, vaginitis, and serious lung diseases.

■ **Rickettsiae** Rickettsiae are parasites that live in lice, fleas, ticks, and mites. When one of these carriers is infected with rickettsiae and bites a person, the disease is transferred to that person. These parasites are responsible for many of the world's worst epidemics, including various types of typhus, spotted fever, and others. Rodent and insect control helps prevent rickettsiae.

host
The organism from which a microorganism takes nourishment. The microorganism gives nothing in return and causes disease or illness.

HOW MICROORGANISMS AFFECT THE BODY

Pathogens cause disease in several different ways. Some microorganisms produce **toxins** that affect the body. For instance, staphylococcus produces an **enterotoxin** that is the cause of food poisoning. The toxin causes fatigue, diarrhea, and vomiting. The tetanus bacilli produce a toxin that enters the bloodstream and attacks the central nervous system, causing severe damage and frequently death. Some microorganisms invade living cells and destroy them; this is called *cell invasion*. For example, there is a protozoan that invades the red blood cells of the host. As the protozoa grow, the cells rupture and cause chills and fever.

The presence of some microorganisms causes a violent *allergic reaction* in the body. A runny nose, watery eyes, and sneezing can be caused by the presence of a microorganism to which the host is allergic.

toxins
Poisonous substances.

enterotoxin
Poisonous substance that is produced in, or originates in, the contents of the intestine.

HOW MICROORGANISMS SPREAD

Now that you know something about microorganisms, you need to know how they are spread and how they enter the body. This helps you protect yourself and your patients/clients from infection. For microorganisms to cause disease or infection, they must have a **susceptible** host. This host is unable to fight off infection because its resistance to the pathogen is low. Low resistance may be caused by poor diet, fatigue, inadequate rest, stress, or poor health. Table 12.1 shows five primary ways microorganisms are spread.

susceptible
Capable of being affected or infected (e.g., body can be attacked by microorganisms and become ill).

Table 12.1 ■ Five Ways Microorganisms Are Spread

Method	Information	Examples	Prevention Guidelines
Direct contact	Occurs when the organisms are transmitted directly from one person to another.	• Physical contact by touch on open or closed skin or body opening • Sexual contact • Breathing in pathogens directly from an infected person	• Abstain from sex. • Do not drink or eat from dishes or utensils used by another person. • Stay an appropriate distance away from individuals who are coughing or sneezing. • Do not, without proper protection, touch objects used by someone who has an infection.
Indirect contact	Occurs when an organism is transferred from one object to another.	• Contaminated substances such as foods, air, soil, feces, clothing, and equipment	• Do not, without proper protection, touch objects used by someone who has an infection. • Hold contaminated linen, belongings, or other items away from your uniform.

Table 12.1 ▪ Continued

Method	Information	Examples	Prevention Guidelines
Airborne	Some microorganisms are carried in the air. Coughing and sneezing project droplets into the air, and these droplets are carried on air currents until they find a place to land. The droplets cling to hair, uniforms, and medical equipment, or they fall on the floor. As you move from place to place, you may spread these organisms.	• Influenza • Chickenpox • Wound infections	• Keep your hair short or tied back so that it does not swing around, spreading microorganisms. • Cover your mouth and nose when you sneeze, then wash your hands. • Change out of your uniform after working and before going anywhere other than home. • Consider anything dropped on the floor as contaminated, DO NOT USE IT. • Stay home when you are sick with an acute respiratory infection.

Oral route	Microorganisms also enter the body through water, **contaminated** food, dirty hands, and from other contaminated objects.	• Food poisoning
		• Polio
		• Hepatitis
		• Salmonellosis
		• Typhoid fever
			• Wash your hands:
			  • before eating or handling food
			  • using the toilet
			  • helping patients
			• Refrigerate food properly to prevent contamination and microorganism growth.
			• Dispose of wound drainage promptly and according to policy.

Insects and pests	Organisms are picked up from contaminated areas and carried to water, food, and people.	• Bubonic plague • Malaria • Amoebic dysentery	• Keep all flies and insects out of the environment. • Report insects or pests immediately.

contaminated   Soiled, unclean, not suitable for use.

PROTECTION FROM MICROORGANISMS

Standard Precautions and Transmission-Based Precautions were created to provide guidelines that prevent the spread of microorganisms. These guidelines are described in Unit 3 of this chapter. Read the guidelines carefully and follow them whenever infectious microorganisms are present.

SIGNS AND SYMPTOMS OF INFECTION

generalized

Affecting all of the body.

localized

Affecting one area of the body.

An infection may be **generalized** or it may be **localized.** If the infection is generalized, there is usually headache, fatigue, fever, and increased pulse and respiration. There may also be vomiting and/or diarrhea. If the infection is localized, you can see and feel one or more of the following: redness, swelling, heat, and/or drainage. There is usually pain at the site of the infection.

SUMMARY

We are surrounded by microorganisms. They are in the air we breathe, on our skin, in our food, and on everything we touch. Some microorganisms are pathogens; others are nonpathogens. Pathogens include some bacteria, viruses, protozoa, fungi, and rickettsiae. Since pathogens cause illness, it is important to understand how they are spread and how they can be controlled. Learning the signs and symptoms of infection will help you provide better patient care.

It is the responsibility of every health care worker to help prevent the spread of infection. Every year thousands of patients have extended stays in the hospital because they have acquired an infection while hospitalized. It is vital that all health care workers practice good techniques to prevent the spread of infection.

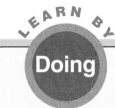

Doing

UNIT 1 ACTIVITY

1. Complete Worksheet 2 and Worksheets/Activities 3 & 4.
2. When you are confident that you can meet each objective, ask your instructor for the unit evaluation.

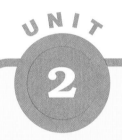

Asepsis

STEPS TO SUCCESS

1. Complete Vocabulary Worksheet 1 in the Student Workbook.
2. Read this unit.
3. Complete the Learn by Doing assignment at the end of this unit.

UNIT RATIONALE

The environment of the health care worker contains larger numbers of microorganisms than do most other environments. The health care worker must acquire the knowledge and skills required to restrict the spread of pathogenic microorganisms. The health care worker who practices good aseptic technique and follows Standard Precautions protects patient, co-workers, and the community from infection.

UNIT OBJECTIVES

When you have completed this unit, you will be able to do the following:

✔ Define *medical asepsis*.

✔ Match terms related to medical asepsis with their correct meanings.

✔ List five aseptic techniques.

✔ List some of the Standard Precaution guidelines concerning the use of protective equipment.

✔ Demonstrate appropriate handwashing techniques.

✔ Explain the difference between *bactericidal* and *bacteriostatic*.

✔ List reasons why asepsis is important.

INTRODUCTION TO ASEPSIS

Health care facilities are filled with people who are ill. Some of their illnesses are caused by body dysfunctions; others are caused by infections or injury. Thus, health care environments are constantly contaminated with pathogenic microorganisms

aseptic technique

Methods used to make the environment, the worker, and the patient as germ-free as possible.

nosocomial infection

An infection acquired while in a health care setting, such as a hospital.

Standard Precautions

Guidelines designed to reduce the risk of trans-mission of microorganisms from recognized and unrecognized sources of infection in the hospital.

transmitting

Causing to go from one person to another person.

carried in by patients, visitors, and staff. This constant presence of pathogens requires the staff to wage an all-out battle against these organisms. This battle is waged by the continual use of medical asepsis, which means to destroy the environment that allows pathogens to live, breed, and spread. Medical asepsis is accomplished by using **aseptic technique.** Aseptic technique is very important when you are working with patients/clients. The practice of aseptic technique helps to prevent

- Cross infection, which is caused by infecting the patient with a new microorganism from another patient or health care worker **(nosocomial infection)**
- Reinfection with the same microorganism that caused the original illness
- Self-inoculation by the patient's own organisms, such as E. coli from the intestines entering the urethra
- An illness passing from the patient to the health care worker or from the health care worker to the patient

Aseptic technique includes

- Employees being clean and neat
- Proper handling of all equipment
- Using sterile procedure when necessary
- Using proper cleaning solutions: *bacteriostatic* solutions, which slow or stop the growth of bacteria, or *bactericidal* solutions, which kill bacteria
- Proper handwashing
- Following **Standard Precautions**

The health care team must strive toward achieving an aseptic environment to reduce the infection rate in the health care setting.

STANDARD PRECAUTIONS

Special precautions are necessary to lower the risk of **transmitting** pathogens from person to person. In 1985, health care isolation practices in the United States changed to defend against the increased risk of exposure to hepatitis B virus (HBV) and human immunodeficiency virus (HIV). For the first time, all blood and body fluids were treated as infected substances. The Occupational Safety and Health Administration (OSHA) of the U.S. Department of Labor established mandatory guidelines published in the Occupational Exposure to Bloodborne Pathogens: Final Rule. These guidelines ensure that all employers provide personal protective equipment to employees at risk of exposure to body fluids. In 1992, OSHA increased its mandate to employers, insisting that training and immunization be provided to all employees within 10 days of hire. This means that employees at risk for exposure to body fluids must

- Be offered hepatitis B vaccine (HBV) at no charge
- Be trained to use the appropriate protective equipment to prevent exposure to body fluids
- Receive an annual update and review

In 1996, the Centers for Disease Control and Prevention (CDC) expanded the bloodborne pathogen guidelines to assist in the prevention of nosocomial infections. These expanded guidelines are known as Standard Precautions. Standard Precautions are appropriate for all patients receiving care or service in a health care environment regardless of their diagnosis. Standard Precautions provide protection from contact with blood, mucous membranes, nonintact skin, and all body fluids. Body fluids include the following:

- Blood
- Vaginal secretions
- Pericardial fluid
- Body fluids containing visible blood
- **Amniotic fluid**
- **Peritoneal fluid**
- Tissue specimens
- **Cerebrospinal fluid**
- **Interstitial fluid**
- **Semen**
- **Pleural fluid**

    Infection with HBV and HIV occur through

- Direct injection of infected blood or a contaminated needle that punctures the skin
- Contact of infected body fluids with mucous membranes such as the eye or inside of the mouth
- Sexual contact
- Pregnancy—when the mother is infected, the infection is transferred to the newborn infant

    The risk of being infected in the health care setting is high. It is important for you to treat all patients as though they were infected. If you provide hands-on care to patients, you must follow all Standard Precaution guidelines (see Table 12.2) to protect yourself and others. Make it a habit to follow each step in the Standard Precaution guidelines.

amniotic fluid
Liquid that surrounds the fetus during pregnancy.

peritoneal fluid
Liquid in the peritoneal cavity.

cerebrospinal fluid
Liquid that flows through and around brain tissue.

interstitial fluid
Liquid that fills the space between most of the cells of the body.

semen
Fluid from the testes, seminal vesicles, prostate gland, and bulbourethral glands.

pleural fluid
Liquid that surrounds the lungs.

Table 12.2 ▪ Standard Precaution Guidelines	
Protective Equipment	**When to Use Personal Protective Equipment (PPE)**

Gloves (see procedure for removing gloves on page 271)	• Wear when in contact with
	  —Any body fluid
	  —Nonintact skin and mucous membrane
	• Wear when your hands are chapped, when a rash is present, or when you have open sores present.

Nonpermeable gowns or aprons (see procedure for removing and discarding gowns on page 271)	• Wear during procedures that are likely to expose you to
	  —Any body fluid
	  —Nonintact skin and mucous membrane

Mask and protective eyewear or face shield	• Wear when
	  —Body fluid droplets or splashes are likely
	  —Patients are coughing continuously

Special masks and eyewear that seal against face	• Wear when assisting with procedures that cause body tissues to be aerosolized (e.g., laser treatments).

Table 12.2 ■ Continued	
Protective Equipment	**When to Use Personal Protective Equipment (PPE)**
Handwashing (see procedure on page 263)	• Wash hands before putting on and after removing gloves and before and after working with each patient with his or her equipment, or both.
Shared equipment/ multiple-use patient care equipment (e.g., blood pressure cuff, stethoscope, aural thermometer)	• Remove all equipment for cleaning immediately upon contact with —Any body fluid —Nonintact skin and mucous membrane

sterilized

Made free from all living microorganisms.

disinfection

Process of freeing from microorganisms by physical or chemical means.

exposed

Left unprotected.

autoclaves

Sterilizers that use steam under pressure to kill all forms of bacteria on fomites (objects that pathogens live on and can transfer infection).

● CONTROLLING THE SPREAD OF INFECTION

Skin and hair cannot be **sterilized** because any solutions or procedures that kill microorganisms are harmful to skin. You use a bacteriostatic solution for cleaning skin. Bacteriocidal solutions are used on equipment. This method of controlling the spread of infection is called **disinfection.** A 10% solution of household bleach can be used to disinfect items that tolerate exposure to mild bleach solution.

CAUTION   Never use bleach on any item that will be put into the body or with any other product (e.g., cleansers, sprays).

Sterilization is the process of killing all microorganisms, even spores (bacteria with a protective hard shell around them). Spores are killed when they are **exposed** to steam under pressure at a high temperature. **Autoclaves** are used to produce steam. Gas autoclaves and chemical baths are used to sterilize equipment that would be damaged by steam. Items needing sterilization are those that are put into the body or around an open wound.

Handwashing is the process of removing microorganisms from contaminated hands. Proper handwashing is the most effective way to prevent infecting yourself or others. See Table 12.3 for proper handwashing guidelines.

Table 12.3 ■ Handwashing Guidelines	
Directions	**Information**
Always wash your hands • Before and after contact with a patient and/or patient's belongings • Before and after eating • After using the bathroom • After handling any contaminated fluid or object	Handwashing is the *most effective way* to reduce the spread of microorganisms.
Use enough soap from dispenser to make a good lather.	A bar of soap is considered contaminated after it is opened.
Interlace your fingers together and rub all sides of fingers and hands to produce friction.	Lather and friction help remove micro-organisms.

Table 12.3 ■ Continued	
Directions	**Information**
Hold hands lower than elbows and rinse thoroughly to remove pathogens.	This prevents lather and water from running over arms and causing contamination.
Turn off faucets with paper towel.	Faucets and sink are considered contaminated.
Rewash your hands if you touch the sink or faucet.	Touching a contaminated area recontaminates your hands.
Dry hands completely.	Reddened and chapped hands easily leave open areas that can become infected.

PROCEDURE 12.1

HANDWASHING

RATIONALE:

Contaminated hands are the most common cause of infection. Proper handwashing technique is the most effective way to prevent the spread of infection.

1. Tear off paper towel to turn off faucets.
2. Turn on water.

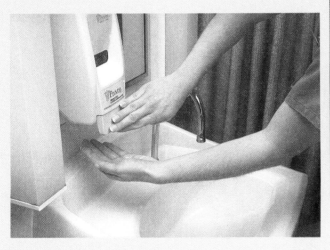

3. Regulate water temperature.
4. Wet hands, fingers pointed downward.

5. Apply soap to hands and wrists.

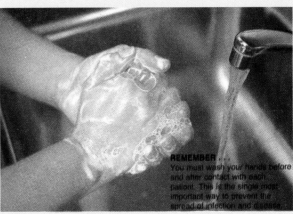

REMEMBER . . .
You must wash your hands before and after contact with each patient. This is the single most important way to prevent the spread of infection and disease.

6. Rub hands in circular motion.
7. Interlace fingers, rub back and forth to create friction (add water when necessary to keep moist).

PROCEDURE 12.1 | HANDWASHING *(Continued)*

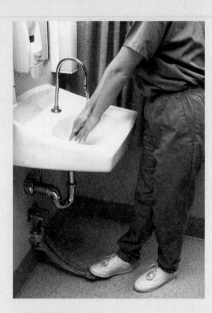

8. Use a nailbrush. If none is available, rub fingernails on palms of hands.

9. Rinse with fingers pointed down.

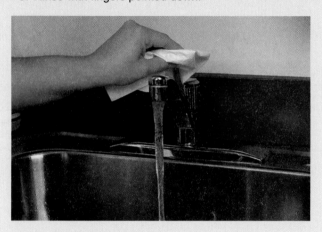

10. Dry hands with paper towel.
11. Turn off faucet with paper towel.
12. Leave area clean and neat.

⬤ SUMMARY

Infection control is critical in health care environments. Asepsis is the method used to destroy the environment that allows pathogens to live, breed, and spread. Major factors in the control of microorganisms are handwashing, disinfection, sterilization, and following Standard Precautions. The effective health care worker always strives to provide an aseptic environment by following aseptic technique procedures and Standard Precautions.

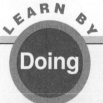

LEARN BY **Doing**

UNIT 2 ACTIVITY

1. Complete Worksheet 2.
2. Practice the procedures.
3. When you are confident that you can meet each objective, ask your instructor for the unit evaluation.

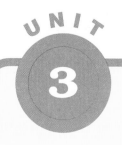

UNIT 3

Standard Precautions and Transmission-Based Precautions

STEPS TO SUCCESS

1. Read this unit.

2. Complete the Learn by Doing assignment at the end of this unit.

UNIT RATIONALE

As a health care worker, you are exposed to patients, equipment, and supplies that are contaminated with pathogens. An estimated 2.4 million hospital-acquired infections occur in the United States each year. It is possible that these infections cause 30,000 deaths annually. Use the techniques taught in this chapter to protect yourself and others and help prevent the spread of infection to patients, co-workers, and the community.

UNIT OBJECTIVES

When you have completed this unit, you will be able to do the following:

✔ Name primary levels of precautions identified in the guidelines developed by the Centers for Disease Control and Prevention (CDC).

✔ Identify three types of Transmission-Based Precautions.

✔ Demonstrate the correct procedure for entering and leaving an area where Transmission-Based Precautions are followed.

✔ Differentiate between Standard Precautions and Transmission-Based Precautions.

⦿ INTRODUCTION TO STANDARD AND TRANSMISSION-BASED PRECAUTIONS

The 1996 guidelines from the CDC established the need for two levels of protection. Standard Precautions, the primary strategy for successful hospital-acquired (nosocomial) infection control, are appropriate for all patients receiving care or service in a health care environment, regardless of their diagnosis. As stated in Unit 2, these precautions provide protection from contact with blood, mucous membranes, non-intact skin, and all body fluids. Transmission-Based Precautions are designed for patients suspected to be infected with pathogens spread by **airborne** or **droplet** transmission, contact with dry skin, or contaminated surfaces.

Transmission-Based Precautions are used in addition to Standard Precautions when some contagious diseases are present. There are three types of Transmission-Based Precautions:

- **Airborne** Precautions
- **Droplet** Precautions
- Contact Precautions

Follow the guidelines in Table 12.4 when working with patients in Transmission-Based Precaution environments.

airborne
Particles that float in the air.

droplet
A small drop of fluid.

Table 12.4 ■ Transmission-Based Precautions

Common Communicable Diseases Requiring Special Precautions	Type of Precautions		Precaution Guidelines				
Chickenpox (varicella) Tuberculosis Herpes zoster (varicella zoster)	**Airborne**	*Reduces the spread of airborne droplet nuclei (5 **microns** or smaller in size) or dust particles containing the pathogen*	Standard Precautions	Private room with specific ventilation criteria	Keep the room door closed	Wear respiratory protection	**Wash hands** • before entering the room • before leaving the room • after leaving the room
Haemophilus influenzae Some forms of meningitis Diphtheria Pertussis Adenovirus Mumps Some forms of pneumonia Severe viral infections	**Droplet**	*Reduces the risk of transmission by contact of the mucous membranes of the eye, nose, or mouth with large-particle droplets*	Standard Precautions	Private room or room with another patient with same microorganism		Wear a mask when working within 3 feet of the patient	**Wash hands** • before entering the room • before leaving the room • after leaving the room
Multidrug-resistant infections of • Gastrointestinal system • Respiratory system • Integumentary (skin) system	**Contact**	*Reduces the risk of transmission through direct or indirect contact*	Standard Precautions	Private room or room with another patient with same microorganism		Expecting contact with the patient or with contaminated surfaces	**Wash hands** • before entering the room • before leaving the room • after leaving the room

microns   Units equaling one millionth of a meter.

TRANSMISSION-BASED PRECAUTION ROOMS

Figures 12.3 and 12.4 illustrate precautions that should be taken within the room when contagious diseases are present. When entering or leaving a Transmission-Based Precaution room, follow the specific directions on the precaution card at the door. The procedures titled *Applying Personal Protective Equipment* and *Removing Personal Protective Equipment* guide you through the steps in applying and removing personal protective equipment. Each medical environment determines the specific order in which to apply each item. Always follow your organization's policies and procedures.

Transmission-Based Precautions

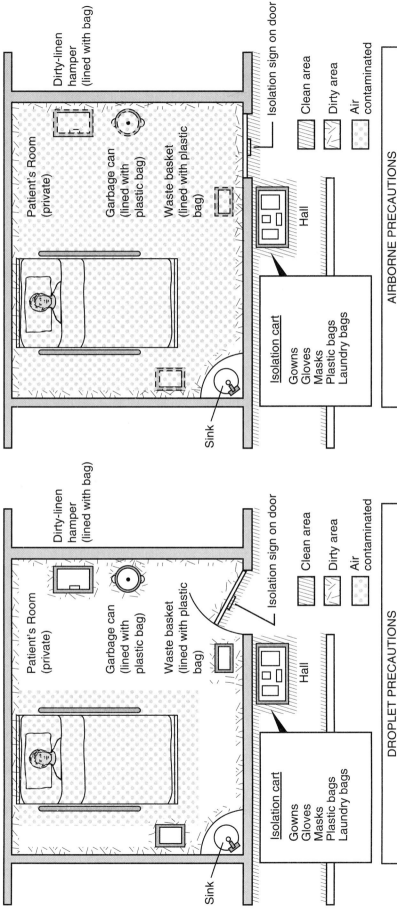

DROPLET PRECAUTIONS
(droplets larger than 5 microns in size)
Visitors – Report to Nurses' Station
Before Entering Room

1. Masks are indicated for those who come within 3 feet of the patient.
2. Gowns are not indicated.
3. Gloves are indicated per Standard Precautions (for contact with blood or body fluids).
4. Hands must be washed after touching the patient or potentially contaminated articles and before taking care of another patient.
5. Articles contaminated with infective material should be discarded or bagged and labeled before being sent for decontamination and reprocessing.

AIRBORNE PRECAUTIONS
(droplets smaller than 5 microns in size)
Visitors – Report to Nurses' Station
Before Entering Room

1. Masks are indicated.
2. Gowns are indicated only if needed to prevent gross contamination of clothing.
3. Gloves are indicated per Standard Precautions (for contact with blood or body fluids).
4. Hands must be washed after touching the patient or potentially contaminated articles and before taking care of another patient.
5. Articles should be discarded, cleaned, or sent for decontamination and reprocessing.

Figure 12.3

Transmission-Based Precautions.

Figure 12.4

Contact precautions.

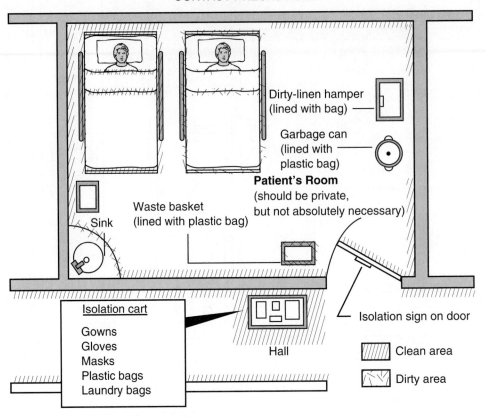

CONTACT PRECAUTIONS

Dirty-linen hamper (lined with bag)

Garbage can (lined with plastic bag)

Patient's Room
(should be private, but not absolutely necessary)

Waste basket (lined with plastic bag)

Sink

Isolation sign on door

Hall

Clean area

Dirty area

Isolation cart

Gowns
Gloves
Masks
Plastic bags
Laundry bags

CONTACT PRECAUTIONS
Visitors – Report to Nurses' Station
Before Entering Room

1. **Masks** are not indicated.
2. **Gowns** are indicated if soiling is likely.
3. **Gloves** are indicated for touching infective material.
4. **Hands must be washed after touching the patient or potentially contaminated articles and before taking care of another patient.**
5. **Articles** contaminated with infective material should be discarded or bagged and labeled before being sent for decontamination and reprocessing.

A private room is indicated for Contact Precautions if patient hygiene is poor. A patient with poor hygiene does not wash hands after touching infective material, contaminates the environment with infective material, or shares contaminated articles with other patients. In general, patients infected with the same organism may share a room.

Psychosocial Issues During Special Precautions

Patients who are placed in special precaution rooms and separated from other patients and health care staff may begin to feel isolated and alone. Prolonged periods in isolation could cause the patient to feel angry, depressed,

Table 12.5 ■ Age-Specific Considerations

RATIONALE: Isolation is difficult for patients of any age. Understanding the special needs of each group gives the patient a sense of security and improves the healing process.

Age	Communication	Comfort	Safety
Birth–5 years	Explain the reason for isolation to the parents and family members.	Keep child with parent or family member to increase feeling of security.	Teach family the procedures that must be followed in an isolation area.
5–12 years	Explain the reason for isolation and the importance of staying in the isolation unit.	Keep child with parent or family member to increase feeling of security.	Teach patient, parent, or family member the procedures.
12+ years	Explain the reason for isolation and the importance of staying in the isolation unit.	Encourage peer, parent, or family member to stay as much as possible.	Teach patient, peer, and family members the procedures for isolation.

and frustrated. It is important for the health care worker to provide time for frequent communication and to assess the patient's comfort level. Taking steps to educate patients and their families on procedures and expectations during special precaution situations could help reduce anxiety for everyone involved. You can make a difference by staying attuned and responding to patients' feelings and moods, always treating each person with dignity, and by providing the very best care. Some age-specific considerations for patients/clients requiring Transmission-Based Precautions are listed in Table 12.5.

⬤ TRANSMISSION-BASED PRECAUTIONS

Transmission-Based Precautions may be difficult for patients. They are alone most of the time. Visitors must wear personal protective wear. Hugs or touching may not be allowed. The health care worker cannot stay and visit because there is other work to do. This may cause the patient to feel angry, depressed, and frustrated. Take as much time as you can to listen to the client's feelings and concerns. Encourage communication and be supportive. If the patient seems unusually upset, report it to your supervisor.

PROCEDURE 12.2 **TRANSMISSION-BASED PRECAUTIONS: APPLYING PERSONAL PROTECTIVE EQUIPMENT**

RATIONALE

A primary responsibility of all health care workers is to prevent the spread of pathogenic microorganisms. Wearing appropriate protective equipment is one way health care workers can protect themselves and others from being infected by pathogenic microorganisms.

1. Assemble equipment.
2. Wash hands.
3. Cover all hair on head with a paper cap.
4. Put on a mask by:
    a. Unfolding mask if appropriate.
    b. Cover mouth and nose with mask.

   c. Secure mask by:
     Pull elastic on each side of mask over ear, or
     Tie top string at sides of mask at back of head and tie lower string at back of neck.

PROCEDURE 12.2 **TRANSMISSION-BASED PRECAUTIONS: APPLYING PERSONAL PROTECTIVE EQUIPMENT** *(Continued)*

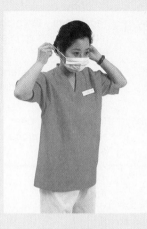

5. Put on gown with opening at back.

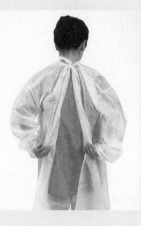

a. Tie bow at back of neck.
b. Overlap gown edges.
c. Tie at waist.

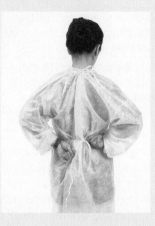

d. Make sure that uniform is completely covered.

PROCEDURE 12.3 TRANSMISSION-BASED PRECAUTIONS: REMOVING PERSONAL PROTECTIVE EQUIPMENT

RATIONALE

A primary responsibility of all health care workers is to prevent the spread of pathogenic microorganisms. Removing and disposing of protective equipment appropriately is one way health care workers prevent the spread of pathogenic microorganisms.

1. Untie waist tie of gown.
2. Remove gloves by:
   a. Pulling the first glove inside out as you remove it from hand.
   b. While holding the inside out glove in remaining gloved hand—pull glove off hand covering the first glove. (The second glove removed surrounds the first and both are inside out.) Discard.
3. Wash hands.
4. Untie gown at neck.
5. Remove gown by:
   a. Crossing arms and grasping shoulder of gown with each hand.
   b. Pull gown forward causing it to fold inside out.
   c. Roll gown so that all contaminated portions are inside of roll and place in dirty hamper marked "*Toxic Waste*" or "*Hazardous Waste*" inside room.
6. Wash hands.
7. Remove cap and mask, and discard.

8. Use paper towel to open door.

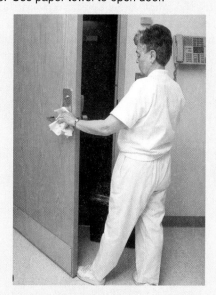

9. Discard towel inside room.
10. Wash hands immediately after leaving the room.

◉ SUMMARY

In this unit you learned about Transmission-Based Precautions, which are designed for patients suspected to be infected with pathogens. In the preceding unit you learned about Standard Precautions, which are required for the care of all patients. Your careful use of these precautions prevents transmission of infectious agents that cause disease and illness in yourself and others.

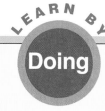

UNIT 3 ACTIVITY

1. Complete Worksheet 1.
2. Practice the procedures.
3. When you are confident that you can meet each objective for this unit, ask your instructor for the unit evaluation.
4. Complete Chapter Review—Your Link to Success at the end of the chapter.

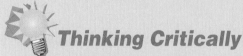

Thinking Critically

1. **Communication** Write a half-page scenario describing how you would explain to a patient the precautionary measures taken daily to control infection in the health care environment. Think in simple terms, such as replacing handkerchiefs with disposable tissues.

2. **Patient Education** A patient in a Transmission-Based Precaution room requests fresh water immediately after you have cleaned her wound. After you wash your hands and return to get the water jug it becomes clear from her distressed silence that she is offended. Think of ways to talk to her about asepsis and passing on infection so that she understands that this is not a personal matter.

3. **Computers** Advances in medicine are continually changing the way health care workers protect themselves and treat infections. Explain how computers help keep the med-

ical community informed about the latest medical progress. Describe ways you can access this information if you do not own a computer.

4. **Patient Satisfaction** Patients in restricted Transmission-Based Precautions feel isolated and locked away from everyday life. They are often avoided by health care workers and family because of the additional, time-consuming procedures required for their care. Mrs. Grey was just admitted for a respiratory tubercle bacillus (tuberculosis—T/B) infection. Her condition requires her to be in Transmission-Based, Airborne Precautions. Write a plan telling how you will provide a sense of comfort and satisfaction while she is in the hospital. Include details about how you will identify and satisfy her special needs.

Portfolio Connection

1. The medical community is constantly finding new information about how microorganisms affect our lives. This constant flow of new information makes it necessary to research how new findings affect us. Conduct your own research and write a research paper about a microorganism. Select a microorganism from those mentioned in this chapter or from another source. Explain how the microorganism affects society and describe its shape, size, color, and pattern of growth. Describe its nature (aerobic or anaerobic), its effect on the body, and the physical symptoms it causes.

2. Contact a local hospital or the County Health Department infection control manager and ask for permission to visit the site and conduct an interview. Develop questions to ask during the interview that will provide insight into the greatest infectious health risks in the hospital or community and find out why the risk is so high. Write a report and place it in the section of your portfolio labeled "Written Reports and Assignments."

Portfolio Tip

Health care levels of cleanliness may be more demanding than some households. Patients are not necessarily dirty when noncompliant and must not be shamed. It is important to show patients and their families respect in all situations. Role-play with a classmate and record for your portfolio the rationales you would give two patients. One patient wants to bathe morning and night while the other patient prefers bathing only once a week. Without quoting facility policy, how would you explain to each patient what the acceptable levels of hygiene are and the reasons for them?

Remember! 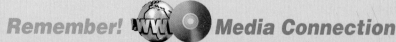 *Media Connection*

Use the Companion Website **www.prenhall.com/badasch** and the CD-ROM for additional interactive learning activities.

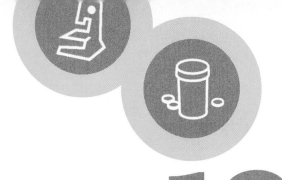

Chapter **13** Patient and Employee Safety

MEDIA CONNECTION

Use the Companion Website
www.prenhall.com/badasch and the CD-ROM
for additional interactive learning activities.

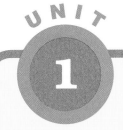

UNIT 1

General Safety and Injury and Illness Prevention

STEPS TO SUCCESS

1. Complete Vocabulary Worksheet 1 in the Student Workbook.
2. Read this unit.
3. Complete the Learn by Doing assignment at the end of this unit.

UNIT RATIONALE

A health care worker is responsible for maintaining a safe environment. You must know your employer's policies and procedures and be able to respond quickly to prevent injury. Your employer is also obligated to provide a safe environment by supplying equipment that protects against injury. The Occupational Safety and Health Ad-

ministration (OSHA) of the U.S. Department of Labor determines, develops, and monitors safe practices for each industry. The Joint Commission on Accreditation of Health Care Organizations (JCAHO) establishes guidelines for the operation of health care facilities. It conducts accreditation surveys that endorse OSHA standards. JCAHO audits look for policy and procedures that follow OSHA guidelines. Health care agencies strive to achieve excellence by meeting OSHA and JCAHO standards. Keeping you and those served by your health care agency safe is a priority for your employer. If you or your employer fails to provide appropriate safety for all, OSHA will penalize your employer with a large fine or lock the doors of the facility until the safety violation is corrected. If you are at fault for not providing safe conditions, you could lose your job.

UNIT OBJECTIVES

When you have completed this unit, you will be able to do the following:

✔ Match vocabulary words to their correct meanings.

✔ Define *OSHA* and explain the agency's role in safety.

✔ Differentiate between IIPP, hazard communication, and exposure control.

✔ Name places to find information about hazards in a facility.

✔ Explain the health care worker's role in maintaining a safe workplace.

✔ Discuss the employer's role in maintaining a safe workplace.

✔ Identify 14 general safety rules.

✔ Summarize the importance of safety in a health care environment.

comply

To follow directions, do what you are asked to do.

OSHA STANDARDS

The Occupational Safety and Health Administration (OSHA) is part of the U.S. Department of Labor. OSHA establishes the guidelines for a safe work environment for all employers and their employees. The OSHA standards say that employees have the "right to know" what hazards are present in their environment. OSHA regulations require employers to train and offer immunization to high-risk employees in the first 10 days of a new job. A committed partnership between the employer and employee is necessary to provide a safe environment for everyone. This unit explains the areas with which health care agencies and facilities must **comply.** They are the

- Ergonomic Program
- Injury and Illness Prevention Program
- Hazard Communication Program
- Exposure Control Plan

Ergonomic Program

ergonomic

Related to the study of the work environment.

Employers are changing the work environment to meet the expected OSHA **ergonomic** standard. You spend a large portion of your day in the work environment. You should be comfortable, use good posture, and learn the exercises to prevent getting stiff and sore. The safety officer where you work will help you adjust your environment to accomplish this. If you sit in a workstation during the day, your chair, desk, and computer must be adjusted to fit your needs. There are exercises in your Student Workbook to help you evaluate your work environment to ensure that you are in good alignment as you work. This prevents physical problems caused by improper working conditions.

Injury and Illness Prevention Program

mandates

Commands, orders.

implement

To accomplish; make it work.

The Injury and Illness Prevention Program (IIPP) **mandates** that every employer establish, **implement,** and maintain an effective IIPP.

As a student or employee, you are responsible for

- Knowing who is responsible in the facility for the IIPP.
- Practicing policy and procedures that ensure safe and healthy work practices.
- Understanding the communication system used to keep you informed of

    • Hazards • Personal protective equipment (PPE) • Knowing how you learn about hazards on the work site
- Knowing what hazards are present and how to prevent injury from them.
- Knowing to whom to report an injury or illness during work hours and what documentation to complete.
- Knowing where the safety bulletin board (or communication book) is in your facility. You are responsible for reading all items posted each month.

Your school or employer will test you for signs of tuberculosis (TB). Exposure to tuberculosis is determined by a TB skin test. If your TB test indicates exposure, additional tests will be necessary. You will also be offered hepatitis B vaccine. This vaccine protects you from getting hepatitis B while working in the health care environment.

Hazard Communication Program

The Hazard Communication Program mandates that employers inform employees of

- Chemicals or hazards in the environment
- Where chemicals or hazards are stored and used

- How to interpret chemical labels and hazard signs
- Methods and equipment for cleaning chemical spills
- Personal protection equipment and its storage location
- The hazard communication system

As a student or employee you are responsible for knowing

- What chemicals or hazards are in your work area
- Where the chemicals or hazards are stored or used
- How to read and interpret container signs and labels
- What to do when a chemical or **biohazard** spills
- What personal protective equipment (PPE) to wear when working with or around chemicals and biohazards
- Your facility's system for informing you of hazards in the work area

biohazard

Substance that has potential to transmit disease.

Hazard Categories

The way that harm is caused determines the hazard category.

- *Physical hazards* cause harm when a chemical is mixed with another chemical, causing a reaction. When a chemical reacts with another substance or because of temperature change, it creates a new chemical. For example: Chlorine bleach mixed with ammonia creates a harmful gas.
- *Health hazards* have the potential to harm a healthy body. For example, acid burns and destroys skin.

Material Safety Data Sheets (MSDSs)

Product manufacturers prepare material safety data sheet (MSDS) forms to provide the information needed to handle chemicals safely. Employers must make the MSDSs available to employees. Figure 13.1 identifies the type of information discussed on the MSDS.

The Hazard Communication Program explains how the employer plans to keep people safe when chemicals are present. The communication system must explain

- What hazards are present and where they are stored and used.
- What precautions to take when hazardous products are present. These precautions include

  • Wearing appropriate personal protective equipment (PPE) • Proper room ventilation • Keeping flammable products away from flames or other heat sources

- How to use potentially hazardous products safely.
- Proper cleanup and disposal of hazardous products.
- First aid if exposure occurs.
- How to label containers with a chemical, by always including

  • Product name • Chemicals in the product • Precautions for use of the product

As a student or employee you are responsible for knowing where hazard communications are kept and how to access them. You find hazard information on manufacturer's literature. You may receive memorandums from your employer

MATERIAL SAFETY DATA SHEET

I   Product Identification

COMPANY NAME: Calgon Vestal Laboratories
ADDRESS: 5035 Manchester Avenue   Nights: 314-802-2000
St. Louis, Missouri 63110   CHEMTREC: (800) 424-9300
PRODUCT NAME: Klenzyme   Product No.:   1103
SYNONYMS: Medical Apparatus and Instrument Presoak

II   Hazardous Ingredients of Mixtures

Material	(CAS#)	% by Wt.	TLV	PEL
Subtilisins (Proteolytic enzymes)	(9014-01-1)	< 5	.06ppb	N/A
Sodium tetraborate, decahydrate	(1303-96-4)	< 5	5mg/m3	10mg/m3

III   Physical Data

Vapor Pressure, mmHg: N/A
Evaporation Rate (ether = 1): N/A
Solubility in H_2O: Complete
Freezing Point F: N/A
Boiling Point F: > 212F
Specific Gravity H_2O = 1 @ 25C: 1.08

Vapor Density (Air = 1) 60–90 F: Undeterm.
% Volatile by wt: N/A
pH @ Undiluted Solution: N/A
pH as Distributed: 7.5–8.0
Appearance: Amber liquid
Odor: Typical, mild odor

IV   Fire and Explosion

Flash Point F: N/A   Flammable Limits: N/A
Extinguishing Media: Not flammable. In event of fire, use water fog, CO_2, and dry chemical.
Special Fire Fighting Procedures: No special requirements given. As with any chemical fire, proper cautions should be taken, such as wearing a self-contained breathing apparatus.
Unusual Fire and Explosion Hazards: None known

V   Reactivity Data

Stability-Conditions to avoid: Stable
Incompatibility: None known
Hazardous Decomposition Products: Propionaldehyde, CO, CO_2 in fire situations
Conditions Contributing to Hazardous Polymerization: Will not occur

VI   Health Hazard Data

Effects of Overexposure (Medical Conditions Aggravated/Target Organ Effects)
A. *Acute* (Primary Route of Exposure)
   Eyes & Skin: Upon contact, mildly irritating to eyes. Prolonged or repeated contact may irritate skin.
   Inhalation: Spray mists or dusts from dried residues may result in respiratory irritation, coughing and/or difficulty in breathing.
   Ingestion: May cause upset to gastrointestinal tract.
B. *Subchronic, Chronic, Other:*   Subtilisins chronic exposure to dusts showed allergic sensitization with respiratory allergic reactions within minutes or delayed up to 24 hours.

VII   Emergency and First Aid Procedures

Eyes: Immediately flush eyes with plenty of water for at least 15 minutes. See a physician.
Skin: Immediately wash with soap and plenty of water for at least 15 minutes while removing contaminated clothing. If irritation develops, seek medical aid.
Inhalation: Remove to fresh air. If not breathing, give artificial respiration. If breathing difficult, give oxygen if available. Seek medical aid and report all inhalation exposures to health and safety personnel.
Ingestion: Do not induce vomiting. Give water to dilute. Call a physician. Never give anything by mouth to an unconscious person.

Figure 13.1

Example of an MSDS form (continued on next page).

VIII Spill or Leak Procedures

Spill Management: Contain spill and absorb material with an inert substance. Collect waste in suitable container.
Waste Disposal Methods: Dispose of in accordance with local, state, and federal regulations.

IX Protection Information/Control Measures

Respiratory: Not required under normal use
Eye: Safety glasses
Glove: Rubber
Other Clothing and Equipment: Clothes sufficient to avoid contact
Ventilation: Local exhaust

X Special Precautions

Precautions to be taken in Handling and Storing: Avoid exposure to high temperature or humidity. Wash hands thoroughly after use. Keep container closed when not in use.
Additional Information: Read and observe all labeled precautions.

Prepared by: R. C. Jente   Revision Date: 08/24/96
Seller makes no warranty, expressed or implied, concerning the use of this product other than indicated on the label.
Buyer assumes all risks of use and/or handling of this material when such use and/or handling is contrary to label instructions.
While Seller believes that the information contained herein is accurate, such information is offered solely for its customers' consideration and verification under their specific use conditions. This information is not to be deemed a warranty or representation of any kind for which Seller assumes legal responsibility.

Figure 13.1

Example of an MSDS form (continued).

alerting you to new hazards in the environment. Most facilities keep hazard communications

- In safety policy and procedure manuals
- In material safety data sheet (MSDS) books
- On the safety bulletin board
- On product labels
- On signs

Exposure Control Program

An exposure control plan provides steps to reduce employee or student exposure to bloodborne pathogens. The plan includes the following:

- Determining the possibility of exposure under each position description
- Developing a schedule and method for ensuring that the plan is enforced
- Postexposure evaluation

See the Occupational Exposure to Bloodborne Pathogens: Final Rule and Standard Precautions in Units 2 and 3 of Chapter 12 for more specific protective guidelines under the Exposure Control Program.

GENERAL SAFETY

Safety is everyone's responsibility. There are rules that are important to all health care workers. To be a safe worker and to protect yourself, co-workers, and patients/clients, learn the rules listed here.

abreast
Side by side.

■ **Walk! Never run in hallways.** If you run, you may fall and injure yourself. You can collide with another person or object. You can injure someone else, or you might create panic.

■ **Walk on the right-hand side of the hall not more than two abreast.** It is important to leave hallways open so that there are no traffic jams. In an emergency, a traffic jam can cause a delay and make the difference between life and death.

■ **Use handrails when using the stairs.** This prevents falling and injuring yourself.

■ **Watch out for swinging doors.** Be certain that someone is not on the other side of a swinging door. You might injure yourself or someone else (see Figure 13.2).

horseplay
Rowdy behavior; acting inappropriately in a work environment.

■ **Horseplay** is not tolerated. It is disturbing to others, may lead to accidents, causes confusion, and shows a lack of respect for patients and personnel.

■ **Always check labels.** Never use anything from containers that are not labeled. Using the wrong contents can cause injury or death to a patient. Using the wrong contents may also damage or ruin equipment.

■ **Wipe up spills and place litter in containers.** A wet floor can cause someone to slip and fall. If there is litter on the floor, someone may trip and be seriously injured.

■ **Follow instructions carefully.** If you do not understand instructions or do not know how to do a task, always ask for instructions. If you do something incorrectly, you may cause a serious problem.

■ **Report any injury to yourself or others to your supervisor immediately.** Reporting an injury ensures treatment for the injured without delay and correction of the potential hazard.

frayed
Worn or tattered (e.g., electrical cords may be worn, causing wires to be exposed).

■ **Do not use electrical cords that are frayed** or damaged. Frayed or damaged cords can cause **shocks,** burns, or fire.

shocks
Convulsion of muscles and extreme stimulation of nerves when an electric current passes through the body.

■ **Report a shock you receive from electrical equipment to your supervisor.** This prevents fire or a shock to someone else.

■ **Do not use malfunctioning** equipment. It is dangerous and may cause serious injury to you or someone else.

malfunctioning
Not working as it is supposed to.

■ **Report unsafe conditions to your supervisor immediately.** Safety is everyone's business. Be aware of your environment. Watch for unsafe conditions.

■ Follow Standard Precaution guidelines.

Figure 13.2

Watch for swinging doors!

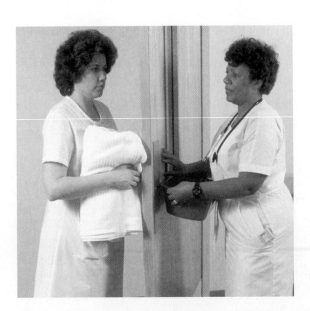

SUMMARY

Safety is the responsibility of all health care workers. OSHA is very strict about enforcement of regulations that keep the work environment safe.

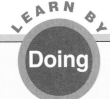

UNIT 1 ACTIVITY

1. Complete Worksheets 2, 3, 7, and 8 and Worksheets/Activities 4, 5, and 6 as assigned.
2. When you are confident that you can meet each objective, ask your instructor for the unit evaluation.

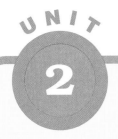

Patient Safety

STEPS TO SUCCESS

1. Read this unit.
2. Complete the Learn by Doing assignment at the end of this unit.

UNIT RATIONALE

Health care workers are responsible for the safety of patients/clients. If you do not follow Standard Precautions and basic safety precautions, patients can be seriously injured. Accidents involving clients are reduced if simple safety measures are followed. In this unit, we explain rules to follow when using ambulation devices, transporting devices, postural supports, and side rails.

UNIT OBJECTIVES

When you have completed this unit, you will be able to do the following:

✔ Explain how to use ambulation devices, transporting devices, postural supports, and side rails safely.

✔ Match descriptions and principles associated with ambulation devices, transporting devices, postural supports, and side rails.

✔ Explain the importance of safety measures.

✔ Follow safe practice guidelines when caring for patients/clients.

IDENTIFYING THE PATIENT

When you work directly with a patient, you must identify him or her to avoid a mistake. Errors are avoided if you follow these *important* steps:

■ Check with the nurse's station for the right room number.

■ Check the requisition or physician's order, which has the patient's name on it, against the patient's identification band.

■ In ambulatory care, confirm chart name and information with each client.

⊙ AMBULATION DEVICES

Ambulation devices are devices used to assist in walking. The most common devices in the health care setting are canes, crutches, and walkers (see Figure 19.1, page 531). These devices give the patient/client additional support and aid in balancing while walking or standing.

Safe Practice Guidelines When Using Ambulation Devices

It is essential that all devices be in good condition, because patients/clients depend on these items.

■ Devices must always be structurally safe, without dents or cracks. For example, wood crutches are unsafe if the wood is split or cracked. A loose joint in a walker allows it to wobble or break, and the patient can fall.

■ Areas touching the ground must be covered with rubber tips to prevent slipping.

■ The devices must always be clean and free of blood or body fluids.

⊙ TRANSPORTING DEVICES

Transporting devices include equipment used to move patients from one place to another. The most common transporting devices are wheelchairs and gurneys. Gurneys and wheelchairs make it easy to move patients who are unable to walk. Follow these basic principles to ensure the patient's safety (see Figure 13.3, page 281).

Safe Practice Guidelines When Using Gurneys and Wheelchairs

■ Always lock the brakes except when you are moving.

■ Back a wheelchair over indented or raised doorways, such as an elevator or any ridges on the floor.

■ Always back a client in a wheelchair or a gurney down a hill.

■ Always secure straps or put side rails up on a gurney.

■ Lock brakes when moving the client on or off a gurney.

■ Always back the patient on a gurney headfirst into an elevator.

■ Never leave a patient on a gurney unattended.

■ Always keep the gurney free of blood and body fluids.

⊙ POSTURAL SUPPORTS

restrict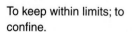

To keep within limits; to confine.

Postural supports are devices that **restrict** a patient's movement. This type of restriction is necessary only when the patient's safety is in jeopardy. Occasionally, patients become disoriented due to a change of environment or as a response to medication. When this occurs, postural supports are used to keep clients safe. Postural supports are more common in long-term care facilities. *Example:* A confused patient may not realize that he is too weak to walk to the bathroom without falling. Use a postural support to remind clients to call for assistance when they need to get out of bed. There are many types of supports. The most common are vest supports, wrist supports, and ankle supports. When you use postural supports, certain principles must be observed. (See Chapter 15, page 424.)

Safe Practice Guidelines When Using Postural Supports

■ A physician's order is required by law.

■ Never use a postural support on a patient in a chair or bed without wheels.

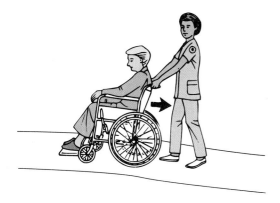

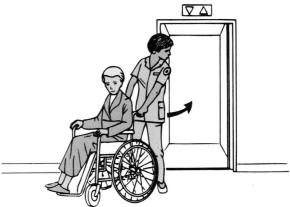

Back a wheelchair over indented or raised doorways, such as an elevator or any ridges on the floor.

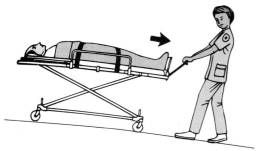

Always back a patient in a wheelchair or a gurney down a hill.

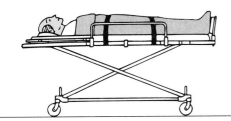

Never leave a patient on a gurney unattended.

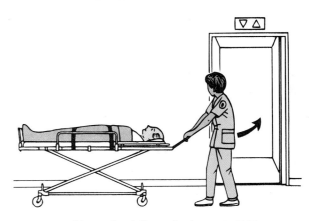

Always back the patient on a gurney headfirst into an elevator.

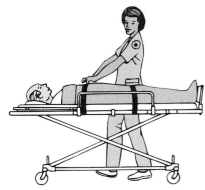

Always secure straps or put side rails up on a gurney.

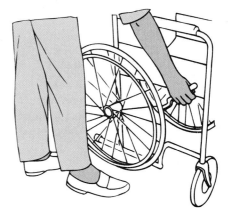

Always lock the brakes except when you are moving.
Lock brakes when moving the patient on or off a gurney.

Figure 13.3

Principles in the use of gurneys and wheelchairs.

- Clients requiring postural supports must be checked frequently. The support must be released or loosened every 2 hours.
- Use a half-bow knot to secure the support.
- Leave at least two fingers' ease between the patient's skin and the support so his or her circulation is not restricted.
- Never secure supports to side rails; always attach to the framework of a bed or gurney.
- Secure the half-bow knot out of the client's reach.
- Discard supports that have touched blood or body fluids, following Standard Precautions.

○ SIDE RAILS

Use side rails on bedsides and gurneys (stretchers) to keep clients from falling. In the hospital, falls from beds are the most common cause of injury. The use of side rails helps reduce the number of falls. Side rails aid in turning or moving patients who are heavily medicated. Patients use them to help lift or turn themselves, and they prevent the patient from falling out of bed.

Safe Practice Guidelines When Using Side Rails

- Side rails are always in place at night. If clients refuse to have them in place, a release must be signed relieving the facility of responsibility.
- Small children, heavily medicated patients, and confused or restless patients require side rails at all times.
- Side rails must be locked securely. Patients often lean on rails for support. If they are not secure, the patient can fall.
- Precautions must be taken when side rails are put up or down. Tubing and the client's legs and arms must be in a safe position.
- If the side rails are up when you begin a procedure, be certain they are up when you leave the room.
- Side rails should always be clean and free of blood or body fluids.

○ SUMMARY

By following each of the simple principles discussed in this unit, you provide safe conditions for your patients/clients. You have learned to identify the patient to prevent errors and to keep your patients safe when using ambulation devices, transporting devices, postural supports, and side rails.

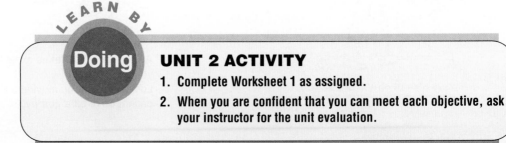

LEARN BY

Doing

UNIT 2 ACTIVITY

1. **Complete Worksheet 1 as assigned.**
2. **When you are confident that you can meet each objective, ask your instructor for the unit evaluation.**

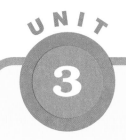

UNIT 3

Disaster Preparedness

STEPS TO SUCCESS

1. Read this unit.

2. Complete the Learn by Doing assignment at the end of this unit.

UNIT RATIONALE

Disasters can occur anywhere and at any moment. As a health care worker, you are expected to respond quickly according to your agency disaster plan. You must be famil-iar with the practices that are detailed in that plan and be able to follow them if a disaster occurs. A disaster is any-thing that causes damage and injury to a group of people. Examples are flood, earthquake, tornado, explosion, fire, and bioterrorism. Be alert to emergency equipment, exits, and the disaster plan. They provide the essentials neces-sary to respond effectively to a disaster. Be particularly aware of instructions in the disaster plan telling you how to cooperate with first responders, police and fire personnel, and disaster-specific instructions from local, state, and federal officials.

UNIT OBJECTIVES

When you have completed this unit, you will be able to do the following:

✔ Define vocabulary words.

✔ Identify what you are responsible for knowing and doing when a disaster occurs.

✔ List the three elements required to start a fire.

✔ Explain four ways to prevent fires.

✔ Summarize all safety requirements that protect the employee/student, patient, and employer.

○ DISASTER PLAN

Your facility is required to have a disaster plan. You are responsible for knowing the plan and responding when a disaster occurs. To be prepared for any type of disas-ter you need to know the following:

■ The floor plan of your facility

■ The nearest exit route

■ The location of alarms and fire extinguishers

■ How to use alarms and fire extinguishers

■ Your role as a health care worker when a disaster occurs

The following are some basic rules to remember when a disaster strikes:

■ Assess the situation; count to 10 to calm yourself.

■ Be sure that you are not in danger. (Placing yourself in danger only makes the situation worse.)

■ Remove those who are in immediate danger, if it is safe to do so.

■ Notify others of the emergency according to facility policy.

■ Use stairs, *not* the elevator.

Fire is often the result of a disaster. It is your responsibility to be alert to causes of fire and act to prevent fire when possible.

Figure 13.4a

The three elements needed to start a fire.

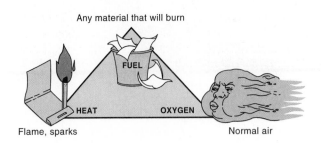

Any material that will burn

FUEL

HEAT   OXYGEN

Flame, sparks   Normal air

Figure 13.4b

Misuses of electricity.

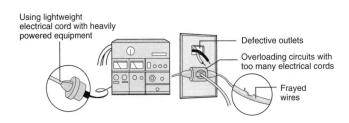

Using lightweight electrical cord with heavily powered equipment

Defective outlets

Overloading circuits with too many electrical cords

Frayed wires

FIRE CAUSES AND PREVENTION

There are three elements that must be present before a fire can start (Figure 13.4a):

■ Oxygen ■ Heat ■ Fuel

Most fires can be prevented if everyone is **observant** and careful. The following are some ways you can help prevent fires:

observant

Quick to see and understand.

■ Provide ashtrays for smokers. Never empty ashtrays into wastebaskets or containers that can burn. Ashtrays must be emptied into separate containers. Smoking is restricted to designated areas.

■ Check electrical equipment for proper functioning and frayed electrical cord. If there is any problem, report it immediately (see Figure 13.4b).

■ When using flammable liquids, take only the amount needed to complete the task. You would spill only the amount you poured, not the whole container. Keep flammable liquids in a container approved by the Underwriters' Laboratories.

■ Post a No Smoking sign when oxygen is in use in an area. If the oxygen is in a **cylinder,** strap the cylinder securely on a cart or stand.

cylinder

Long, narrow, circular container.

BIOTERRORISM

Everyone must be aware of the dangers of chemical or biological disasters. Facilities have plans to provide for the safety of patients, physicians, staff, and visitors. These plans include shelter-in during a possible exposure. Shelter-in is a nationally accepted term indicating the need to remain inside of the facility during a potential exposure to chemical and biological hazards. These plans include securing entrances and exits to the building and securing outside air sources. Your responsibility is to learn what your facility plan is and to follow the procedures that are in place.

SUMMARY

potential

Possible.

Disaster preparedness is everyone's responsibility. Each person is responsible for responding to a disaster and being alert to **potential** hazards.

There are three elements required to start a fire: oxygen, heat, and fuel. There are at least four ways to help prevent fires. These include following the rules for smoking, checking for frayed electrical cords and malfunctioning equipment, careful handling of flammable liquids, and following proper oxygen procedures.

Know the disaster plan of your agency or facility. Move patients to safety if they are in danger. Know where to find the fire extinguishers and which exits to use. Do not use an elevator. Be calm. Do not panic!

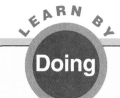

Doing — LEARN BY

UNIT 3 ACTIVITY

1. **Complete Worksheet 1 as assigned.**
2. **When you are confident that you can meet each objective, ask your instructor for the unit evaluation.**

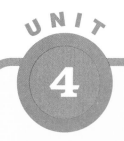

UNIT 4

Principles of Body Mechanics

STEPS TO SUCCESS

1. Read this unit.
2. Complete the Learn by Doing assignment at the end of this unit.

UNIT OBJECTIVES

When you have completed this unit, you will be able to do the following:

✔ Define vocabulary words.

✔ Define *body mechanics.*

✔ List six rules of correct body mechanics.

UNIT RATIONALE

As a health care worker, you lift, move, and carry many different objects and patients. It is important to use your body correctly to prevent both fatigue and injury. If you injure yourself, you then become ineffective in your job.

✔ List six principles of body mechanics.

✔ Demonstrate correct lifting and moving of objects.

⬤ BODY MECHANICS

Health care workers move, lift, and carry all types of equipment and supplies. They also help position or move patients. When you use proper body mechanics, you save energy, prevent muscle strain, and increase your **efficiency.** Body mechanics is the coordination of body alignment, balance, and movement. When you use your body and your muscles properly, you are practicing good body mechanics.

efficiency

Ability to accomplish a job with the least possible difficulty.

Principles of Body Mechanics

1. Stoop. Do not bend.

• Stand close to the object. • Create a base of support by placing your feet wide apart. • Place one foot slightly forward. • Bend at your hips and knees with your back straight, lower your body, and bring your hands down to the object. • Use the large muscles in your legs to return to a standing position.

2. Lift firmly and smoothly after you size up the load.

• If you cannot easily pull the object to you (i.e., the load is too heavy), *get help!* • Grasp the load firmly. • Lift by using the large muscles of your legs (see Figure 13.5). • Keep the load close to your body. • Do not twist your body (see Figure 13.6). • To change direction, shift your feet in the direction you want to go.

gravity

Natural force or pull toward the earth. In the body, the center of gravity is usually the center of the body.

3. Always use the center of **gravity** when carrying a load.

• Keep your back as straight as possible. • Keep the weight of the load close to the body and centered over your hips. • Put down the load by bending at the hips and knees. Keep your back straight and the load close to your body. • If the load is too heavy, *get help!* • When two or more people carry the load, assign one person as the leader so that he or she can give commands.

4. Pulling: Push or pull rather than lift the load.

• Place your feet apart with one foot slightly forward. Keep close to the object you are moving. • Grasp the object firmly, close to its center of gravity.

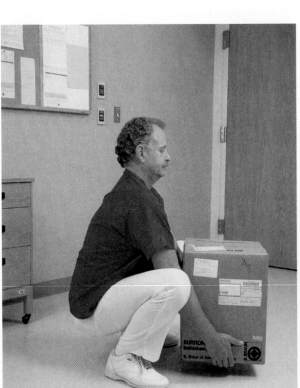
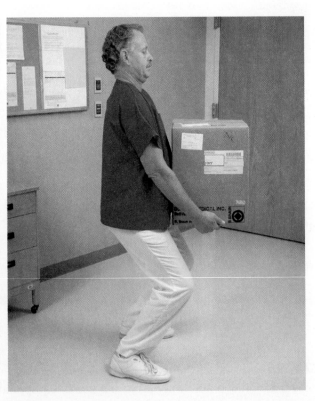

Figure 13.5

Use large muscles of legs when lifting, and keep your back straight.

• **Crouch;** lean away from the object. • Pull by straightening your legs. Keep your back straight. • Walk backwards. Your leg muscles should do all the work.

5. Pushing: Push or pull rather than lift the load.

• Stand close to the object to be moved. • Crouch down with your feet apart. • Bend your elbows and put your hands on the load at chest level. • Lean forward with your chest and shoulders near the object. • Keep your back straight. • Push with your legs.

6. Reaching: Carefully evaluate the distance.

• Always use a stool or a ladder to reach objects that are too high. • Stand close to the object. • If you are standing on the floor, place your feet wide apart, one foot slightly forward. • Maintain good body alignment. Move close to the object. Do not reach to the point of straining. • When reaching for an object that is above your head, grip it with your palms up, and lower it. Keep it close to your body on the way down.

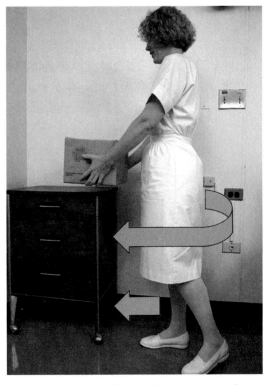

Figure 13.6

Do not twist your body when lifting—turn it.

crouch

To stoop, using the large muscles of the legs to help maintain balance.

SUMMARY

In this unit, you learned that by following basic principles, you prevent fatigue and injury.

There are six important rules to remember when following the basic principles of body mechanics.

Six Rules to Remember

■ Keep your back straight.

■ Bend at the hips and knees.

■ Keep your feet approximately 6 to 8 inches apart to provide a wide base of support.

■ Use the strongest muscles of your legs.

■ Do not twist your body.

■ Use the weight of your body to help push or pull.

When you learn to lift and move correctly, you protect yourself and others from injury.

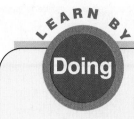

UNIT 4 ACTIVITY
1. **Complete Worksheet 1 as assigned.**
2. **When you are confident that you can meet each objective ask your instructor for the unit evaluation.**

First Aid

STEPS TO SUCCESS

1. Read "Unit Rationale" through "General Principles of First Aid."
2. Complete the Learn by Doing assignment at the end of this reading.

UNIT RATIONALE

In or out of the clinical setting, the health care worker is expected to respond quickly and effectively when there is a sudden illness or injury. As a health care worker you are responsible for seeking information and becoming competent in first-aid skills. This knowledge enables you to be a well-prepared and effective health care worker.

UNIT OBJECTIVES

When you have completed this unit, you will be able to do the following:

✔ Match vocabulary words with their correct meanings.
✔ Demonstrate the procedures for:
  • Mouth-to-mouth breathing
  • Obstructed airway
  • Serious wounds
  • Preventing shock
  • Splints
  • Slings
  • Bandaging

cardiopulmonary
Having to do with the heart and lungs.

definitive
Clear, without question, exacting (e.g., when giving emergency care, each treatment should be done in a definitive manner).

⬤ INTRODUCTION TO FIRST AID

This unit is an overview of commonly used first-aid techniques. The authors of this book strongly advise that everyone attend a basic first-aid class and a heart saver or **cardiopulmonary** resuscitation (CPR) class in order to become proficient. These classes are given by the American Red Cross and the American Heart Association. Appropriate first aid can save a life and prevent a permanent disability. Most situations requiring first aid need prompt, **definitive** action. To gain understanding and a high skill level, you need supervised practice for each of the procedures listed.

First aid is the emergency care given to a victim of an accident or a sudden illness. This treatment is required immediately and continues as needed until advanced medical care is available.

GENERAL PRINCIPLES OF FIRST AID

1. Never panic; always remain calm. Unfortunately, this statement is easier said than done. Here are some basic rules that help you remain calm:

• Take a few slow, deep breaths. • Survey the surrounding area and ensure that it is safe before approaching. • Determine what resources are available and what is needed.

2. Evaluate the situation by

• Checking the victim's level of consciousness • Opening the victim's airway • Checking for breathing • Checking circulation, including pulse and bleeding

3. Determine if the victim is in a safe environment, free from danger.

4. Determine **priorities** of treatment (i.e., decide which condition requires the most immediate care).

• Urgent care is required in life-threatening situations, such as stopped breathing, heart attack, shock, serious wounds, poisoning, burns. • A victim may need first aid, but the situation may not be life threatening. Non-life-threatening conditions include **fracture** of an arm or leg and a minor **contusion** or **laceration.**

5. Decide how to provide the care that is needed and begin providing any care you are trained of permitted to give.

6. Call or send for help as soon as possible.

LIFE-THREATENING SITUATIONS

Most cities have an emergency medical system (EMS) that responds immediately with emergency care providers. The most common number used to alert the EMS system is 911. The following situations are considered life threatening and require emergency medical care.

Oxygen is necessary for brain cells to live. Permanent brain damage can occur if oxygen is not present for 4 to 6 minutes. You have only a few minutes to save the life of a person who has stopped breathing.

Obstructed Airway (Closed Airway, Stopped or Not Breathing)

An obstructed airway occurs when an object blocks the airway leading to the lungs. This occurs when a piece of food or other object lodges in the back of the throat or in the windpipe. Early detection of an airway obstruction is important in determining your plan of action. There are two types of obstructions:

■ *Partial obstruction* occurs when some air can be exchanged. There may be *good air exchange* when the victim coughs forcefully or wheezes between coughs. *Do not* interfere with the victim's attempt to cough the object out. If there is *poor air exchange* and the victim

• Becomes weak • Has an ineffective cough • Has a crowing or high-pitched noise during inhalation • Has increased difficulty breathing • Turns bluish around the mouth and fingernails

priorities
Those things that are most important.

fracture
Broken bone.

contusion
Condition in which the skin is bruised, swollen, and painful, but is not broken.

laceration
Wound or tear of the skin.

RESCUE BREATHING—ADULT

1. Put on disposable gloves.
2. Check for consciousness by shaking victim's shoulder gently and asking if he or she is OK. If there is no response, activate EMS system.
3. Open airway by placing one hand at victim's chin and the other hand on victim's forehead; gently lift chin by supporting jawbone with fingertips and lifting upward

ALERT: Follow Standard Precautions.

to open mouth. (Do not put pressure on throat; this may block airway.) This is called the *head tilt/chin lift.*

4. Check for breathing by placing your ear near victim's mouth and nose. Turn your head so that you can see his or her chest. Look to see if chest is rising or falling. Listen for breathing. Feel for air from victim's mouth or nose on your cheek. If breathing is *not* present:

5. Ventilate. Place a pocket mask over mouth and nose. Put apex (point) over bridge of nose and base between lip and chin. Give two breaths (1½ to 2 seconds per breath) through the one-way valve. Allow lungs to empty between each breath. (If dentures obstruct the airway, remove them.) If air does *not*

inflate lungs: Retilt head to ensure an open airway and repeat the two breaths. Watch for chest to rise, allow for exhalation between breaths. (If lungs still do not inflate, treat victim for an obstructed airway; see the Obstructed Airway procedures.)

6. Check carotid pulse.

7. If breathing is absent and pulse is present, keep the airway open and give one breath to victim every 5 seconds. If there is no pulse, cardiopulmonary resuscitation (CPR) is needed to circulate oxygenated blood through body. To learn CPR, take a course given by a qualified instructor approved by American Heart Association or American Red Cross.

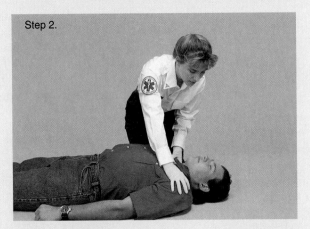

Step 2.

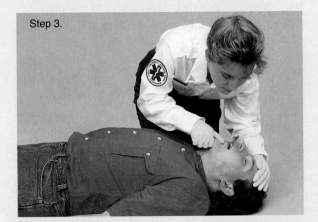

Step 3.

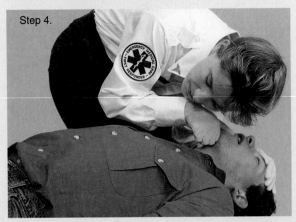

Step 4.

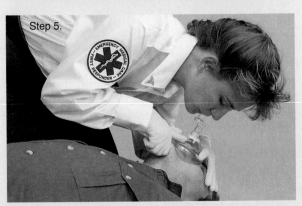

Step 5.

PROCEDURE 13.2 — OBSTRUCTED AIRWAY IN A CONSCIOUS VICTIM—ADULT

When signs of choking are present:

1. Ask "Are you choking?" Observe victim for coughing or wheezing. *Do not interfere* if good air exchange is present.

2. Give **abdominal thrust,** sometimes called the **Heimlich maneuver.** Stand in back of victim; put your arms around victim's waist. Make a fist with one hand and put your thumb between breastbone and

ALERT: Follow Standard Precautions.

navel. Take your other hand and grasp fist; pull into victim's abdomen with quick upward thrust. Repeat separate, rapid inward and upward thrusts until

airway is cleared or patient becomes unconscious. (Use chest thrusts for a pregnant or obese victim.)

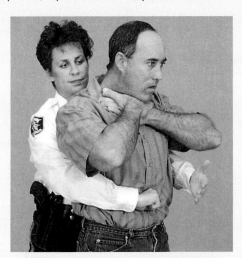

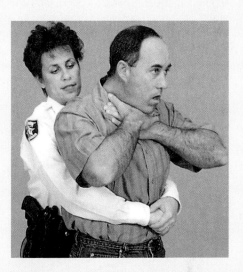

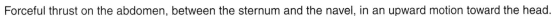

abdominal thrust or Heimlich maneuver

Forceful thrust on the abdomen, between the sternum and the navel, in an upward motion toward the head.

Treat the victim for complete airway obstruction (conscious victim).

- *Complete obstruction* occurs when there is no air exchange or there is poor air exchange. The signs of complete obstruction are present when the victim

  - Is suddenly unable to breathe, cough, or speak • Clutches neck (see photograph in procedure box above) • Is struggling to breathe

When you observe these signs, follow the procedure for obstructed airway.

Heart Attack

The first two hours after the onset of a heart attack are the highest-risk period. Recognition of early warning signs alerts you to an impending heart attack. Early warning signs are

- Squeezing feeling in the chest ("feels like a band is around my chest"), pressure, or tightness ("feels like an elephant is sitting on my chest")

- Persistent discomfort that spreads to shoulders, arms, neck, jaw, or across the chest

- Sweating, nausea, vomiting, shortness of breath, or feeling faint

If the victim becomes unconscious:

1. Activate the EMS system.

2. Put on disposable gloves.

3. Open airway. Place one hand at victim's chin and the other hand on victim's forehead; gently tip head back. Lift chin in head tilt/chin lift position.

ALERT: Follow Standard Precautions.

4. Attempt to ventilate. Open the airway and ventilate through a pocket face mask with a one-way valve. If no air enters, retilt head and try to ventilate again. If air enters, give two breaths and continue rescue breathing. If air does not inflate lungs, give abdominal thrusts.

5. Abdominal thrust. Straddle victim's legs and place heel of your hand between breastbone and navel. Then push quickly and sharply straight upward and inward up to five times.

6. Finger sweep. On an unconscious victim, use the finger sweep to remove objects from the mouth that may be, loosened during the abdominal thrusts. Use your index finger to sweep from one side of the mouth to the back of the throat and out the other side of the mouth. Perform a sweep only if an object is visible and be careful not to push the object deeper into the throat.

7. Attempt to ventilate using pocket face mask again. If lungs do not inflate, repeat entire procedure. Reposition head and attempt to ventilate again, then do up to five abdominal thrusts; sweep mouth if an object is seen; attempt to breathe for victim again, and repeat until the airway is clear and air enters. Give two breaths and follow steps 6 and 7 of Rescue Breathing.

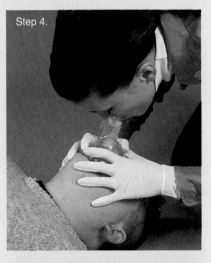

Step 4.

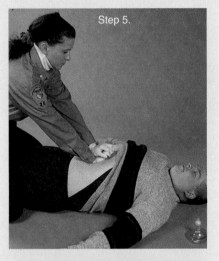

Step 5.

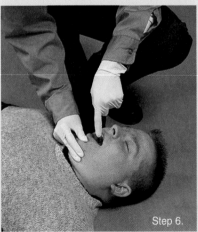

Step 6.

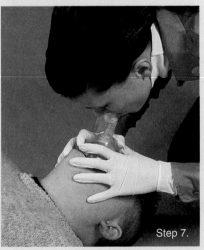

Step 7.

PROCEDURE 13.4

STOPPED BREATHING IN AN INFANT

1. Put on disposable gloves.
2. **Check for consciousness.** Shake baby's shoulders gently and speak baby's name. If no response, shout for help.

ALERT: Follow Standard Precautions.

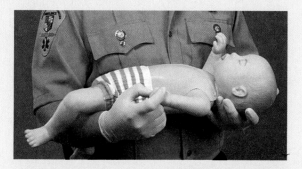

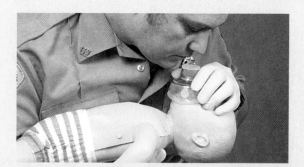

3. **Open airway.** Use head tilt/chin lift method. Do not overtilt head or neck.

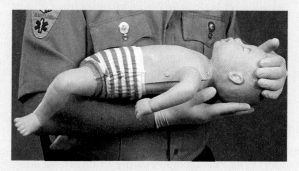

4. **Check for breathing.** Look, listen, and feel.

If not breathing:

5. Place an infant-sized barrier device on the infant's face.* Ventilate through the one-way valve and give rescue breathing. Give two slow breaths using only

air in your cheeks. (Too much air may overinflate an infant's lungs.) Watch for chest to rise and allow chest to fall or deflate between each breath. If air does not inflate lungs:

6. Retilt head to ensure open airway. Repeat the two breaths. If lungs still do not inflate, treat infant for an obstructed airway.

If lungs do inflate:

7. **Keep airway open,** and give one breath to infant every 3 seconds. After 1 minute activate EMS.

8. **Check pulse.** Place three fingers over brachial artery/pulse. The baby's heart may have stopped. In this event, only cardiopulmonary resuscitation (CPR) will help to circulate oxygenated blood throughout the body. CPR can be learned by taking a course offered by an instructor who is certified by the American Heart Association or the American Red Cross. We strongly recommend you complete such a program.

*Adult-sized pocket face masks can be adapted by inverting (reversing) them. See manufacturer's guidelines.

When one or all of these signs are present, call for advanced life support systems (doctor or paramedics depending upon the health care setting). If signs continue, the heart and breathing may stop, and it will be necessary to start CPR.

Serious Wounds

Serious wounds are life threatening because heavy bleeding is frequently present. Bleeding that pulsates or **spurts** with each heartbeat is from an artery. The victim

spurts

To force out in a burst; to squirt.

PROCEDURE 13.5

OBSTRUCTED AIRWAY IN A CONSCIOUS INFANT

1. Put on disposable gloves
2. Observe to determine infant's ability to cry, cough, or breathe. If there is no evidence of air exchange, shout for help.

ALERT: Follow Standard Precautions.

3. Give five back blows. Place infant face down, supporting head and neck and tilting infant so that the head is lower than rest of body. Give five firm hits with heel of your hand over backbone and between shoulder blades.

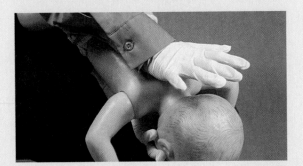

4. Give five chest thrusts by turning infant on its back with head lower than rest of body. Using two to three fingers, push five times on midsternum, which is about one finger's width below nipple line at midchest.

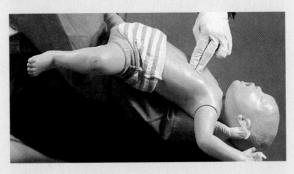

5. Continue procedure until obstruction is clear or infant becomes unconscious.

will bleed to death if the bleeding is not controlled. Venous bleeding is also serious and must be controlled. An open wound allowing a constant flow of blood from a vein can also cause death. The open area is also susceptible to infection and needs to be covered.

To stop bleeding and minimize infection, apply direct pressure with your gloved hand and some type of dressing or pad. Sterile gauze pads/gauze **dressings** are very effective. If gauze dressings are not available, use a piece of clean cloth, a handkerchief, or toweling. Even though the cloth is not sterile, it aids in controlling the bleeding.

dressings

Gauze pads that are used to cover a wound.

LEARN BY Doing

UNIT 5 ACTIVITY

1. Complete Worksheets 2 through 4 as assigned.
2. Practice the procedures.
3. Read "Serious Wounds" through "Preventing Shock."
4. Complete the Learn by Doing assignment at the end of this reading.

PROCEDURE 13.6

OBSTRUCTED AIRWAY IN AN UNCONSCIOUS INFANT

Follow steps 1 to 5 above, then . . .

6. If second rescuer is available, instruct him or her to activate EMS system.

ALERT: Follow Standard Precautions.

7. Attempt to see the obstruction. Open infant's mouth. Place your thumb over infant's tongue, and lift jaw by grasping jawbone with your fingers. If object *is* visible, use your little finger to hook it and sweep it from the mouth; then attempt to ventilate. If object is *not* visible:

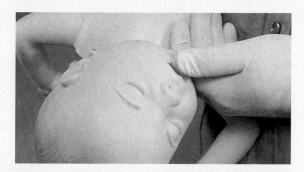

8. Try to ventilate as described on page 293. If lungs do not inflate, reposition head and try to ventilate again.

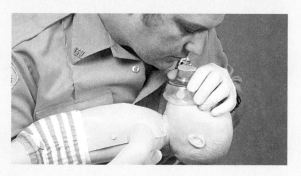

9. If air still does not enter, repeat steps 6 and 7.
10. Repeat five back blows; then:

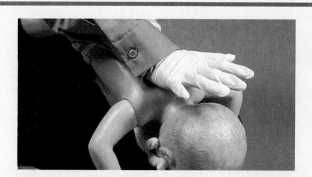

11. Repeat five chest thrusts.

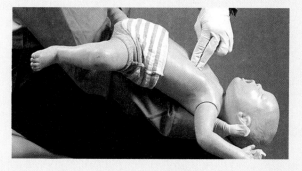

12. Open mouth to attempt to see object. Sweep mouth if object is visible. If not visible:
13. Continue procedure until obstruction is expelled. If the obstruction is not relieved after 1 minute, activate EMS system.
14. Once the airway is clear, ventilate once every 3 seconds.

NOTE Carry disposable gloves. Always wear them to prevent exposure to body fluids. Always follow Standard Precautions.

Figure 13.7

Combine elevation and direct
pressure to treat serious
wounds.

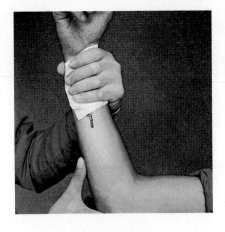

saturated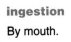

Soaked; filled to capacity.

How to Treat Serious Wounds

1. Follow the procedure for preventing shock (page 298).
2. Apply direct pressure over the wound with your gloved hand. Apply a pressure dressing and secure with a bandage.
3. Elevate the wounded area if you do not think there are broken bones (see Figure 13.7).

If direct pressure and elevation do not control bleeding:

1. Apply pressure to the appropriate pressure point above the wound (see Figure 13.8). The pressure point must be on the same limb or the same side of the body.
2. Continue to apply direct pressure and maintain elevation to the wound. Do not remove the dressings and bandages when they are **saturated**. Apply dry dressings over the saturated bandage.
3. When bleeding is under control, gradually release pressure at the pressure point. Keep applying direct pressure over the pressure dressing.
4. Call or send for help as soon as possible.

Shock

Shock is life threatening. Shock is usually caused by major loss of body fluids or blood: it can be caused by vomiting and diarrhea. If it is due to major blood loss, body cells and organs are deprived of oxygen, which is carried by the blood. Shock slows body functions and keeps the major organs from functioning normally. Anyone with a serious injury should seek advanced medical care immediately. A victim can be treated appropriately for an injury, yet die from shock because of the fluid or blood and oxygen loss. Treat every victim for a life-threatening injury until the victim is stabilized and emergency care providers or doctors arrive. Follow the procedure to prevent shock.

Poisoning

ingestion

By mouth.

Poisoning often causes sudden collapse, vomiting, and difficult breathing. Poisoning can occur in various ways—for example, **ingestion,** inhalation, which is breathing in a poisonous substance, absorption through the skin, or by injection, insect stings or animal bites, or from needles that puncture the skin. Look for items near the victim that may be the source of poisoning, such as an empty container or a needle. To care for a poisoning victim follow the procedure for a *conscious* victim.

An *unconscious victim* who is suffering from poisoning may be convulsing and vomiting. Follow the procedure for an unconscious poison victim.

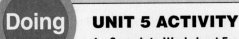

LEARN BY

Doing   **UNIT 5 ACTIVITY**

1. **Complete Worksheet 5 as assigned.**
2. **Practice the procedures.**
3. **Read "Poisoning" through "Treating Burns."**
4. **Complete the Learn by Doing assignment at the end of this reading.**

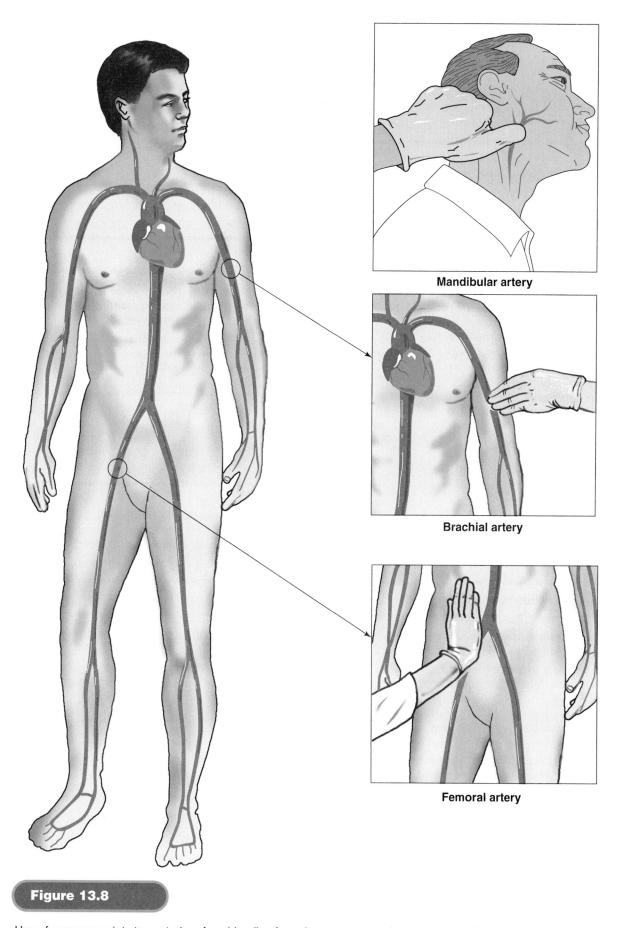

Mandibular artery

Brachial artery

Femoral artery

Figure 13.8

Use of pressure points to control profuse bleeding from the upper extremity, lower extremity, and neck.

PROCEDURE 13.7

PREVENTING SHOCK

1. Put on disposable gloves.
2. Provide comfort, quiet, and warmth.
3. Maintain normal body temperature by covering with blanket.
4. Keep victim calm.
5. Keep victim lying down on back if possible. Elevate feet and arms. Do not elevate an unsplinted arm or leg that is fractured.

ALERT: Follow Standard Precautions.

6. If victim is vomiting, bleeding from mouth, or feels like vomiting, position victim on side. Do not move the victim if there is any possibility of a spinal injury or if the victim complains of numbness, tingling, lack of sensation, or inability to move limbs.
7. If person has a head injury, neck injury, or breathing problem, feet should not be elevated and the victim should not be turned on his or her side.
8. Provide oxygen as soon as possible if you have the training and equipment to do so; otherwise, call immediately for someone who does.

PROCEDURE 13.8

TREATING A CONSCIOUS POISON VICTIM

1. Put on disposable gloves.
2. Try to locate poison container (try to identify source of poisoning); **do not waste time.**
3. For some ingested poisons, give victim water or milk to dilute the poison. Do *not* give fluids if the poison was gasoline or a caustic substance. Additional fluids

ALERT: Follow Standard Precautions.

may spread the damage and cause vomiting and aspiration into the airway.

4. Call 911 to get an ambulance* as soon as possible; then call the nearest poison center, hospital, or physician. (Directions on poison containers and for ingested substances are *not* always correct.) When you call, state that you have a poisoning emergency.

If you have the container, be prepared to read ingredients.

5. Be alert for breathing problems. If breathing stops, you will perform mouth-to-mask (rescue breathing) resuscitation as discussed at beginning of unit.
6. Follow procedure for preventing shock.

*Ambulance personnel can communicate directly with the hospital and the poison control center. They can start lifesaving procedures with special equipment and poison treatment medications.

Burns

The seriousness of a burn is determined by the degree or depth of the burn (see Figure 13.9):

Severity of Burns

■ Superficial or *first-degree burns* are surface burns.

PROCEDURE 13.9

TREATING AN UNCONSCIOUS POISON VICTIM

1. Put on disposable gloves.
2. Do *not* give any fluids.
3. Position victim on his or her side in a safe place.

ALERT: Follow Standard Precautions.

4. Try to identify the poison source; **do not waste time.**

5. Call 911 to get an ambulance* as soon as possible; then call the nearest poison center, hospital, or physician.

6. Be alert for breathing problems.

7. Follow procedure for preventing shock.

*Ambulance personnel can communicate directly with the hospital and the poison control center. They can start lifesaving procedures with special equipment and poison treatment medications.

■ Partial thickness or *second-degree burns* are deeper or just below the surface of the skin, and blistering occurs.

■ Full thickness or *third-degree burns* are even deeper, destroying both surface and underlying tissue.

Burns around the mouth or nose may indicate that the airway is burned. This can cause swelling that may obstruct the airway. If breathing stops, follow the procedure for rescue breathing as discussed at the beginning of this unit. However, if the airway is swollen causing breathing to stop, rescue breathing may be ineffective. Call emergency care providers immediately. Blistering and swelling may not appear until later. A full thickness burn destroys nerve endings, so a burn victim may not feel pain in that

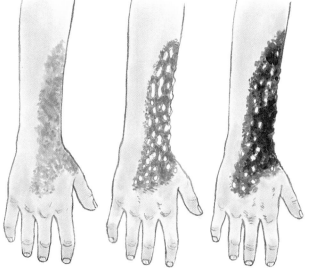

Figure 13.9

Severity of burns.

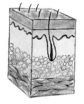
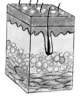

Superficial
First Degree

Partial thickness
Second Degree

Full thickness
Third Degree

Epidermis
Dermis
Fat
Muscle

Skin reddened

Blisters

Charring

PROCEDURE 13.10

TREATING BURNS

FIRST-DEGREE BURN

1. Put on disposable gloves.
2. Apply cool water to burn area, or submerge burn site in cool water; this will reduce pain.

ALERT: Follow Standard Precautions.

discomfort. Partial thickness or deeper burns (full thickness) require the following procedure.

SECOND- AND THIRD-DEGREE BURNS

1. Put on disposable gloves.
2. Stop the burning process by smothering or dousing with water and removing smoldering or hot clothing.

3. Large surface burns should never be wet as this causes shock. Large burns may be dried with sterile dressing. Apply a cold pack over dressing to reduce

3. Cover burned area with dry sterile dressing to help prevent infection. Do not pull away clothing that is stuck to burn site.
4. Place a dry cold pack over dressing if it does not cause discomfort to the victim.
5. Follow procedure to prevent shock.
6. Call or send for advanced medical assistance as soon as possible.

area, but surrounding areas may be painful. The absence of pain *does not* indicate a mild burn. Do the following for a burn victim as described in the following procedure:

- Relieve pain
- Minimize the chance of infection
- Prevent shock (page 298)

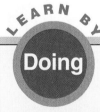

UNIT 5 ACTIVITY

1. **Complete Worksheets 6 and 7 as assigned.**
2. **Practice the procedures.**
3. **Read "Non-Life-Threatening Situations" through to the end of this unit.**
4. **Complete the Learn by Doing assignment at the end of this unit.**

NON-LIFE-THREATENING SITUATIONS

The bone fractures described below are examples of non-life-threatening conditions. Such conditions require first aid or medical care but not urgent care.

Bone Fractures

There are two main types of fractures: closed and open.

- A *closed fracture* is difficult to determine. The following are signs and symptoms of closed fractures:

• Swelling • Pain •
Change in the color of the
skin • Deformity

■ An *open fracture* is present
when the skin over the
fracture site is broken or
open and/or the broken
bone protrudes through
the skin.

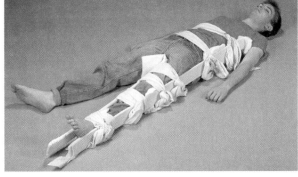

Long-board splinting for a
fractured hip or for any bone
in the leg.

Call or send for advanced
medical help if you believe a
fracture is present. If medical help is not available or the victim must be taken to a
medical facility, splint the fracture (see Figure 13.10 for a leg or hip fracture).

A fracture of the arm usually requires a sling. Apply a triangle sling so that the
victim's hand and forearm are slightly higher than the elbow. This helps to minimize
the swelling. A sling is a triangular bandage used to support the arm. Once the patient's arm is placed in a sling, a **swathe** can be used to hold the patient's arm
against the side of the chest. Commercial slings are available. Roller bandage can
be used to form a sling and swathe. Velcro straps can be used to form a swathe. Use
whatever materials you have on hand, provided that they will not cut into the patient as will narrow cords or wire. Remember: Shirts, ties, and wide belts can be
used to make both sling and swathe.

swathe

Bandage.

⬤ DRESSINGS AND BANDAGES

Dressings cover wounds and help prevent infectious bacteria from entering a
wound. Also use dressing to apply direct pressure over a wound to control bleeding.
There are many types of dressings used for various body locations. Bandages hold
dressings in place.

Principles of Bandaging

■ Always wear disposable gloves and follow Standard Precautions.

■ Never tie a bandage around the neck; taping a dressing to the neck is safer. Anything that encircles the neck could strangle the victim.

■ The bandage needs to be snug enough to hold the dressing in place but not tight
enough to stop the circulation.

■ When applying dressings and bandages to wounds on arms or legs, leave fingers
and toes exposed so that you can watch for discoloration of the skin or swelling.

■ Check the skin temperature. Cold skin may indicate poor circulation caused by
a bandage that is too tight. Check the bandage to be certain it is not too tight.
You should be able to insert a finger under the bandage.

■ Loosen bandages if the patient complains of numbness or a tingling feeling.

■ Do not remove a dressing once it has been applied. If blood soaks through, add
another layer of dressings and secure with a bandage.

PROCEDURE 13.11

APPLYING A SPLINT

1. Put on disposable gloves.
2. Move fractured area as little as possible.

ALERT: Follow Standard Precautions.

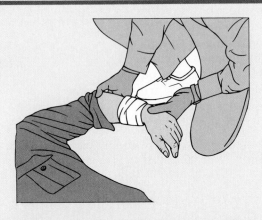

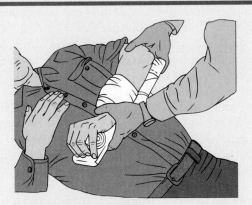

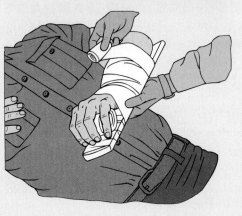

3. Splint area with a firm object, such as newspapers, magazines folded flat, wood, or a commercially made splint. The **splint** should extend from the fingertips to the elbow. Place padding or roller gauze in the hand for support and comfort.

4. Secure splint in place using roller gauze, wrapping it snugly and overlapping about two-thirds each wrap, or secure splint to extremity with strips of cloth at distal and proximal ends of the arm. You can wrap roller gauze over the fracture site.

5. If it is an open fracture, apply dressing over wound and secure in place with tape or with roller gauze that holds splint in place.

splint   Firm object used to support an unstable body part.

APPLYING A TRIANGULAR SLING

1. Put on disposable gloves.
2. Make a sling from a piece of cloth, clothing, towel, or sheet; fold or cut this material into shape of a triangle.

The ideal sling is about 50 to 60 inches long at its base and 36 to 40 inches long on each side.

ALERT: Follow Standard Precautions.

3. Position triangular material over top of patient's chest opposite the injured arm, as shown in Figure A. Fold patient's arm across chest. If patient cannot hold his or her own arm, have someone assist you, or provide support for client's arm until you are ready to tie sling. Note that one point of triangle should extend beyond patient's elbow on injured side.
4. Take bottom point of triangle and bring this end up over patient's arm. When you are finished, take this bottom point over top of patient's shoulder on the side of injured arm. (See Figure B.)
5. Draw up on ends of sling so that patient's hand is about 4 inches above elbow. Tie the two ends of the sling together, making sure that the knot does not press against back of client's neck. Place a flat pad of dressing

or a handkerchief under the knot. Leave patient's fingertips exposed so that you can see any color changes that indicate lack of circulation. Check for radial pulse. If pulse is absent, take off sling and attempt to reposition arm to regain pulse, then repeat procedure.

6. Take point of material at patient's elbow and fold it forward. Pin it to front of sling. This forms a pocket for patient's elbow. If you do not have pin, twist excess material and tie knot in point. This will provide a shallow pocket for patient's elbow. (See Figure C.)
7. Create a swathe by folding a triangular bandage in half and then folding it to a 4-inch width. This swathe is tied around chest and injured arm, over sling. Do not place this swathe over patient's arm on uninjured side. (See Figure D.)

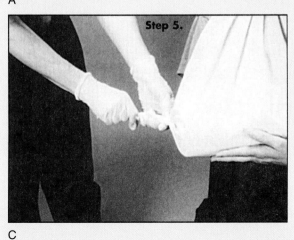

Step 2.

A

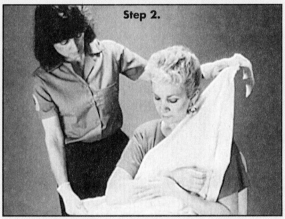

Step 3.

B

Step 5.

C

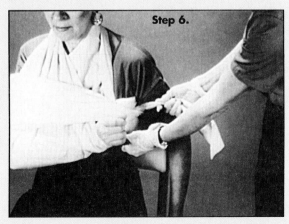

Step 6.

D

1. Put on disposable gloves.
2. Fold triangular bandage to make 2-inch hem along base.

ALERT: Follow Standard Precautions.

3. Apply gauze pad over wound. With folded edge face out, position bandage on patient's forehead, just above eyes. Make certain that point of bandage hangs down behind patient's head.

4. Draw ends of bandage behind patient's head and tie them.

5. Next, pull ends to front of client's head and tie them together.

6. Tuck in the tail at back.

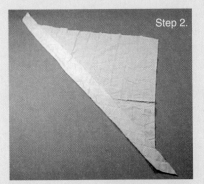

Step 2.

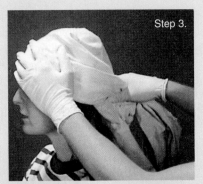

Step 3.

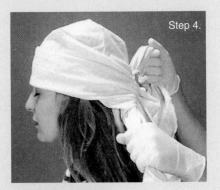

Step 4.

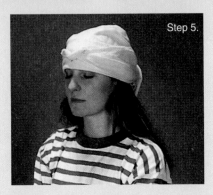

Step 5.

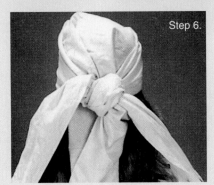

Step 6.

PROCEDURE 13.14

CIRCULAR BANDAGING OF A SMALL LEG OR ARM WOUND

1. Put on disposable gloves.
2. Apply dressing to wound and elevate extremity.

3. Place end of gauze roll (1 to 2 inches wide) on dressing. Anchor end of gauze roll over dressing with two

ALERT: Follow Standard Precautions.

CIRCULAR BANDAGING OF A SMALL LEG OR ARM WOUND *(Continued)*

initial wraps. (Place end of gauze over the dressing. Wrap gauze around the area once. Fold angled corner of gauze back over wrapped gauze.) Continue to wrap from distal (far) end of extremity to proximal (near the torso) end until entire dressing is covered.

Bandage will overlap dressing on both sides. Pull bandage snug as you wrap. Overlap each wrap by about two-thirds. Cut gauze and tape end or tie gauze to secure in place.

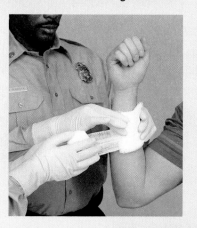
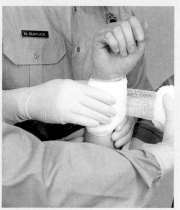

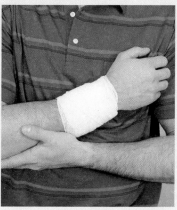

SPIRAL BANDAGING OF A LARGE WOUND

1. Put on disposable gloves.
2. Apply dressing to wound.

3. Place end of gauze roll (3 to 6 inches wide) on lower edge of dressing.

ALERT: Follow Standard Precautions.

4. Anchor end.
5. Wrap gauze around arm or leg at an angle and overlap the edges.

6. If you use up the gauze, continue the wrap with another roll.
7. Secure end by taping or tying off.

PROCEDURE 13.16

BANDAGING OF AN ANKLE OR FOOT WOUND

1. Put on disposable gloves.
2. Apply dressing to wound.

3. Place end of gauze roll (1 to 2 inches wide) on top of foot just above toes, and anchor ends.

ALERT: Follow Standard Precautions.

4. On second wrap around foot, bring gauze around back of ankle and over top of foot. Bring gauze under foot and over top of foot again. Wrap around ankle and over top of foot, then under foot. Continue these steps until dressing is covered, and secure gauze by tying off or taping.

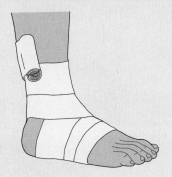

⬤ SUMMARY

In this unit, you learned very basic first-aid skills. You have been introduced to the general principles of handling both life-threatening and non-life-threatening situations. You have learned about rescue breathing, obstructed airway, and heart attack. We have discussed the treatment for shock, poisoning, serious wounds, and burns. It is very important for you to become proficient in first aid. To do this, you should attend a class given by a qualified American Red Cross instructor.

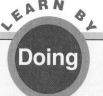

Doing

UNIT 5 ACTIVITY

1. Complete Worksheet 8 as assigned.
2. Practice the procedure.
3. Prepare responses to each item listed in Chapter Review—Your Link to Success at the end of this chapter.
4. When you are confident that you can meet each objective, ask your instructor for the unit evaluation.

Thinking Critically

1. **Legal and Ethical** When you stop to help those involved in an accident, do the laws of your state protect you against legal action if something goes wrong? What is the law called? Give an example of a recent case in which the law protected a rescuer or did not protect a rescuer.

2. **Case Study** The facility you work in is being evacuated for a bomb threat. When the fire department arrives, they find a patient who was not evacuated from an examination room. The patient panics, starts screaming, and then faints. Later, in the parking lot, the patient complains of chest pain and is transferred to the hospital. A week later, it is determined that the patient suffered a heart attack during the evacuation episode. The patient and family are threatening to sue your employer.

Can you justify leaving the patient in a room during the evacuation? Can you predict the outcome of the lawsuit?

3. **Patient Education** Mrs. Green is the most cheerful patient in the facility and a pleasure to work with. She is fond of telling everyone that whatever is in the cards will happen, whatever you do. How will you get her to cooperate with the facility's safety policies and procedures, such as fire drills? Describe how you would talk to her about safety requirements and what is necessary for patients to understand and to do.

4. **Customer Service** In a home care environment you notice that your client is very careless with the kitchen stove. Describe how you could demonstrate safer stove use while assisting the client with meal preparation.

Portfolio Connection

Reading product labels correctly is a key component of many of our daily projects. We need to know if products will do what we want them to do. We need to know if there is a risk in using a product. In this chapter, we discussed MSDS (material safety data sheet) forms. You learned that MSDSs provide all the primary information needed for any product in the work environment. If you become a home health aide, you work in clients' homes. There will not be an MSDS book to refer to. You will have to read the labels on products for the information you need. Choose three household products from home—for example, toothpaste, a cleaning product, White-Out, a synthetic food product—and create your own MSDS form for each of these three products. Use the following headings in your forms.

1. Product Identification
2. Hazardous Ingredients of Mixture
3. Physical Data
4. Fire and Explosion
5. Reactivity Data
6. Health Hazard Data
7. Emergency and First-Aid Procedures
8. Spill or Leak Procedures
9. Protection Information/Control Measures
10. Special Precautions

Portfolio Tip

Always keep good body mechanics in mind as you work so that you stay strong and limber. Make notes for your portfolio identifying the most enjoyable ways of staying in shape. Interview family and friends and keep the emphasis on fun and relaxation: how many types of dancing could you learn? Line dancing, tap, ballroom?

Completion of this assignment for your portfolio shows your ability to assimilate information and transfer your knowledge into a usable format for your daily use. When you appropriately apply each step of your learning, you show others that you are capable of taking responsibility in a work environment. Place these three forms in the section of your portfolio labeled "Written Reports and Assignments."

Remember! Media Connection

Use the Companion Website **www.prenhall.com/badasch** and the CD-ROM for additional interactive learning activities.

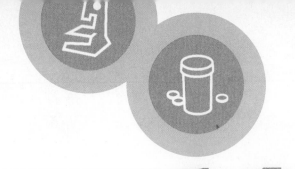

Chapter 14

Employability and Leadership

MEDIA CONNECTION

Use the Companion Website
www.prenhall.com/badasch and the CD-ROM
for additional interactive learning activities.

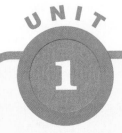

UNIT 1

Job-Seeking Skills

STEPS TO SUCCESS

1. Read this unit.
2. Complete the Learn by Doing assignment at the end of this unit.

UNIT OBJECTIVES

When you have completed this unit, you will be able to do the following:

✔ List seven places to seek employment opportunities and explain the benefits of each.

✔ Explain four ways to contact an employer.

✔ Name three occasions when a cover letter is used.

✔ List eight items required on a résumé.

UNIT RATIONALE

Before you apply the skills you have learned, you must find a job and be hired as an employee. It is important to learn the skills needed to find a job and to keep a job. This enables you to practice the health care career that you worked so hard to learn.

✔ Identify seven items generally requested on a job application form.

✔ Write a cover letter and a résumé.

✔ Complete a job application.

✔ List five do's and five don'ts of job interviewing.

⬤ FINDING A JOB

Looking for and finding a job takes planning and requires the use of many skills. In this chapter, you learn the steps to follow when you are ready to find a job. These skills give you the tools to be successful in job seeking and save you a lot of time.

⬤ YOUR VOCATIONAL PORTFOLIO

As time approaches to begin your search for a job, review your portfolio notebook. Obtain a new cover and section dividers so your finished portfolio has a clean, crisp look. Identify the items that best reflect your knowledge level, skills, and personality. When you complete your résumé and other portfolio requirements place them in the appropriate section of your new portfolio.

○ PLACES TO SEEK EMPLOYMENT

■ **Newspaper ads.** Jobs in health care careers appear in newspaper ads. When you look for a job in the newspaper, turn to the classified ads and look under "Help Wanted." There are different ways of listing jobs. Some papers list all health care positions under "Medical." Others list them under a particular job. See Figure 14.1 for some examples of ads from several newspapers. You also need to become familiar with some of the abbreviations used by newspapers.

Common Abbreviations

appl.	applicant	immed.	immediately
asst.	assistant	incl.	included
cert.	certified	lic.	licensed
exp.	experience	N.A.	nurse aide
FT	full time	PT	part time

■ **Directly to the employer.** If you are looking for a position in a laboratory, you might apply directly to a medical laboratory. If you want to work in a hospital, you go to the **personnel** department. The Yellow Pages of your phone book offer an excellent resource of possible employers.

■ **Friends and relatives.** You may know of someone working in the health care field who can suggest a place to apply or who can introduce you to a possible employer.

■ **School counselors.** Many schools have career counselors and/or work experience counselors. They are a good resource for the types of jobs available in your community.

■ **School bulletin boards.** If you have a career center or a bulletin board where jobs are listed, be sure to check it daily.

■ **Employment agencies.** There are both public and private employment agencies. Employers call these agencies to list the job openings that they have. A public agency does not charge a fee; however, a private agency charges either the employer or the person seeking a position. The Yellow Pages list employment agencies, and some of them specialize in health care careers. The public agencies are listed in the white pages under "Government Agencies."

■ **Internet.** If you have access to a computer that is connected to the Internet, go to Search and type in the words *"job search"* or *"job link."*

personnel 🔊

People who work in an establishment; a personnel office is where a worker goes to apply for a job.

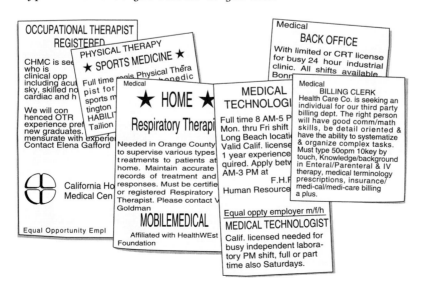

Figure 14.1

Examples of newspaper advertisements for health care jobs.

⚪ WAYS TO CONTACT AN EMPLOYER

Now that you know where to look for a job, you need to know how to make the contact and how to present yourself.

Telephone

If you have a lead on a possible job, you may choose to call for an appointment. Give your name and the job you are interested in and ask when you may come in to apply.

Cover Letter

You may be asked to send a letter in order to apply for a particular position. You need a cover letter when

- You are applying for a job that is out of town.
- You are answering a newspaper advertisement.
- A potential employer requests a letter.

Your cover letter is a sales letter. You want to sell yourself to the employer in order to get an interview. (A sample cover letter is shown in Figure 14.2.) Your letter should

- Be neat
- Have all the words spelled correctly
- State where you heard about the job opening
- State what you are applying for and why you are qualified for this specific position
- Give a brief overview of your education, experience, and qualifications
- Refer to your portfolio with work samples, skills checkoff lists, and evaluations
- Request an interview
- Give your address and phone number

Résumé

In addition to your cover letter, it is helpful for a potential employer to have more details about you and your qualifications. This is accomplished by preparing a résumé. (See the example in Figure 14.3.) A résumé includes the following:

- Your name, address, phone number, and message number
- Career plans
- Details about your education
- Your past work experience—paid or unpaid
- What honors you have earned
- What activities you like
- Skills, strengths, and abilities
- References (always ask permission to use someone as a reference)

Job Application

Most employers require that you fill out an application. When you fill out a job application, you give the employer needed information and also have an opportunity to demonstrate that you are neat and well organized. Use the information in your vocational portfolio to fill out an application. Included should be

888 Whitegate Avenue
Los Angeles, CA 90820

January 25, 2003

Mr. E. B. Burns
Director of Nurses
St. Joseph's Hospital
P.O. Box 123
Los Angeles, CA 90880

Dear Mr. Burns:

I am responding to your advertisement in Nurses World on January 14, 2003. I am interested in applying for the position of nurse assistant. I graduated from Medical Technologies High School on December 15, 2002. I studied nursing assisting and am well qualified for this position. My course work included communication, CPR, and a core of courses that prepared me to be employed as a nursing assistant. I also worked in a hospital setting eight hours a week for sixteen weeks. My attendance is excellent, and I am very reliable. My goal is to use my skills as a nursing assistant and to be an exemplary employee.

My résumé is enclosed. Also included is a list of skills I have mastered. I know that I am well qualified for this position. I am looking forward to an opportunity to interview for this position. I will call on Monday, February 3, at 9:00 a.m. and hope to arrange an interview at that time.

If you require additional information, or want to contact me, please call me at (123) 456-7890 after 3:00 p.m.

Sincerely,

Mark Adams, CNA

Figure 14.2

Sample cover letter to potential employer.

- Your complete address with the zip code.
- Your Social Security number.
- Your phone number or a number where you can be reached.
- A list of the schools you have attended, with dates.
- A list of any special training that you have.
- A prepared list of any past jobs, the address of the employer, the dates you worked there, and what your duties were.
- A list of people who can give you a reference. Be certain that you have their addresses and phone numbers. Also be certain that you have asked permission to use them as a reference.

There are also other ways that you can prepare. Be sure that you

- Carry a pen—do not use a pencil.
- Read the application all the way through.

800 N. Euclid   Home: 220-666-8340
New York, New York 00333   Message: 220-620-9180

Mary Jane Rodgers

Career Plans	Complete 2-year Associate of Science Nursing Program

Short-range: Nursing assistant

Long-range: Complete a Bachelor of Science Program as a registered nurse

Experience

2002–present	Henry's Hamburger Shop	New York, NY

Sales Clerk

- Food preparation
- Counting inventory
- Customer service
- Operating a cash register and making change
- Maintaining health standards

2000–2002	June Allison	New York, NY

Babysitter

- Meal preparation
- Overnight care of two children, 8 and 10 years of age
- Planning recreation

Family Responsibilities

- Prepare dinner 2–3 times a week
- Weekly gardening
- Perform minor household tasks

Experience

Diploma candidate 2003 Hoover High School	New York, NY

Interests

Dancing, classical music, reading, skiing, member of Explorer Scouts Medical Post and Health Occupation Students of America

Skills and Strengths

Fluent in oral and written Spanish communication

Proficient in Windows programs including Word, WordPerfect, Excel, and Lotus applications

Figure 14.3

Sample résumé.

- Print unless you are told to write.
- Spell accurately.
- Answer every question. Put "NA" (not applicable) in the space to show that you did not overlook the question.
- Recheck for errors.

◯ INTERVIEW

The interviewer wants to be sure that you are the best fit for the job. She is assessing your skills from the time she receives your résumé. Her focus during the interview is to determine if your explanations and behaviors match the job requirements. This evaluation occurs throughout the interview process, even when conversation is about the weather or hobbies. It is important to make a good first impression. The following guidelines tell you what to do and what not to do during an interview.

Interview Guidelines

Follow these guidelines for a positive interview experience.

- Be well groomed.
- Dress neatly and appropriately (no jeans).
- Be on time.
- Greet the interviewer by name, and smile.
- Shake hands firmly.
- Stand until asked to sit.
- Answer questions truthfully and sincerely.
- Be enthusiastic.
- Do not chew gum.
- Do not criticize former employers or teachers.
- Look at the interviewer when you talk.
- Do not talk about personal problems.
- When the interview is over, thank the interviewer and leave quickly.

Interview Preparation

The interviewer expects you to answer a variety of questions pertinent to the job you are applying for. Be prepared to give at least three examples of your behavior in various situations. Each experience should describe the

- **Situation.** What exactly happened?
- **Behavior.** What did you do?
- **Outcome.** What were the results?

Read the following questions and determine how to answer them.

- Tell me about the most difficult decision you made at school or work in the last few months.
- Tell me how you get along with people at school or work.
- Tell me about the most difficult job or school task you've done. Why was it difficult? How did you get past the difficulties?
- Explain a recent situation that demonstrates your ability to be a team player.

- Describe a situation in which you had to work under pressure. What kind of pressure were you facing? How did you handle the situation? What was the outcome?

- Describe a situation where you had to be very flexible. How did your actions demonstrate your flexibility?

After the Interview

The interviewer will do a reference check to verify that your résumé and application are honest and accurate. She will also rate your responses to help her make a decision about which candidate is best for the job. The following is an example of an interview rating scale with topics.

	Excellent	Average	Not Acceptable
Appearance			
Manner			
Qualifications			
Experience			
Job fit			

After the interview, send a letter of thanks to the interviewer. (See the example in Figure 14.4.) This lets the interviewer know that you are interested in the position, and it may increase your chance of getting the job.

Finding a job and then getting a job take effort on your part. Careful planning is the key to your success, and you will be glad that you took time to prepare yourself.

Figure 14.4

Sample thank-you letter to interviewer.

888 Whitegate Avenue
Los Angeles, CA 90820

February 10, 2003

Mr. E. B. Burns
Director of Nurses
St. Joseph's Hospital
P.O. Box 123
Los Angeles, CA 90880

Dear Mr. Burns:

Thank you for interviewing me yesterday afternoon. The position interests me very much, and I know that I will do a good job for you. I hope that you will give me an opportunity to work for the nursing department at St. Joseph's.

Sincerely,

Mark Adams, CNA

SUMMARY

Finding a job requires effort on your part. When you decide to look for a job, check the newspaper; go to a personnel department; ask friends, relatives, and your school counselor if they know of an opening; check employment agencies and bulletin boards; and search the Internet. After finding a possible opening, contact the employer. Call for an appointment, or send a cover letter with your résumé. You will also have to fill out a job application.

The last step is your interview with the employer. There are some important rules to follow when you go to an interview. After your interview, send a thank-you note to the interviewer.

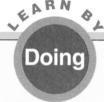

UNIT 1 ACTIVITY

1. **Complete Worksheet 1.**
2. **Ask your instructor for directions to complete Worksheets/ Activities 2 through 7.**
3. **When you are confident that you can meet each objective, ask your instructor for the unit evaluation.**

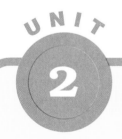

Keeping a Job

STEPS TO SUCCESS

1. Complete Vocabulary Worksheet 1 in the Student Workbook.
2. Read this unit.
3. Complete the Learn by Doing assignment at the end of this unit.

UNIT RATIONALE

You spend a lot of time and effort learning the skills for a career in health care. You also spend a lot of time and effort finding a job and then getting the job. Now that you have the job, you want to keep it. Employers have very specific things that they are looking for in an employee. The information in this unit tells what these things are and how you can be a good employee.

UNIT OBJECTIVES

When you have completed this unit, you will be able to do the following:

✔ Define vocabulary words.

✔ List four employer responsibilities.

✔ List four responsibilities of a good employee.

⬤ RESPONSIBILITIES

The Good Employer

An employer has responsibilities to you, and you have responsibilities to the employer. The good employer demonstrates

- *Dignity,* by respecting each employee as an important member of the health care team. Providing a safe, clean working environment is an example of treating employees and patients with dignity.

- *Excellence,* by encouraging personal and professional development, accountability, teamwork, and a commitment to quality health care. Employers who support routine activities and provide the necessary materials that allow you to do the best possible job show a dedication to excellence.

- *Service,* by establishing standards and guidelines directing appropriate, caring, compassionate health care to those dependent on the health care services. Providing clear guidelines for employees to follow gives the direction necessary to accomplish the job in a caring, compassionate manner.

- *Fairness and justice,* by establishing employee salaries and benefits that are fair and reliable. An employer who provides a reasonable salary for agreed-upon work and establishes a standard salary and benefit structure for all employees is striving to be a fair, equitable employer.

The Good Employee

As a good employee, you demonstrate

- *Dignity* through communication and interpersonal effectiveness, by

  • Being open, honest, and respectful • Listening actively and seeking understanding • Providing positive, helpful feedback

- *Excellence* through teamwork and accountability, by

  • Creating an environment of continuous improvement • Trying new ways to improve performance, processes, and service • Seeking growth and development opportunities for you and others • Taking responsibility for individual and team actions, decisions, and results • Adapting to changing needs and learning new skills, knowledge, and behaviors

- *Service* through being flexible and customer focused, by

  • Responding to the needs of those served and showing concern for meeting those needs • Responding quickly and effectively to problems that arise while providing service

- *Fairness and justice* by

  • Using equipment and supplies in an appropriate manner • Treating and responding to all people in the work environment with the same dignity, excellence, and service standards

Teamwork and team building are essential if you and your fellow workers expect to accomplish your goals (see Figure 14.5). When you follow these guidelines, your job gives you a sense of accomplishment. Being able to keep a job until you are ready to leave builds your references for the future. Remember that each job you have becomes an important part of your professional experience, and you want it to be a positive experience.

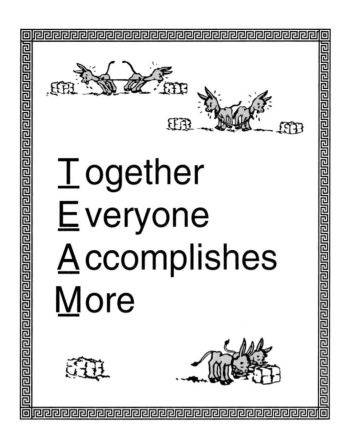

Figure 14.5

Together everyone
accomplishes more.

SUMMARY

Once you acquire a job, you and your employer agree to work together to accomplish the job you are hired to do. Your behavior reflects your attitude and values. Continually evaluate your actions using the Dignity, Excellence, Service, and Fairness/Justice criteria as a measure of your progress in the work environment. Be a team player by respecting your co-workers and encouraging them to do the best job they can do.

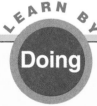

LEARN BY

Doing **UNIT 2 ACTIVITY**

1. **Ask your instructor for directions to complete Worksheet/
   Activity 2.**

2. **When you are confident that you can meet each objective, ask your instructor for the
   unit evaluation.**

Becoming a Professional Leader

STEPS TO SUCCESS

1. Read this unit.

2. Complete the Learn by Doing assignment at the end of this unit.

UNIT RATIONALE

Student and professional health care organizations enhance the delivery of compassionate, high-quality care by providing knowledge, skill, and leadership development. Committed students and professionals seek opportunities provided by these organizations to keep current and to provide patients with good-quality care.

UNIT OBJECTIVES

When you have completed this chapter, you will be able to do the following:

✔ Define vocabulary words.

✔ Name the three main benefits of being a member of a student health vocational organization.

✔ Name six benefits of being a member of a professional organization.

✔ Identify ways to find a professional organization.

✔ Identify steps to becoming a leader.

✔ Define *HOSA* and *SkillsUSA*.

✔ Summarize why you plan to participate in a student and professional organization.

◯ MEMBERSHIP IN AN ORGANIZATION

Membership in your student or professional organization gives you an opportunity to gain occupational knowledge and skills. It also provides opportunities to develop leadership skills. Some of the skills that you learn include the following:

■ Professional ethics

■ Communication and interpersonal relations

■ Leadership skills

■ Ability to recognize and initiate change

■ How to organize activities and people

■ Time management

■ Establishing priorities

■ Budgeting

■ Fund raising

■ Current health issues

Health Occupations Students of America (HOSA)

Health Occupations Students of America (HOSA) is the student organization for health occupation students at the secondary, postsecondary, adult, and college level (See HOSA's emblem in Figure 14.6). Among HOSA's primary goals are to

■ Promote career opportunities in the health care industry

■ Enhance and promote the delivery of quality health care to all people

■ Encourage all health occupations students and instructors to be actively involved in current health care issues

Skills Competitions

HOSA provides many opportunities for students to learn and achieve. One such opportunity is the skills competitions. Competitions are at three levels—local, state, and national—with students advancing on to the next levels by winning the previous ones. HOSA offers 44 different events divided into categories based on the curriculum. Competitive event categories include:

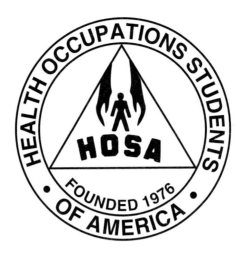

Figure 14.6

Emblem of HOSA. (Reprinted by permission of Health Occupations Students of America.)

■ Category I: Health occupations related to

• Medical math • Medical spelling • Medical terminology • Dental spelling • Dental terminology

■ Category II: Health occupations skills such as

• Medical assisting—clerical • Medical assisting—clinical • Dental assisting • Nursing assisting • Practical/vocational nursing • CPR/first aid

■ Category III: Individual leadership skills including

• **Extemporaneous** speaking • Extemporaneous health display • Extemporaneous writing • Job-seeking skills • Prepared speaking

extemporaneous
Completed with little preparation.

■ Category IV: Team leadership demonstrated by

• Community awareness • HOSA Bowl participation

■ Category V: Recognition

• Outstanding HOSA chapter • National recognition program

Competition requirements include the following:

■ Student must be an active HOSA member.

■ Student must be identified as either a secondary student (currently enrolled in a high school) or a postsecondary student (graduate from high school or over 18 years of age).

Students attending HOSA functions follow a strict code of conduct and official HOSA uniform and competitive event dress codes. Experiencing the challenges, structure, and competition in HOSA teaches students how to reach for and achieve their highest potential.

Vocational Industrial Clubs of America (VICA)

SkillsUSA-VICA is a national organization serving more than 250,000 high school and college students and professional members who are enrolled in training programs in technical, skilled, and service occupations, including health occupations. SkillsUSA has more than a quarter million student members annually, organized into 13,000 chapters and 54 state and territorial associations (including the District of Columbia, Puerto Rico, Guam and the Virgin Islands). See the SkillsUSA-VICA emblem in Figure 14.7. For additional information see the Website at www.skillsUSA.org.

Figure 14.7

Emblem of SkillsUSA-VICA.

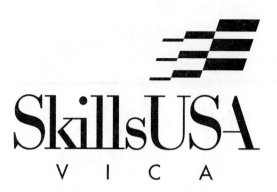

Purpose Statement

SkillsUSA prepares America's high performance workers. It provides quality educational experiences for students in leadership, teamwork, citizenship and character development. It builds and reinforces self-confidence, work attitudes and communications skills. It emphasizes total quality at work, high ethical standards, superior work skills, life-long education and pride in the dignity of work. SkillsUSA also promotes understanding of the free enterprise system and involvement in community service activities.

Programs

SkillsUSA programs include local, state and national competitions in which students demonstrate occupational and leadership skills. During the annual national-level SkillsUSA Championships, more than 4,100 students compete in 73 occupational and leadership skill areas. SkillsUSA programs also help to establish industry standards for job skill training in the classroom.

The Total Quality Curriculum enhances SkillsUSA's Quality at Work movement by preparing students for the world of work starting in the classroom. The curriculum emphasizes the competencies and essential workplace basic skills identified by employers and the U.S. Secretary of Labor's Commission on Achieving Necessary Skills (SCANS). The Professional Development Program is a self-paced curriculum for secondary and college students. It teaches skills such as effective communication and management, teamwork, networking, workplace ethics, job interviewing and more. The curriculum involves local industry and academics and can be used in day-trades, apprenticeship training, cooperative education, school-to-work, academic and special needs programs.

National Program of Work

The National Program of Work sets the pace for SkillsUSA-VICA nationwide. All programs are in some way related to the following seven major goals. The expectation is that each chapter will carry out this program of work.

Professional development

To prepare each SkillsUSA-VICA member for entry into the work force and provide a foundation for success in a career. Becoming a professional does not stop with acquiring a skill, but involves an increased awareness of the meaning of good citizenship and the importance of labor and management in the world of work.

Community service

To promote and improve good will and understanding among all segments of the community through services donated by SkillsUSA-VICA chapters, and to instill in its members a lifetime commitment to community service.

Employment

To increase student awareness of quality job practices and attitudes, and to increase the opportunities for employer contact and eventual employment.

Ways and means

To plan and participate in fund-raising activities to allow all members to carry out the chapter's projects.

SkillsUSA Championships

To offer students the opportunity to demonstrate their skills and be recognized for them through competitive activities in occupational areas and leadership.

Public relations

To make the general public aware of the good work that students in career and technical education are doing to better themselves and their community, state, nation and world.

Social activities

To increase cooperation in the school and community through activities that allow SkillsUSA-VICA members to get to know each other in something other than a business or classroom setting.

PROFESSIONAL ORGANIZATIONS

Professional organizations help professionals keep current in the latest technology and trends. Being aware of the advantages offered through involvement in such organizations motivates health care workers to become active in the professional group for their chosen occupation.

There are numerous professional organizations for the health care worker. Most organizations have a local chapter, state chapter, and national chapter. Each supports the other, and all work toward common goals. Belonging to a professional organization provides the following benefits:

- Updates on new technological advances
- Communication with other geographical areas
- Shared resources
- Resources for employment opportunities
- Current legislative issues
- Interaction with other health professionals
- Pooled money to accomplish changes for the good of the occupation/profession
- Power as a united group to encourage positive change
- Development of new ideas that support growth

When your classes are complete, find your professional organization by

- Referring to Chapter 2 of this book
- Asking fellow employees
- Reading the bulletin boards at work
- Reading your professional journals
- Reading brochures
- Attending occupationally related inservice programs
- Checking the *Occupational Outlook Handbook*

LEADERSHIP

Becoming a leader in your occupational area takes time and patience. To become a leader you must take several important steps. These include the following:

- Developing a superior skill level
- Becoming a decision maker

- Being a good communicator
- Developing a balanced focus on tasks and people

Tom Peters, author of *A Passion for Excellence*, says:

"A leader is a . . .	**A leader is not a . . .**
cheerleader	cop
enthusiast	referee
nurturer	devil's advocate
coach	naysayer
facilitator	pronouncer"

A true leader unites people and works toward positive outcomes.

⬤ SUMMARY

Participation in HOSA or SkillsUSA is an important part of your career development and professionalism. As a member, you are introduced to various health careers, develop a responsible attitude toward your community, develop knowledge and skills for the work world, and gain self-confidence.

Membership prepares you to be a leader in your chosen occupation; it also helps you prepare to become a valuable member of your professional organization when you join the workforce.

To become a leader you must develop superior skill levels, become a decision maker, be a good communicator, and develop a balanced focus on tasks and people.

For more information, write

National HOSA
6021 Morriss Road
Suite 111
Flower Mound, TX 75028
(800) 321-4672
FAX (972) 874-0063
Website: http://www.hosa.org
e-mail: info@hosa.org

SkillsUSA-VICA
P.O. Box 3000
Leesburg, VA 20177-0300
(703) 777-8810
FAX (703) 777-8999
Website: http://www.skillsusa.org
e-mail: anyinfo@skillsusa.org

UNIT 3 ACTIVITY

1. Complete Worksheet 1.
2. Ask your instructor for directions to complete Worksheet/ Activity 2.
3. Prepare responses to each item listed in Chapter Review—Your Link to Success at the end of this chapter.
4. When you are confident that you can meet each objective, ask your instructor for the unit evaluation.

Thinking Critically

1. **Communication** Preparing for an interview requires time and practice. To prepare adequately for an interview,
   - Write answers to the questions on pages 313–314.
   - Think through how you want to use your tone of voice to emphasize certain points.
   - Practice saying your answers to questions in front of the mirror.
   - Ask another person (a professional who interviews in his or her work setting is best) to ask you these questions and to hear your responses.
   - Ask the questioner to evaluate you and make recommendations.
   - Find a partner and role-play a job interview. Write a full job description and plan at least a 15-minute interview. Decide your roles; record the interview and then switch roles. Play back your sessions and critique one another.

2. **Computers** Go to the Web sites for HOSA and SkillsUSA to learn more about them. Do these organizations offer information to members on continuing education? Do they further members' rights as practicing professionals? Print out and keep a copy of any relevant information.

3. **Medical Math** Concepts in medical math apply in calculating values pertinent to choosing a job. You make the best job choice when you take all of the benefits of a job into consideration. Some jobs pay less but have excellent benefits. Other jobs pay a high salary and provide only minimum benefits. Calculate the full value of three different jobs by determining the dollar value of health insurance, paid vacation time, stock or retirement benefits, and life insurance benefits. Compare your findings and evaluate which job is best for you.

 Portfolio Connection

The cover letter, résumé, and thank-you letter are the primary tools for acquiring a job. There are ways to make your application packet stand out from others. Here are some of them:

- Prepare each item perfectly so that it presents you as the best possible candidate.

- Include a job objective at the top of your résumé— use key phrases that indicate your special talents and desires. *Example:* "I am seeking the position of a Clinical Medical Assistant in the ambulatory care setting. I am qualified for this position because it provides an opportunity to use my skills and training as a Clinical Medical Assistant."

- Add a statement to your cover letter that tells about your values concerning client-centered care and about teamwork. *Example:* "My school and work experience reflects a dedication to excellence through teamwork and responsibly carrying out assignments. My grades demonstrate an ability to focus on learning and to apply the learning in a clinical area."

- Add a statement to your thank-you letter that indicates your confidence in being capable of doing the job and your interest in the position. *Example:* "I am confident that my skill level as a Medical Assistant is appropriate for your office and that our

Portfolio Tip

First impressions last: greet everyone cheerfully and directly so that it becomes a habit.

common goals to serve patients and families through providing responsible health care will make me an asset to your team."

Rewrite your cover letter, résumé, and thank-you letter samples with these additional elements. Place them in your portfolio behind the appropriate tabs. When you complete training in a specific occupation, refer back to these documents and adapt them to focus specifically on the job you are applying for.

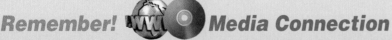

Remember! **Media Connection**

Use the Companion Website **www.prenhall.com/badasch** and the CD-ROM for additional interactive learning activities.

Part 2

Multidisciplinary Skills

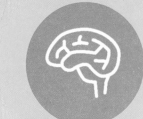
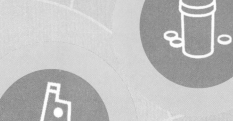

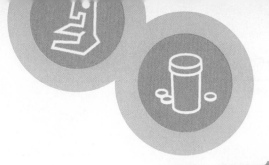

Chapter 15

Nurse Assistant/ Patient Caregiver

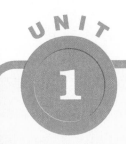

UNIT 1

Basic Care Skills/OBRA Standards/ Long-Term Care

STEPS TO SUCCESS

1. Complete Vocabulary Worksheet 1 in the Student Workbook.

2. Read this unit.

3. Complete the Learn by Doing assignment at the end of this unit.

UNIT OBJECTIVES

When you have completed this unit, you will be able to do the following:

✔ Complete all objectives in Part One of this book.

✔ Match vocabulary words with their correct meanings.

✔ Identify the following:
  • Responsibilities of the nurse assistant
  • Personal care equipment used by residents
  • Four skin conditions requiring special attention
  • Areas on the body where pressure sores usually develop
  • Antipressure aids
  • Occupied bed, closed bed, and open bed
  • Causes and symptoms of dehydration
  • Common types of specimens collected for analysis
  • Six common prosthetic devices

✔ List the following:
  • Four types of bathing
  • Two body areas requiring special attention during the bathing process

  • Four changes in the skin that may indicate the beginning of a pressure sore
  • Four techniques for positioning residents
  • Seven reasons why ambulation is important
  • Signs of diabetic coma and insulin shock
  • Nine steps to preparing a resident for a meal
  • Six ways to prevent pressure sores
  • Causes and symptoms of edema
  • Ways to help residents who have a colostomy, ileostomy, or ureterostomy
  • Symptoms that indicate a resident is about to faint, and precautions that prevent injury
  • Five conditions that may develop when using postural supports
  • Five things you must do when using postural supports
  • Five rules for oxygen safety

✔ Explain the following:
- Four important reasons to give mouth care
- Six important reasons for routine bathing
- Nine conditions poor body alignment causes
- Why residents with diabetes must have their toenails cut by a podiatrist
- Why a urinary drainage bag is not raised above the level of insertion
- Six causes of incontinence
- Procedures for bowel and/or bladder training
- Important observations about urine
- Important observations about stool

✔ Define the following terms:
- *AM* and *PM care*
- *Good body alignment*
- Seizure

- Syncope
- *Soft postural supports*
- *Guarding technique* and *guarding belt* from Chapter 19

✔ Match range-of-motion vocabulary words with their meanings.

✔ Calculate in cc's and record fluid intake properly.

✔ Evaluate and determine appropriate action for a given situation.

✔ Demonstrate each procedure in this chapter.

✔ Demonstrate the following in
- Chapter 19: Ambulating with a walking belt
  Walking with crutches
  Walking with a walker

○ RESPONSIBILITIES OF A LONG-TERM CARE NURSE ASSISTANT

Nurse assistants are important members of the health care team. They are responsible for giving personal care to the resident. They spend more time with the resident than the other members of the team. This gives them an opportunity to give extra support and understanding to the resident. They may work in an acute care hospital or in long-term care. Long-term care nurse assistants are required to complete training that meets the Omnibus Budget Reconciliation Act (OBRA) 1987 guidelines. They must also pass a test and receive a nursing assistant certification. (See pages xxiii–xxv.) Many long-term care nurse assistants choose to learn additional skills and work in the long-term care/rehabilitation sub-acute care area. These additional skills are described in Unit 2 of this chapter. The acute care and assistive personnel care skills are in your teacher's Instructors Guide. If you are interested in these areas, talk to your instructor about your interest (see Figure 15.1).

As a long-term nurse assistant you will

- **Admit,** discharge, and transfer residents.
- Provide AM and PM care.
- Provide oral hygiene.
- Offer the bedpan and urinal.
- Understand the seriousness of **impaction.**
- Understand the use of **enemas.**
- Assist with dressing and undressing.
- Bathe residents.
- Give **perineal** care.
- Give good skin care.
- Follow the patient care plan (see Figure 15.2).
- Perform range of motion.
- Provide body alignment and positioning.
- Care for hair and nails.
- Shave the resident.

admit
To let someone in, take in.

impaction
Being tightly wedged into a part (e.g., fecal material wedged into the bowel that requires mechanical means to remove).

enemas
Solution introduced into the rectum.

perineal
Region between the vulva and anus in a female, or between the scrotum and anus in a male.

Figure 15.1

The interdisciplinary team is made up of professionals and nonprofessionals from many health care fields.

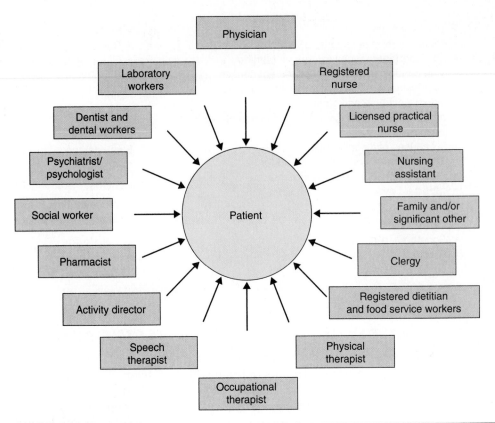

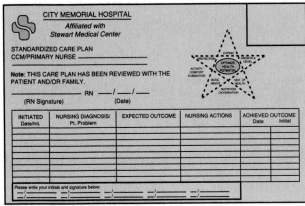

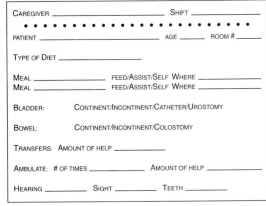

Figure 15.2

Components of the patient care plan.

- Apply hot and cold applications.
- Make the bed.
- Assist residents to move and ambulate.
- Apply prosthetic devices and supports.
- Assist with feeding the resident.
- Record intake and output.
- Care for the **incontinent** resident.
- Understand tubes and **catheters.**

incontinent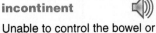

Unable to control the bowel or bladder.

catheters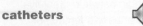

Tubes inserted into body opening or cavity.

■ Collect specimens.

■ Measure height and weight.

■ Take seizure precautions.

■ Give **stoma** care.

■ Do **postmortem** care.

◯ ADMISSION

You are one of the first people the resident and family see (see Figure 15.3). Be pleasant and try to put everyone at ease. The facility where you work has a procedure for you to follow when you admit the resident. Do not rush the resident. Give the person time to adjust to the new environment. When a resident is admitted to the hospital, there are some basic procedures that are followed. (See Figure 15.4 for a sample of an admission checklist.) These include the following:

■ Making a clothing list

■ Making a list of personal items

■ Requesting that the family take home valuables or see that they are put in a safe place

■ Taking vital signs

■ Weighing the resident

■ Explaining the call light and routine

■ Collecting urine specimens if required

NOTE: Always remember to record date, time, personal care or treatment given, any complaints, problems reported to the team leader/head nurse, and any other required information. Always sign with your name and certification.

Charting Flow Sheet

Many facilities provide a printed flow sheet for charting. The sheet includes activities of daily living (ADL), vital signs, diet, liquids, and type of care given. This checkoff list (see Figure 15.5) helps the charter provide all of the necessary information about patient care. If your facility doesn't have a flow sheet, use the charting examples.

stoma

Opening, e.g., opening in abdomen in an ostomy.

postmortem

After death.

Figure 15.3

Admitting a resident.

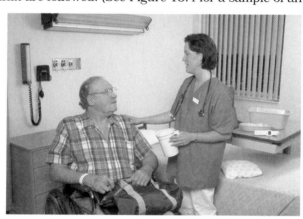

Figure 15.4

Sample admission checklist.

A SAMPLE ADMISSION CHECK LIST
(Fill in every statement and check every appropriate item)

Resident's name _____ Room number _____

Time of admission _____ a.m./p.m.   Date of admission _____
Unit ready to receive resident? Yes☐No☐ Equipment ready? Yes☐No☐
Admitted by stretcher _____ wheelchair _____ walking _____
Check identification bracelet? Yes☐No☐ Bed tag in place? Yes☐No☐
Did the resident need help to get undressed? Yes☐No☐
Is the resident in bed at this time? Yes☐No☐ Time _____ a.m./p.m.
Siderails up? Yes☐No☐
Bruises, marks, rashes, or broken skin noted? Yes☐No☐
    If yes, describe _____
Weight _____ Height _____ Scale Used? Yes☐No☐
Temperature_____ Pulse _____ Respirations _____ Blood Pressure _____
Admission urine specimen collected? Yes☐No☐ Sent to lab? Yes☐No☐
Unusual behavior noted? Yes☐No☐ Unusual appearance noted? Yes☐No☐
    If yes, describe_____
Does the resident have any difficulty with the English language? Yes☐No☐
Is the resident allergic to food? Yes☐No☐ Allergic to drugs? Yes☐No☐
Reason for admission _____
Complaints_____
Dentures? Yes☐No☐ Partial? Yes☐No☐ Full? Yes☐No☐ Denture cup? Yes☐No☐
Vision problems? Yes☐No☐ Does the resident wear glasses? Yes☐No☐ Contact lenses? ☐
Valuables: Money? Yes☐No☐ Describe_____
    Jewelry? Yes☐No☐ Describe_____
Is the resident hard of hearing? Yes☐No☐ Hearing aid? Yes☐No☐ Contact lenses? Yes☐No☐
    Artificial limb? Yes☐No☐ Brace? Yes☐No☐
Is the resident calm? Yes☐No☐ Is the resident very anxious? Yes☐No☐
    Angry? Yes☐No☐ Is the resident agitated or very excited? Yes☐No☐
Has the resident been admitted to this hospital before? Yes☐No☐
Is the clothing list completed? Yes☐No☐ Signed by _____
Is the signal cord attached to the bed? Yes☐No☐
Have drugs brought into the hospital by the resident been given to the charge nurse? Yes☐No☐
Name of the nurse drugs were given to _____
Additional comments _____
Admitted by _____

PROCEDURE 15.1

ADMITTING A RESIDENT

RATIONALE

Carefully following the admitting procedure gives the patient a sense of well-being and security. It also protects the facility from errors in identification and loss of patients' belongings.

ALERT: Follow Standard Precautions.

1. Wash hands.
2. Assemble equipment.
   a. Admission checklist
   b. Admission pack (may be all disposable depending on facility)
      (1) Bedpan
      (2) Urinal
      (3) Emesis basin
      (4) Wash basin
      (5) Tissues
   c. Gown or pajamas
   d. Portable scale
   e. Thermometer
   f. Blood pressure cuff
   g. Stethoscope
   h. Clothing list
   i. Envelope for valuables
3. Fan-fold bed covers to foot of bed. (See the procedure "Making an Open Bed.")
4. Put away resident's equipment.
5. Put gown or pajamas on foot of bed.
6. Greet resident and introduce yourself.
7. Identify resident by looking at arm band and asking name (see top figure at right).
8. Introduce resident to roommates.
9. Explain
   a. How call signal works
   b. How bed controls work (see bottom figure at right).
   c. Hospital regulations
   d. What you will be doing to admit him or her
10. Provide privacy by pulling privacy curtains.
11. Ask resident to put on gown or pajamas.
12. Check weight and height.
13. Help to bed if ordered. (Check with nurse.)

14. Put up side rails if required.
15. If resident has valuables:
   a. Make a list of jewelry, money, wallet, etc.
   b. Have resident sign list
   c. Have relative sign list
   d. Either have relative take home valuables or send to cashier's office in valuables envelope

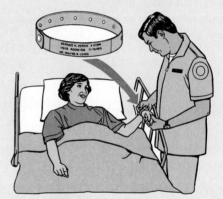

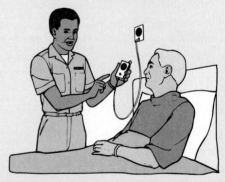

16. Take and record the following:
   a. Temperature, pulse, respiration
   b. Blood pressure
   c. Urine specimen, if required

17. Complete admission checklist noting
    a. Allergies
    b. Medications being taken
    c. Food preferences and dislikes
    d. Any prosthesis
    e. Skin condition
    f. Handicaps (e.g., deafness, sight, movement)
18. Orient resident to meal times, visiting hours, etc.

19. Wash hands.
20. Record information according to your facility's policy.

> 10/04/03 1500
> VS 98–76–18 120/80
> Admitted and oriented to facility.
> Admission checklist completed.
> Sitting in chair.
> States "Wish I could stay at home."
> _____ S. Gomez CNA

Figure 15.5

Example of a flow chart.

ACTIVITIES OF DAILY LIVING CHECKLIST

SELF —Done by patient
ASSIST —Patient assisted by nursing staff
TOTAL —Done by nursing staff
✔ —Check procedure performed.
Include time if appropriate.

DATE															
DIET	B'fast	Dinner	Supper	B'fast	Dinner	Supper	B'fast	Dinner	Supper	B'fast	Dinner	Supper	B'fast	Dinner	Supper
Ate all food served															
Ate approx. 1/2 food served															
Refused to eat															
PROCEDURE	11-7	7-3	3-11	11-7	7-3	3-11	11-7	7-3	3-11	11-7	7-3	3-11	11-7	7-3	3-11
A.M. or H.S. Care															
Oral Hygiene															
Bath–Bed bath complete															
Bed bath partial															
Shower															
Tub															
Self Care															
Back Care															
Bed Made															
ELIMINATION															
Bowel movement															
Involuntary B.M.															
Voided															
Incontinent															
Foley cath.															
Sitz Bath @															
ACTIVITY															
Bed rest complete															
Dangle															
Bed rest–B.R.P.															
Up in chair															
Up in room															
Walk in hall															
Ambulatory															
POSITION CHANGED															
Flat in bed															
Semi–Fowler's															
Deep breathe, cough															
Range of motion															
Turn from side to side															
Side Rails–Up															
Down															
Fresh Water @															
SIGNATURE & TITLE															

◯ HEIGHT AND WEIGHT

Residents are weighed and measured for height when they are admitted. These measurements provide a baseline during the resident's stay. Measurements must be accurate, as they are important to the well-being of the resident. The resident's weight is important because it indicates

- Nutritional status
- Any change (weight loss or gain) in condition

There are several different types of scales. Each is designed for ease in weighing residents with varying problems. The three types of scales are the

- Standing scale
- Scale with mechanical lift
- Wheelchair scale (Figure 15.6)

Figure 15.6

Chair scale.

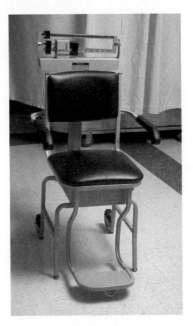

Residents who are wheelchair-bound can be left in the wheelchair and weighed. Allowance is made for the weight of the wheelchair and platform by subtracting a certain amount from the weight or by having the scale adjusted to allow for the extra weight. You can also use a mechanical lift that has a scale. It is operated by using a hydraulic pump to raise and lower the resident. This makes weighing a bedfast resident much easier.

Height is used as an indicator of the ideal weight of the resident. You may have to measure the resident with a measuring tape if the person is unable to stand. If the resident can stand, use the measure on the standing scale.

PROCEDURE 15.2 | **MEASURING WEIGHT ON A STANDING BALANCE SCALE**

RATIONALE

Weighing the patient provides a weight baseline. This baseline is used to compare decreases or increases in the patient's weight. Changes in body weight may indicate a change in the patient's health.

ALERT: Follow Standard Precautions.

1. Wash hands.
2. Assemble equipment.
   a. Portable balance scale
   b. Paper towel
   c. Paper and pencil/pen
3. Identify resident.
4. Explain what you are going to do.
5. Take resident to scale or bring scale to resident's room.

6. Place paper towel on platform of scale (with standing scale).
7. Put both weights to the very left on zero.
8. Balance beam pointer must stay steady in middle of balance area. (If pointer does not center, turn balance screw until it remains centered.)
9. Have resident remove shoes and stand on scale.

NOTE   The balance bar raises to top of bar guide and pointer is not centered.

PROCEDURE 15.2 | MEASURING WEIGHT ON A STANDING BALANCE SCALE *(Continued)*

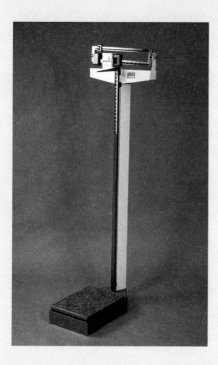

10. Move large weight to estimated weight of resident.

11. Move small weight to right until balance bar hangs free halfway between upper and lower bar guide.

12. The largest (lower) weight is marked in increments of 50 pounds; the smaller (upper weight) is marked in single pounds. The even-numbered pounds are marked with numbers (e.g., 2, 4, 6). The uneven pounds are unmarked long lines and the short line is one-fourth of a pound.

13. Write down weight on a notepad.

14. Help resident with shoes and make him or her comfortable.

15. Replace scale.

16. Wash hands.

17. Chart weight. Report any unusual increases or decreases in weight.

10/05/03 0900

Standing scale weight 125; 10 pounds less than last weight.

No complaints of loss of appetite, pain, or other problems.

Weight change reported to head nurse.

_____ S. Gomez CNA

PROCEDURE 15.3

MEASURING WEIGHT ON A CHAIR SCALE

RATIONALE

The chair scale provides a safe way to weigh a nonambulatory patient. Weighing the patient provides a weight baseline. This baseline is used to compare decreases or increases in the patient's weight. Changes in body weight may indicate a change in the patient's health.

ALERT: Follow Standard Precautions.

1. Place wheelchair on scale or transfer resident to chair on scale.
2. Follow the directions in the procedure "Measuring Weight on a Standing Balance Scale."

3. Write down weight on notepad.
4. Make resident comfortable.
5. Wash hands.
6. Chart weight.

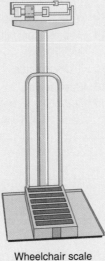

Wheelchair scale

> 10/05/03 0800
> Chair scale weight 125; no weight change.
> ———— S. Gomez CNA

PROCEDURE 15.4

MEASURING WEIGHT ON A MECHANICAL LIFT

RATIONALE

The mechanical lift provides a safe method for weighing a bedridden patient. Weighing the patient provides a weight baseline. This baseline is used to compare decreases or increases in the patient's weight. Changes in body weight may indicate a change in the patient's health.

ALERT: Follow Standard Precautions.

1. Wash hands.
2. Assemble equipment.
   a. Mechanical lift
   b. Sling
   c. Clean sheet

3. Identify resident.
4. Explain what you are going to do.
5. Pull privacy curtain.
6. Lower side rail on side you are working on.

7. Cover sling with clean sheet.

8. Help resident roll on side and place sling with top at shoulders and bottom at knees.

9. Fan-fold remaining sling.

10. Help resident roll to other side onto one half of sling and pull other half of sling through.

11. Broaden base of lift.

12. Wheel lift to side of bed with base beneath bed.

13. Position lift over resident.

14. Attach sling using chains and hooks provided. *(Keep open end of hook away from resident to avoid injury.)*

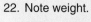

Scale with mechanical lift

15. Use hand crank or pump handle to raise resident from bed. Make certain that buttocks are not touching bed.

16. Check to be certain that resident is in center of sling and is safely suspended.

17. To weigh resident:

    a. Swing feet and legs over edge of bed; move lift away from bed so that no body part contacts bed.

    b. If bed is low enough, raise resident above bed so that no body part contacts bed.

18. Adjust weights until scale is balanced. (See the procedure "Measuring Weight on a Standing Balance Scale.")

19. Return resident to bed by reversing steps.

20. Replace mechanical lift.

21. Wash hands.

22. Note weight.

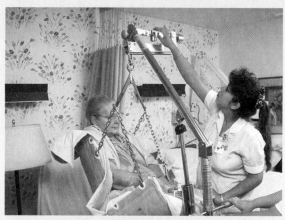

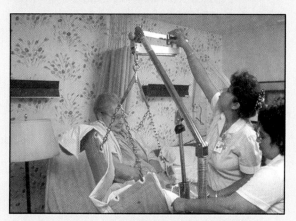

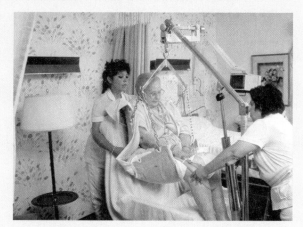

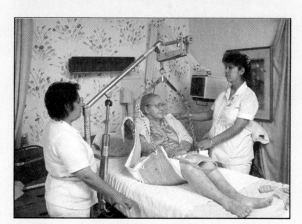

10/07/03 1000

Chair scale weight 250

No changes since last weighing

Tolerated well.

Noted reddened area on left shoulder

Reported to head nurse

S. Gomez CNA

PROCEDURE 15.5

MEASURING HEIGHT

RATIONALE

Accurately measuring height provides a baseline to help determine the patient's ideal weight. A loss in height over a period of time may indicate osteoporosis.

ALERT: Follow Standard Precautions.

1. Wash hands.
2. Assemble equipment.
   a. Balance scale with height rod
   b. Paper towels
3. Identify resident.
4. Explain what you are going to do.
5. Have resident remove shoes.
6. Raise measuring rod above head.
7. Have resident stand with back against measuring rod.
8. Instruct resident to stand straight, with heels touching measuring rod.
9. Lower measuring rod to rest on resident's head.
10. Check number of inches indicated on rod. This number is found where the sliding rod enters the hollow post.
11. Record in meters, centimeters, or feet and inches according to hospital policy.
12. Help resident with shoes.
13. Chart height.

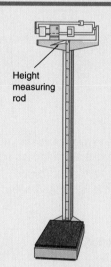

Height measuring rod

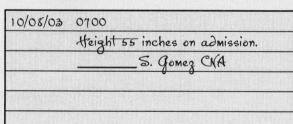

10/08/03 0700

Height 55 inches on admission.
S. Gomez CNA

⬤ TRANSFER

When you assist in transferring the resident to another area, the resident may be unhappy about the move. Be calm and pleasant, and explain that you will make the move as easy as possible. Be certain that all of the resident's belongings are transferred to the new area and that the nurse assistant who is responsible for the resident knows that the resident has arrived. Follow the policies and procedures of your facility for transferring residents.

⬤ DISCHARGE

A resident cannot be discharged without an order from his or her physician. If your resident plans to leave when it has not been ordered, report it to the head nurse immediately. Each facility has a policy and procedure for discharging the resident.

PROCEDURE 15.6 MOVING RESIDENT AND BELONGINGS TO ANOTHER ROOM

RATIONALE

Following the transfer procedure provides a sense of security for the patient and ensures that personal belongings are not lost. Introduction to the new area, roommate, and caregiver reduces the stress and provides continuing care.

ALERT: Follow Standard Precautions.

1. Wash hands.
2. Assemble equipment.
   a. Resident's chart
   b. Nursing care plan
   c. Medications
   d. Paper bag
3. Identify resident.
4. Explain what you are going to do.
5. Determine location to which resident is being transferred.
6. Gather resident belongings. (Check admission list.)
7. Determine how resident is to be transported.
   a. Wheelchair
   b. Stretcher
   c. Entire bed
   d. Ambulation
8. Transport resident to new unit.
9. Introduce to staff on new unit.
10. Introduce to new roommate.
11. Make resident comfortable.
12. Put away belongings.
13. Wash hands.
14. Give transferred medications, care plan, and chart to nurse.
15. Before leaving unit, record the following:
   a. Date and time of transfer
   b. How transported (e.g., wheelchair)
   c. How transfer was tolerated by resident
16. Return to original unit and report completion of transfer.

10/04/03   1430
Transferred in bed to room 20
Introduced to roommate and caregiver
Resting quietly in bed
_____ S. Gomez CNA

PROCEDURE 15.7 DISCHARGING A RESIDENT

RATIONALE

Carefully following the discharge procedure ensures that the patient takes all medications and personal belongings and that final arrangements are completed.

ALERT: Follow Standard Precautions.

1. Check chart for discharge order.
2. Wash hands.
3. Identify resident.
4. Explain what you are going to do.
5. Provide privacy by pulling the privacy curtain.
6. Help resident dress.
7. Collect resident's belongings.
8. Check belongings against admission list.

PROCEDURE 15.7 | DISCHARGING A RESIDENT *(Continued)*

9. Secure and return valuables.

    a. Verify with resident that all valuables are there.

    b. Have resident sign for them.

10. Check to see if resident has medications to take home.

11. Check to see if any equipment is to be taken home.

12. Help resident into wheelchair.

13. Help resident into car.

14. Return to unit.

    a. Remove all items left in unit (e.g., basins, disposable items).

    b. Clean unit according to your facility's policy.

15. Wash hands.

16. Record discharge.

    a. Date and time

    b. Method of transport

    c. Whom resident left with

10/04/03   1100

Discharged by wheelchair with son, personal belongings, medications, and instructions

———— S. Gomez CNA

Know what you are expected to do if you are asked to assist in discharging the resident. Be sure that the resident has all of his or her personal belongings. If the resident has valuables that were put away for safekeeping, remind the person to take them home. This is usually a happy time for the resident.

STANDARD PRECAUTIONS

Always follow Standard Precautions when caring for a resident. You must evaluate the situation before you start a procedure to determine when you must wear protective gear. The following procedures indicate when to put on gloves and when to discard them. However, you are responsible for determining when to wear gloves. There are times when you need gloves to protect yourself from body fluids that may not be addressed in a procedure. Carefully think through the care you are giving and protect yourself and others.

MORNING AND EVENING CARE (AM AND PM CARE)

The beginning of the day is very important. How you care for the resident when he or she first awakens sets the tone for the entire day. This care is called AM care and is given before breakfast. Awaken the resident quietly; never be loud or abrupt. Do not shake the person by the shoulder. Touch him or her on the arm and say the person's name. After the person is awake, there are several steps in the care you give. Follow the AM care procedures.

The PM care given to residents just before sleep is also important. Use this time to make residents comfortable for the night. Unhurried care allows the residents to feel relaxed, and they sleep better. If you take care of all their needs before you leave the room, it gives you time to finish your other duties. If you do not make them comfortable (e.g., see if they need to go to the bathroom), you have to return frequently to their rooms. Follow the PM care procedures.

PROCEDURE 15.8

AM CARE

RATIONALE

AM care refreshes the patient. Clean teeth, clean hands, morning elimination, and other comfort measures help improve appetite and enjoyment of breakfast.

ALERT: Follow Standard Precautions.

1. Wash hands.
2. Gently awaken resident.
3. Assemble equipment.
    a. Washcloth and towel
    b. Toothbrush and toothpaste
    c. Emesis basin
    d. Glass of water
    e. Denture cup if needed
    f. Clean gown if necessary
    g. Clean linen if necessary
    h. Comb and brush
    i. Disposable gloves (two pair)
4. Explain what you plan to do.
5. Provide privacy by pulling privacy curtain.
6. Elevate head of the bed if allowed.
7. Put on disposable gloves.
8. Provide a bedpan or urinal if needed, or escort resident to bathroom.
9. Empty bedpan or urinal, rinse it, and dispose of gloves.
10. Put bedpan or urinal out of sight.
11. Allow resident to wash hands and face.
12. Put on disposable gloves.
13. Provide oral hygiene.
14. Provide a clean gown if necessary.
15. Smooth sheets if resident remains in bed.
16. Transfer to a chair if resident is allowed out of bed.
17. Allow resident to comb hair; assist if necessary.
18. Prepare the overbed table.
    a. Clear tabletop.
    b. Wipe off.
19. Position overbed table if resident is to remain in the room, or transport resident to dining room.
20. Remove and discard gloves.
21. Wash hands.

10/06/03   0630

AM care given

Patient looking forward to breakfast

No complaints

_____ S. Gomez CNA

PROCEDURE 15.9

PM CARE

RATIONALE

PM care refreshes, relaxes, and comforts a patient, providing a quiet time before sleep.

ALERT: Follow Standard Precautions.

1. Wash hands.
2. Tell resident what you are going to do.
3. Provide privacy.
4. Assemble equipment.
   a. Washcloth and towel
   b. Toothpaste and toothbrush
   c. Glass of water
   d. Emesis basin
   e. Denture cup, if necessary
   f. Night clothes
   g. Lotion
   h. Linen as needed
   i. Disposable gloves
5. Encourage resident to do his or her own care if capable.
6. Assist if unable to do his or her own care.
7. Put on disposable gloves.
8. Provide bedpan or urinal if necessary, or escort to bathroom.

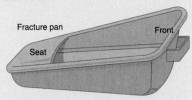

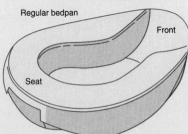

9. Empty bedpan or urinal.
10. Rinse and place in a convenient place for nighttime use.
11. Remove and dispose of gloves.
12. Wash resident's hands and face.
13. Put on gloves.

14. Provide for oral hygiene.
15. Change resident into night clothes.

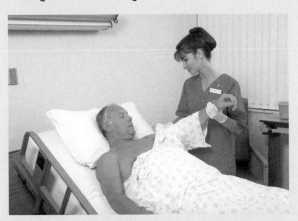

16. Transfer resident from chair or wheelchair into bed, if out of bed.
17. Give back rub with lotion.
18. Observe skin for irritations or breakdown.
19. Smooth the sheets.
20. Change draw sheets if necessary.
21. Provide extra blankets if necessary.
22. Position side rails as ordered after resident is in bed.
23. Remove and discard gloves.
24. Wash hands.
25. Provide fresh drinking water.
26. Place bedside table within resident's reach.
27. Secure call light within resident's reach.

8/30/03   2045
PM care given
No complaints
_____ S. Gomez CNA

⊙ SKIN MANAGEMENT

Skin is the first defense against infection. When you bathe your residents, you have an opportunity to observe their skin. You should look for

- Dryness
- Bruising
- Any unusual condition
- Broken area (pressure sore/decubitus)

Pressure sores/*decubiti* are very serious. Residents must be moved to help remove pressure on the skin, or pressure sores develop. This pressure can occur when residents are in bed or when they are sitting. They must be moved at least every 2 hours. The following areas are very sensitive to pressure:

- Shoulders
- Elbows
- Hips
- Sacrum
- Heels
- Ankles
- Ears
- Toes

Watch these areas carefully (see Figures 15.7 and 15.8). The bones press against the skin and stop circulation of blood. This causes the skin and tissue to break down. Pressure sores/decubiti are very painful and are difficult to heal. They can become quite deep and require a surgical procedure to help them heal. They can be prevented! Report any changes, such as redness, heat, tenderness, or broken skin, to the charge nurse.

To help prevent pressure sores/decubiti:

- Change the resident's position at least every 2 hours.
- Keep skin clean.
- Massage reddened areas over sharp, bony areas to increase circulation.
- Provide back rubs to increase circulation and relax the resident.
- Keep linen dry and free of wrinkles.
- Use foam padding, fiber-filled overlay, gel-filled pads, or sheepskin.
- Use a foot cradle to keep linen off feet.

Residents who are stationary for long periods can be protected by using special cushions on beds. For example:

- An egg-crate cushion made of foam rubber can be placed on a bed or cut to fit a chair.
- Rotating air mattresses circulate air through canals. The circulating air allows pressure from mattress to alternate. This alternating pressure allows blood circulation to keep skin healthy.

Places to Check for Signs of Bedsores

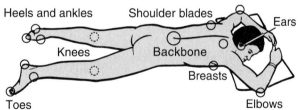

Heels and ankles — Shoulder blades — Ears — Knees — Backbone — Breasts — Toes — Elbows

Figure 15.7

Places to check for signs of pressure sores.

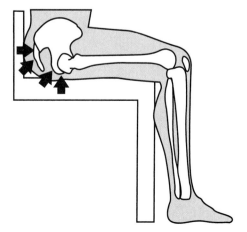

Figure 15.8

Pressure from the ischial bones and sacrum with the resident in the sitting position.

- Turning beds are used when a resident cannot move freely or easily. There are a variety of types of beds that allow a resident to be sandwiched between two mattresses. The bed is then turned and the top mattress is removed until the resident is repositioned.

- Water mattresses conform to the body weight and shape. The water redistributes with movement to prevent pressure.

PROCEDURE 15.10

SKIN CARE—GIVING A BACK RUB

RATIONALE

Giving a back rub provides an opportunity to help the patient relax and to check for any skin changes. It is also a good time to listen to any complaints or concerns the patient might have.

CAUTION: Check with team leader for permission to give a back rub.

1. Wash hands.
2. Assemble equipment.
   a. Lotion
   b. Powder
   c. Towel
   d. Washcloth
   e. Soap
   f. Water (105°F)
   g. Disposable gloves
3. Tell resident what you are going to do.

ALERT: Follow Standard Precautions.

4. Provide privacy by pulling privacy curtains.
5. Place lotion container in warm water to help warm it.
6. Raise bed to a comfortable working height.
7. Lower side rail on the side you are working on.
8. Put on disposable gloves.
9. Position resident on side or in prone position.
10. Place a towel along back to protect linen if resident is in a side-lying position.
11. Wash back thoroughly.
12. Rub a small amount of lotion into your hands.
13. Begin at base of spine and apply lotion over entire back.
14. Use firm, long strokes, beginning at buttocks and moving upward to neck and shoulders.

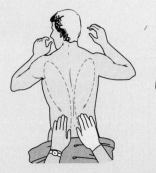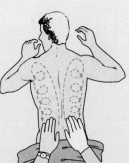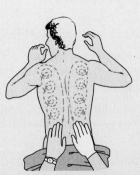

PROCEDURE 15.10 | SKIN CARE—GIVING A BACK RUB *(Continued)*

15. Use firm pressure as you stroke upward, and light circular strokes returning to buttocks.

NOTE Pay special attention to bony prominences.

16. Use a circular motion over each area (shoulder blades, backbone).

17. Observe skin for irritation or breakdown.

NOTE Do not rub or apply lotion to any open area on the skin.

18. Repeat several times (3 to 5 minutes).

19. Dry back.

20. Adjust gown for comfort.

21. Remove towel.

22. Position resident comfortably.

23. Return bed to lowest height.

24. Put up side rail if required.

25. Secure call light in reach of resident.

26. Remove and discard gloves.

27. Wash hands.

28. Record procedure and any observations (e.g., redness, broken areas, dry skin).

> 7/15/03   1350
> Back rub given
> No shin change noted
> Rails up
> _____ R. Johnson CNA

⊙ ORAL HYGIENE

Good mouth care should be provided at least three times a day: before breakfast when you give AM care, after lunch, and after dinner. It is important because it

- ■ Reduces odor
- ■ Helps prevent tooth decay
- ■ Is refreshing
- ■ Relieves dry lips and mouth, especially if the resident has an elevated temperature or breathes through the mouth

Some residents may have **dentures.** Often residents are sensitive about removing their dentures. Provide privacy and encouragement for oral care. Learn the correct method of handling dentures so that you do not break them.

dentures
False teeth.

PROCEDURE 15.11 | ORAL HYGIENE - SELF-CARE

RATIONALE

A clean mouth and clean teeth help prevent oral problems, freshen the breath, and give an overall feeling of well-being.

ALERT: Follow Standard Precautions.

1. Wash hands.
2. Assemble equipment.
   a. Toothbrush
   b. Toothpaste
   c. Mouthwash
   d. Cup of water with straw, if needed
   e. Emesis basin
   f. Bath towel
   g. Tissues

PROCEDURE 15.11 | ORAL HYGIENE - SELF-CARE *(Continued)*

3. Identify resident and explain what you are going to do.

4. Screen resident by pulling privacy curtain around bed.

5. Raise head of the bed if resident is allowed to sit up.

6. Place towel over blanket and resident's gown.

7. Place toothbrush, toothpaste, mouthwash, emesis basin, and glass of water on overbed table.

8. Remove overbed table when resident has completed brushing.

9. Put away towel and make resident comfortable.

10. Put up side rails if required.

11. Secure call bell within resident's reach.

12. Put away all equipment and tidy unit.

13. Wash hands.

14. Chart procedure.

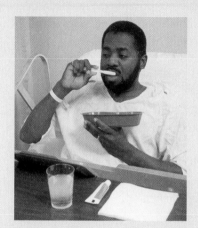

6/14/03   0640
Set up equipment on overbed table
Brushed teeth without assistance
_____ S. Gomez CNA

PROCEDURE 15.12 | ORAL HYGIENE—BRUSHING THE RESIDENT'S TEETH

RATIONALE

A clean mouth and clean teeth help prevent oral problems, freshen the breath, and give an overall feeling of well-being.

ALERT: Follow Standard Precautions.

1. Wash hands.

2. Assemble equipment.

   a. Toothbrush
   b. Toothpaste
   c. Mouthwash
   d. Cup of water with straw, if needed
   e. Emesis basin
   f. Bath towel
   g. Tissues
   h. Disposable nonsterile gloves

3. Identify resident and explain what you are going to do.

4. Screen resident by pulling privacy curtain around bed.

5. Raise head of bed if resident is allowed to sit up.

6. Place a towel over blanket and resident's gown.

7. Put on gloves.

8. Pour water over toothbrush; put toothpaste on brush.

9. Insert brush into the mouth carefully.

10. Place brush at an angle on upper teeth and brush in an up-and-down motion starting at rear of mouth.

11. Repeat on lower teeth.

PROCEDURE 15.12	ORAL HYGIENE—BRUSHING THE RESIDENT'S TEETH *(Continued)*

12. Give resident water to rinse mouth. If necessary, use a straw.

13. Hold emesis basin under chin. Have resident expectorate (spit) water into the basin.

14. Offer tissues to resident to wipe mouth and chin. Discard tissues.

15. Provide mouthwash if available. Use emesis basin and tissues as above.

16. Return all equipment.

17. Remove gloves and put in hazardous waste.

18. Wash hands.

19. Tidy up unit.

20. Put up side rails if required.

21. Secure call bell within resident's reach.

22. Make resident comfortable before leaving the room.

23. Chart procedure and how resident tolerated it.

5/14/03   0825
Brushed teeth, provided oral hygiene
Tolerated well
No oral problems noted
_____ R. Johnson CNA

PROCEDURE 15.13	ORAL HYGIENE—AMBULATORY RESIDENT

RATIONALE

A clean mouth and clean teeth help prevent oral problems, freshen the breath, and give an overall feeling of well-being.

ALERT: Follow Standard Precautions.

1. Wash hands.

2. Tell resident what you are going to do.

3. Set up equipment at sink.

    a. Toothbrush

    b. Toothpaste

    c. Tablets or powder to soak dentures in

    d. Towel

    e. Glass

4. Rinse equipment and put away.

5. Wash hands.

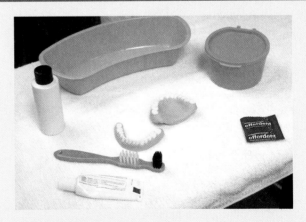

5/24/03   0745
Brushed teeth without assistance
_____ S. Gomez CNA

PROCEDURE 15.14

ORAL HYGIENE—DENTURE CARE

RATIONALE

Food and bacteria collect under dentures causing discomfort due to tissue breakdown and mouth odor. Clean dentures protect against oral problems and refresh the mouth.

ALERT: Follow Standard Precautions.

1. Wash hands.
2. Assemble equipment.
   a. Tissues
   b. Paper towel or gauze squares
   c. Mouthwash
   d. Disposable denture cup
   e. Toothbrush or denture brush
   f. Denture paste or toothpowder
   g. Towel
   h. Disposable nonsterile gloves
3. Identify resident.
4. Explain what you are going to do.
5. Pull privacy curtain.
6. Lower side rails.
7. Raise head of bed if allowed.
8. Place towel across resident's chest.
9. Prepare emesis basin by placing tissue or paper towel in bottom of basin.
10. Put on gloves.
11. Have resident remove his or her dentures.
12. Remove dentures if resident cannot.

Upper Denture
   a. Explain what you are going to do.
   b. Use a gauze square to grip upper denture.
   c. Place your index finger between top ridge of denture and cheek.
   d. Gently pull on denture to release suction.
   e. Remove upper denture.

Lower Denture
   a. Use a gauze square to grip lower denture.
   b. Place your index finger between lower ridge and cheek.
   c. Gently pull on denture to release suction.
   d. Remove lower denture.

13. Place dentures in lined emesis basin and take to sink or utility room.
14. Hold dentures firmly in palm of hand.
15. Put toothpowder or toothpaste on toothbrush.

16. Hold dentures under cold running water and brush dentures until clean.

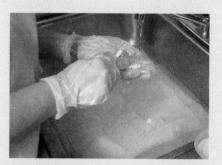

17. Rinse dentures under cold running water.

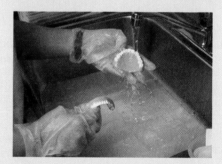

18. Place in denture cup.
19. Place a solution of mouthwash and cool water in cup.
20. Help resident rinse mouth with mouthwash; if food particles are between cheek and gumline, gently swab away with gauze.
21. Have resident replace dentures.
22. Place dentures in labeled denture cup next to bed, if dentures are to be left out.
23. Rinse equipment and put away.
24. Remove gloves; dispose of in hazardous waste.
25. Wash hands.
26. Position resident.
27. Raise side rails if required.

| PROCEDURE 15.14 | **ORAL HYGIENE—DENTURE CARE** *(Continued)* |

28. Secure call bell within resident's reach.
29. Chart procedure and how it was tolerated.

NOTE The resident may want to soak dentures overnight after PM care has been given. Place dentures in a solution in a denture cup and store in a safe place.

7/07/03	0725
	Set out equipment for denture care
	Able to clean dentures
	Or: Removed dentures, cleaned,
	and freshened
	Provided oral hygiene
	No oral problems noted
	_____ R. Johnson CNA

| PROCEDURE 15.15 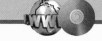 | **ORAL HYGIENE—FOR THE UNCONSCIOUS RESIDENT** |

RATIONALE

The unconscious patient often mouth breathes causing very dry lips and mucous membrane. Careful care and observation help prevent oral problems.

ALERT: Follow Standard Precautions.

1. Wash hands.
2. Tell resident what you are going to do. When resident is unconscious he or she may hear even if he or she cannot respond.
3. Provide privacy.
4. Assemble equipment.
   a. Emesis basin
   b. Towel
   c. Lemon glycerin swabs
   d. Tongue blades
   e. 4 × 4 gauze
   f. Lip moisturizer
   g. Disposable nonsterile gloves
5. Position bed at a comfortable working height.
6. Put on gloves.
7. Position resident's head to side and place towel on bed under resident's cheek and chin.
8. Secure emesis basin under resident's chin.
9. Wrap a tongue blade with 4 × 4 gauze and slightly moisten. Swab mouth being certain to clean gums, teeth, tongue, and roof of mouth.
10. Apply lip moisturizer to lips and swab mouth with lemon and glycerin if available.

11. Remove towel and reposition resident.
12. Discard disposable equipment in hazardous waste.
13. Clean basin and put away.
14. Remove gloves and put in hazardous waste.
15. Wash hands.
16. Report and document resident's tolerance of procedure.

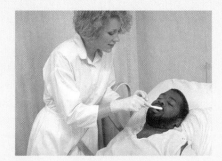

6/16/03	1040
	Cleaned teeth, moistened lips,
	provided oral hygiene
	Noted small canker sore on palate
	Reported to team leader
	_____ S. Gomez CNA

Figure 15.9

Cleansing enema.

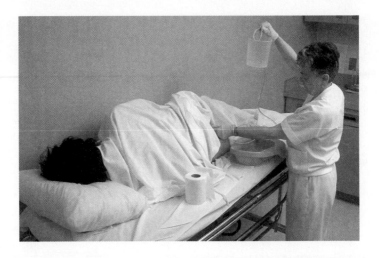

OFFERING THE URINAL AND/OR BEDPAN

Eliminating waste products from the body is necessary for good health. When residents are confined to bed, they must use a bedpan or urinal. Male residents use urinals to empty the bladder. Women use the bedpan for both urine and the elimination of solid waste (bowel movement). Men also use a bedpan for the elimination of solid waste. Solid waste is called *feces* or *stool*. When residents eliminate liquid waste, we call it *urinating* or *voiding*.

If your resident does not eliminate liquid waste from the bladder, he or she may develop a urinary tract infection. This is very painful and serious. Small amounts of liquid elimination may indicate infection, dehydration, or fluid retention in the body. If solid waste is not eliminated, large amounts of stool may cause an impaction. When a large amount of stool stays in the bowel it causes discomfort, and the resident experiences nausea and sometimes vomiting. This can be prevented by carefully recording bowel movements and letting the charge nurse know if a resident has not had a bowel movement. The charge nurse will give the resident a **laxative, suppository,** or enema (see Figure 15.9), which is discussed later in this chapter.

laxative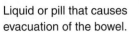

Liquid or pill that causes evacuation of the bowel.

suppository

Bullet shaped mass inserted into rectum to stimulate bowel movement.

PROCEDURE 15.16 — ELIMINATION—OFFERING THE BEDPAN

RATIONALE

Carefully placing the bedpan prevents discomfort. This procedure allows observations for skin breakdown and elimination.

ALERT: Follow Standard Precautions.

1. Wash hands.
2. Assemble equipment.
   a. Bedpan with cover
   b. Toilet tissue
   c. Soap and water
   d. Towel
   e. Disposable nonsterile gloves (two pairs)
3. Ask visitors to wait outside room.
4. Provide privacy for resident.
5. Remove bedpan from storage space.

PROCEDURE 15.16   ELIMINATION—OFFERING THE BEDPAN *(Continued)*

6. Warm metal bedpans by running warm water over them and drying.

7. Lower head of bed if it is elevated.

8. Put on gloves.

9. Fold top covers back enough to see where to place the pan. Do not expose resident.

10. Ask resident to raise hips off bed. Help support resident by placing your hand at resident's midback.

    a. Roll the resident onto his or her side if the resident is unable to lift the hips.

    b. Place bedpan on buttocks.

    c. Hold in place with one hand and help resident roll back onto bedpan.

11. Slide bedpan into place.

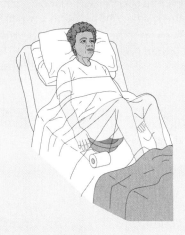

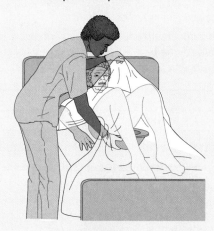

14. Remove gloves.

15. Wash your hands.

16. Leave call light with resident.

17. Leave room to provide privacy.

18. Watch for call light to signal resident's readiness to be removed from bedpan.

19. Put on gloves.

20. Assist resident as necessary to ensure cleanliness.

21. Remove bedpan and empty.

22. Measure urine if on I & O.

23. Remove gloves.

24. Wash hands.

25. Provide washcloth, water, and soap for resident to wash hands.

26. Provide comfort measures for resident.

27. Secure call light in resident's reach.

28. Open privacy curtain.

29. Chart the following:

    a. Bowel movement amount, color, consistency

    b. Amount voided if on I & O

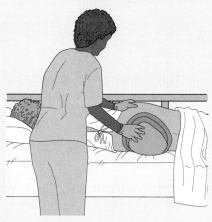

12. Cover resident again.

13. Raise head of bed for comfort.

4/10/03	0830
	Small, light brown, dry bowel
	Complained of discomfort when eliminating
	Noted small amount bright red blood
	Reported to team leader
	_____ R. Johnson CNA

ELIMINATION—OFFERING THE URINAL

RATIONALE

Offering a urinal at the time of elimination allows the patient/resident who is not able to go into the bathroom, a way to stay in bed or in a chair and eliminate liquid waste. Remember to provide privacy to maintain the patient's dignity.

ALERT: Follow Standard Precautions.

1. Wash hands.
2. Assemble equipment.
   a. Urinal with cover
   b. Soap and water
   c. Towel
   d. Disposable nonsterile gloves
3. Ask visitors to wait outside room.
4. Provide privacy for resident.
5. Hand urinal to resident.
   a. Place call light at resident's side.
   b. Wash your hands.
   c. Leave room until resident signals with the call light.

   (If the resident is unable to place urinal, place penis in urinal. If necessary, stand and hold urinal until resident has finished voiding.) Wear gloves for this step.
6. Return to room when resident has finished voiding.
7. Put on gloves.
8. Place cover over urinal and carry it into bathroom.
9. Check to see if resident is on I & O or if a urine specimen is needed. (See I & O and specimen collection in this chapter.)
10. Observe urine color, consistency, and odor.
11. Empty into toilet.
12. Rinse urinal with cold water.
13. Cover and place in a convenient location for the resident.
14. Remove gloves.
15. Wash hands.
16. Secure call light in reach of resident.
17. Report and document unusual color, odor, or consistency of urine.
18. Record amount if on I & O.

> 4/10/03   1030
>
> Voided 250 cc.
>
> Recorded on I + O sheet
>
> ———— R. Johnson CNA

ELIMINATION—BEDSIDE COMMODE

RATIONALE

A bedside commode allows patients/residents who cannot ambulate to the toilet to eliminate body waste by sitting on a chairlike device at the bedside. Patients generally have less difficulty eliminating waste when they use a commode instead of a bedpan.

ALERT: Follow Standard Precautions.

1. Wash hands.
2. Assemble equipment.
   a. Bedside commode
   b. Toilet tissue
   c. Washcloth
   d. Warm water
   e. Soap
   f. Towel
   g. Disposable nonsterile gloves

PROCEDURE 15.18 | ELIMINATION—BEDSIDE COMMODE *(Continued)*

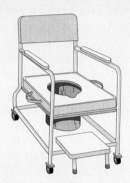

3. Identify resident.
4. Explain what you are going to do.
5. Place commode chair next to bed facing head of bed. *Lock wheels!*
6. Check to see if receptacle is in place under seat.
7. Provide privacy by pulling privacy curtains.
8. Lower bed to lowest position.
9. Lower side rail.
10. Help resident to sitting position.
11. Help resident swing legs over side of bed.
12. Put on resident's slippers and assist to stand.
13. Have resident place hands on your shoulders.
14. Support under resident's arms, pivot resident to right, and lower to commode. (See the procedure "Transferring—Pivot Transfer from Bed to Wheelchair.")
15. Place call bell within reach.
16. Place toilet tissue within reach.
17. Remain nearby if resident seems weak.
18. Return immediately when resident signals.

19. Put on gloves.
20. Assist resident to stand.
21. Clean anus or perineum if resident is unable to help self.
22. Remove gloves and put in hazardous waste.
23. Help resident wash hands.
24. Assist back to bed and position comfortably.
25. Put up side rail if required.
26. Put on gloves.
27. Put down cover on commode chair and remove receptacle.
28. Empty contents, measuring if on I & O.
29. Empty and clean per hospital policy.
30. Remove gloves and put in hazardous waste.
31. Wash hands.
32. Replace equipment and tidy unit.
33. Record the following:
    a. Bowel movement
       (1) Amount
       (2) Consistency
       (3) Color
    b. Any unusual observations, such as
       (1) Weakness
       (2) Discomfort

11/24/03   1030

Eliminated moderate amount of brown, formed stool and 200 cc of urine

Returned to bed, positioned for comfort.

Tolerated activity well

————— S. Gomez CNA

● MOVEMENT AND AMBULATION OF THE RESIDENT

You are responsible for moving your resident in many different ways:

- Into a chair or wheelchair
- Into bed from a chair or wheelchair
- From bed to gurney
- From gurney to bed
- Transferring into a wheelchair

Figure 15.10

Mechanical lift.

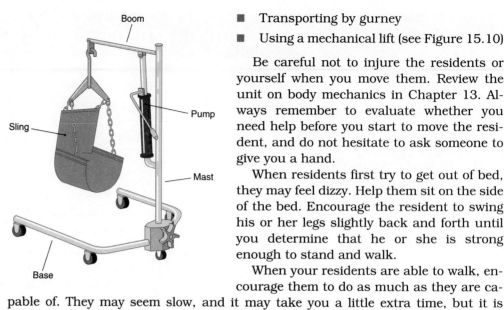

Boom

Pump

Sling

Mast

Base

- Transporting by gurney
- Using a mechanical lift (see Figure 15.10)

Be careful not to injure the residents or yourself when you move them. Review the unit on body mechanics in Chapter 13. Always remember to evaluate whether you need help before you start to move the resident, and do not hesitate to ask someone to give you a hand.

When residents first try to get out of bed, they may feel dizzy. Help them sit on the side of the bed. Encourage the resident to swing his or her legs slightly back and forth until you determine that he or she is strong enough to stand and walk.

When your residents are able to walk, encourage them to do as much as they are capable of. They may seem slow, and it may take you a little extra time, but it is important for them. Walking (**ambulation**)

ambulation

Walking.

- Helps maintain stamina
- Increases joint mobility
- Improves muscle tone
- Helps prevent lung congestion
- Improves circulation
- Helps maintain independence
- Provides a sense of accomplishment

Your residents may need a device such as a cane, crutches, or walker. They may need a wheelchair much of the time but still be able to ambulate in a limited way. Learn the procedures for ambulation in Chapter 19.

Before residents are moved, check to see if there are tubes or catheters in place. You must be careful not to pull them out, crimp them, or put a strain on them. If residents have drainage equipment (e.g., Foley bag [urine drainage bag]), do not raise the tubing above the level of insertion into the body. If they have an IV, do not allow the tubing to drop below the bed level. Never let any tubing touch the floor. If you have any question about moving residents, *ask your instructor or the charge nurse before moving them.*

PROCEDURE 15.19

TRANSFERRING—PIVOT TRANSFER FROM BED TO WHEELCHAIR

RATIONALE

Pivot transfer allows you to move the patient/resident in one easy, safe motion into or out of a wheelchair. Use good body mechanics, explain each step, and reassure the patient/resident of his or her safety.

ALERT: Follow Standard Precautions.

1. Wash hands.
2. *Lock* wheels on chair.
3. Lift foot rests or swing leg supports out of way.
4. Position wheelchair alongside bed. (See instructor for directions in working with stroke residents.) *Lock* wheels.
5. Move resident to edge of bed, with legs over side.

6. Have resident dangle legs for a few minutes. Encourage some slow, deep breaths and observe for dizziness. (See the section on syncope in this chapter.)
7. Support him or her at midriff and ask resident to stand, if resident is not dizzy.
8. Once standing, have resident pivot (turn) and hold onto armrest of wheelchair with both arms or one strong arm.

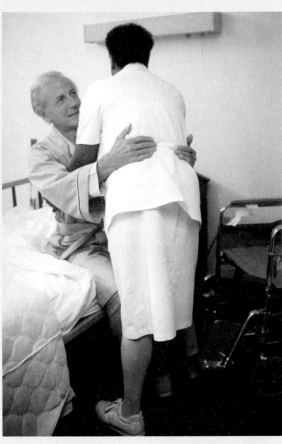

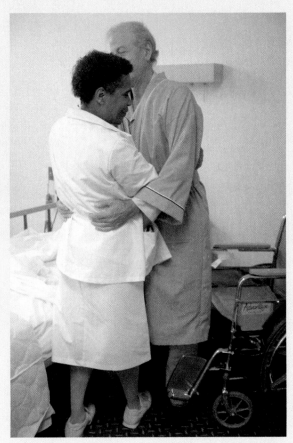

PROCEDURE 15.19   **TRANSFERRING—PIVOT TRANSFER FROM BED TO WHEELCHAIR** *(Continued)*

9. Gently ease resident into a sitting position.

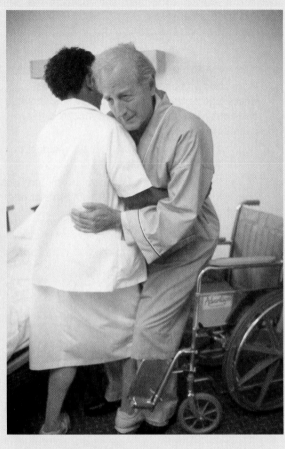

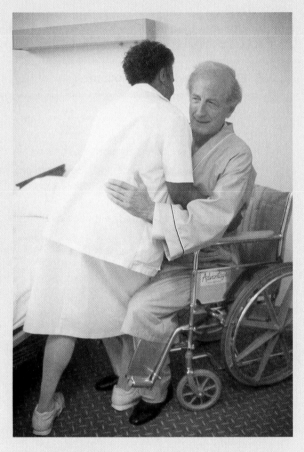

10. Position yourself at back of wheelchair. Ask resident to push on the floor with feet as you lift gently under each arm to ease resident into a comfortable position against backrest.

11. Return foot rests to normal position and place feet and legs in a comfortable position on rests.

12. Do not leave a resident who requires a postural support until it is in place.

13. Reverse above procedure to return resident to bed.

14. Wash hands.

4/4/03	0930
	Transferred from wheelchair
	into bed
	Positioned for HS comfort
	Resident was not able to bear
	weight on right leg during
	pivot transfer Weakness in right leg
	reported to charge nurse
	_____ R. Johnson CNA

PROCEDURE 15.20

TRANSFERRING—SLIDING FROM BED TO WHEELCHAIR AND BACK

RATIONALE

Sliding transfer allows you to assist the patient/resident who is paralyzed from the waist down to easily move in and out of a wheelchair. Use good body mechanics, explain each step, and reassure the patient/resident of his or her safety.

ALERT: Follow Standard Precautions.

1. Wash hands.
2. Assemble equipment: wheelchair with removable arms.
3. Position wheelchair at bedside with back parallel to head of bed. *Lock* wheels.
4. Remove wheelchair arm nearest to bedside.
5. Place bed level to chair seat height if possible. *Lock* bed wheels.
6. Raise head of bed so that resident is in sitting position.

7. Position yourself beside wheelchair and carefully assist resident to slide from bed to wheelchair.
8. Position resident for comfort and apply postural supports PRN.
9. Wash hands.

5/30/03	0945

Transferred from bed into
wheelchair
Tolerated sliding transfer well
———— R. Johnson CNA

PROCEDURE 15.21

TRANSFERRING—TWO-PERSON LIFT FROM BED TO CHAIR AND BACK

RATIONALE

A person who is unable to bear his or her weight during a pivot transfer can be lifted by two people. Use good body mechanics, explain each step, and reassure the patient/resident of his or her safety.

ALERT: Follow Standard Precautions.

1. Wash hands.
2. Assemble equipment: chair.
3. Ask one other person to help.
4. Tell resident what you are going to do.
5. Position chair next to bed with back of chair parallel with head of bed. *Lock* wheels.
6. Position resident near edge of bed.
7. Position co-worker on side of bed near feet.
8. Position yourself behind chair at head of bed.
9. Place your arms under resident's axillae and clasp your hands together at resident's midchest.
10. Co-worker places hands under resident's upper legs.

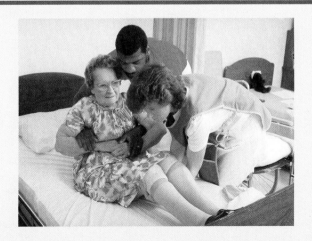

TRANSFERRING—TWO-PERSON LIFT FROM BED TO CHAIR AND BACK *(Continued)*

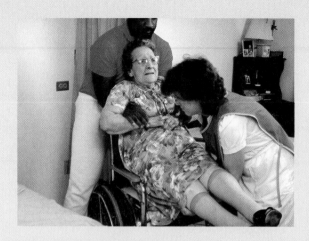

11. Count to three. On the count of three, lift resident into chair.

12. Position for comfort and secure postural supports PRN.

13. Wash hands.

11/20/03   2100
    Transferred per two-person lift from
chair into bed, positioned for HS
comfort
    Tolerated transfer well
              _____ A. Chaplin, CNA

TRANSFERRING—SLIDING FROM BED TO GURNEY AND BACK

RATIONALE

A sliding transfer of a patient/resident on and off a guerney is easily and safely accomplished with two people using a pull sheet. Use good body mechanics, explain each step, and reassure the patient/resident of his or her safety.

ALERT: Follow Standard Precautions.

1. Wash hands.

2. Assemble equipment.
   a. Gurney
   b. Cover sheet

3. Ask a co-worker to help.

4. Explain what you are going to do and *lock* wheels on bed.

5. Cover resident with sheet and remove bed covers.

6. Raise bed to gurney height: lower side rail and move resident to side of bed.

7. Loosen draw sheet on both sides so it can be used as a pull sheet.

8. Position gurney next to bed and *lock* wheels on gurney.

9. Position yourself on outside of gurney—one arm at the head, the other at the hips. Co-worker is on other side of bed.

10. Reach across gurney and securely hold edge of draw sheet. Pull resident onto gurney and cover. (If resident is large, a third person on the opposite side of bed may be necessary.)

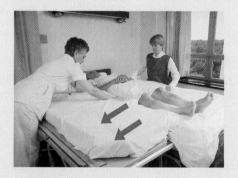

11. Position resident for comfort.

12. Secure with safety straps or raise side rails.

13. Wash hands.

9/10/03   0900
    Transferred to radiology via gurney
following a sliding transfer from bed
    Tolerated transfer well
              _____ A. Chaplin CNA

PROCEDURE 15.23

TRANSFERRING—LIFTING WITH A MECHANICAL LIFT

RATIONALE

Residents who are paralyzed can be easily transferred with a mechanical lift. Mechanical lifts allow patients who would otherwise be bedridden to be placed into a bathtub or chair. Your ability to use the lift safely will provide important environmental and physical stimulation for the resident. Remember to ask a co-worker to double-check all connections and positions before moving the patient to ensure their safety.

ALERT: Follow Standard Precautions.

1. Wash hands.
2. Gather equipment.
   a. Mechanical lift
   b. Sheet or blanket for resident comfort
   c. Sling
3. Check all equipment to be sure it is in good working order and that the sling is not damaged or torn.
4. Ask one other person to help.
5. Prepare resident's destination.
   a. Chair
   b. Gurney
   c. Bathtub
   d. Shower
6. *Lock* wheels on bed and explain what you are going to do.
7. Roll resident toward you.
8. Place sling on bed behind resident.
   a. Position top of sling at shoulders.
   b. Position bottom of sling under buttocks.
   c. Leave enough of sling to support body when the body is rolled back. Fan-fold remaining sling next to body. It will be pulled through when resident is rolled back.
9. Roll resident to other side of bed and pull fan-folded portion of sling flat. Remove all wrinkles and allow resident to lie flat on back.
10. Position lift over resident, being sure to broaden base of lift. This stabilizes the lift while raising resident.
11. Raise head of bed to a semi-Fowler's position.
12. Attach straps on lift to sling loops. Shorter straps must be attached to shoulder loops. Longer straps are attached to loops at hips. *(Important: If you reverse the strap attachment, the resident's head will be lower than his or her hips.)*
13. Reassure resident. Let resident know you will keep him or her from falling. Gently raise resident from bed with hand crank or pump handle.
14. Keep resident centered over base of lift as you move lift and resident to his or her destination. (It is helpful to have a helper stand by and steady resident while moving so that resident doesn't swing.)
15. Position resident over chair, commode, bathtub, shower chair, etc. Ask a co-worker to steady chair.
16. Slowly lower resident into chair using foot-pedal positioning.
17. Unhook sling from lift straps and carefully move lift away from resident.
18. Provide all comfort measures for resident.
19. Secure postural supports if necessary.
20. Return lift to storage area.
21. Wash hands.
22. Reverse procedure when returning resident to bed.

NOTE The mechanical lift is an expensive item. Depending on the size of the facility you are in, there may be a limited number available. Always return the lift to its storage area so that it will be available for others to use.

4/20/03   0830
Transferred via mechanical lift to bathtub
Tolerated bath well
Positioned in day chair and taken to patio
——— S. Gomez CNA

PROCEDURE 15.24

TRANSFERRING—MOVING A RESIDENT ON A GURNEY

RATIONALE

Patients who are medicated or who must stay in a reclined position can be moved throughout a facility on a gurney. It is important to secure safety rails and wheel them in a safe manner.

ALERT: Follow Standard Precautions.

1. Position bed to gurney height.
2. *Lock* all the brakes on gurney and bed.
3. Follow the procedure for transferring to and from a gurney.
4. Stand at the resident's head and push the gurney with resident's feet moving first down the hallway.
5. Slow down when turning a corner. Always check the intersection mirrors for traffic.
6. Enter an elevator by standing at resident's head and pulling gurney into elevator. The feet will be the last to enter elevator.
7. Leave elevator by carefully pushing the gurney out of elevator into corridor.
8. Position yourself at resident's feet, and back a resident on a gurney down a hill.
9. Never leave a resident unattended on a gurney.
10. Raise side rails and secure a safety strap.

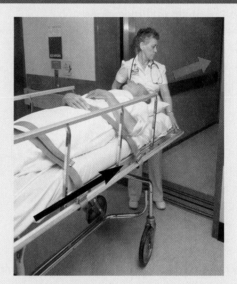

12/14/03   1320

Transferred via gurney to surgery
_____ R. Johnson CNA

● POSITIONING AND BODY ALIGNMENT

alignment

Keeping a resident in proper position.

Always position your residents with the head in a straight line with the spine and the body in a comfortable, normal **alignment.** If a resident is bent in an unnatural position (slumped forward, rolled in a ball) the resident may experience

- Breathing problems
- Added pressure to the bony areas, causing skin breakdown (decubiti)
- Strain on the lumbar spine
- Contractures
- Decreased circulation
- Discomfort and pain
- Edema
- Foot drop

TRANSFERRING—MOVING A RESIDENT IN A WHEELCHAIR

RATIONALE

Patients can easily be transferred from place to place in a wheelchair. It is important to move them safely and secure their transfer in and out of the wheelchair.

ALERT: Follow Standard Precautions.

1. Position wheelchair.
2. *Lock* all brakes on wheelchair and bed.
3. Follow procedure for transferring resident to and from a wheelchair.
4. Push wheelchair carefully into hallway, watching for others who may be near doorway.
5. Move cautiously down hallway, being especially careful at intersections.
6. Always back a resident in a wheelchair over bumps, doorways, and into or out of elevators.
7. Always back a resident in a wheelchair down a hill.
8. Check resident for comfort measures before leaving.
9. Always notify appropriate person that resident has arrived.

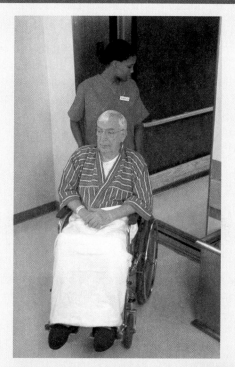

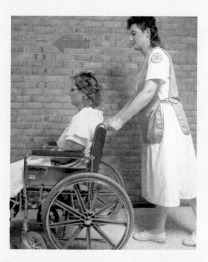

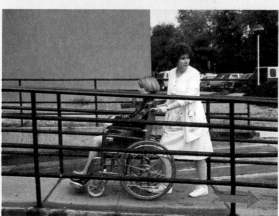

10/10/03 1730

Transferred via wheelchair to radiology

——— S. Gomez CNA

When the resident is confined to bed, the side-lying position is best. This allows for drainage of mucus from the nose and mouth and reduces the areas of pressure on the skin. If a resident must be on his or her back, check frequently for reddened areas, and be certain that antipressure aids are under them (egg-crate mattress, flotation mattress, sheepskin). Some of the techniques you can use are

- Pillow support at back for side lying
- Pillow support from the knee to ankle to support upper leg
- Trochanter support to prevent outward rotation
- Footboard and padded splints to prevent foot drop

Good body alignment is important at all times. This includes when the resident is lying in bed, sitting in a chair, and sitting in a wheelchair. When your residents are positioned in good body alignment, they look comfortable.

PROCEDURE 15.26

MOVING—HELPING THE HELPLESS RESIDENT TO MOVE UP IN BED

RATIONALE

Keeping patients in good alignment helps prevent a decubitus, respiratory problems, and general discomfort. Following correct procedures when lifting and moving the patient prevents injury to the patient and the nurse assistant(s).

ALERT: Follow Standard Precautions.

1. Wash hands.
2. Ask a co-worker to help move resident. (Co-worker will work on opposite side of bed.)
3. Identify resident and explain what you are going to do. (Even if the resident seems unresponsive, he or she may be able to hear.)
4. Lock wheels of bed. Raise bed to comfortable working position, and lower side rails.
5. Remove pillow and place it at head of bed or on a chair.
6. Loosen both sides of draw sheet.
7. Roll edges toward side of resident's body.
8. Face head of bed and grasp rolled sheet edge with hand closest to resident.
9. Place your feet 12 inches apart with foot farthest from the edge of bed in a forward position.
10. Place your free hand and arm under resident's neck and shoulders, supporting head.
11. Bend your hips slightly.
12. On the count of three, you and your co-worker will raise resident's hips and back with draw sheet,

supporting head and shoulders, and move resident smoothly to head of bed.

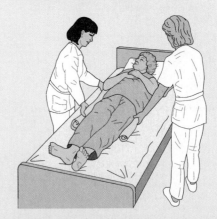

13. Replace pillow under resident's head and check for good body alignment.
14. Tighten and tuck in draw sheet and smooth bedding.
15. Raise side rails and lower bed.
16. Wash hands.

MOVING—ASSISTING RESIDENT TO SIT UP IN BED

RATIONALE

Some patients are too weak to adjust themselves in bed. Sitting up comfortably helps prevent fatigue and poor body alignment. Using correct procedure prevents injury to the patient and the nurse assistant(s).

ALERT: Follow Standard Precautions.

1. Wash hands.
2. Identify resident and explain what you are going to do.
3. Lock bed and lower all the way down.
4. Face head of bed, keeping your outer leg forward.
5. Turn your head away from resident's face.
6. Lock your arm nearest resident with resident's arm. To lock arms, place your arm between resident's arm and body, and hold upper arm near shoulder. Have resident hold back of your upper arm.
7. Support resident's head and shoulder with your other arm.
8. Raise resident to sitting position. Adjust head of bed and pillows.
9. Wash hands.

5/10/03	0850
Helped to sitting position	
No complaints of discomfort	
	R. Johnson CNA

MOVING—LOGROLLING

RATIONALE

Maintaining alignment is essential to prevent injury. Logrolling helps prevent movement of the back following surgery.

ALERT: Follow Standard Precautions.

1. Wash hands.
2. Identify resident and explain what you are going to do.
3. Provide privacy by pulling privacy curtain.
4. Lock wheels of bed. Raise bed to a comfortable working position.
5. Lower side rail on side you are working on.
6. Be certain that side rail on opposite side of bed is in up position.
7. Leave pillow under head.
8. Place a pillow lengthwise between resident's legs.
9. Fold resident's arms across chest.
10. Roll resident onto his or her side like a log, turning body as a whole unit, without bending joints.
11. Check for good body alignment.
12. Tighten and tuck in draw sheet and smooth bedding.
13. Tuck pillow behind back for support.
14. Raise side rails and lower bed.
15. Secure call light in resident's reach.
16. Wash hands.
17. Chart position of resident and how procedure was tolerated.

10/24/03	1145
Logrolled to left side	
Moved every 2 hours	
Skin in good condition	
Complained of slight pain in left leg when moved	
Pillows placed behind back to maintain alignment	
Made comfortable with rails up	
	A. Chaplin CNA

PROCEDURE 15.29

MOVING—TURNING RESIDENT AWAY FROM YOU

RATIONALE

Following correct procedure for turning patients away from you when bed changing, bathing, and positioning provides good alignment and prevents injury.

ALERT: Follow Standard Precautions.

1. Wash hands.
2. Identify resident and explain what you are going to do.
3. Lock bed and elevate to a comfortable working height.
4. Lower side rail on side you are working from.
5. Have resident bend knees. Cross arms on chest.
6. Place arm nearest head of bed under resident's shoulders and head. Place other hand and forearm under small of the resident's back. Bend your body at hips and knees, keeping your back straight. Pull resident toward you.
7. Place forearms under resident's hips and pull resident toward you.
8. Place one hand under ankles and one hand under knees and move ankles and knees toward you.

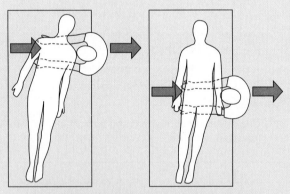

As a safety measure, this procedure must be done before turning a patient onto his side. It ensures that the patient, when turned, is located in the center of the mattress.

9. Cross resident's leg closest to you over other leg at ankles.

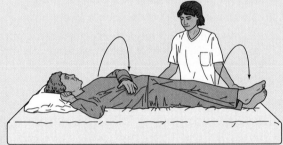

A Bend the resident's farthest arm next to her head and place the other arm across her chest. Cross her near leg over the other leg.

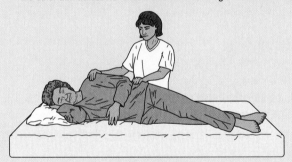

B Place one hand on the resident's shoulder and the other on her hip. Turn her away from you onto her side.

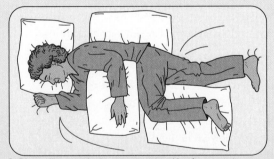

C Place pillows under her upper arm and leg for support.

10. Roll resident away from you by placing one hand under hips and one hand under shoulders.
11. Place one hand under resident's shoulders and one hand under resident's head. Draw resident back toward center of bed.

12. Place both hands under resident's hips and move hips toward center of bed.

13. Put a pillow behind resident's back to give support and keep resident from falling onto his or her back.

14. Be certain resident is in good alignment.

15. Place upper leg on a pillow for support.

16. Replace side rail on near side of bed and return bed to lowest height.

17. You may place a turning sheet under a helpless or heavy resident to help with turning. Use a folded large sheet or half sheet and place it so that it extends just above shoulders and below hips.

18. Wash hands.

8/04/03	1145
	Turned to left side
	Pillows placed behind back to
	maintain good body alignment
	Resting comfortably
	Side rails up
	_____ A. Chaplin CNA

RATIONALE

Following correct procedure for turning patients toward you when bed changing, bathing, and positioning provides good alignment and prevents injury.

ALERT: Follow Standard Precautions.

1. Wash hands.

2. Identify resident and explain what you are going to do.

3. Lock bed and elevate to a comfortable working height.

4. Lower side rail on side you are working from.

5. Cross resident's far leg over leg that is closest to you.

6. Place one hand on resident's far shoulder. Place your other hand on the hip.

7. Brace yourself against side of bed. Roll resident toward you in a slow, gentle, smooth movement.

8. Help resident bring upper leg toward you and bend comfortably (Sims position).

9. Put up side rail. Be certain it is secure.

10. Go to other side of bed and lower side rail.

11. Place hands under resident's shoulders and hips. Pull toward center of bed. This helps maintain side-lying position.

12. Be certain to align resident's body properly.

13. Use pillows to position and support legs if resident is unable to move self.

14. *Check tubing to make certain that it is not caught between legs or pulling in any way if resident has an indwelling catheter.*

15. Tuck a pillow behind resident's back. This forms a roll and prevents resident from rolling backward onto back.

16. Return bed to low position.

17. Secure call light in resident's reach.

18. Wash hands.

5/05/03	1000
	Repositioned on right side
	Skin care given
	Skin is clean and dry
	_____ S. Gomez CNA

range of motion (ROM)

Moving all joints of the body; can be active or passive.

flexibility

Ability to bend easily.

contraction

Drawing up.

RANGE OF MOTION

Range-of-motion (ROM) exercises are very important for the resident who has limited movement. ROM exercises are given to

- Stimulate circulation
- Encourage **flexibility** and mobility of the joints
- Prevent contractures (permanent **contraction** of the muscle)

Residents are encouraged to move each joint to the best of their ability. This is active ROM. When you do passive ROM for your residents, you move the joints for them.

PROCEDURE 15.31

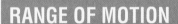

RANGE OF MOTION

RATIONALE

Correct ROM provides exercise to the joints and muscles, preventing contractures and immobility.

NOTE The use of passive and active range of motion (ROM) is related to resident's ability level.

- **Active ROM.** Resident is able to perform all movements without assistance.
- **Passive ROM.** Health care worker moves body parts for resident.

ALERT: Follow Standard Precautions.

---

1. Wash hands.
2. Assemble equipment.
   a. Sheet or bath blanket
   b. Treatment table or bed
   c. Good lighting
3. Identify resident.
4. Explain what you are going to do.
5. Ask visitors to wait outside, and provide privacy.
6. Place resident in a supine position on bed or treatment table and cover with sheet or bath blanket. *Instruct resident to do the following movements at least five times each or to tolerance.*

Head Flexion and Extension

7. Bend head until chin touches chest (flexion), then gently bend backward (extension).

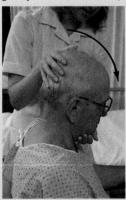 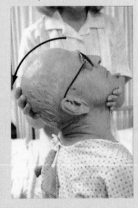

Right/Left Rotation

8. Turn head to right (right rotation), then turn head to left (left rotation).

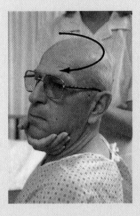 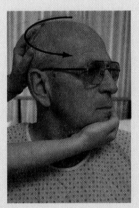

PROCEDURE 15.31 | RANGE OF MOTION *(Continued)*

Right/Left Lateral Flexion

9. Move head so that right ear moves toward right shoulder (right lateral flexion), then move head to central position and continue moving head so that left ear moves toward left shoulder (left lateral flexion).

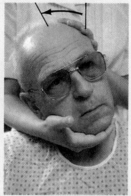
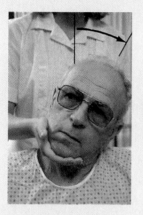

Shoulder Flexion and Extension

10. Raise one arm overhead keeping elbow straight. Return to side position. Repeat with other arm.

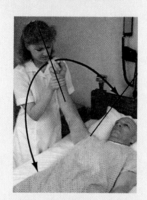

Shoulder Abduction and Adduction

11. Raise arm overhead, then lower, keep arm out to side. Repeat with other arm.

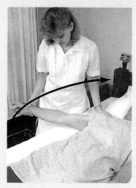

Elbow Flexion and Extension

12. Bend one hand and forearm toward shoulder (flexion) and straighten (extension). Repeat with other arm.

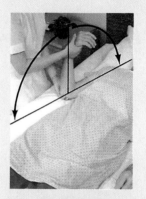

Forearm Pronation and Supination

13. Bend arm at elbow and rotate hand toward body (pronation), then rotate away from body (supination). Repeat with other arm.

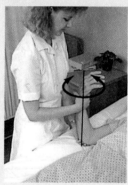

Wrist Flexion and Extension

14. Bend hand at wrist toward shoulder (flex), then gently force backward past a level position with arm (extension) to below arm level (hyperextension). Repeat with other hand.

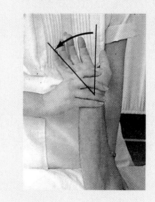
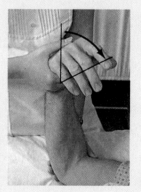

PROCEDURE 15.31 | RANGE OF MOTION *(Continued)*

Ulnar and Radial Deviation

15. Holding hand straight, move toward thumb (radial deviation), then move hand toward little finger (ulnar deviation). Repeat with other hand.

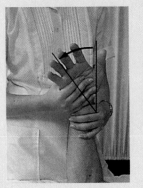
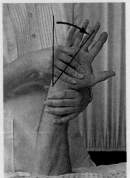

Finger Flexion and Extension

16. Bend thumb and fingers into hand making a fist (flexion), then open hand by straightening fingers and thumb (extension). Repeat with other hand.

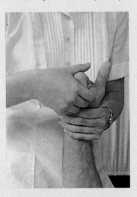
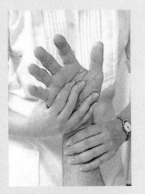

17. Move thumb away from hand (abduct), then toward hand (adduct). Repeat with other hand.

Finger/Thumb Opposition

18. Move thumb toward little finger, touch tips. Touch tip of thumb to each finger. Open hand each time. Repeat with other hand.

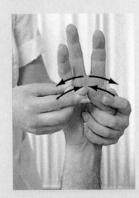

Finger Adduction and Abduction

19. Keeping fingers straight, separate them (abduction), then bring them together (adduction). Repeat with other hand.

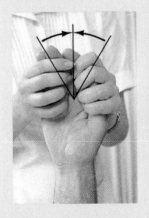
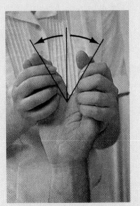

Hip/Knee Flexion and Extension

20. Raise leg, bend knee, then return to bed straightening knee. Repeat with other leg.

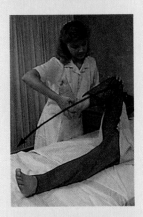

Straight Leg Raising

21. Keep knee straight. Slowly raise and lower leg. Repeat with other leg.

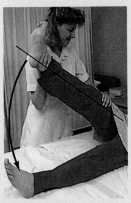

Hip Abduction and Adduction

22. Separate legs (abduction), then bring back together (adduction). Then turn both legs so knees face outward. Turn legs so knees face inward.

PROCEDURE 15.31 | **RANGE OF MOTION** *(Continued)*

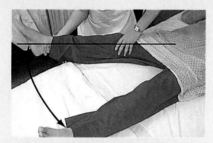

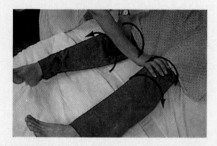

23. Rotate one foot toward other foot (internal rotation), then rotate away from other foot (external rotation). Repeat with other foot.

Ankle Dorsiflexion and Plantar Flexion

24. Move foot so that toes move toward knee (dorsi flexion), then move foot so that toes point away from head (plantar flexion). Repeat with other foot.

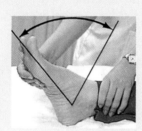

Toe Flexion and Extension

25. Spread toes apart (abduction) on one foot, then bring toes together (adduction). Repeat on other foot.

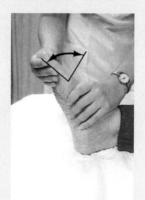 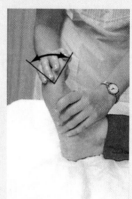

26. Turn resident in a prone position.

Arm Abduction and Adduction

27. Move arm toward ceiling; do not bend elbows (hyperextension), then return to bed. Repeat with other arm.

Leg Flexion and Extension

28. Bend leg so that foot moves toward resident's back (flexion), then straighten leg (extension). Repeat with other leg.

29. Position resident for comfort.

30. Place bath blanket or sheet in laundry basket.

31. Wash your hands.

32. Report and document resident's tolerance of procedure.

12/06/03   1510

Passive ROM to all joints
Complained of some discomfort
in left elbow
Noted some increased stiffness in
fingers of the right hand
Reported to charge nurse
ROM tolerated well
———— S. Gomez CNA

BATHING THE RESIDENT

Providing for your residents' cleanliness is an important responsibility. Bathing is important because it

■ Removes perspiration and dirt

■ Removes odor

■ Increases circulation

■ Allows for some exercise

■ Gives you an opportunity to observe the residents' skin

■ Provides relaxation

You may be asked to give several different types of baths. This depends on the resident's condition. Always check the chart to see what type of bath is ordered. The following are types of baths:

■ Bed bath

■ Tub bath

■ Whirlpool bath

■ Shower

Residents may not have a complete bath every day. Sometimes they are bathed only twice a week. This is especially true of elderly residents, who have drier skin, less subcutaneous fat, and more fragile tissues. Always wash the perineum (pericare) and the underarms every day. These areas tend to develop an odor because they have more bacteria and are not open to the air. Good pericare is especially important when there is a urinary catheter in place. Good pericare helps prevent infection.

PROCEDURE 15.32   GIVING A BED BATH

RATIONALE

Providing a bed bath improves circulation, relaxes the patient, provides an opportunity to examine the skin, and enables you to interact with the patient.

ALERT: Follow Standard Precautions.

1. Wash hands.
2. Assemble equipment.

   a. Soap and soap dish
   b. Face towel
   c. Bath towel
   d. Washcloth
   e. Hospital gown or resident's sleepwear
   f. Lotion or powder
   g. Nailbrush and emery board
   h. Comb and brush
   i. Bedpan or urinal and cover
   j. Bed linen
   k. Bath blanket

   l. Bath basin, water at 105° F
   m. Disposable nonsterile gloves

3. Place linens on chair in order of use and place towels on overbed table.

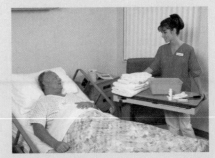

PROCEDURE 15.32 | GIVING A BED BATH *(Continued)*

4. Identify resident.

5. Explain what you are going to do.

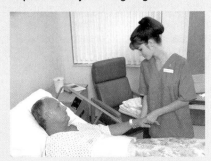

6. Provide for privacy by pulling the privacy screen.

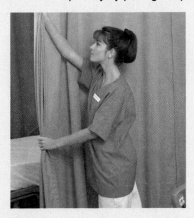

7. Raise bed to a comfortable working height.

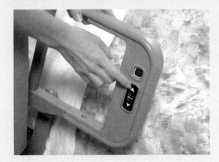

8. Offer bedpan or urinal. Empty and rinse before starting bath. Wash your hands. (Remember to wear gloves when handling urine.)

9. Lower headrest and knee gatch (raised knee area/bed) so that bed is flat.

10. Lower the side rail only on side where you are working.

11. Put on gloves.

12. Loosen top sheet, blanket, and bedspread. Remove and fold blanket and bedspread, and place over back of chair.

13. Cover resident with a bath blanket.

14. Ask resident to hold bath blanket in place. Remove top sheet by sliding it to foot of bed. *Do not expose resident.* (Place soiled linen in laundry container.)

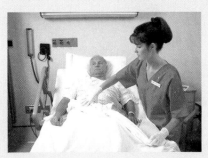

15. Leave a pillow under resident's head for comfort.

16. Remove resident's gown and place in laundry container. If nightwear belongs to resident, follow hospital policy (i.e., send home with family or to hospital laundry).

17. To remove gown when the resident has an IV:

   a. Loosen gown from neck.
   b. Slip gown from free arm.
   c. Be certain that resident is covered with a bath blanket.
   d. Slip gown away from body toward arm with IV.
   e. Gather gown at arm and slip downward over arm and tubing. *Be careful not to pull on tubing.*
   f. Gather material of gown in one hand and slowly draw gown over tip of fingers.
   g. Lift IV free of standard with free hand and slip gown over bottle.
   h. *Do not lower bottle! Raise gown.*

18. Fill bath basin two-thirds full with warm water.

19. Help resident move to side of bed nearest you.

20. Fold face towel over upper edge of bath blanket. This will keep it dry.

21. Form a mitten by folding washcloth around your hand.

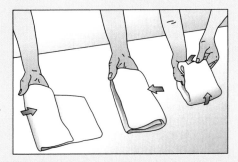

PROCEDURE 15.32   GIVING A BED BATH (Continued)

22. Wash resident's eyes from nose to outside of face. Use different corners of washcloth.

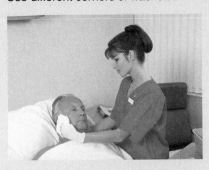

23. Ask resident if he or she wants soap used on the face. Gently wash and rinse face, ears, and neck. Be careful not to get soap in eyes.

24. To wash resident's arms, shoulders, axilla:
    a. Uncover resident's far arm (one farthest from you).

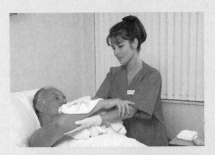

    b. Protect bed from becoming wet with a bath towel placed under arm. Wash with long, firm, circular strokes, rinse, and dry.
    c. Wash and dry armpits (axillae). Apply deodorant and powder.

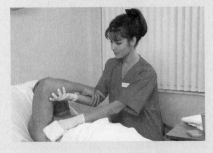

25. To wash hand:
    a. Place basin of water on towel.
    b. Put resident's hand into basin.
    c. Wash, rinse, and dry and push back cuticle gently.

26. Repeat on other arm.

27. To wash chest:
    a. Place towel across resident's chest.
    b. Fold bath blanket down to resident's abdomen.
    c. Wash chest. Be especially careful to dry skin under female breasts to prevent irritation. Dry area thoroughly.

28. To wash abdomen:
    a. Fold down bath blanket to pubic area.
    b. Wash, rinse, and dry abdomen.

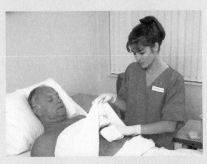

    c. Pull up bath blanket to keep resident warm.
    d. Slide towel out from under bath blanket.

29. To wash thigh, leg, and foot:
    a. Ask resident to flex knee if possible.
    b. Fold bath blanket to uncover thigh, leg, and foot of leg farthest from you.
    c. Place bath towel under leg to keep bed from getting wet.
    d. Place basin on towel and put foot into basin.
    e. Wash and rinse thigh, leg, and foot.

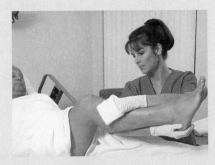

    f. Dry well between toes. Be careful to support the leg when lifting it.

30. Follow same procedure for leg nearest you.

31. Change water. You may need to change water before this time if it is dirty or cold.

32. Raise side rail on opposite side if it is down.

PROCEDURE 15.32 | **GIVING A BED BATH** *(Continued)*

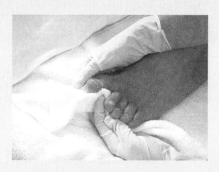

33. To wash back and buttocks:
    a. Help resident turn on side away from you.
    b. Have resident move toward center of bed.
    c. Place a bath towel lengthwise on bed, under resident's back.
    d. Wash, rinse, and dry neck, back, and buttocks.

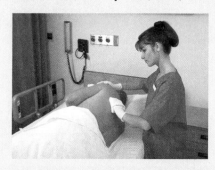

   e. Give resident a back rub. Massage back for at least a minute and a half, giving special attention to shoulder blades, hip bones, and spine. *Observe for reddened areas.* (See the procedure "Skin Care—Giving a Back Rub.")

34. To wash genital area:
    a. Offer resident a clean, soapy washcloth to wash genital area.
    b. Give the person a clean, wet washcloth to rinse with and a dry towel to dry with.

35. Clean the genital area thoroughly if resident is unable to help. To clean the genital area:
    a. When washing a female resident always wipe from front to back.
    b. When washing a male resident, be sure to wash and dry penis, scrotum, and groin area carefully.
    c. Remove gloves and put in hazardous waste.

36. If range of motion is ordered, complete at this time. (See the procedure "Range of Motion.")

37. Put a clean gown on resident.

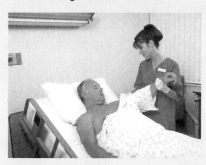

38. If resident has an IV:
    a. Gather the sleeve on IV side in one hand.
    b. Lift bottle free of stand. *Do not lower bottle.*
    c. Slip bottle through sleeve from inside and rehang.
    d. Guide gown along the IV tubing to bed.
    e. Slip gown over the resident's hand. Be careful not to pull or crimp tubing.
    f. Put gown on arm with IV, then on opposite arm.

39. Comb or brush hair.

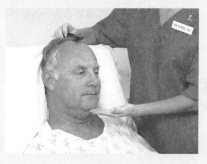

40. Follow hospital policy for towels and washcloths. (Some have you hang them for later use; others have you place them in the laundry containers immediately.)

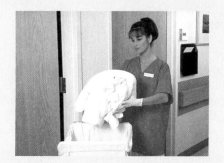

PROCEDURE 15.32 | GIVING A BED BATH *(Continued)*

41. Leave resident in a comfortable position and in good body alignment.

42. Place call bell within reach. Replace furniture and tidy unit.

43. Wash hands.

44. Chart procedure and how resident tolerated it. Note any unusual skin changes or resident complaints.

> 10/24/03   0945
> Completed bed bath
> Dime-sized red area on sacrum
> Reported to charge nurse
> No complaints of discomfort
> Resting quietly with rails up
>   A. Chaplin CNA

PROCEDURE 15.33 | GIVING A PARTIAL BATH (FACE, HANDS, AXILLAE, BUTTOCKS, AND GENITALS)

RATIONALE

Providing a partial bath relaxes the patient and prevents odors. The interaction with the patient is important through communication and touch.

ALERT: Follow Standard Precautions.

1. Wash hands.

2. Assemble equipment.

   a. Soap and soap dish
   b. Face towel
   c. Bath towel
   d. Washcloth
   e. Hospital gown or resident's sleepwear
   f. Lotion or powder
   g. Nail brush and emery board
   h. Comb and brush
   i. Bedpan or urinal and cover
   j. Bath blanket
   k. Bath basin, water at 105°F
   l. Clean linen, as needed
   m. Disposable gloves

3. Identify resident.

4. Explain what you are going to do.

5. Provide privacy by pulling privacy screen.

6. Offer bedpan or urinal. Empty and rinse before starting bath. (Wear gloves if handling body fluid.)

7. Raise headrest to a comfortable position, if permitted.

8. Lower side rails if permitted. If they are to remain up, lower only side rail on side where you are working.

9. Put on gloves.

10. Loosen top sheet, blanket, and bedspread. Remove and fold blanket and bedspread and place over back of chair.

11. Cover resident with a bath blanket.

12. Ask resident to hold bath blanket in place. Remove top sheet by sliding it to the foot of bed: *Do not expose resident.* (Place soiled linen in laundry container.)

13. Leave a pillow under the resident's head for comfort.

14. Remove resident's gown and place in laundry container. If nightwear belongs to resident, follow hospital policy (i.e., send home with family or to hospital laundry).

15. To remove gown when resident has an IV, see the procedure "Giving a Bed Bath."

16. Fill bath basin two-thirds full with warm water and place on overbed table.

17. Put overbed table where resident can reach it comfortably.

PROCEDURE 15.33	**GIVING A PARTIAL BATH (FACE, HANDS, AXILLAE, BUTTOCKS, AND GENITALS)** *(Continued)*

18. Place towel, washcloth, and soap on overbed table.

19. Ask resident to wash as much as he or she is able to and tell the person that you will return to complete bath.

20. Place call bell where resident can reach it easily. Ask resident to signal when ready.

21. Remove gloves, wash your hands, and leave unit.

22. When resident signals, return to unit, wash your hands, and put on gloves.

23. Change water. Complete bathing areas the resident was unable to reach. Make sure that face, hands, axillae, genitals, and buttocks are dry. To wash the genital area:

    a. Offer the resident a clean, soapy washcloth to wash genital area. Provide a clean, wet washcloth to rinse with and a dry towel to dry with. If resident is unable to help, you will need to clean the genital area thoroughly.

    b. When washing a female resident, always wipe from front to back.

    c. When washing a male resident, be sure to wash and dry penis, scrotum, and groin area carefully.

    d. Remove gloves and put in hazardous waste. If range of motion is ordered, complete it at this time. (See the procedure "Range of Motion.")

24. Give a back rub. (See the procedure "Skin Care—Giving a Back Rub.")

25. Put a clean gown on resident.

26. If resident has an IV, see the procedure "Giving a Bed Bath."

27. Assist resident in applying deodorant and putting on a clean gown.

28. Change bed according to hospital policy. Not all facilities change linen every day.

29. Put up side rails if required.

30. Leave resident in a comfortable position and in good body alignment.

31. Remove and discard gloves.

32. Wash hands.

33. Place call bell within reach. Replace furniture and tidy unit.

34. Chart procedure and how it was tolerated.

9/23/02	0730
	Partial bath
	No skin breakdown noted
	Complained of headache
	Reported to charge nurse
	S. Gomez CNA

PROCEDURE 15.34	**TUB/SHOWER BATH**

RATIONALE

Providing a relaxing tub/shower bath gives one-on-one time to the patient. It is an opportunity to check for skin and other problems. Careful observation is essential.

ALERT: Follow Standard Precautions.

1. Wash hands.

2. Assemble equipment on a chair near the tub. Be certain the tub is clean.

    a. Bath towels
    b. Washcloths
    c. Soap

    d. Bath thermometer
    e. Wash basin
    f. Clean gown
    g. Bathmat
    h. Disinfectant solution
    i. Shower chair if necessary

3. Identify resident and explain what you are going to do.

4. Provide privacy by pulling privacy curtain.

5. Help resident out of bed.

6. Help with robe and slippers.

7. Check with head nurse to see if the resident can ambulate or if a wheelchair or shower chair is needed. If a shower chair is used, always do the following:

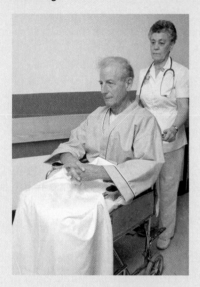

a. Undress resident in room so that shower is not tied up for long periods while residents are dressing or undressing.

b. Cover resident with a bath blanket or sheet so that resident is not exposed in any way.

c. Before leaving room with resident, step back and walk around resident to see if he or she is exposed from any view.

8. Take resident to shower or tub room.

9. For tub bath, place a towel in bottom of tub to help prevent falling.

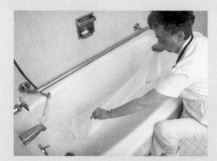

10. Fill tub with water or adjust shower flow (95–105°F).

11. Help resident undress. Give a male resident a towel to wrap around his midriff.

12. Assist resident into tub or shower. If shower, leave weak resident in shower chair.

13. Wash resident's back. Observe carefully for reddened areas or breaks in skin.

14. Resident may be left alone to complete genitalia area if feeling strong.

NOTE If resident shows signs of weakness, remove plug from tub and drain water, or turn off shower. Allow resident to rest until feeling better.

15. Assist resident from tub or shower.

16. Wrap bath towel around resident to prevent chilling.

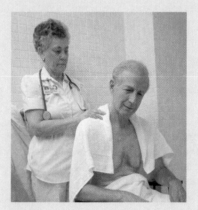

17. Assist in drying and dressing.

18. Return to unit and make comfortable.

19. Put away equipment.

20. Clean bathtub with disinfectant solution.

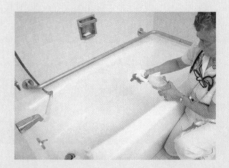

21. Wash hands.

22. Chart procedure and how resident tolerated it.

Use gloves if you are in contact with body fluids.

7/07/03	0900
	Assisted with shower
	Taken to shower on shower chair
	No skin problems noted
	Tolerated well
	_____ A. Chaplin CNA

PROCEDURE 15.35

RESIDENT GOWN CHANGE

RATIONALE

Changing a resident's gown makes the resident feel clean and refreshed. It also allows you to visually examine the skin.

ALERT: Follow Standard Precautions.

1. Wash hands.
2. Assemble equipment: clean resident gown.
3. Tell resident what you are going to do.
4. Provide privacy by pulling privacy curtain.
5. Untie strings of gown at neck and midback. (It may be necessary to assist resident onto side.)
6. Pull soiled gown out from sides of resident.
7. Unfold clean gown and position over resident.
8. Remove soiled gown one sleeve at a time.
9. Leave soiled gown laying over resident's chest; insert one arm into sleeve of clean gown.
10. Fold soiled gown to one side as clean gown is placed over resident's chest.
11. Insert other arm in empty sleeve of gown.
12. Tie neck string on side of neck.
13. Tie midback tie if resident desires.
14. Remove soiled gown to linen hamper.
15. Slip gown under covers, being careful not to expose resident.
16. Position resident for comfort.
17. Raise side rails when necessary.
18. Place bedside stand and call light in resident's reach.

Use gloves if you are in contact with body fluids.

PROCEDURE 15.36

PERINEAL CARE

RATIONALE

Perineal care provides cleansing around areas where body waste is eliminated. The perineal area is dark, warm, and moist, providing an environment for bacterial growth. Keeping the perineum free of drainage and bacteria is an important preventive health measure and helps patients feel more comfortable.

ALERT: Follow Standard Precautions.

1. Wash hands.
2. Assemble equipment.
   a. Bath blanket
   b. Bedpan and cover
   c. Graduate pitcher
   d. Solution, water, or other if ordered
   e. Cotton balls
   f. Waterproof protector for bed
   g. Disposable gloves
   h. Perineal pad and belt if needed
   i. Bag to dispose of cotton balls
3. Identify resident.
4. Explain what you are going to do.
5. Provide privacy by pulling privacy curtain.
6. Put warm water in graduate pitcher (about 100° F).
7. Raise bed to a comfortable working height.
8. Lower side rail.
9. Put on disposable gloves.
10. Remove spread and blanket.
11. Cover resident with bath blanket.
12. Have resident hold top of bath blanket, and fold top sheet to bottom of bed.

PROCEDURE 15.36 | **PERINEAL CARE** *(Continued)*

13. Place waterproof protector under resident's buttocks.

14. Pull up bath blanket to expose perineal area.

15. Provide male and female pericare.

   a. Circumcised male:

     (1) Wipe away from urinary meatus as you wash with soap and water, rinse, and dry.

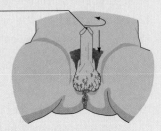

Urethra (start here and wipe downward)

   b. Uncircumcised male:

     (1) Gently move foreskin back away from tip of penis. Wash as directed in step a. After drying, gently move foreskin back over tip of penis.

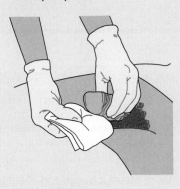

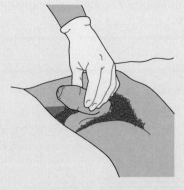

   c. Female:

     (1) Instruct resident to bend knees with feet flat on bed.

     (2) Separate resident's knees.

     (3) Separate the labia and wipe from front to back away from the urethra as you wash with soap and water, rinse, and dry.

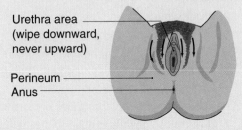

Urethra area (wipe downward, never upward)

Perineum

Anus

16. Remove waterproof protector from bed and dispose of gloves.

17. Cover resident with sheet and remove bath blanket.

18. Return top covers.

19. Return bed to lowest position and put up side rails if required.

20. Secure call bell within resident's reach.

21. Put on gloves.

22. Clean equipment; dispose of disposable material according to hospital policy.

23. Discard gloves and wash hands.

4/14/03   1045

Perineal care provided

Observed a dime-sized reddened area

on the interior left thigh approximately

2 inches below the groin

_____ R. Johnson CNA

RATIONALE

Vaginal douching helps remove excessive discharge and reduce inflammation caused by infection. Your careful practice in following the procedure will help provide comfort and promote healing.

ALERT: Follow Standard Precautions.

1. Wash your hands.
2. Assemble equipment.
   a. Disposable douche kit
      (1) Tubing clamp
      (2) Douche nozzle
      (3) Irrigating container
   b. Cleansing solution
   c. Cotton balls
   d. Bedpan and cover
   e. Waterproof bed protector
   f. Disposable gloves
3. Identify patient.
4. Explain what you are going to do.
5. Provide privacy by pulling privacy curtains.
6. Put on gloves and offer bedpan; empty after use.
7. Remove and discard gloves; wash hands.
8. Raise bed to comfortable working height.
9. Place waterproof protector under patient's buttocks.
10. Open douche kit.
11. Clamp tubing and pour solution into douche container.
12. Put on gloves.
13. Place bedpan under patient.
14. Pour cleansing solution over cotton balls.
15. Cleanse vulva with cotton balls by spreading lips (labia) and wiping one side from front to back.
16. Discard cotton balls into bedpan. Wipe other side and discard cotton ball.
17. Open clamp to expel air from tubing.
18. Allow solution to flow over vulva. Do not touch vulva with nozzle.
19. Insert douche nozzle into vagina as solution is flowing. Insert about 2 inches with an upward, then downward, and backward gentle movement.
20. Allow solution to flow into vagina while holding douche container no more than 18 inches above mattress.
21. Rotate nozzle until all solution has been used.
22. Clamp tubing and remove nozzle gently.
23. Place nozzle and tubing in douche container for disposal.
24. Assist patient to upright position on bedpan to help drain solution from vagina.
25. Help patient dry perineal area.
26. Remove bedpan.
27. Remove waterproof protector.
28. Empty bedpan; rinse, and put away.
29. Remove gloves and discard according to facility policy.
30. Wash hands.
31. Lower bed to lowest position.
32. Position patient comfortably.
33. Put up side rails if required.
34. Secure call bell within patient's reach.
35. Wash hands.
36. Record procedure.

| 9/14/03 1600 |
| Vaginal douche completed |
| No vaginal discharge noted |
| Resident tolerated well |
| _____ S. Gomez CNA |

Vaginal Douche

The doctor may order a vaginal douche for your patient. A vaginal douche is given by flowing a solution into the vagina and letting it flow back out. A douche is given only when the doctor orders it. Douching often removes the normal, protective (good) secretions and can cause increased inflammation or infection. A vaginal douche is used to cleanse the vagina

- To remove excessive discharge.
- To reduce inflammation caused by infection.

CARE OF HAIR AND NAILS

Hair and nail care helps residents feel good about themselves. Good grooming adds to a feeling of well-being. Hair is always kept clean and neatly arranged. Style hair appropriately for the age of the client. For example, ponytails are not a hairstyle that an elderly person would normally select. If residents can have a tub bath or shower, shampoo their hair at bath time.

It is important to keep your residents' hair clean even when they are on bed rest. Today there are chemical shampoos that remove oil and refresh the scalp. You will need a physician's order together with a facility policy that says you can use a chemical shampoo. To use a packaged chemical on the hair, always follow the directions on the package. To wash hair in bed with water and shampoo, carefully follow the steps below.

PROCEDURE 15.38 SHAMPOOING THE HAIR IN BED

RATIONALE

Clean hair makes a patient feel fresh and provides a sense of well-being. Your careful attention to the steps below will make this a pleasant experience for the resident and yourself.

ALERT: Follow Standard Precautions.

1. Wash hands.
2. Assemble equipment.
   a. Chair
   b. Basin of water (105° F)
   c. Pitcher of water (115° F)
   d. Paper or Styrofoam cup
   e. Large basin
   f. Shampoo tray or plastic sheet
   g. Waterproof bed protector
   h. Pillow with waterproof cover
   i. Bath towels
   j. Small towel
   k. Cotton balls
3. Identify resident.
4. Explain what you are going to do.
5. Provide privacy by pulling privacy curtain.
6. Raise bed to a comfortable working position.
7. Place a chair at side of bed near resident's head.
8. Place small towel on chair.
9. Place large basin on chair to catch water.
10. Put cotton in resident's ears to keep water out of ears.
11. Have resident move to side of bed with head close to where you are standing.
12. Remove pillow from under head. Cover pillow with waterproof case.

13. Place pillow under resident's back so that when he or she lies down the head will be tilted back.
14. Place bath blanket on bed.
15. Have resident hold top of bath blanket, and pull top covers to foot.
16. Place waterproof protector under head.
17. Put shampoo tray under resident's head (i.e., plastic bag with both ends open).
18. Place end of plastic in large basin.
19. Have resident hold washcloth over eyes.
20. Put basin of water on bedside table with paper cup. Have pitcher of water for extra water.
21. Brush resident's hair thoroughly.
22. Fill cup with water from basin.
23. Pour water over hair; repeat until completely wet.
24. Apply small amount of shampoo; use both hands to massage the resident's scalp with your fingertips. Be careful not to scratch the scalp with your fingernails.
25. Rinse soap off hair by pouring water from cup over hair. Have resident turn head from side to side. Repeat until completely rinsed.
26. Dry resident's forehead and ears.
27. Remove cotton from ears.
28. Lift resident's head gently and wrap with bath towel.
29. Remove equipment from bed.

30. Change resident's gown and be certain resident is dry.
31. Gently dry resident's hair with towel. (Use a hair dryer if allowed by your facility.)
32. Comb or brush hair and arrange neatly.
33. Remove bath blanket and cover resident with top covers.
34. Make resident comfortable.
35. Lower bed to its lowest position.
36. Put up side rail if required.
37. Return equipment.
38. Tidy unit.
39. Wash hands.
40. Record procedure.

9/06/03	1130

Hair washed while in bed

There is a dime-sized red scaly area on scalp directly above left ear

Resident denies pain or itching at site

Notified charge nurse

Hair dried with hair dryer and styled to suit resident

_____ R. Johnson CNA

PROCEDURE 15.39 | **SHAMPOOING IN SHOWER OR TUB**

RATIONALE

Clean hair makes a patient feel fresh and provides a sense of well-being. Your careful attention to the steps below will make this a pleasant experience for the patient/resident and yourself.

ALERT: Follow Standard Precautions.

1. Assemble equipment.
   a. Shampoo
   b. Washcloth
   c. Towel
   d. Cream rinse, if desired
2. Explain what you are going to do.
3. Instruct resident to tip head back.
4. Wet hair with water, being careful not to get eyes wet.
5. Give resident a washcloth to wipe his or her face as needed.
6. Apply a moderate amount of shampoo to hair. Massage head and hair until a lather develops. (Be careful not to use fingernails.)
7. Rinse hair with clean, clear water until shampoo has disappeared.
8. Repeat shampooing procedure a second time. When rinsing, be sure to remove all shampoo.
9. If a cream rinse is used, apply a small amount to hair, paying special attention to ends of hair.
10. Allow rinse to remain on hair for a few seconds before rinsing.
11. Rinse thoroughly with clean, clear water.
12. Towel dry.
13. Gently comb or brush hair to remove tangles.
14. Use a hair dryer to dry hair.
15. Arrange in an appropriate hairstyle for the resident's age and manner. (Remember that ponytails, pigtails, etc. are not appropriate for a 70-year-old resident.)

10/13/03	0830

Hair washed while in shower

Scalp is clean and there is no evidence of sores or scratches present

Upon return to room, hair styled according to resident's preference

_____ A. Chaplin CNA

PROCEDURE 15.40

ARRANGING THE HAIR

RATIONALE

A patient's outward appearance plays a significant role in his or her self-image. Arranging the hair is a key part of the daily grooming routine for every resident. It is important to arrange your resident's hair according to their preferences.

ALERT: Follow Standard Precautions.

1. Wash hands.
2. Assemble equipment.
   a. Comb and/or brush
   b. Towel
3. Identify resident.
4. Explain what you are going to do.
5. Provide privacy by pulling privacy curtain.
6. Raise bed to a comfortable working height.
7. Assist as needed.
8. If total assistance is needed:
   a. Section the hair, starting at one side, working around to other side.

   b. Comb or brush hair thoroughly, being careful not to pull it.
   c. Arrange hair neatly.
9. Lower bed to lowest position.
10. Put up side rail if required.
11. Secure call light in resident's reach.
12. Clean and replace all equipment.
13. Wash hands.
14. Report procedure and observations (e.g., dry scalp, reddened areas).

Keep nails trimmed and clean. Long nails may scratch the resident or someone else. They break more easily and are more difficult to clean when they are not kept short. Toenails may become very thick and hard. Often it is necessary to have a podiatrist (foot doctor) cut them. If the resident has diabetes, *do not cut the nails.* Diabetic residents tend to have poor circulation and do not heal well. This results in severe **ulcerations** if their skin is knicked or broken. Whenever you cut fingernails or toenails, check first with the charge nurse.

ulcerations

Open areas, or sores.

⬤ SHAVING THE RESIDENT

Men usually shave every day when they are able to care for themselves. Encourage them to shave themselves when possible. They will feel much better about themselves. If they are unable to shave themselves, take time to shave them. Women tend to have facial hair when they age. This can be very distressing to the resident. Follow the procedures that your facility has to remove the facial hair. In some facilities it is plucked; in others it is shaved. Be certain to look in the procedure book.

PROCEDURE 15.41 NAIL CARE

RATIONALE

A patient's outward appearance plays a significant role in his or her self-image. Nail care is a key part of the daily grooming routine for every resident. Keeping nails clean and trimmed prevents sores from developing around the nail beds and eliminates unintentional scratches that could become infected.

ALERT: Follow Standard Precautions.

1. Wash hands.
2. Assemble equipment.
   a. Warm water
   b. Orange sticks
   c. Emery board
   d. Nail clippers

NOTE Do not clip a diabetic resident's nails.

3. Identify the resident.
4. Cleanse nails by soaking in water.
5. Use slanted edge of orange stick to clean dirt out from under nails.
6. File nails with emery board to shorten. (Clip if permitted by your facility.)
7. Use smooth edge of emery board to smooth.
8. Apply lotion to help condition cuticle.
9. Massage hands and feet with lotion.
10. Make resident comfortable.

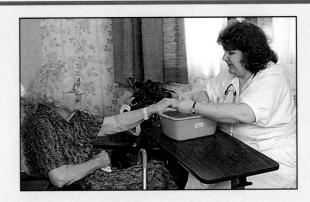

11. Raise side rail if required.
12. Return equipment.
13. Wash hands.
14. Record procedure and any unusual conditions (e.g., hangnails, broken nails).

PROCEDURE 15.42 SHAVING THE RESIDENT

RATIONALE

A patient's outward appearance plays a significant role in his or her self-image. Shaving facial hair is a key part of the daily grooming routine for many residents. Carefully follow the steps below as you groom your resident each day.

ALERT: Follow Standard Precautions.

1. Wash hands.
2. Assemble equipment.
   a. Electric shaver or safety razor
   b. Shaving lather or an electric preshave lotion
   c. Basin of warm water
   d. Face towel
   e. Mirror
   f. Aftershave
   g. Disposable gloves

3. Identify resident and explain what you are going to do.
4. Provide privacy by pulling privacy curtains.
5. Raise head of bed if permitted.
6. Place equipment on overbed table.
7. Place a towel over resident's chest.
8. Adjust light so that it shines on resident's face.

PROCEDURE 15.42 | **SHAVING THE RESIDENT** *(Continued)*

9. Shave resident.

   a. If you are using a safety razor:

      (1) Put on gloves.
      (2) Moisten face and apply lather.
      (3) Start in front of ear; hold skin taut and bring razor down over cheek toward chin. Use short firm strokes. Repeat until lather on cheek is removed and skin is smooth.
      (4) Repeat on other cheek.
      (5) Wash face and neck. Dry thoroughly.
      (6) Apply aftershave lotion or powder if desired.
      (7) Discard gloves according to facility policy.

   b. If you are using an electric shaver:

      (1) Put on gloves.
      (2) Apply preshave lotion.
      (3) Gently shave until beard is removed.
      (4) Wash face and neck. Dry thoroughly.
      (5) Apply aftershave lotion or powder if desired.
      (6) Remove gloves.

10. Wash hands.

11. Chart procedure and how procedure was tolerated.

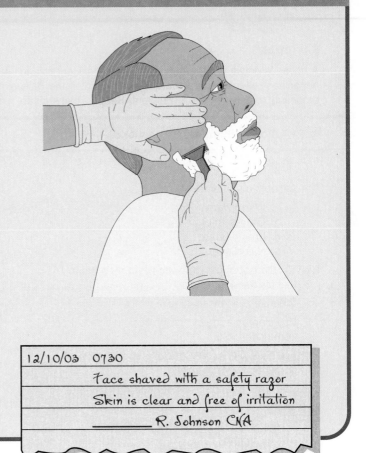

12/10/03   0730

    Face shaved with a safety razor

    Skin is clear and free of irritation

             R. Johnson CNA

⬤ DRESSING AND UNDRESSING THE RESIDENT

It is very important for the resident to be up and dressed. Residents must not remain in bed unless the doctor orders bedrest. Being up and dressed creates an attitude of wellness. Staying in bedclothes presents an attitude of "being sick." Be certain that residents are dressed nicely and that their clothes are in good repair. Match the clothing rather than just throwing on "anything that's handy."

For residents who have a handicap, take special care in how you put on their clothes. This is also true of residents who have an IV. The following are some rules to follow:

limb

Arm, leg.

■ Always dress the weak or most involved side first. A **limb** that does not function well slides into a sleeve or pant leg if you start on that side.

■ Always undress the weak or most involved side last.

■ If the resident has an IV, be very careful not to disturb or dislodge it. Ask your instructor how to do this.

⬤ PROSTHETIC DEVICES

A prosthesis or prosthetic device replaces or aids a body part that is injured, lost, or not working correctly. These include

- Dentures
- Glasses/contact lenses
- Hearing aids
- Artificial limbs
- Artificial eyes
- Artificial breasts (after mastectomy)
- Pacemaker

These devices are very important to the well-being of the resident and are treated carefully. You need to learn the correct way to put them on. Your resident is an excellent source of information on how they fit. Always put them in the same place when the resident is not using them so that they are not lost and the resident can find them.

BEDMAKING

When bedding is wrinkled or wet it causes irritation to the skin and is very uncomfortable. Keeping the bed smooth and dry prevents a decubitus, a severe breakdown of the skin (see the section "Skin Management"). The number of times that you change the bed depends on whether or not the resident is continent. When the resident is in bed, check to be sure that the wrinkles are smoothed out and that the bed is dry.

The hospital bed has a small sheet, called a draw sheet, that is placed in the midsection of the bed between the resident's knees and shoulders. This provides protection to the bottom sheet and can be changed easily without having to change the entire bottom sheet. Often, a plastic cover is placed over the bottom sheet and under the draw sheet to prevent soiling. Be certain that the plastic sheet is always smooth.

There are several ways that hospital beds are made. If the resident is up and around, you make a closed bed. If the resident must remain in bed, you have to make an occupied bed. When the resident is in and out of bed during the day you make an open bed.

PROCEDURE 15.43 — MAKING A CLOSED BED

RATIONALE

Clean linens help prevent the spread of bacteria in the health care environment. A closed bed is made ready for new admissions or when a resident is not expected to return to bed until evening. Neatly made beds create a sense of order.

ALERT: Follow Standard Precautions.

1. Wash hands.
2. Assemble equipment.
   a. Mattress pad and cover
   b. Plastic or rubber draw sheet (if used in your facility)
   c. Two large sheets or fitted bottom sheet and one large sheet
   d. Draw sheet or half-sheet
   e. Blankets as needed
   f. Spread
   g. Pillow
   h. Pillowcase

PROCEDURE 15.43 | **MAKING A CLOSED BED** *(Continued)*

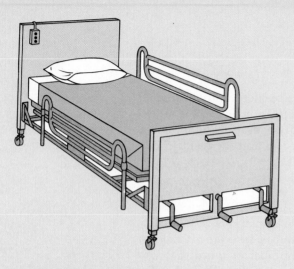

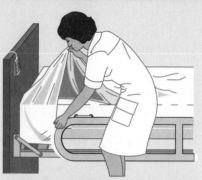

Grasp the edge of the sheet 10–12 inches from the top of the bed and fold it onto the mattress.

3. Raise bed to a comfortable working height. Lock wheels on bed.

4. Place a chair at the side of bed.

5. Put linen on chair in the order in which you will use it. (First things you will use go on top.)

6. Position mattress at head of bed until it is against head board.

7. Place mattress cover even with top of mattress and smooth it out.

8. Work on one side of bed until that side is completed. Then go to other side of bed. This saves you time and energy.

9. Bottom sheet is folded lengthwise. Place it on bed with center fold in center of mattress from head to foot. Place large hem to head of bed and narrow hem even with foot of mattress.

10. Open sheet. Check to see that it hangs the same distance over each side of bed.

11. Leave about 18 inches of sheet to tuck under head of mattress.

12. To make a mitered corner:

   a. Pick up edge of sheet at side of bed approximately 12 inches from head of bed.

   b. Place folded corner (triangle) on top of mattress.

   c. Tuck hanging portion of sheet under the mattress.

   d. While you hold the fold at the edge of mattress, bring folded section down over side of mattress.

   e. Tuck sheet under mattress from head to foot. Start at head and pull toward foot of bed as you tuck.

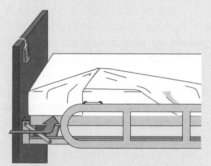

Tuck the part of the sheet that is hanging down under the mattress.

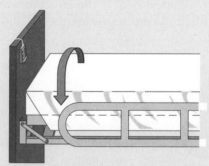

Bring the folded part down over the mattress.

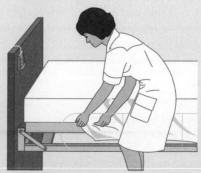

Tuck the entire side of the sheet under the mattress.

PROCEDURE 15.43 | MAKING A CLOSED BED *(Continued)*

13. Fold draw sheet in half and place about 14 inches down from top of mattress. Tuck it in. Check to be sure that each piece of linen is straight and even as you tuck it in.

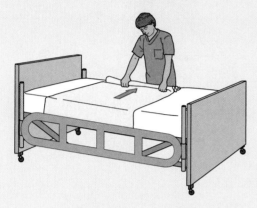

14. Top sheet is folded lengthwise. Place on bed.

    a. Place the center fold at center of bed from head to foot.
    b. Put large hem at head of bed, even with top of mattress.
    c. Open the sheet. Be certain rough edge of hem is facing up.
    d. Tightly tuck the sheet under at foot of bed.
    e. Make a mitered corner at foot of bed.
    f. Do not tuck in sheet at side of bed.

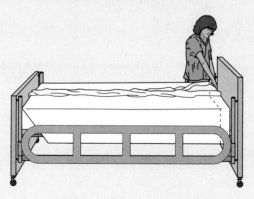

15. Blanket is folded lengthwise. Place it on bed.

    a. Place center fold of blanket on center of bed from head to foot.
    b. Place upper hem 6 inches from top of mattress.
    c. Open blanket and tuck it under foot tightly.
    d. Make a mitered corner at foot of bed.
    e. Do not tuck in at sides of bed.

16. Bedspread is folded lengthwise. Place it on bed.

    a. Place center fold in center of bed from head to foot.

b. Place upper hem even with upper edge of mattress.
    c. Have rough edge down.
    d. Open spread and tuck it under at foot of bed.
    e. Make a mitered corner.
    f. Do not tuck in at sides.

17. Go to other side of bed. Start with bottom sheet.

    a. Pull sheet tight and smooth out all wrinkles.
    b. Make a mitered corner at top of bed.
    c. Pull draw sheet tight and tuck it in.
    d. Straighten out top sheet. Make a mitered corner at foot of bed.
    e. Miter foot corners of blanket and bedspread.

18. Fold top hem of spread over top hem of blanket.

19. Fold top hem of sheet back over edge of spread and blanket to form cuff. The hem should be on the underside so that a rough surface does not come in contact with resident's skin and cause irritation.

20. Put pillowcase on pillow.

    a. Hold pillowcase at center of end seam.
    b. With your other hand, turn pillowcase back over hand holding end seam.
    c. Grasp pillow through case at center of end of pillow.

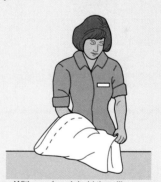

With one hand, hold the pillowcase at the center of the seamed end.

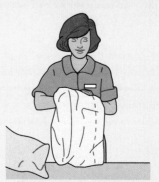

Turn the pillowcase back over that hand with your free hand.

PROCEDURE 15.43 | MAKING A CLOSED BED *(Continued)*

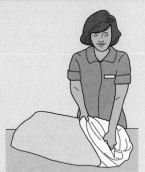

Grasp the pillow at the center of one end
with the hand that is inside the pillowcase.

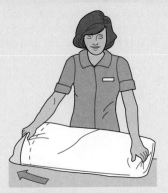

Straighten the pillowcase.

d. Bring case down over pillow and fit pillow into
   corners of case.
e. Fold extra material over open end of pillow and
   place it on bed with open end away from door.

21. Put bed in lowest position.
22. Wash hands.

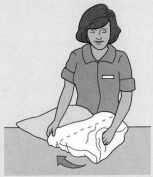

Pull the pillowcase down over the
pillow with your free hand.

PROCEDURE 15.44 | MAKING AN OCCUPIED BED

RATIONALE

Clean linens help prevent the spread of bacteria in the
health care environment. Making an occupied bed with
fresh linen will provide cleanliness, comfort, and will help
the resident maintain a healthy skin condition.

ALERT: Follow Standard Precautions.

1. Wash hands.
2. Assemble equipment.
   a. Draw sheet
   b. Two large sheets or fitted bottom sheet and
      one large sheet

   c. Two pillowcases
   d. Blankets as needed
   e. Bedspread (if clean one is needed)
   f. Pillow
   g. Disposable gloves if needed

3. Identify resident and explain what you are going to do.

4. Raise bed to comfortable working height. Lock wheels on bed.

5. Place chair at side of bed.

6. Put linen on chair in the order in which you will use it. (First things you will use go on top.)

7. Provide for privacy by pulling privacy curtain.

8. Lower headrest and kneerest until bed is flat, if allowed.

9. Loosen linens on all sides by lifting edge of mattress with one hand and pulling out bedclothes with the other. *Never shake linen: This spreads microorganisms.*

10. Push mattress to top of bed. Ask for assistance if you need it.

11. Remove bedspread and blanket by folding them to the bottom, one at a time. Lift them from center and place over back of chair.

12. Place bath blanket or plain sheet over top sheet. Ask resident to hold top edge of clean cover if he or she is able to do so. If resident cannot hold the sheet, tuck it under resident's shoulders.

13. Slide soiled sheet from top to bottom and put in dirty linen container. Be careful not to expose resident.

14. Ask resident to turn toward the opposite side of bed. Have resident hold onto the side rail. Assist resident if he or she needs help. Resident should now be on far side of bed from you.

15. Adjust pillow for resident to make him or her comfortable.

16. Fan-fold soiled draw sheet and bottom sheet close to resident and tuck against resident's back. This leaves mattress stripped of linen.

17. Work on one side of bed until that side is completed. Then go to other side of bed. This saves you time and energy.

18. Take large clean sheet and fold it lengthwise. Be careful not to let it touch floor.

19. Place sheet on bed, still folded, with fold on middle of mattress. Small hem should be even with foot of mattress.

20. Fold top half of sheet toward resident. Tuck folds against resident's back.

21. Miter corner at head of mattress. Tuck clean sheet on your side from head to foot of mattress.

22. Place clean bottom draw sheet that has been folded in half with fold along middle of mattress. Fold top half of sheet toward resident. Tuck folds against resident's back.

23. Raise side rail and lock in place.

24. Lower side rail on opposite side.

25. Ask resident to roll away from you to other side of bed and onto clean linen. Tell resident that there will be a bump in the middle. (Be careful not to let resident become wrapped up in bath blanket.)

26. Remove old bottom sheet and draw sheet from bed and put into laundry container.

27. Pull fresh linen toward edge of mattress. Tuck it under mattress at head of bed and make mitered corner.

28. Tuck bottom sheet under mattress from head to foot of mattress. Pull firmly to remove wrinkles.

29. Pull draw sheet very tight and tuck under mattress.

30. Have resident roll on back, or turn resident yourself. Loosen bath blanket as resident turns.

31. Change pillowcase.

    a. Hold pillowcase at center of end seam.
    b. With your other hand turn pillowcase back over hand, holding end seam.
    c. Grasp pillow through case at center of end of pillow.
    d. Bring case down over pillow and fit pillow into corners of case.
    e. Fold extra material over open end of pillow and place pillow under resident's head.

32. Spread clean top sheet over bath blanket with wide hem at the top. Middle of sheet should run along middle of bed with wide hem even with top edge of mattress. Ask resident to hold hem of clean sheet. Remove bath blanket by moving it toward foot of bed. Be careful not to expose resident.

33. Tuck clean top sheet under mattress at foot of bed. Make toepleat in top sheet so that resident's feet can move freely. To make a toepleat, make 3-inch fold toward foot of bed in topsheet before tucking in sheet. Tuck in and miter corner.

34. Place blanket over resident, being sure that it covers the shoulders.

35. Place bedspread on bed in same way. Tuck blanket and bedspread under bottom of mattress and miter corners.

36. Make cuff.

    a. Fold top hem edge of spread over blanket.
    b. Fold top hem of top sheet back over edge of bedspread and blanket, being certain that rough hem is turned down.

37. Position resident and make comfortable.

38. Put bed in lowest position.

39. Open privacy curtains.

40. Raise side rails, if required.

41. Place call light where resident can reach it.

42. Tidy unit.

43. Wash hands.

44. Chart linen change and how the resident tolerated procedure.

PROCEDURE 15.45   MAKING AN OPEN BED

RATIONALE

Clean linens help prevent the spread of bacteria in the health care environment. An open bed provides easy access for residents returning to bed within a short period.

1. Wash hands.
2. Grasp cuff of bedding in both hands and pull to foot of bed.

Fan-fold to foot of bed.

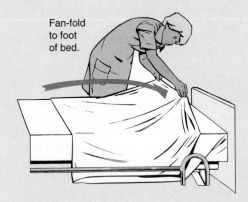

3. Fold bedding back on itself toward head of bed. The edge of cuff must meet fold. (This is called fan-folding.)

Fold sheet back toward head of bed.

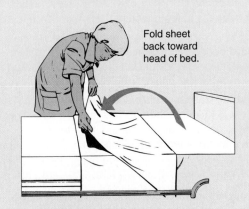

4. Smooth the hanging sheets on each side into folds.
5. Wash hands.

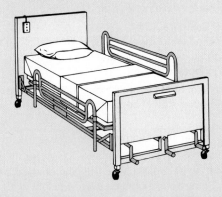

FEEDING THE RESIDENT

Mealtime is a pleasant time for residents. It is often the most pleasurable event of the day. This should be an unhurried, enjoyable experience. Be certain that the resident is prepared for meals before the food arrives. The preparation for the meal includes the following:

■ Assisting residents or reminding them to wash their hands

■ Removing any unpleasant items from the area, such as **emesis** basins and bedpans

■ Offering the opportunity to use the bedpan or the bathroom

emesis

Vomit.

- Providing for the resident's comfort:

  • Raise the head of the bed. • Position the resident in a chair. • Transport the resident to the dining area.

- Checking to be certain that you have the right tray for the resident and that it is the correct diet

- Always placing the food within reach

- Checking the tray to be certain that everything is there

- Preparing any item that the resident cannot manage

- Telling the resident where each item is according to the face of a clock if the resident is blind

PROCEDURE 15.46

PREPARING THE RESIDENT TO EAT

RATIONALE

Meals are an important part of every culture. Preparing residents for a meal by providing clean, neat surroundings and encouraging toileting and washing hands before eating can help residents enjoy their meal and promote their appetites.

ALERT: Follow Standard Precautions.

1. Wash hands.
2. Assemble equipment.
   a. Bedpan or urinal
   b. Toilet tissue
   c. Washcloth
   d. Hand towel
3. Assist resident as needed to empty bladder and wash hands and face.
4. Explain that you are getting ready to give resident a meal.
5. Clear bedside table.
6. Position resident for comfort and a convenient eating position.
7. Wash your hands.
8. Identify resident and check name on food tray to ensure that you are delivering the correct diet to resident.
9. Place tray in a convenient position in front of resident.

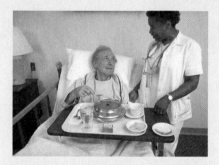

10. Open containers if resident cannot.
11. If resident is unable to prepare food, do it for resident.
    a. Butter the bread
    b. Cut meat
    c. Season food as necessary
12. Follow the procedure for feeding a resident if resident needs to be fed.
13. Wash hands.

PROCEDURE 15.47

PREPARING THE RESIDENT TO EAT IN THE DINING ROOM

RATIONALE

Eating in the dining room provides a more normal environment for residents, creating an opportunity to visit with others during the meal.

ALERT: Follow Standard Precautions.

1. Wash hands.
2. Help resident take care of toileting needs.
3. Assist with handwashing.
4. Take resident to dining room.
5. Position resident in wheelchair at table that is proper height for wheelchair.
6. Be certain resident is sitting in a comfortable position in wheelchair.
7. Provide adaptive feeding equipment if needed.
8. Bring resident tray.
9. Identify resident.
10. Serve tray and remove plate covers.
11. Provide assistance as needed (e.g., cut meat, butter bread, open containers).
12. Remove tray when finished, noting what resident ate.
13. Assist with handwashing and take resident to area of choice.

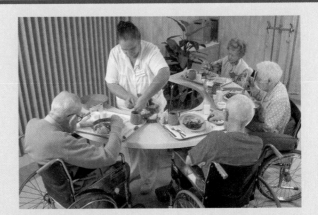

14. Wash hands.
15. Record what resident ate.
16. Record I & O if necessary. (See the section "Measuring Intake and Output" later in the unit.)

8/10/03	0800
	Taken by wheelchair to dining room
	80% of breakfast eaten, and
	tolerated well
	_____ S. Gomez CNA

ASSISTING THE RESIDENT WITH MEALS

RATIONALE

Food is essential to maintain health. As a health care worker you are responsible to encourage residents to maintain their health by eating routine meals. Your attitude and willingness to assist residents who require your attention during meals can encourage their intake of a balanced diet.

ALERT: Follow Standard Precautions.

1. Wash hands.
2. Check resident's ID band with name on food tray to ensure that you will be feeding correct diet to resident.

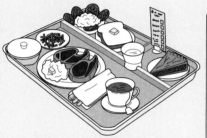

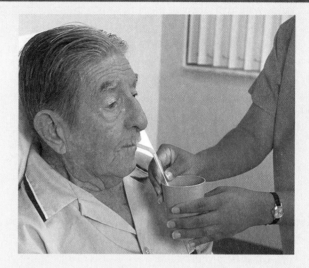

DINNER MENU

JONES, MARY MRS.
PATIENT'S NAME   EAST - 1
F-EL 1-78640   WARD
IDENTIFICATION NO.   E 1010
REGULAR   ROOM NO.
TYPE OF DIET

BREAD ☑   ROLLS ☐   BUTTER ☑

SOUP
VEGETABLE   ☑
CREAM OF MUSHROOM   ☐

SALAD
COTTAGE CHEESE, TOMATO   ☑
TOSSED SALAD (FRENCH DRESSING) ☐

ENTREES
ROAST BEEF   ☐
ROAST CHICKEN   ☐
BROILED PORK CHOPS   ☑

VEGETABLES
STRING BEANS   ☑
PEAS AND CARROTS   ☐
SPINACH   ☐
BAKED POTATOES   ☐
MASHED POTATOES   ☑

DESSERTS
ICE CREAM (CHOCOLATE)   ☐
FRUIT JEL (LIME)   ☐
CHERRY PIE   ☑

BEVERAGES
COFFEE ☐   TEA ☑   MILK ☐

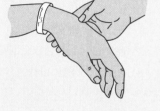

3. Tell resident what food is being served.
4. Ask resident how he or she prefers food to be prepared (e.g., salt, pepper, cream or sugar in coffee).
5. Position resident in a sitting position, as allowed by physician. If ordered to lie flat, turn resident on side.
6. Position yourself in a comfortable manner so that you won't be rushing resident because you are uncomfortable. (Do not sit on bed.)
7. Cut food into small bite-sized pieces.
8. Place a napkin or small hand towel under resident's chin.
9. Put a flex straw in cold drinks. Hot drinks tend to burn mouth if taken through a straw.
10. Use a spoon to feed resident small to average-sized bites of food. (Encourage resident to help self as much as possible.)

11. Always feed resident at a slow pace. It may take more time for him or her to chew and swallow than you think is necessary.
12. Always be sure that one bite has been swallowed before you give another spoonful to resident.
13. Tell resident what is being served and ask which item he or she prefers first, if resident cannot see food.
14. Encourage resident to finish eating, but do not force.
15. Assist resident in wiping face when resident is finished eating.
16. Observe amount of food eaten.
17. Remove tray from room.
18. Position resident for comfort and safety.
19. Place call light in a convenient place.
20. Wash hands.
21. Record amount of food eaten (half, three-fourths, one-fourth, etc.) on chart, and indicate if food was tolerated well or not.

10/10/03   1800
50% of meal taken with assistance and tolerated well.
Resident stated that he doesn't like beef. Dietitian notified of resident's request for meat other than beef.
_____ R. Johnson CNA

PROCEDURE 15.49

SERVING FOOD TO THE RESIDENT IN BED (SELF-HELP)

RATIONALE

As a health care worker you are required to identify the right diet for each resident and recognize what they need assistance with. Your opening packages and cartons or cutting food into bite-sized pieces may make the difference between a resident eating or refusing his or her food.

ALERT: Follow Standard Precautions.

1. Wash hands.
2. Assemble equipment.
    a. Food tray with diet card
    b. Flex straws
    c. Towel
3. Assist resident with bedpan or urinal.
4. Place in a sitting position if possible.
5. Help resident wash hands and face.
6. Remove unsightly or odor-causing articles.
7. Clean overbed table.
8. Check tray with diet card for
    a. Resident's name
    b. Type of diet
    c. Correct foods according to diet (e.g., diabetic, puréed, chopped, regular)
9. Set up tray and help with foods if needed (e.g., cut meat, butter bread, open containers). *Do not add foods to the tray until you check on diet.*
10. Encourage resident to eat all foods on tray.
11. Remove tray when finished and note what resident ate.
12. Help resident wash hands and face.
13. Position resident comfortably.
14. Remove tray.
15. Be certain that water is within reach.
16. Wash hands.
17. Record I & O if required.
18. Record amount eaten.

> 11/03/03　1230
>
> Lunch served with meat and vegetables cut into bite-sized pieces.
> Mr. Axel struggled to butter the bread without assistance. He said, "I knew I could butter it without help." 90% of lunch eaten, tolerated well.
> —————— S. Gomez CNA

PROCEDURE 15.50

FEEDING THE HELPLESS RESIDENT

RATIONALE

Residents must routinely eat a balanced diet. You are required to feed patients who are not able to feed themselves. Your patience and willingness to feed them in a gentle, caring, compassionate manner could make the difference in their eating or not eating.

ALERT: Follow Standard Precautions.

1. Wash hands.
2. Bring resident's tray.
3. Check name on card with resident ID band.
4. Explain to resident what you are going to do.
5. Tuck a napkin under resident's chin.
6. Season food the way resident likes it.
7. Use a spoon and fill only half full.
8. Give food from tip, not side of spoon.

PROCEDURE 15.50 | FEEDING THE HELPLESS RESIDENT *(Continued)*

9. Name each food as you offer it, if resident cannot see food.

10. Describe position of food on plate (e.g., hot liquids in right corner, peas at the position of 3 o'clock on a clock) if resident cannot see but can feed self.

11. Tell resident if you are offering something that is hot or cold.

12. Use a straw for giving liquids.

13. Feed resident slowly and allow time to chew and swallow.

14. Note amount eaten and remove tray when finished.

15. Help with washing hands and face.

16. Position resident comfortably.

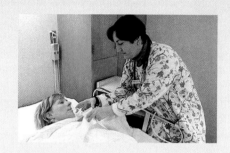

17. Wash hands.

18. Record amount eaten and I & O if required. See following pages for directions on recording I & O.

INTAKE AND OUTPUT SHEET							
Hospital #				Patient Name			
Date				Room #			
INTAKE				OUTPUT			
				URINE		GASTRIC	
Time 7-3	BY MOUTH	TUBE	PARENTERAL	VOIDED	CATHETER	EMESIS	SUCTION
TOTAL							
Time 3-11							
TOTAL							
Time 11-7							
TOTAL							
24 HOUR TOTAL							
24 Hour Grand Total • Intake				24 Hour Grand Total • Output			

12/12/03   1830
Ate 60% of food and drank
240cc of tea
Chokes easily when drinking liquids
Reported choking incidents to team
leader
_____ A. Chaplin CNA

PROCEDURE 15.51

SERVING NOURISHMENTS

RATIONALE

Between-meal nourishments are served to people who need additional nutrients to maintain or improve their health. People with diabetes need nourishments to maintain balanced glucose levels. Some may need protein to build and repair body tissue and others may need specific vitamins.

ALERT: Follow Standard Precautions.

1. Wash hands.
2. Assemble equipment.
   a. Nourishment
   b. Cup, dish, straw, spoon
   c. Napkin
3. Identify resident.
4. Take nourishment to resident.
5. Help if needed.
6. After resident is finished, collect dirty utensils.
7. Return utensils to dietary cart or kitchen.
8. Record intake on I & O sheet if required.
9. Wash hands.
10. Record nourishment taken.

9/15/03   1500
Took 50% of afternoon nourishment
_____ R. Johnson CNA

Additional Nourishments

Nourishments are usually served to residents who require additional nutrition. You are required to identify the right nourishment for residents and to recognize what they need assistance with. Telling the resident that the nourishment is served, making it ready to drink or eat, or feeding him or her if necessary makes it possible for the resident to receive the needed nourishment.

You may have a resident with a nasogastric (N/G) tube. The nasogastric tube is used when the resident has difficulty swallowing or has no swallow reflex. It is a soft, plastic tube that is inserted in the nostril and goes down the back of the throat through the esophagus to the stomach. The tube is taped to the resident's nose. Fluids such as liquid food and medication are put into the tube. Another type of tube is the gastric tube. This tube enters the stomach through the abdominal wall. It is left in place and capped after each feeding. Be very careful not to pull out these tubes.

⬤ MEASURING INTAKE AND OUTPUT

One of your most important responsibilities is helping the resident with fluid balance. Normally, our bodies maintain this balance without our thinking about it. We take in fluids in our foods and liquids. About the same amount is eliminated by the kidneys (urine), respiration, and perspiration. However, in some residents, fluid balance becomes a very serious problem (see Figure 15.11). Fluid imbalance occurs when fluid stays in the tissues, causing edema, or when there is excessive loss of fluid (dehydration).

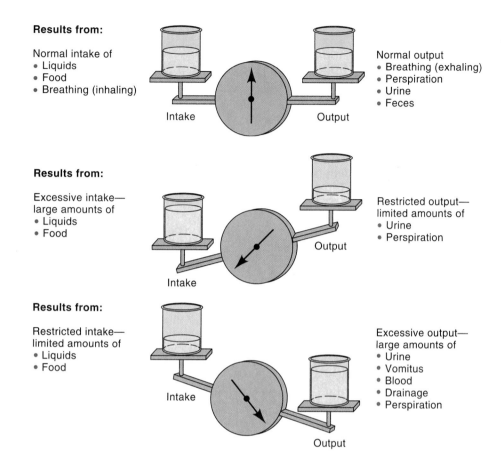

Results from:

Normal intake of
- Liquids
- Food
- Breathing (inhaling)

Intake   Output

Normal output
- Breathing (exhaling)
- Perspiration
- Urine
- Feces

Results from:

Excessive intake—
large amounts of
- Liquids
- Food

Output

Intake

Restricted output—
limited amounts of
- Urine
- Perspiration

Results from:

Restricted intake—
limited amounts of
- Liquids
- Food

Intake

Output

Excessive output—
large amounts of
- Urine
- Vomitus
- Blood
- Drainage
- Perspiration

Figure 15.11

Fluid balance and imbalance.

Dehydration is caused by

- Diarrhea
- Vomiting
- Bleeding
- Excessive perspiration (diaphoresis)
- Poor fluid intake

If you notice any of the following symptoms of dehydration, report them immediately:

- Fever is present.
- There is a decrease in urine.
- Urine is concentrated.
- Weight loss occurs.
- Membranes are dry, and patient has difficulty swallowing.
- Tongue is coated and thickened.
- Skin becomes hard and cracks and is dry and warm.

Edema is serious; it is caused by

- High salt intake
- Infections
- Injuries or burns

dehydration

Severe loss of fluid from tissue and cells.

Figure 15.12

Fluid intake.

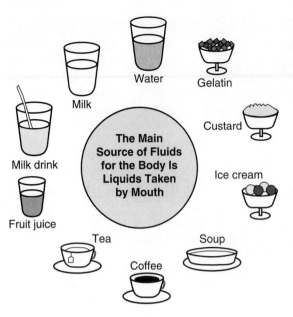

- Certain kidney diseases
- Certain heart diseases or heart inefficiencies
- Sitting too long in one position
- Infiltration of IV fluid

If you notice any of the symptoms of edema, report them immediately:

- Decrease in urine output
- Gain in weight
- Puffiness or swelling
- Sometimes shortness of breath

When any of these situations occur, the doctor writes an order to record intake and output (I & O). You record any fluid taken in and any fluid that is eliminated. To measure intake, record the amount of fluid consumed by mouth (see Figure 15.12). Be sure to include the following:

- All liquid taken by mouth
- Any food item that turns to liquid at room temperature (e.g., gelatin, ice cream)
- All fluid taken by IV or tube feeding

Your facility has a charting method for you to use. Record the amount of liquid taken at the time it is taken. This way, you do not forget this important task. You are probably most familiar with measuring liquid in ounces. When you record liquid intake, you record it in cubic centimeters (cc's). This is a metric measure and is used in medical facilities. Most facilities have a chart that helps you determine how many cubic centimeters are in a serving (see Table 15.1). If you need to change ounces to cubic centimeters, use the formula below.

$$30 \times (\text{number of ounces}) = \text{number of cc}$$

For example:

$$30 \times 8 \text{ ounces} = 240 \text{ cc}$$

To measure resident output, measure all

Figure 15.13

Nasogastric suction.

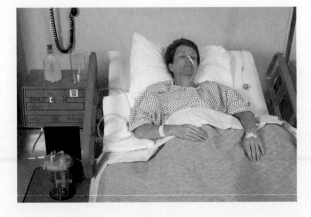

- Urine
- Emesis (vomit)
- Suctioned secretion
- Drainage
- Excessive perspiration

Suctioned secretion (see Figure 15.13) and perspiration are estimated. It is a good idea to have an experienced person help you determine the amount. When you have measured input and output, record them on the chart

Table 15.1 ■ Customary Liquid Measures and Their Equivalents*

1 cc/1 mL	15 drops
1 cc/1 mL	1/4 teaspoon
5 cc/mL	1 teaspoon
15 cc/mL	1 tablespoon
30 cc/mL	1 oz
60 cc/mL	2 oz
120 cc/mL	4 oz
180 cc/mL	6 oz
240 cc/mL	8 oz (1 cup)
500 cc/mL	16 oz (1 pint)
1,000 cc/mL	32 oz (1 quart)
4,000 cc/mL	64 oz (1 gallon)

*cc, cubic centimeter; mL, milliliter; oz, ounce.

PROCEDURE 15.52

MEASURING URINARY OUTPUT

RATIONALE

All body systems rely on fluid balance to maintain normal functioning. By measuring urinary output, you can determine the body's ability to maintain fluid balance and observe characteristics of urine that indicate normalcy or potential abnormalities.

ALERT: Follow Standard Precautions.

1. Wash hands.
2. Assemble equipment.
   a. Bedpan, urinal, or special container
   b. Graduate or measuring cup
   c. Disposable nonsterile gloves
3. Put on gloves.
4. Pour urine into measuring graduate.
5. Place graduate on flat surface and read amount of urine.
6. Observe urine for
   a. Unusual color
   b. Blood
   c. Dark color
   d. Large amounts of mucus
   e. Sediment
7. Save the specimen and report to nurse immediately if you notice any unusual appearance.
8. Discard if urine is normal.
9. Rinse graduate or pitcher and put away.
10. Remove gloves and discard according to facility policy.
11. Wash hands.
12. Record amount of urine in cc's on I & O sheet.

11/11/03   1200
Voided 300 cc dark,
amber-colored urine
——— S. Gomez CNA

11/11/03   1600
Voided 100 cc pink-tinged urine
Complained of pain upon urination
Team leader notified
——— S. Gomez CNA

provided. You may be asked to empty a urinary bag and measure the urine at the end of your shift. The totals are taken each 24 hours. If you notice any unusual recordings, be absolutely certain that you report it.

● SPECIAL PROCEDURES

Enemas

You may have the responsibility of giving the resident an enema. Fluid is run into the rectum to remove feces and gas from the bowel. The solution in the bowel causes the resident to feel uncomfortable and want to force the fluid out. Encourage him or her to retain the fluid as long as possible. This gives better results. An enema is given only when there is a doctor's order. There are several different kinds of enemas. These include tap water, soap suds, saline, and prepackaged enemas. An oil retention enema is held in the bowel longer than the cleansing enema. Encourage the resident to retain the oil solution for 20 to 30 minutes. See pages 398–402 for enema procedures.

PROCEDURE 15.53 | OIL RETENTION ENEMA

RATIONALE

Oil retention enema solutions stimulate the bowl and lubricate the colon and rectum, which facilitates the release of stool from the colon.

ALERT: Follow Standard Precautions.

1. Wash your hands.
2. Assemble equipment.
   a. Prepackaged oil retention enema
   b. Bedpan and cover
   c. Waterproof bed protector
   d. Toilet tissue
   e. Towel, basin of water, and soap
   f. Disposable gloves
3. Identify patient.
4. Ask visitors to leave the room.
5. Explain what you are going to do.
6. Put on gloves.
7. Cover patient with a bath blanket, and fan-fold linen to foot of bed.
8. Put bedpan on foot of bed.
9. Place bed protector under buttocks.
10. Help patient into the Sims' position.
11. Tell patient to retain enema as long as possible.
12. Open a prepackaged oil retention enema.
13. Lift patient's upper buttock and expose anus.

14. Tell patient when you are going to insert prelubricated tip into anus. (Instruct patient to take deep breaths and try to relax.)
15. Squeeze container until all solution has entered rectum.
16. Remove container; place in original package to be disposed of in contaminated waste according to facility policy and procedure.
17. Instruct patient to remain on side.
18. Remove gloves and discard according to facility policy.
19. Check patient every 5 minutes until fluid has been retained for at least 20 minutes.
20. Position patient on bedpan or assist to bathroom. Instruct patient not to flush toilet.
21. Raise head of bed, if permitted, if using a bedpan.
22. Place toilet tissue and call bell within easy reach.
23. Stay nearby if patient is in bathroom.
24. Put on gloves.

25. Remove bedpan or assist patient to return to bed. Observe contents of toilet or bedpan for
    a. Color, consistency, unusual materials, odor
    b. Amount of return
26. Cover bedpan and dispose of contents.
27. Remove gloves and discard.
28. Replace top sheet and remove bath blanket and plastic bed protector.
29. Give patient soap, water, and towel for hands and face.
30. Wash your hands.
31. Chart the following:
    a. Type of enema given
    b. Consistency and amount of bowel movement
    c. How the procedure was tolerated

5/13/03	1930
	16 oz oil retention enema administered
	and retained 12 minutes
	Passed large amount of dark brown
	formed stool
	———— R. Johnson CNA
6/07/03	0800
	Tolerated enema well
	Resting quietly
	———— S. Gomez CNA

PROCEDURE 15.54 | **PREPACKAGED ENEMAS**

RATIONALE

Prepackaged enema solutions stimulate the bowel and facilitate the release of stool from the colon.

ALERT: Follow Standard Precautions.

1. Wash your hands.
2. Assemble equipment.
    a. Prepackaged enema
    b. Bedpan and cover
    c. Waterproof bed protector
    d. Toilet tissue
    e. Towel, basin of water, and soap
    f. Disposable gloves
3. Identify patient.
4. Ask visitors to leave room.
5. Explain what you are going to do.
6. Cover patient with a bath blanket, and fan-fold linen to foot of bed.
7. Put on gloves.
8. Place bed protector under buttocks.
9. Put bedpan on foot of bed.
10. Help patient into the Sims' position.

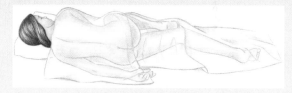

11. Tell patient to retain enema as long as possible.
12. Open a prepackaged enema.
13. Lift patient's upper buttock and expose anus.

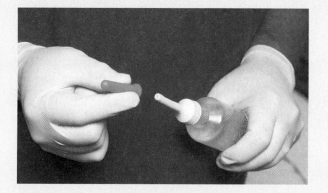

PROCEDURE 15.54 | PREPACKAGED ENEMAS *(Continued)*

14. Tell patient when you are going to insert prelubricated tip into anus. (Have patient take deep breaths and try to relax.)

15. Squeeze container until all the solution has entered the rectum.

16. Remove container; place in original package to be disposed of according to facility policy.

17. Remove gloves.

18. Instruct patient to remain on side and to hold solution as long as possible.

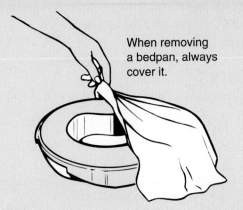

When removing a bedpan, always cover it.

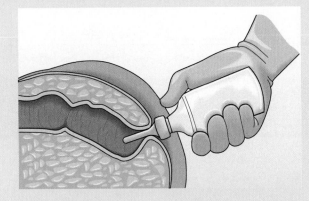

19. Put on gloves.

20. Position patient on bedpan or assist to bathroom. Instruct patient not to flush toilet.

21. Raise head of bed if permitted if patient is using a bedpan.

22. Place toilet tissue and call bell within easy reach.

23. Stay nearby if patient is in bathroom.

24. Remove bedpan or assist patient to return to bed.

25. Observe contents of toilet or bedpan for
    a. Color, consistency, unusual materials, odor
    b. Amount of return

26. Cover bedpan and dispose of contents.

27. Remove gloves and dispose of according to facility policy.

28. Replace top sheet and remove bath blanket and plastic bed protector.

29. Give the patient soap, water, and towel for hands and face.

30. Wash hands.

31. Chart the following:
    a. Type of enema given
    b. Consistency and amount of bowel movement
    c. How the procedure was tolerated

9/10/03	1430
	12 oz prepackaged enema administered and retained 5 minutes Complained of severe abdominal cramps Passed 12 oz watery, tan-colored fluid. Reported to team leader _____ A. Chaplin CNA
9/10/03	1515
	Restless Continues to complain about abdominal cramps Team leader notified _____ A. Chaplin CNA

PROCEDURE 15.55

TAP WATER, SOAP SUDS, SALINE ENEMAS

RATIONALE

Tap water, soap suds, and saline solutions stimulate the bowel and facilitate the release of stool from the colon.

ALERT: Follow Standard Precautions.

1. Wash your hands.
2. Assemble equipment.
   a. Disposable gloves
   b. Disposable enema equipment
      (1) Plastic container
      (2) Tubing
      (3) Clamp
      (4) Lubricant
   c. Enema solution as instructed by the head nurse, e.g.:
      (1) Tap water, 700–1,000 cc water (105°F)
      (2) Soap suds, 700–1,000 cc (105°F), one package enema soap
      (3) Saline, 700–1,000 cc water (105°F), 2 teaspoons salt
   d. Bedpan and cover
   e. Urinal, if necessary
   f. Toilet tissue
   g. Waterproof disposable bed protector
   h. Paper towel
   i. Bath blanket
3. Identify patient.
4. Ask visitors to leave room.
5. Tell patient what you are going to do.
6. Attach tubing to irrigation container. Adjust clamp to a position where you can easily open and close it. Close clamp.
7. Fill container with warm water (105° F).
   a. Add one package enema soap for soap suds enema.
   b. Add 2 teaspoons salt for saline enema.
   c. For tap water enema, do not add anything.
8. Provide privacy by pulling privacy curtain.
9. Cover patient with a bath blanket. Remove upper sheet by fan-folding to foot of bed. *Be careful not to expose patient.*
10. Put on gloves.
11. Put waterproof protector under patient's buttocks.
12. Place bedpan on foot of bed.
13. Place patient in the Sims position.

14. Open clamp on enema tubing and let a small amount of solution run into bedpan. (This eliminates air in tubing and warms tube.) Close clamp.
15. Put a small amount of lubricating jelly on tissue. Lubricate enema tip. Check to be certain that the opening is not plugged.
16. Expose buttocks by folding back bath blanket.
17. Lift the upper buttock to expose anus.
18. Tell patient when you are going to insert lubricated tip into anus.
19. Hold rectal tube about 5 inches from tip and insert slowly into rectum.
20. Tell patient to breathe deeply through mouth and to try to relax.
21. Raise container 12 to 18 inches above patient's hip.

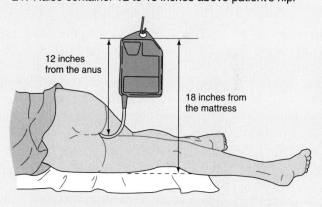

12 inches from the anus

18 inches from the mattress

22. Open clamp and let solution run in slowly. If patient complains of cramps, clamp tubing for a minute and lower can slightly.
23. When most of solution has flowed into rectum, close clamp. Gently withdraw rectal tube. Wrap tubing with paper towel and place into enema can.
24. Ask patient to hold solution as long as possible.
25. Help patient onto bedpan and raise head of bed if permitted.
26. Assist patient to bathroom and stay nearby if patient can go to bathroom. Ask patient not to flush toilet.
27. Place call light within reach and check patient every few minutes.

PROCEDURE 15.55 | TAP WATER, SOAP SUDS, SALINE ENEMAS *(Continued)*

28. Dispose of enema equipment while you are waiting for patient to expel enema. *Follow hospital policy.*

29. Remove bedpan or assist patient back to bed.

30. Observe contents for

    a. Color, consistency, unusual materials
    b. Note amount (i.e., large or small)

31. Cover bedpan and remove bed protector.

32. Remove gloves and dispose of according to facility policy. Wash hands.

33. Replace top sheet and remove bath blanket.

34. Give patient soap, water, and a towel to wash hands.

35. Secure call light in patient's reach.

36. Clean and replace all equipment used and wash your hands.

37. Chart the following:

    a. Date and time
    b. Type of enema given

    c. Results (amount, color, consistency) of bowel movement
    d. How the procedure was tolerated

4/14/03	1800
	1,000 cc soap suds enema
	administered and retained 15 minutes
	Complained about severe abdominal
	cramps
	Passed large amount of brown, formed
	stool, brown-colored liquid, and loose
	brown stool particles
	———— S. Gomez CNA
4/14/03	1845
	Resting quietly in bed, no pain
	———— S. Gomez CNA

distension

Stretched out; bloated.

Harris Flush

Excess gas in the bowel causes **distension** and is very painful. To relieve the excess gas, a Harris flush may be ordered by the doctor. A small amount of water is introduced into the rectum and allowed to flow out. When the irrigation can is lowered, the water runs out of the bowel and gas is removed. This can be repeated several times until the patient is more comfortable and the distension is relieved.

PROCEDURE 15.56 | HARRIS FLUSH

RATIONALE

A Harris flush helps evacuate flatus (gas) from the colon which releases abdominal distention and discomfort.

ALERT: Follow Standard Precautions.

1. Wash your hands.

2. Assemble equipment.

    a. Disposable gloves
    b. Disposable enema equipment

        (1) Plastic container
        (2) Tubing

        (3) Clamp
        (4) Lubricant

    c. 500 mL of tap water (105° F)
    d. Toilet tissue
    e. Waterproof disposable bed protector
    f. Bath blanket

PROCEDURE 15.56 HARRIS FLUSH *(Continued)*

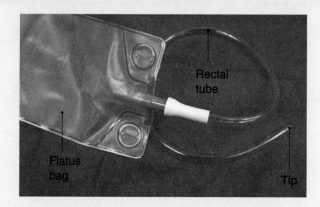

Rectal tube

Flatus bag

Tip

3. Identify patient.

4. Ask visitors to leave room.

5. Tell patient what you are going to do.

6. Attach tubing to irrigation container. Adjust clamp to a position where you can easily open and close it. Close clamp.

7. Fill container with warm water (105°F).

8. Provide for privacy by pulling privacy curtain.

9. Cover patient with a bath blanket. Remove upper sheet by fan-folding to foot of bed. *Be careful not to expose patient.*

10. Put on gloves.

11. Put waterproof protector under patient's buttocks.

12. Place patient in a left Sims' position.

13. Place bedpan on foot of bed.

14. Open clamp on enema tubing and let a small amount of solution run into bedpan. (This eliminates air in tubing and warms tube.) Close clamp.

15. Put a small amount of lubricating jelly on tissue. Lubricate enema tubing tip. Check to make certain that opening is not plugged.

16. Expose buttocks by folding back bath blanket.

17. Lift upper buttock to expose anus.

18. Tell patient when you are going to insert lubricated tip into anus.

19. Hold rectal tube about 5 inches from tip and insert slowly into rectum.

20. Tell patient to breathe deeply through mouth and to try to relax.

21. Raise container 12 to 18 inches above patient's hip.

22. Open clamp and let 200 mL of solution run in slowly.

23. Lower irrigating can about 12 inches below level of bed and allow fluid to flow out of rectum into can.

24. Continue process until gas is expelled. When all fluid has returned, clamp tube, and gently withdraw rectal tube. Wrap tubing with paper towel and place in enema can.

25. Position patient for comfort.

26. Dispose of equipment according to facility policy.

27. Remove gloves and dispose according to facility policy.

28. Replace top sheet and remove bath blanket. Straighten bed and make patient comfortable.

29. Put up side rails if required.

30. Secure call bell within patient's reach.

31. Wash your hands.

32. Chart the following:
    a. Date and time
    b. Type of procedure (Harris flush)
    c. Amount of flatus expelled
    d. How procedure was tolerated by patient

11/08/03   0900
600 cc Harris flush administered with moderate amount of flatus returned
Tolerated well
———— A. Chaplin CNA
11/08/03   0920
Ambulating in hall, no pain
———— R. Johnson CNA

Rectal Suppositories

A rectal suppository is ordered to

■ Help relieve constipation

■ Soften the feces

■ Help regulate the bowel

■ Give medications

PROCEDURE 15.57

INSERTING A RECTAL SUPPOSITORY

RATIONALE

As a nurse assistant/patient caregiver you may be asked to insert a suppository to facilitate evacuation of the bowel and relieve constipation.

ALERT: Follow Standard Precautions.

1. Wash your hands.
2. Assemble equipment.
   a. Ordered suppository
   b. Lubricant
   c. Disposable gloves
   d. Toilet tissue
   e. Bedpan with cover
3. Identify patient.
4. Ask visitors to leave the room.
5. Explain what you are going to do.
6. Provide privacy by pulling privacy curtain.
7. Raise bed to comfortable working position.
8. Position patient on left side with one knee bent toward chest (left Sims' position).
9. Put on gloves.
10. Lift sheet and expose buttocks.
11. Apply lubricant to gloved finger.
12. Apply lubricant around anus.
13. Hold suppository between thumb and index finger. Insert gently into anus as far as lubricated index finger will reach.
14. Remove finger and hold toilet tissue against anus for short time.
15. Remove gloves by turning inside out, and discard in hazardous waste.
16. Reposition patient and ask him or her to hold suppository as long as possible.
17. When patient signals for assistance, lower bed and assist to bathroom. Ask patient not to flush toilet.
18. Put on gloves.
19. Provide privacy and assist patient onto bedpan.
20. Raise head of bed to a comfortable position.
21. Provide toilet tissue and place call bell within patient's reach.
22. Remove gloves and discard according to facility policy.
23. Wash hands.
24. Return every few minutes until patient has expelled suppository or had a bowel movement.
25. Put on gloves to help patient clean self.
26. Dispose of waste.
27. Clean bedpan, cover, and place in storage area.
28. Remove gloves and discard, and wash hands.
29. Reposition bed to lowest position (if bed patient).
30. Put up side rail if required.
31. Secure call bell within patient's reach.
32. Wash your hands.
33. Record time suppository given and results.

9/10/03   2200

Glycerin suppository inserted

Tolerated well

_____ S. Gomez CNA

Ostomy

A patient may require an ostomy (Figure 15.14). When the bowel is diseased or injured, it may be necessary to operate and create a new passage for feces. A part of the bowel is brought through the abdominal wall. Sometimes this is permanent. Often the bowel can be reconnected after it has healed. The new opening is called a *stoma,* and fecal material is expelled through it. This can cause irritation and an unpleasant odor. Patients often feel depressed and may have difficulty accepting the new ostomy. Be careful not to show any reaction that might make them feel worse about themselves. The registered nurse cares for a new ostomy. However, you may be asked to care for one that is not new. The patient needs an ostomy bag to collect the drainage. Skin care around the stoma is very important, and proper placement of the bag requires careful attention. Check the hospital policy before you care for an ostomy.

Some illnesses, injuries, and diseases may require surgery that leaves an opening in the wall of the digestive or urinary tract (see Figure 15.15), such as:

- Into the colon: colostomy
- Into the ileum: ileostomy
- Into the ureter: ureterostomy

These openings may be temporary or permanent. Be aware that the resident suffers a change in self-image, which can be very difficult for him or her. Give help by

- Being a good listener
- Giving support
- Keeping the ostomy (opening) clean and dry
- Being alert for odor that is unpleasant
- Observing the skin for irritation or breakdown
- Notifying the charge nurse about any change, pain, or discomfort

Ileostomy

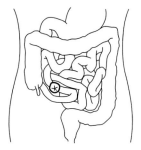

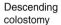
Descending colostomy

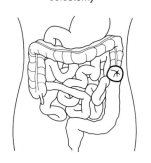

Figure 15.14

Common ostomies.

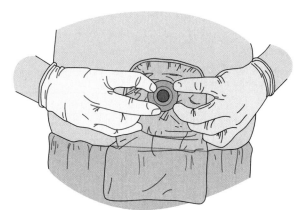

Place the wafer over the stoma and attach a clean bag.

Figure 15.15

Ostomy appliance in place over the stoma.

CHANGING AN OSTOMY BAG

RATIONALE

Ostomy bags collect body waste from a surgically created opening in the skin. The bags require changing to prevent leakage of body waste, keep skin at site healthy, provide comfort, and prevent embarrassment for the resident.

ALERT: Follow Standard Precautions.

1. Wash your hands.
2. Assemble equipment.
   a. Bedpan
   b. Waterproof bed protector
   c. Disposable gloves
   d. Basin of water and soap
   e. Washcloth
   f. Towel
   g. Skin protector (ordered by doctor)
   h. Biohazard waste bag
3. Identify patient.
4. Ask visitors to leave room.
5. Explain what you are going to do.
6. Raise bed to comfortable working height.
7. Position patient on back with head elevated, if allowed.
8. Put waterproof protector on bed next to stoma (opening to ostomy).
9. Fill basin with water (105°F).
10. Put on gloves.
11. Place bedpan where you can reach it easily.
12. Expose abdomen; keep genital area covered.
13. Carefully open ostomy belt.
14. Remove soiled or full ostomy bag by gently peeling away from skin. (Use toilet tissue to protect skin from feces.)
15. Put soiled ostomy bag in bedpan.
16. Check contents of ostomy bag for undigested food, blood, or any change in consistency of feces.
17. Remove belt if soiled.
18. Apply lubricant, skin protector, or skin cream around stoma.
19. Carefully observe surrounding area for redness, tenderness, or sores.
20. Place a clean bag over stoma.
21. Remove gloves and discard according to facility policy.

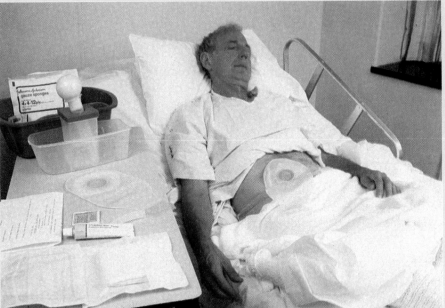

22. Wash hands. Position patient comfortably.
23. Put a clean belt around patient.
24. Lower bed to lowest position.
25. Put up side rail if required.
26. Secure call bell within patient's reach.
27. Put on gloves.
28. Dispose of bag according to your facility's policy.
29. Wash bedpan and return to storage.
30. Remove gloves and dispose of according to facility procedure.
31. Wash your hands.
32. Document procedure.
33. Report any unusual observations.

8/08/03	1500
	300 cc liquid brown stool discarded with colostomy bag
	Skin around colostomy stoma is pink with no evidence of irritation
	New ostomy bag applied
	_____ R. Johnson CNA

⊙ INCONTINENT RESIDENT

When a resident is incontinent, he or she loses the ability to control the bowel or bladder or both. This is embarrassing to most residents. They are often irritable and depressed. You can help them by having a positive attitude and by being patient and kind. Some of the causes of incontinence are

- Infections
- Surgical problems (e.g., prostate surgery)
- Spinal cord injuries
- Loss of sphincter control (muscle control)
- Some diseases, such as multiple sclerosis and central nervous system damage
- Disorientation

Bladder training is one method that is used to help relieve incontinence. This requires the cooperation of the health care workers and the resident. Your part in helping with the retraining of the bladder is to follow instructions carefully. They include the following:

- Keeping a careful intake and output record
- Giving fluids at specific times
- Taking the resident to void at specific intervals
- Watching for symptoms of bladder distension:

   • Restlessness • Dribbling • Distended lower abdomen • Sensation of pressure • **Residual** urine

 residual
Left over.

Staying on a schedule is the only way that bladder training can be successful. Everyone who cares for the resident must cooperate.

When bladder training is not successful and urinary incontinence continues, the doctor may order an indwelling catheter (see Figure 15.16). This is a sterile tube that is inserted into the bladder and drains the urine into a bag. Use of the catheter helps keep the resident dry and prevents skin irritation. However, careful technique is absolutely

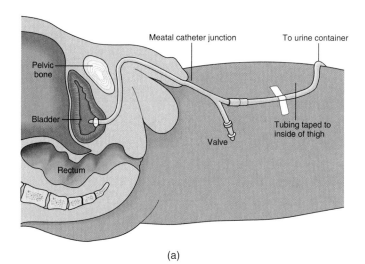

(a)

How to Loosely Tape Tubing in Place
(b)

Figure 15.16

Urinary catheter.

DISCONNECTING AN INDWELLING CATHETER

RATIONALE

Disconnecting an indwelling catheter from the drainage bag and plugging the catheter keeps urine from draining out of the body. This procedure is commonly followed when

- The physician wants to remove the catheter and bladder retraining is necessary; or
- To allow the resident to participate in activities without the urinary drainage bag.

ALERT: Follow Standard Precautions.

1. Wash hands.
2. Assemble equipment.
   a. Disinfectant
   b. Sterile gauze sponges
   c. Sterile cap or plug
   d. Disposable gloves
3. Identify resident.
4. Explain what you are going to do.
5. Put on gloves.
6. Disinfect connection between catheter and drainage tubing where it is to be disconnected by applying disinfectant with cotton or gauze.
7. Disconnect catheter and drainage tubing. *Do not allow catheter ends to touch anything!*
8. Insert a sterile plug in end of catheter. Place sterile cap over exposed end of drainage tube.
9. Carefully secure drainage tube to bed.
10. Remove gloves and discard according to facility policy.
11. Wash hands.
12. Record procedure. *Reverse procedure to reconnect.*

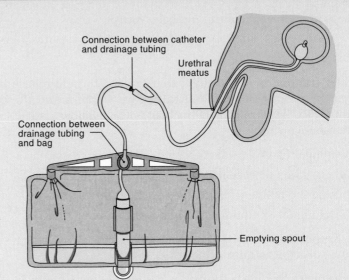

Connection between catheter and drainage tubing

Urethral meatus

Connection between drainage tubing and bag

Emptying spout

5/11/03	1000
	Urinary catheter disconnected and
	plugged with a sterile plug
	S. Gomez CNA
5/11/03	1130
	Lower abdominal pain
	Catheter drained 400 cc of urine
	Plug reinserted
	S. Gomez CNA

essential, because the catheter also increases the chances of infection. When you are caring for the resident, notice the urine that is in the bag. It should be

- Clear, not cloudy
- Straw-colored, pale yellow (not deep in color)
- 1,200 to 1,500 cc per day; if less than 30 cc per hour, notify the charge nurse

If you notice anything unusual about the urine, report it immediately. This includes blood, mucus, or deep color.

NOTE Never allow the urinary drainage bag to be higher than the hips of the resident. Keeping the bag lower provides drainage away from the urinary bladder. If the drainage bag were higher, urine could flow back into the bladder and cause an infection.

PROCEDURE 15.60

GIVING INDWELLING CATHETER CARE

RATIONALE

Giving indwelling catheter care helps to prevent infection and provides an opportunity to observe the insertion site for irritation and to adjust catheter position to maximize efficient drainage.

ALERT: Follow Standard Precautions.

1. Wash hands.
2. Assemble equipment.
    a. Antiseptic solution
    b. Waterproof bed protector
    c. Disposable nonsterile gloves
3. Identify resident.
4. Explain what you are going to do.
5. Provide privacy by pulling the privacy curtains.
6. Put on gloves.
7. Put waterproof protector on bed.
8. Carefully clean perineum.
9. Observe around catheter for sores, leakage, bleeding, or crusting. Report any unusual observation to nurse.
10. For females, separate labia with forefinger and thumb. Apply antiseptic solution around area where catheter enters the urethra.
11. For males, pull back foreskin on uncircumcised resident and apply antiseptic to entire area.
12. Apply antiseptic ointment (if allowed in your facility).
13. Position resident so catheter does not have kinks and is not pulling. *Be sure the tubing is free of kinks and is draining!*
14. Remove waterproof protector.
15. Cover resident.
16. Dispose of supplies according to facility policy.
17. Remove gloves.
18. Position resident comfortably.
19. Secure call light within resident's reach.
20. Wash hands.
21. Record procedure.

11/02/03 0920
Perineal care complete
Catheter insertion site clean and free
from irritation
Catheter secured to left inner thigh to
allow drainage
_____ R. Johnson CNA

PROCEDURE 15.61

EXTERNAL URINARY CATHETER

RATIONALE

An incontinent resident may use an external urinary catheter to control the flow of urine into a drainage bag in place of wearing a diaper.

ALERT: Follow Standard Precautions.

1. Wash hands.
2. Assemble equipment.
    a. Basin warm water
    b. Washcloth
    c. Towel
    d. Waterproof bed protector
    e. Gloves
    f. Plastic bag

PROCEDURE 15.61 | EXTERNAL URINARY CATHETER *(Continued)*

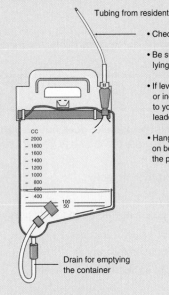

Tubing from resident

• Check tubing for kinks.

• Be sure patient is not lying on tubing.

• If level remains the same or increases rapidly, report to your head nurse or team leader.

• Hang plastic urine container on bed frame below level of the patient's urinary bladder.

CC
2000
1800
1600
1400
1200
1000
800
600
400
100
50

Drain for emptying the container

g. Tincture of benzoin
h. Condom with drainage tip
i. Paper towels

3. Identify resident.

4. Explain what you are going to do.

5. Provide privacy by pulling privacy curtain.

6. Raise bed to comfortable working height.

7. Cover resident with bath blanket. Have resident hold top of blanket, and fold cover to bottom of bed.

8. Put on gloves.

9. Place waterproof protector under resident's buttocks.

10. Pull up bath blanket to expose genitals only.

11. Remove condom by rolling gently toward tip of penis.

12. Wash and dry penis.

13. Observe for irritation, open areas, bleeding.

14. Report any unusual observations.

15. Check condom for "ready stick" surface. If there is none, apply a thin spray of tincture of benzoin. *Do not spray on head of penis.*

16. Apply new condom and drainage tip to penis by rolling toward base of penis.

17. Reconnect drainage system.

18. Remove and dispose of gloves.

19. Pull up top bedding and remove bath blanket.

20. Replace equipment.

21. Lower bed to lowest position.

22. Put up side rail if required.

23. Secure call light within resident's reach.

24. Tidy unit.

25. Wash hands.

26. Record procedure.

4/10/03	0730
Shower taken and tolerated well
Urinary condom drainage system
applied and drains well
_____ A. Chaplin CNA

Bowel Incontinence

The resident may be incontinent of stool. This can be more embarrassing for the resident and more unpleasant for you than bladder incontinence. The same principles apply to bowel training as to bladder training:

■ Everyone must participate.

■ A specific time to evacuate the bowel is identified.

■ Avoid between-meal snacks.

■ Give 2,000 cc of fluid intake per day.

There are additional aids for stimulating the bowel and helping to time evacuation. The nurse is responsible for giving these aids, but she relies on the reports of everyone caring for the resident. Mechanical aids used include the following:

■ Suppositories (medication)

PROCEDURE 15.62

EMPTYING THE URINARY DRAINAGE BAG

RATIONALE

Emptying the urinary drainage bag provides an opportunity to

■ Measure urinary output for a specific period of time
■ Observe characteristics of urine

ALERT: Follow Standard Precautions.

1. Wash hands.
2. Assemble equipment.
    a. Graduate or measuring cup
    b. Disposable gloves
3. Put on disposable gloves.
4. Carefully open drain outlet on urinary bag. *Do not allow container outlet to touch floor!* This will introduce microorganisms into bag and can cause infection.
5. Drain bag into graduate and reattach drainage outlet securely.
6. Observe urine for
    a. Dark color
    b. Blood
    c. Unusual odor
    d. Large amount of mucus
    e. Sediment
7. Report any unusual observations to nurse immediately (do not discard urine).
8. Hold graduate at eye level and read amount of urine on measuring scale.
9. Discard urine if normal.
10. Rinse graduate and put away.
11. Remove gloves and discard in hazardous waste.

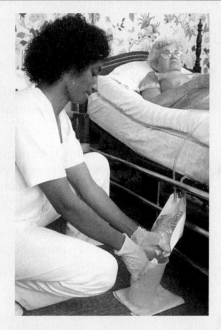

12. Wash hands.
13. Record amount of urine in cc's on the I & O record.

10/10/03   0700
              15.00 Urinary drainage, 1,290 cc
                       _____ A. Chaplin CNA

■ Laxatives (medication)
■ Enemas

Observe the stool for

■ **Color:** brown, light or dark (may be black from certain medications)— this is reported because black stool can also indicate bleeding.
■ **Consistency:** usually soft and formed (report dry, hard stool and stool that is watery, runny, frequent, or has mucus in it).
■ **Odor.**

Always report a bowel movement and/or any unusual changes.

consistency
Thickness.

● SPECIMEN COLLECTION

Specimens that you collect from your residents are sent to the laboratory and tested. These tests give the physician information that helps him or her treat the resident. It is important that specimens be collected carefully and properly. They must also be labeled correctly.

Urine specimens are collected in different ways. The following are five common urine specimen collection procedures:

- Routine urine specimen
- Clean-catch urine specimen
- Fresh fractional urine
- 24-hour urine specimen
- Strained urine

When obtaining urine specimens, always observe and record

- **Color:** may range from light straw color to dark amber
- **Clearness, cloudiness, or particles**
- **Odor:** normal, strong, or unusual

Use the urine specimen collection procedures to guide you in the correct way to collect useful specimens.

Other specimens commonly collected for testing include stool and sputum (see Figure 15.17). The stool samples are examined for occult (hidden) blood and for microorganisms. Sputum samples help the physician determine what is causing an illness of the respiratory system.

When obtaining these specimens always observe and record

- Color
- Consistency
- Odor

Use the correct specimen collection procedures to guide you when obtaining these specimens.

PROCEDURE 15.63

ROUTINE URINE SPECIMEN

RATIONALE

To evaluate the chemical structure of urine and determine the need for further testing.

ALERT: Follow Standard Precautions.

1. Wash hands.
2. Assemble equipment.
   a. Graduate (pitcher)
   b. Bedpan or urinal
   c. Urine specimen container
   d. Label
   e. Paper bag
   f. Disposable nonsterile gloves
3. Identify resident.
4. Explain what you are going to do.

PROCEDURE 15.63 | ROUTINE URINE SPECIMAN *(Continued)*

5. Label specimen carefully:
   a. Resident's name
   b. Date
   c. Time
   d. Room number
6. Provide privacy by pulling privacy curtain.
7. Put on gloves.
8. Have resident void (urinate) into clean bedpan or urinal.
9. Ask resident to put toilet tissue into paper bag.
10. Pour specimen into graduate.
11. Pour from graduate into specimen container until about three-quarters full.

12. Place lid on container.
13. Discard leftover urine.
14. Clean and rinse graduate, bedpan, or urinal, and put away.
15. Remove gloves.
16. Position resident comfortably.
17. Assist resident to wash hands.
18. Wash hands.
19. Store specimen according to direction for lab pickup.
20. Report and record procedure and observation of specimen.

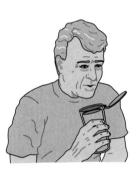

(a)

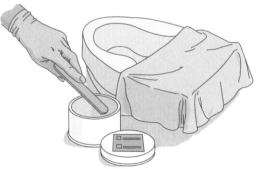

(b)

Figure 15.17

(a) Collecting the sputum specimen; (b) collecting a stool specimen; (c) straining the urine; (d) collecting a 24-hour specimen.

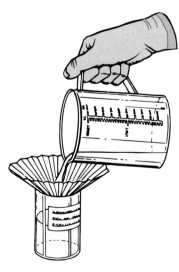

(c)

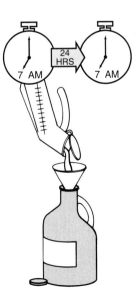

(d)

PROCEDURE 15.64

MIDSTREAM CLEAN-CATCH URINE, FEMALE

RATIONALE

A midstream clean-catch urine procedure provides a way to collect urine free of bacteria present

- ■ at the urethral meatus at the beginning of urination, and
- ■ in sediment in the urinary bladder which drains at the end of urination.

ALERT: Follow Standard Precautions.

1. Wash hands.
2. Assemble equipment.

   a. Antiseptic solution or soap and water or towelettes
   b. Sterile specimen container
   c. Tissues
   d. Nonsterile gloves

3. Identify resident.
4. Explain what you are going to do.
5. Label specimen:

   a. Resident's name
   b. Time obtained
   c. Date

6. If resident is on bedrest:

   a. Put on gloves.
   b. Lower side rail.
   c. Position bedpan under resident.

7. Have resident carefully clean perineal area if able; if not, you will be responsible for cleaning perineum:

   a. Wipe with towelette or gauze with antiseptic solution from front to back.
   b. Wipe one side and throw away wipe.
   c. Use a clean wipe for other side.
   d. Use another wipe down center.
   e. Then proceed with collecting midstream urine.

8. Explain procedure if resident is able to obtain own specimen.

   a. Have resident start to urinate into bedpan or toilet.
   b. Allow stream to begin.
   c. Stop stream and place specimen container to collect midstream.
   d. Remove container before bladder is empty.

9. Wipe perineum, if on bedpan.

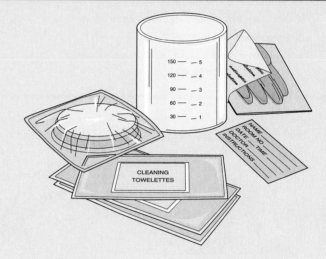

10. Remove bedpan.
11. Rinse bedpan and put away.
12. Remove gloves and discard according to facility policy and procedure.
13. Raise side rail.
14. Secure call light in resident's reach.
15. Dispose of equipment. Never handle contaminated equipment without gloves.
16. Wash hands.
17. Record specimen collection.
18. Report any unusual

    a. Color
    b. Consistency
    c. Odor

7/14/03   1300

Clean-catch urine collected

Urine was straw colored

Labeled and sent to the laboratory

_____ R. Johnson CNA

PROCEDURE 15.65

MIDSTREAM CLEAN-CATCH URINE, MALE

RATIONALE

A midstream clean-catch urine procedure provides a way to collect urine free of bacteria present
■ at the urethral meatus at the beginning of urination, and

■ in sediment in the urinary bladder which drains at the end of urination.

ALERT: Follow Standard Precautions.

1. Wash hands.
2. Assemble equipment.
   a. Antiseptic solution or soap and water or towelettes
   b. Sterile specimen container
   c. Tissues
   d. Disposable gloves
3. Identify resident.
4. Label specimen:
   a. Resident's name
   b. Date
   c. Time obtained
5. Explain procedure (if possible allow resident to obtain his own specimen).
   a. Put on gloves.
   b. Cleanse head of penis in a circular motion with towelette or gauze and antiseptic. (If resident is uncircumcised, have him pull back foreskin before cleaning.)

   c. Have resident start to urinate into bedpan, urinal, or toilet. (If he is uncircumcised, have resident pull back foreskin before urinating.)
   d. Allow stream to begin.
   e. Stop stream and place specimen container to collect midstream.
   f. Remove container before bladder is empty.
6. Dispose of equipment according to facility policy.
7. Remove and discard gloves according to facility policy and procedure.
8. Wash hands.
9. Record specimen collection.

5/16/03   1300
Clean-catch urine collected
Urine was dark amber in color with
white sediment
Labeled and sent to the laboratory
_____ A. Chaplin CNA

PROCEDURE 15.66

HEMACOMBISTIX

RATIONALE

HemaCombistix detects the presence of blood in urine.

ALERT: Follow Standard Precautions.

1. Wash hands.
2. Assemble equipment.
   a. Bottle of HemaCombistix
   b. Nonsterile gloves

3. Identify resident.
4. Explain what you are going to do.
5. Put on gloves.

PROCEDURE 15.66 HEMACOMBISTIX *(Continued)*

6. Secure fresh urine sample from resident.

7. Take urine and reagent to bathroom.

8. Remove cap and place on flat surface. Be sure top side of cap is down.

9. Remove strip from bottle by shaking bottle gently. *Do not touch areas of strip with fingers.*

10. Dip reagent stick in urine. Remove immediately.

11. Tap edge of strip on container to remove excess urine.

12. Compare reagent side of test areas with color chart on bottle. Use time intervals that are given on bottle.

NOTE Do not touch reagent strip to bottle.

13. Remove gloves and discard according to facility policy and procedure.

14. Replace equipment.

15. Wash hands.

16. Record results.

    a. Date and time

    b. Name of procedure used

    c. Results

> 10/04/03 1800
>
>   Urine specimen tested with a
>
>   hemacombistix
>
>   Results negative for blood
>
>   _____ R. Johnson CNA

PROCEDURE 15.67 STRAINING URINE

RATIONALE

Pouring urine through a strainer allows calculi (kidney stones) to be collected.

ALERT: Follow Standard Precautions.

1. Wash hands.

2. Assemble equipment.

    a. Paper strainers or gauze

    b. Specimen container and label

    c. Bedpan or urinal and cover

    d. Laboratory request for analysis of specimen

    e. Sign for resident's room or bathroom explaining that all urine must be strained

    f. Nonsterile gloves

3. Identify resident.

4. Tell the resident to urinate into a urinal or bedpan and that the nurse assistant must be called to filter each specimen. Tell resident not to put paper in specimen.

5. Put on gloves.

6. Pour voided specimen through a paper strainer or gauze into a measuring container.

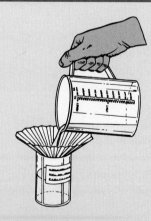

7. Place paper or gauze strainer into a dry specimen container if stones or particles are present after pouring urine through.

PROCEDURE 15.67 | STRAINING URINE *(Continued)*

NOTE Do not attempt to remove the particles from strainer.

8. Measure the amount voided and record on intake and output record.
9. Discard urine and container according to facility policy and procedure.
10. Clean urinal or bedpan and put away.
11. Remove gloves and discard according to facility policy and procedure.
12. Wash hands.
13. Label specimen:
    a. Resident's name
    b. Date
    c. Room number
    d. Time

14. Return resident to comfortable position.
15. Place call button within reach of resident.
16. Provide for resident safety by raising side rails when indicated or using postural supports as ordered.
17. Wash hands.
18. Report collection of specimen to supervisor immediately.
19. Record specimen collection.

6/20/03	1400
	300 cc strained
	Two small stones collected
	Given to team leader
	_____ S. Gomez CNA

PROCEDURE 15.68 | STOOL SPECIMEN COLLECTION

RATIONALE

Stool specimens are collected most frequently to determine if blood or parasites are present in the stool.

ALERT: Follow Standard Precautions.

1. Wash hands.
2. Assemble equipment.
    a. Stool specimen container with label
    b. Wooden tongue depressor
    c. Disposable gloves
    d. Bedpan and cover
3. Identify resident.
4. Explain what you are going to do.
5. Be certain container is properly labeled with
    a. Resident's name
    b. Time
    c. Date
    d. Room number
6. Provide privacy by pulling privacy curtains.
7. Put on gloves.
8. Take bedpan into bathroom after resident has had bowel movement.

9. Use tongue depressor to remove about 1 to 2 tablespoons of feces from bedpan.
10. Place specimen in specimen container.
11. Cover container immediately.
12. Wrap tongue depressor in paper towel and discard.

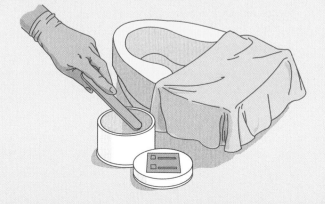

PROCEDURE 15.68 | **STOOL SPECIMAN COLLECTION** *(Continued)*

13. Remove gloves and dispose of according to facility policy.
14. Wash hands.
15. Follow instruction for storage of specimen for collection by lab.
16. Position resident comfortably.

17. Report and record procedure.

12/14/03   1000

Soft, brown stool collected,

labeled, and sent to laboratory

R. Johnson CNA

PROCEDURE 15.69 | **OCCULT BLOOD HEMATEST**

RATIONALE

Occult blood Hematest reveals the presence of blood in a stool specimen.

ALERT: Follow Standard Precautions.

1. Wash hands.
2. Assemble equipment.
   a. Hematest Reagent filter paper
   b. Hematest Reagent tablet
   c. Distilled water
   d. Tongue blade
   e. Disposable gloves
3. Identify resident.
4. Explain what you are going to do.
5. Put on gloves.
6. Secure stool specimen from resident.
7. Place filter paper on glass or porcelain plate.
8. Use tongue blade to smear a thin streak of fecal material on filter paper.
9. Place Hematest Reagent tablet on smear.

10. Place 1 drop distilled water on tablet.
11. Allow 5 to 10 seconds for water to penetrate tablet.
12. Add second drop, allowing water to run down side of tablet onto filter paper and specimen.
13. Gently tap side of plate to knock water droplets from top of tablet.
14. Observe filter paper for color change (2 minutes). Positive is indicated by blue halo on paper.
15. Dispose of specimen and equipment according to your facility's policy.
16. Remove gloves and dispose of according to your facility's policy.
17. Wash hands.
18. Report and record results (e.g., date, time, procedure, and results).

PROCEDURE 15.70

SPUTUM SPECIMEN COLLECTION

RATIONALE

Sputum is collected to determine if disease-causing bacteria
are present.

ALERT: Follow Standard Precautions.

1. Wash hands.
2. Assemble equipment.
   a. Sputum container
   b. Disposable
      nonsterile gloves
3. Identify resident.
4. Explain what you are
   going to do.
5. Label container:
   a. Resident's name
   b. Date
   c. Time taken
   d. Room number
6. Put on gloves.
7. Help resident rinse
   mouth if he or she has
   just eaten.
8. Ask resident to take three
   deep breaths. On the third
   breath tell resident to
   cough deep from lungs
   and try to bring up thick
   sputum. (Saliva is not
   adequate for this test.)
9. Have resident try several
   times until you get a good specimen. (You need 1 to
   2 tablespoons.)
10. Cover container immediately.
11. Remove gloves and discard according to facility
    policy.
12. Wash hands.
13. Report to nurse that specimen has been collected. (It
    needs to go to lab immediately.)

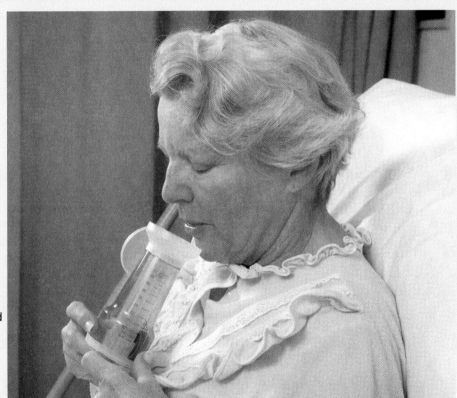

14. Record that specimen has been taken and record
    color, amount, odor, and consistency.

> 3/05/03   1600
>
> Sputum specimen collected,
> clear and unremarkable
> Specimen labeled and sent to
> the laboratory
> _____ A. Chaplin CNA

insulin shock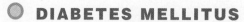

Condition caused by too
much insulin.

◉ DIABETES MELLITUS

Diabetes mellitus is an endocrine problem. This disease is caused when the islets
(islands) of Langerhans in the pancreas do not produce enough insulin. When there
is an insulin imbalance, you must watch the resident carefully for signs of diabetic
coma or **insulin shock.** Diabetic coma occurs when the diabetic resident does not
have enough insulin, when there is an infection, or if there is increased stress. The
following are symptoms of diabetic coma:

- Loss of appetite
- Abdominal discomfort or pain
- Dry skin
- Flushed skin
- Sweet or fruity odor of the breath
- Soft eyeballs
- Generalized aches
- Increased urination
- Air hunger, increased respiration, labored breathing
- Nausea and/or vomiting
- Dulled senses
- Weakness
- Excessive thirst

   Insulin shock occurs when the resident receives too much insulin, misses a meal,
or exercises too much. *Remember to report a missed meal to the head nurse.* The following are symptoms of insulin shock:

- Excessive sweating, perspiration
- Hunger
- Numbness of tongue and lips
- Faintness, weakness, dizziness
- Headache
- Irritability, personality change, nervousness
- Inability to awaken, stupor, unconsciousness, coma
- Tremors, trembling
- Blurred or impaired vision

   Your responsibility in caring for the diabetic resident includes securing a fresh
urine sample to test for sugar and acetone. These tests are usually done ½ hour before meals and again at bedtime. A reagent stick test is dipped into the fresh urine
to measure glucose, acetone, and protein in the blood. Follow the procedure in
Chapter 18, "Using Reagent Sticks to Test Urine." Report any reading on the dipstick above negative to your supervisor. The most common test for glucose levels is
the blood test. This test is performed with a glucose meter. The procedure for glucose monitoring with a meter is in Chapter 18, "Monitoring Glucose." These tests
are essential for the health of the resident. Errors in testing can result in diabetic
coma or insulin shock.

⬤ THERAPIES

Oxygen Therapy

Some residents require oxygen to help them breathe. Concentrated oxygen helps these residents breathe more easily. The following are common ways to give oxygen therapy:

- **Nasal cannula:** A two-pronged tube that fits into the nostrils and is secured with an elastic strap that stretches around the back of the head
- **Nasal catheter:** A small tube that fits into a nostril and is secured with tape on the nose and side of the face
- **Mask:** A plastic see-through mask that fits over the nose and mouth and is secured with an elastic strap that stretches around the back of the head

You have specific responsibilities when you care for a resident on oxygen therapy, including the following:

- Ensuring that all oxygen safety rules are followed. Review Chapter 13, Unit 3.
- Checking the elastic strap for chafing and a firm fit.
- Cleaning the cannula, catheter, or mask and checking the skin for irritation.
- Providing oral hygiene by moistening the lips and mouth frequently. Encourage fluid intake if allowed.
- Keeping tubing free of kinks or blockage.
- Checking flow rate and oxygen humidifier frequently.
- Immediately reporting to supervisor any changes or problems, e.g., cyanosis, dyspnea, shortness of breath.

Hot and Cold Applications

You may give hot or cold applications. Be certain that this is allowed by your facility and by state law. These applications help provide healing but must be done correctly. Read the information in Chapter 19 of this text on thermotherapy and cryotherapy and be certain that you have demonstrated competency before giving any treatments.

⬤ SPECIAL PRECAUTIONS

Seizure Precautions

Seizures are caused by

- Strokes
- Poisoning
- Infection with high temperature
- **Epilepsy**

A seizure is serious; the resident can be hurt. A seizure is an involuntary contraction and relaxation of the muscles. There are two common types:

- **Grand mal:** The entire body becomes stiff, followed by the muscles jerking. This lasts several minutes.
- **Petit mal:** The eyes roll back and the muscles may quiver. The resident seems to be daydreaming. This lasts about 30 seconds.

seizure
Involuntary muscle contraction and relaxation.

epilepsy
Chronic disease of the nervous system.

PROCEDURE 15.71

SEIZURE PRECAUTIONS

RATIONALE

Seizure precautions explain safeguards that protect residents from injury if a seizure should occur.

ALERT: Follow Standard Precautions as needed.

If you are with a resident who has a seizure:

1. Use call signal or shout to get help. *Do not leave resident.*
2. Assist resident to lie down to prevent falling.
3. Protect head with pillow or soft cushion.
4. Move furniture to prevent limbs from bumping into it.
5. Turn resident on side to allow secretions to drain from mouth.
6. Observe resident for
   a. Length of time of seizure
   b. Part of body where seizure began
   c. Incontinence
   d. Injury (where and severity)
   e. Severity of convulsions
7. Help resident to bed when seizure is over.
8. Make resident comfortable.
9. Put up side rails.
10. Wrap side rails with blanket, sheet, or soft material to pad them.
11. Wash hands.
12. Chart seizure and observations.
13. Report seizure to charge nurse.

You cannot stop the seizure, but you can follow seizure precautions to help protect the resident from injury. The dangers to the resident include

- Physical injury to limbs and body parts
- Aspiration
- Biting cheeks and tongue if the jaws clamp closed

Syncope

syncope
Fainting.

Syncope is another term for fainting. It is caused when the brain does not have an adequate supply of blood. Symptoms of syncope include the following:

- Feeling of uneasiness
- Lightheadedness
- Pale, cool, **clammy** skin
- Dilated pupils

clammy
Moist, cold skin.

Several different things can cause this:

- Fear of pain
- Sight of blood or needles
- Emotional disturbance
- Pain
- Long periods without movement, causing poor blood circulation
- Dehydration
- Standing up too fast may cause dizziness

If a resident complains of any of these symptoms, take proper precautions to prevent an accident or injury to the resident or to yourself. You should

■ Have the resident put his or her head between the knees, with arms hanging loose at his or her sides. Place your hands on the back of the resident's head. Instruct resident to apply upward pressure with the head.

■ Break open a spirits of ammonia ampule and place under the resident's nose.

■ Have the resident lie down, with the head lower than the legs, if possible.

■ Place a cold towel on the forehead.

■ Loosen any tight clothing.

■ Have resident remain quiet until you are sure he or she has adjusted and is not dizzy.

⬤ SPECIAL CARE DEVICES

Antiembolism Hose

Antiembolism hose are used to prevent blood from pooling in the legs. This reduces the possibility of developing phlebitis and blood clots. Elasticized hose are called TEDS or antiembolism hose. Sometimes elastic bandages are used. These extend from the ankle or foot to calf or midthigh. They are applied after surgery and when there is danger of a clot forming and causing thrombophlebitis. They must be applied so that they are smooth and even and do not cut off the circulation. Be certain to remove them and reapply them at least once every 8 hours.

PROCEDURE 15.72 ELASTIC HOSE (ANTIEMBOLISM HOSE)

RATIONALE

Elastic hose help prevent blood from pooling in the legs, thus reducing the possibility of developing phlebitis.

ALERT: Follow Standard Precautions as needed.

1. Wash hands.
2. Select elastic hose. Check to be sure that they are the correct size and length.

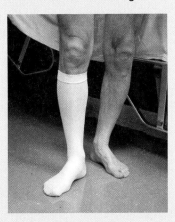

3. Identify resident.
4. Have resident lie down; expose one leg at a time.
5. Hold the hose with both hands at top and roll toward toe end.
6. Place hose over toes, positioning opening at base of toes unless toes are to be covered. The raised seams should be on outside.
7. Check to be sure that the stocking is applied evenly and smoothly. There must be no wrinkles.
8. Repeat on opposite leg.
9. Record the following in the medical record
   a. Date and time applied
   b. Any skin changes, temperature change, or swelling

PROCEDURE 15.72   ELASTIC HOSE (ANTIEMBOLISM HOSE) *(Continued)*

10. Remove and reapply at least once every 8 hours, or more often if necessary.

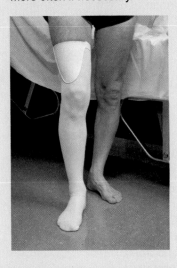

4/14/03   0700
Elastic hose applied to both legs before transferring resident into wheelchair
R. Johnson CNA

Postural Supports

postural supports 🔊

Soft restraints used to protect resident.

Soft postural supports (soft cloth ties used on arms and legs, or vests are used to protect elderly or disoriented residents from hurting themselves or someone else (see Figure 15.18). It is much better if you do not have to use them. They can be used only if they are ordered by the doctor. Precautions must be taken when they are used as they may create the following conditions:

- Increased agitation
- Immobilized resident
- Increased risk of pneumonia
- Skin breakdown
- Decreased circulation

When postural supports are used, you must

- Anticipate elimination needs.
- Check for swelling above, below, and at the site of supports.
- Release the supports periodically.
- Provide for hydration by offering fluids.
- Change position frequently.

There are times when postural support must be used:

- To prevent resident from pulling out tubes and catheters
- To prevent resident from scratching or injuring self and others
- To keep resident from falling out of bed or chair

However, there must be a valid reason for using the supports. Do not use them just because you are annoyed that the resident takes too much of your time.

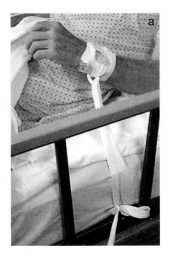
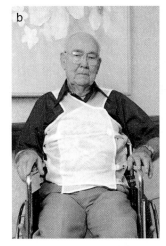

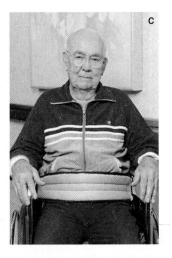
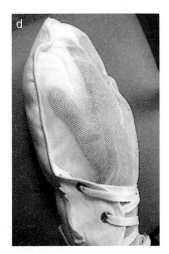

Figure 15.18

Soft protective devices:
(a) limb, (b) vest, (c) body,
(d) mitten

PROCEDURE 15.73

HOW TO TIE POSTURAL SUPPORTS

RATIONALE

Postural supports must be secured with a quick-release knot that allows the resident to be moved quickly in the event of an emergency.

ALERT: Follow Standard Precautions.

1. Wash hands.
2. Assemble equipment: a postural support that has been ordered.
3. Tie a half-bow knot or quick-release knot. Tie the same way you tie a bow on a shoe. Once bow is in place, grasp one loop and pull end of tie through knot.
4. Knot can be easily released pulling end of loop.

NOTE Half-bow knot/quick-release knot is always used when a restraint is attached to wheelchair or mattress support. This allows quick release if it is necessary to move resident in a hurry.

9/09/03	0930
	Transferred to wheelchair
	Vest postural support applied and
	secured with a quick-release knot
	at back of chair
	————— S. Gomez CNA

PROCEDURE 15.74 POSTURAL SUPPORTS: LIMB

RATIONALE

Postural supports for the limbs are necessary to prevent some residents from causing injury to themselves or others.

ALERT: Follow Standard Precautions.

1. Wash hands.
2. Assemble equipment: a limb support.
3. Identify resident.
4. Explain what you are going to do.
5. Place soft side of limb support against skin.
6. Wrap around limb and put one tie through opening on other end of support (see Figure 15.18a).
7. Gently pull until it fits snugly around limb.
8. Buckle or tie in place so that support stays on limb.
9. Tie out of resident's reach. (See the procedure "How to Tie Postural Supports.")
   a. Tie to bed frame (not side rails).
   b. Tie to wheelchair (not to stationary chair).
10. Check for proper alignment and comfort of resident.
11. Check to be certain that knots or wrinkles are not causing pressure.
12. Check to be certain that support is snug but does not bind. (You should be able to put two fingers under edges.)
13. Place call light where it can be easily reached.
14. Check resident frequently and move at least every 2 hours.
15. Chart the following:
    a. Reason for use of support
    b. Type of support used
    c. When it was applied
    d. When it was released
    e. Times of repositioning
    f. How resident tolerated it

> 10/14/03   0200
> Resident disoriented; swinging arms and legs against side rails
> Limb postural supports applied and secured with a quick-release knot to legs and arms, to prevent injury per physician's order
> _____ R. Johnson CNA

PROCEDURE 15.75 POSTURAL SUPPORTS: MITTEN

RATIONALE

Mitten postural supports prevent the hands from grasping objects.

ALERT: Follow Standard Precautions.

1. Wash hands.
2. Assemble equipment: a soft cloth mitten.
3. Identify resident.
4. Explain what you are going to do.
5. Slip mitten on hand with padded side against palm and net on top of hand.
6. Lace mitten (see Figure 15.18d).
7. Gently pull until it fits snugly around wrist.

8. Tie with a double bow knot so that support stays on hand.

NOTE Double bow knot helps secure the restraint to the resident. Use only a half-bow/quick-release knot to tie a postural support to a bed, wheelchair, or other furniture.

9. Check for proper alignment and comfort of resident.
10. Check to be certain knots or wrinkles are not causing pressure.
11. Check to be certain support is snug but does not bind. *(You should be able to put two fingers under edges.)*
12. Place call light where it can be easily reached.
13. Check resident frequently and move at least every 2 hours.

14. Chart the following:
    a. Reason for use of support
    b. Type of support used
    c. When it was applied
    d. When it was released
    e. Times of repositioning
    f. How resident tolerated it

11/07/03   1400
Bilateral mitten postural supports applied and secured with a quick-release knot to prevent the resident from removing abdominal dressing and IV per physician's order
S. Gomez CNA

RATIONALE

Vest postural support is necessary to prevent some residents from injuring themselves.

1. Wash hands.
2. Assemble equipment: a vest support.
3. Identify resident.
4. Explain what you are going to do.
5. Put arms through armholes of vest with opening to back (see Figure 15.18b).
6. Cross back panels by bringing tie on left side over to right and right tie to left.
7. Carefully smooth material so that there are no wrinkles.
8. Tie where resident cannot reach. (See the procedure "How to Tie Postural Supports.")
    a. Tie to bed frame *(not side rails)*.
    b. Tie to wheelchair *(not stationary chair)*.
9. Check for proper alignment and comfort of resident.
10. Check to be certain that knots or wrinkles are not causing pressure.

11. Check to be certain that support is snug but does not bind. *(You should be able to put two fingers under edges.)*
12. Place call light where it can be easily reached.
13. Check resident frequently and move at least every 2 hours.
14. Chart the following:
    a. Reason for use of support
    b. Type of support used
    c. When it was applied
    d. When it was released
    e. Times of repositioning
    f. How resident tolerated it

9/14/03   1700
Vest postural support applied to protect resident from getting out of bed and falling, per physician's order
A. Chaplin CNA

⊙ TERMINAL AND POSTMORTEM CARE

You may be called upon to provide care for someone who is dying. Refer to Chapter 9, Unit 4, "End of Life Issues." This helps you understand the stages the resident goes through. Always be gentle and respectful both before and after death. Before death occurs, gently wash away discharges that have accumulated. As death approaches, the muscles lose their tone and the body openings drain. Gently straighten the limbs and make the resident as comfortable as possible. After death occurs, you may be asked to prepare the body. Check the procedures of the facility you work in and follow the steps your facility provides.

PROCEDURE 15.77   **POSTMORTEM CARE**

RATIONALE

Provides direction for the preparation of the body following death.

ALERT: Follow Standard Precautions.

---

1. Wash hands.
2. Assemble equipment.
   a. Wash basin with warm water
   b. Washcloth and towel
   c. Shroud/postmortem set:
      (1) Sheet or plastic container
      (2) Strap to tie chin (to keep mouth closed)
      (3) Identification tags
      (4) Large container for personal belongings
      (5) Plastic pad
   d. Gurney or morgue cart
   e. Nonsterile disposable gloves

Plastic bag
(for personal belongings)

The Morgue Kit

Ties

Plastic shroud (body bag)

Chin strap

Tags

Cellu-cotton pads

3. Close privacy curtains.
4. Put on gloves.
5. Position body in good alignment in supine position.
6. Keep one pillow under head.
7. Straighten arms and legs.
8. Gently close each eye. Do not apply pressure to eyelids.

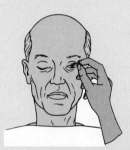

9. Put dentures in mouth or in a denture cup. If placed in a denture cup, put cup inside shroud so that mortician can find.
10. Secure chin with a chin strap. Use pads under straps along side of face to prevent marking.
11. Remove all soiled dressings or clothing.
12. Bathe body thoroughly.
13. Apply clean dressings where needed.
14. Tie wrists loosely together over abdomen. Use pads under ties to prevent marking.

PROCEDURE 15.77 | POSTMORTEM CARE *(Continued)*

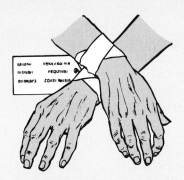

15. Tie ankles loosely together. Use pads under ties to prevent marking.

16. Attach identification tags to wrists and ankles. Fill in tags with

   a. Name
   b. Sex
   c. Hospital ID number
   d. Age

17. Place body in a shroud, sheet, or other appropriate container. Do this in the following way:

   a. Ask for assistance from a co-worker.
   b. Logroll body to one side. Place shroud behind body leaving enough material to support body when rolled back. Fan-fold remaining shroud next to body.
   c. Place a plastic protection pad under buttocks.
   d. Roll body on its back and then to the other side.
   e. Pull fan-folded portion of shroud until flat.

   f. Roll body on its back.
   g. Cover entire body with shroud.
   h. Tuck in all loose edges of cover.
   i. Position a tie above elbows and below knees and secure around body.
   j. Attach ID tag to tie just above elbows.

18. Remove gloves and discard according to facility policy and procedure.

19. Wash hands.

20. Place all personal belongings in a large container. Label container with

   a. Resident's name
   b. Age
   c. Room number

21. Place list of belongings in container and on resident's chart.

22. Follow your facility's procedure for transporting body and belongings through hallways.

23. Remove all linen and other supplies from room.

24. Wash hands.

25. Report procedure completed to charge nurse.

12/07/03 0430
Postmortem care completed
Belongings listed and placed in
bag, given to family
Charge nurse notified
_____ R. Johnson CNA

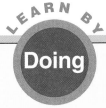

Doing   UNIT 1 ACTIVITIES

1. **Complete Worksheets/Activities 2, 6, 7, and 8 and Worksheets 3 through 5 and 9 through 13 as assigned.**

2. **Practice all procedures.**

3. **When you are confident that you can meet each objective, ask your instructor for the unit evaluation.**

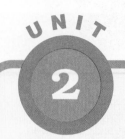

Advanced Roles/Sub-Acute Care

STEPS TO SUCCESS

1. Complete Vocabulary Worksheet 1 in the Student Workbook.

2. Read this unit.

3. Complete the Learn by Doing assignment at the end of this unit.

UNIT OBJECTIVES

When you have completed this unit, you will be able to do the following:

✔ List types of services in the sub-acute area.

✔ Explain transitional care.

✔ Describe the nurse assistant's role in the sub-acute area.

✔ List 11 observations for the postoperative patient.

✔ Explain why proper body alignment is important.

✔ List five devices used to align the body and explain how they work.

SUB-ACUTE CARE

Patients are often well enough to leave the acute care hospital but not well enough to return to their homes. Many long-term care facilities have a sub-acute area where these patients receive the care and rehabilitation they require. The goal in these units is to provide transitional care at a lower cost than acute care. The lower cost allows care to be provided with less time restraint, allowing the patient to progress according to his or her level of ability. The goal of transitional care is to help the patient regain physical and living skills through physical therapy and occupational therapy, allowing a return to an independent lifestyle when possible. The nurse assistant is an important part of the interdisciplinary rehabilitation team. The sub-acute area also provides residents in long-term care with additional services when needed. Patients in this specialized care area usually require treatment or services for

■ Postoperative care

■ Complex wound care

■ Intravenous infusions

■ Tracheostomy care

■ Ventilator/respiratory care

■ Multiple trauma and head injuries

■ Stroke care

■ Physical, occupational, and speech therapy

RESPONSIBILITIES OF A SUB-ACUTE NURSE ASSISTANT

Nurse assistants in the sub-acute area use all of their CNA skills. They must also learn some additional specialized skills:

■ Organize patient care so that it does not interfere with treatment.

■ Observe, recognize, and report vital signs, symptoms, and complications.

- Perform neurological checks.
- Protect intravenous lines or Port-a-caths from pulling or dislodging.
- Prevent infection at insertion sites.
- Recognize problems related to intravenous infusions.
- Observe wounds and recognize symptoms of infection.
- Clean the area around tracheostomies.
- Participate on rehabilitation team.
- Observe, recognize, and report problems related to intravenous infusions.
- Observe, recognize, and report problems related to tracheostomy care.
- Observe, recognize, and report changes in patients with head and brain injuries.

NOTE You may use additional or expanded skills. Chapter 25 in the Instructor's Guide provides these skills.

POSTOPERATIVE CARE

Patients are in the sub-acute area for monitoring of vital signs and neurological status, pain management, infection control, and rehabilitation. The nurse assistant's role is to monitor the patient carefully and report any changes to the charge nurse. Use Table 15.3 on page 435 as a checklist for monitoring the postoperative patient.

Supportive Devices and Equipment

Fractures and joint replacement are two major areas in sub-acute postoperative care. Keeping the patient in good **alignment** is very important. Poor alignment can cause a new hip joint to move out of the socket and cause improper healing of fractures. The following are some of the common supportive devices:

- **Trochanter roll:** A towel or small blanket is rolled and put next to the greater trochanter (femur). It keeps the hip from rotating outward and prevents permanent disability or difficulties with walking.
- **Abduction splint:** This is a device that keeps the thighs apart and keeps the hip joints in proper alignment.
- **Abductor wedge:** A wedge-shaped, spongy material is placed between the legs. The wedge is used to keep the hip that has been replaced or fractured away from the center of the body. This prevents excessive strain on the hip and prevents a dislocation of the repair.
- **Footboard:** A padded board is placed at the feet when the patient is in a prone or supine position. The feet naturally extend when lying in this position. If the feet are not aligned correctly, contractures occur and cause problems with walking.
- **Pillows:** Pillows of different sizes and shapes are placed to support joints and provide support for proper body alignment.

Ambulatory Devices

There are many different ambulatory devices, such as walkers, crutches, and canes. These are discussed in Chapter 19.

WOUND CARE AND OBSERVATION

Patients who have suffered a trauma or surgery have very specific needs. Their wounds may be life threatening and must be cared for properly. As a nurse assistant, your primary responsibility in caring for wounds includes careful, specific observations and reporting.

You must understand wounds in order to make good observations and reports. Always observe and report the location, size, appearance, and odor of the wound; the condition of the surrounding skin; and the type and amount of drainage. Wounds often have drainage, and there are other complications to watch for. Refer to Table 15.3 for help with observation and charting.

Types of Wounds

Wounds are described as being either *open* or *closed.*

- **Closed wounds:** Tissue is injured, but the skin is not broken. These wounds can be caused by bruising, sprains, and twists.
- **Open wounds:** The skin or mucous membrane is broken. These wounds can be caused by bites, cuts, and incisions. Whenever there is an open wound there is a chance of infection.

Open wounds can be either partial thickness or full thickness wounds.

- **Partial thickness wounds:** The dermis and epidermis are broken.
- **Full thickness wounds:** The dermis, epidermis, and subcutaneous tissue are penetrated. Muscle and bone may be involved.

The following are some common types of wounds.

- **Abrasion:** partial thickness wound caused by scraping the skin away
- **Contusion:** closed wound caused by a blow to the body
- **Incision:** intentional wound made with a scalpel
- **Laceration:** open wound with jagged edges and torn tissue
- **Penetrating wound:** open wound caused by piercing the underlying tissues of the skin
- **Puncture wound:** open wound caused by a sharp object entering the skin and underlying tissues

⬤ HOW WOUNDS HEAL

Types of Healing

Wounds are allowed to heal in different ways.

- **Primary (first) intention:** The wound is pulled together by suturing, stapling, taping, clipping, or gluing. This is a clean wound that usually heals quickly.
- **Secondary (second) intention:** The wound edges are not brought together. The wound is cleaned, and dead tissue is removed. This method is often used in infected and contaminated wounds.
- **Third intention:** The wound is left open and may be closed at a later time. Poor circulation and infection are common reasons for using this method.

Medical Emergencies in Wound Healing

Wound healing is dependent on many factors, including the type of wound and the patient's age, nutrition, and lifestyle. The patient's medical history is also very important. Poor circulation, diabetes, some medications, and a weakened immune system can cause complications. The following are major complications:

- **Dehiscence:** The skin layer and/or the underlying tissues separate, reopening the wound. Stress to the wound from coughing, vomiting, and abdominal distension is usually the cause of dehiscence. This is a surgical emergency. Notify your supervisor immediately.

- **Evisceration:** The skin layer is separated by the **protrusion** of an internal organ through the wound. The causes are the same as in dehiscence. This is also a surgical emergency. Notify your supervisor immediately.

- **Hemorrhage:** Excessive bleeding that is life threatening. *Hemorrhage is a medical emergency and must be reported to your supervisor immediately.* The patient is in immediate danger.

  • *External hemorrhage* is easily seen. Dressings soak with blood and blood may flow under the body. Always check under the patient for pooling blood when you see saturated dressings. • *Internal hemorrhage* cannot be seen. The bleeding is in the tissue of the body and in the body cavities. Signs of internal bleeding include the patient's vomiting blood or coughing up blood, shock, and loss of consciousness. A hematoma may form (i.e., blood collects under the skin, causing swelling and discoloration).

protrusion

Pushing through.

Types of Drainage

Wound drainage occurs during the inflammatory stage of healing when healing fluid and cells escape from the surrounding tissues. The overlying skin heals, but the underlying tissue does not. Drainage that is trapped in the wound and underlying tissue causes swelling and pain and may cause infection. The doctor puts in a drainage tube when large amounts of drainage are expected.

There are several different types of drainage, including the following:

- **Purulent drainage:** thick green, yellow, or brown drainage.
- **Sanguineous drainage:** bloody drainage. Large amounts may indicate hemorrhage.
- **Serous drainage:** watery, clear drainage.
- **Serosanguineous drainage:** thin, watery, blood-tinged drainage.

Remember always to follow Standard Precautions when in contact with any type of drainage.

● INTRAVENOUS THERAPY

When a needle or catheter is inserted into a vein it is called intravenous (IV) therapy. IV therapy is ordered to provide fluids when the patient is not allowed to drink or eat; to replace needed vitamins and minerals lost in injury or illness; to administer medications and blood; and to replace sugar for energy.

The following equipment is used for IV therapy:

- **IV pole:** May be attached to the bed or stand alone. It is used to hang the IV solution.
- **Solution container:** Plastic bags are most common. You may also see a glass bottle. The containers come in different sizes from 50 to 1,000 mL.
- **Infusion pump:** This is a device that controls the rate of infusion.
- **Catheters and needles:** These come in different sizes and are inserted into the vein to allow the solution to circulate through the body. A catheter may be implanted in the upper chest area when repeated use is necessary. This is called a peripherally inserted central catheter (PICC line) or Port-a-cath.

TRACHEOSTOMY CARE

Tracheostomies may be permanent or temporary. They are permanent when the patient's airway structure is removed due to disease or injury. They are temporary when the patient requires only temporary ventilation. The tracheostomy tube is inserted through an incision in the trachea. Normally, foreign bodies are filtered as they pass through the nose. The patient with a tracheostomy, or "trache," does not have this protection, and foreign bodies such as bacteria enter directly into the lungs. This causes mucus and secretions that make it difficult for the patient to breathe. These secretions must be removed by suction through the tracheostomy. A licensed nurse does suctioning. The patient may be on mechanical ventilation, which means that a machine is moving the air in and out of the lungs to maintain the oxygen supply to the body.

As a nurse assistant, you are responsible for making good observations and reporting them. Use Table 15.3 as a guideline for observing the patient with a tracheostomy.

MULTIPLE TRAUMA AND HEAD INJURIES

cerebrovascular accidents (CVA)

Complete or partial loss of blood flow to brain tissue caused by blood vessel spasms, intracranial bleeding, and/or obstruction of the blood vessels in the brain.

irreversible

Cannot be changed; condition will remain the same.

intracranial

Inside the skull.

Accidents and sports injuries cause head and brain injuries. Brain tumors and **cerebrovascular accidents (CVA)** also cause brain trauma. They happen at any age and can cause paralysis, seizures, **irreversible** coma, loss of bowel and bladder control, and mental retardation. Most nerve pathways cross inside the brain. This means that signs and symptoms will appear on the opposite side of the body. The type of impairment depends on which side of the brain is injured and on the severity of the damage (see Table 15.2). Recovery may be very slow, and the patient often has to relearn how to speak, to perform simple tasks, and to function as normally as possible.

A major problem with head and brain injuries is increased **intracranial** pressure caused by bleeding and cerebrospinal fluid. The increased pressure can cause permanent brain injury and brain death. As a nurse assistant, you are responsible for making good observations and reporting them. Use Table 15.3 as a guideline for observing the patient with a head or brain injury.

| Table 15.2 ■ Possible Results of Left and Right Brain Injuries ||
Left Brain Injury	Right Brain Injury
Causes partial or complete paralysis of the right side of body, with loss of feeling (e.g., touch, temperature, and pain).	Causes partial or complete paralysis of the left side of body, with loss of feeling (e.g., touch, temperature, and pain).
Affects speech and communication centers; causes aphasia, an inability to communicate verbally.	Affects thought processes, memory, written computation, ability to tell time, judgment of movement, size, and distance.
Patient may act cautiously and slowly.	Patient may act impulsively and unsafely.

Table 15.3 ■ Guidelines for the Nurse Assistant in Sub-Acute Care

POSTOPERATIVE OBSERVATIONS	Loose dressing or dressing with drainage showing through. IV fluid that is not flowing and tubing that is crimped. IV that is beginning to run out. Skin where the needle is placed is swelling, red, or wet. Drainage tubes or catheters that are bent or plugged, or that have unusual-looking drainage. Pulse rate over 100 or below 60. Respirations that are labored, shallow, above 30, or below 14. Changes in blood pressure. Nausea or vomiting. Cyanosis of the skin, lips, or nailbeds. Bleeding. Complaints of pain, or moaning.
WOUND CARE	Location (e.g., lower-left abdominal quadrant). Size: Measure in centimeters. Measure side to side. Appearance: Is wound red, swollen, discolored, warm to touch? Wound edge parted or closed? Odor: Is it foul or unusual? Surrounding skin: Is it swollen, discolored, intact? Drainage: Observe type and amount.
INTRAVENOUS CARE	Alarm ringing on infusion pump. Changes in flow rate. Empty or near-empty bottle or bag. Bleeding at site. Puffiness, redness, and swelling at site. Changes in skin temperature, blood pressure. Pulse change (e.g., tachycardia, bradycardia, arrhythmia). Respiration change (e.g., rapid or shallow breathing, shortness of breath, or dyspnea). Confusion or mental changes. Pain (e.g., headache, chest pain). Skin color (e.g., paleness or cyanosis).
TRACHEOSTOMY CARE	Dislodged tracheostomy tube. Bleeding at site. Bubbling of mucus at site. Respiratory change: rapid, slow, labored. Changes in skin, nailbed color (e.g., cyanosis or grayness). Alarm ringing on mechanical respirator. Any equipment that is loose or kinked.
HEAD AND BRAIN INJURIES	Complaints of headache, blurred or double vision, dizziness. Vomiting. Loss of sensation. Change in ability to move (weakness, paralysis). Changes in vital signs. Slurred or changed speech pattern. Change in alertness. Disorientation and/or confusion. Pupils not equal in size. Pupils do not react to light (i.e., pupil does not become smaller when flashlight is directed at eye). Convulsions.

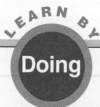

UNIT 2 ACTIVITY

1. Complete Worksheet 2 as assigned.
2. Practice all procedures.
3. Prepare responses to each item listed in Chapter Review—Your Link to Success at the end of this chapter.
4. When you are confident that you can meet each objective, ask your instructor for the unit evaluation.

Thinking Critically

1. **Cultural Competency** You notice that Mr. Brown never touches fruit or vegetables on his meal tray. When you suggest he might want to try a salad, he tells you he doesn't eat rabbit food. How could you talk to him about the importance of adding fruits and vegetables to his diet?

2. **Medical Terminology** Mrs. Sherman experienced a stroke four months ago. Using appropriate medical terms, describe each passive range-of-motion exercise performed on her weak side and what you will say to instruct Mrs. Sherman in how to do active range of motion on her stronger side.

3. **Legal** When you answer Mr. Sikorski's call signal, he tells you that he wants the side bed rails lowered immediately: he refuses to stay in a crib like a baby. How will you explain why you cannot do that? What are the legal issues that relate to what he sees as an insult to his maturity?

4. **Patient Education** You are assigned to a new patient who just arrived for admission to the facility. Write a list of things you will explain about safety, daily routine, and meeting the patient's needs. Describe how you will educate the patient and family about each of these items.

5. **Medical Math** Calculate how many cc's of fluid Miss White ate during her lunch. She ate the following: turkey sandwich with lettuce and tomato, 8 ounces of cream of mushroom soup, 6 ounces of tea, two chocolate chip cookies, and 4 ounces of sherbet.

Portfolio Connection

Write a description of two patient care events with which you feel you really helped the patient or the patient's family during your training. Include details about how staff and/or instructors were involved in the event.

Write a paper describing your doubts and realizations and the barriers that you were able to overcome during your nurse assistant experience. For example, were you afraid that you couldn't learn to use the equipment? Describe the ways you plan to use the skills, information, and insights that you gained about people and about this job. This assignment must be in standard report format.

Portfolio Tip

A nurturing atmosphere makes a positive difference to a patient's recovery and is something you can practice in your personal life. Greet your residents cheerfully and inquire about their interests.

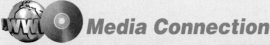

Remember! Media Connection

Use the Companion Website **www.prenhall.com/badasch** and the CD-ROM for additional interactive learning activities.

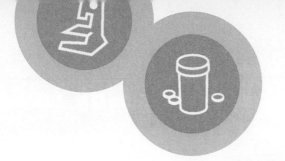

Home Health Aide

Chapter 16

STEPS TO SUCCESS

1. Complete Vocabulary Worksheet 1 in the Student Workbook.

2. Read this chapter.

3. Complete the Learn by Doing assignment at the end of this unit.

OBJECTIVES

When you have completed this chapter, you will be able to do the following:

✔ Complete all objectives in Part One of this book.

✔ Complete all objectives in Chapter 15.

✔ Define vocabulary words.

✔ List the following:

- Five causes of mental impairment

- Items included when charting

- Six rights to check when assisting a patient/client with medication

- Seven basic rules to follow when using household cleaners

- Ten safety concerns specific to the patient's/client's home

- Eight elements to remember when planning food/menus

✔ Explain the following:

- Why correct charting is important

- Proper care of a sterile and nonsterile dressing

- The basic guidelines to follow when storing medications

- Why deep breathing is important for bedridden clients

- The elements of an escape plan to use in case of fire

- The basic guidelines for food storage

- The definition of *sterile*

- The home health aide's responsibilities when there are children in the home

✔ Develop an action plan to use when caring for

- Children

- Aging persons

- Dying persons

✔ Demonstrate all procedures in this chapter.

✔ Demonstrate all procedures in Chapter 15.

✔ Complete the following objectives in Chapter 20:

- List three methods of packaging items.

- Demonstrate envelope wrap and square wrap.

✔ Apply medical terminology when charting and discussing the patient's/client's condition.

✔ Demonstrate putting on a nonsterile dressing.

RESPONSIBILITIES OF A HOME HEALTH AIDE

Home health aides are the members of the health care team who provide personal care for patients/clients at home. They perform a variety of tasks under the supervision of a registered nurse.

As a home health aide, you perform the following skills:

- Transfer patients/clients from place to place.
- Assist with bathing.
- Help patients/clients with walking and prescribed exercise.
- Help with braces or artificial limbs.
- Check and record temperature, pulse, and respiration.
- Check and record blood pressure.
- Change surgical dressings.
- Change bed linens.
- Provide emotional support.
- Do laundry.
- Clean patients'/clients' living quarters.
- Plan and prepare meals.
- Shop for patients'/clients' food.
- Report findings and observations to supervisors.
- Document daily activities and observations.

HOME HEALTH CARE AGENCIES

Home health care agencies are the major employers of home health aides. The goal of most home health care agencies is to promote the highest level of function for their patients/clients. As a home health aide, you are the major personal care provider for your patient/client. A registered nurse will instruct you about the procedures to follow and decide the best plan to follow for the client's care. The home care team includes the following caregivers:

- Physicians
- Therapists
- Social worker
- Nutritionist/dietitian
- Registered nurse
- Licensed vocational/licensed practical nurse
- Home health aide
- Homemaker
- Housekeeper
- Sitter/companion

WORKING WITH CLIENTS IN THE HOME

Mentally Impaired Patients/Clients

Review Unit 2, "Understanding Human Needs," in Chapter 4. When we understand basic needs and the reasons that people react to situations in different ways, we understand some occasional unacceptable behavior in people. In some cases, people

psychotherapy

Method of treatment using mental applications, such as hypnotherapy.

heredity

Characteristics passed from parent to child.

coping

Handling difficult situations.

who behave in socially unacceptable ways may have some type of mental impairment. Some of these behaviors can be changed through **psychotherapy.** Usually, psychotherapy helps patients/clients who are reacting to their environment, stress, or a lack of problem-solving abilities. Other types of mental impairments may be caused by

- **Heredity**
- Extreme high body temperature
- Impaired circulation
- Drugs
- Venereal disease

Your role in providing care is focused on basic personal care needs and protecting patients/clients from harming themselves and others.

Ill and Disabled Patients/Clients

To fully understand the implications of illness and disability, review Unit 3, "Disabilities and Role Changes," in Chapter 9. An ill or recently disabled person in the home may cause many disruptions. The family unit has longstanding methods for **coping** with all kinds of situations. Do not try to change the coping devices that each family member is using to survive during a difficult situation. As a health care provider, you may observe behaviors and attitudes that create tension and stress. Report these observations to your supervisor. Be a good listener, and use your best health care techniques. This provides a sense of caring and trust. When you establish trust, you help ease unnecessary worry about your ability to give the client or the family proper care.

Children

Review Unit 1, "Development and Behavior," in Chapter 9. Ask your instructor for a copy of *The Pediatric Patient.* As a home health aide, you interact with children of the patients/clients you are caring for. You also interact with children who are assigned to you as patients. Your responsibility in each of these situations differs from household to household. Always discuss with your supervisor your primary responsibility to all family members. When a child is present in the home of a patient, always be sensitive to the implications of the patient's condition and the environment the child is exposed to. Noise and activity may be restricted for a child. A few positive comments about how much their cooperation is appreciated are helpful. When it is possible, answer children's questions truthfully and openly. If you are uncomfortable discussing questions children ask, *do not ignore them* but refer them to your supervisor or another adult in the household. Remember, children usually like to be helpful, so, when appropriate, include them in teaching about the patient's care or condition.

If the child is the patient, he or she will be most interested in his or her own care. Do not talk behind his or her back or just outside his or her room. Fears may develop when the child feels that secrets are being kept from him or her. Always remember that you are in a patient's home. Do not overstep your bounds with children by disciplining them before you discuss it with the patient or other adult in the home.

Aging Patients/Clients

Review Unit 2, "Aging and Role Change," in Chapter 9. It provides information on attitudes and physical changes of aging persons. It is important when you are working in patients' homes to respect their wishes about when and how you perform each task. Try to make arrangements that are acceptable to both of you. However, these arrangements should not affect the treatment. Your overall attitude about elderly people affects the way you interact with geriatric patients. It is important to evaluate your thinking about older people in general. Consider the following:

■ How do you picture an older person?

■ What is "old?"

■ When does a person stop being of value?

■ Does the amount of money a person has make a difference in deciding that person's value?

■ When does a person stop wanting to have fun?

■ Is there a time when a person would not be worth your giving of time and energy?

Answer these questions honestly, and then discuss your answers with others. When you discuss the various responses to the same questions, you become more aware of your attitude toward aging.

Dying Patients/Clients

Many people are choosing to die at home rather than in the hospital. They are comfortable in their own environment and feel that they have more control at home. Remember to review the five stages of dying discussed in Chapter 9. These help you understand your patients' many needs and desires. Try to provide a sense of normalcy by keeping the routine standard. Encourage activity as tolerated. Remember, humor and laughter can be the best medicine.

Continued relationships with others are an important part of each day. These relationships provide a sense of being cared about and feeling worthwhile. Take time just to be there for patients (e.g., sit quietly with them, listen to them, have a conversation with them). When you perform your duties in a professional manner and with confidence, your patients and their families maintain a sense of security knowing that all that can be done is being done.

As the moment of death draws near, a spiritual leader may be requested. At this time, ensuring privacy and quiet may be the most important task you perform. Remember that you do not have to agree with the spiritual belief of the household to provide good care at this time. The time of death may be difficult for you as the caregiver, especially if you have provided care for the same patient and family for a long period. It is all right to express your own sadness, but do not become an extra burden. When providing personal care for the patient, always be respectful both before and after death. As death approaches, the muscles lose their tone and the body openings may drain. Before death occurs, gently wash away discharges that have accumulated around the orifices of the body. Gently straighten the limbs and make the patient as comfortable as possible.

When death occurs, the physician must be notified. Before the body is moved to a funeral home, the physician must establish that the client has died. If the cause of death is not certain, an **autopsy** may be required. The agency you work for will have specific procedures to guide you at this time. Usually, you will need to bathe the body and change the bed. This is especially important if family or friends will be viewing the body before it is taken from the home. Always notify your supervisor as soon as possible when a client dies.

Recording Observations

Insurance companies and other third-party payers **reimburse** for care you provide only when appropriate documentation is prepared in a timely manner. It is essential

autopsy
Medical procedure after death to determine the cause of death.

reimburse
To pay back for something given or spent.

that you document each procedure you provide for the patient's needs. You must keep your records accurate and up to date. Each agency has specific terms and phrases that it requires for reimbursement purposes. Be sure you use your agency's guidelines when recording observations and procedures. Do not hesitate to ask your supervisor for assistance. Review "Charting and Observation" in Unit 2 of Chapter 5.

When charting about care given in the home, include the following for each visit:

- Caregiver's name, title, and Social Security number
- Patient's name and case number
- Date and time care was provided
- Reason for the visit
- Statements describing the patient's condition when you arrived
- Statements describing the time, treatment, or activity done and the patient's tolerance of the activity or procedure
- Description of teaching completed
- Your signature
- The patient's signature, which is often required

It is important to remember that no matter how efficient you are as a home health aide, if your records are not properly prepared, you may be fired.

Patient/Client Movement and Ambulation in the Home

See the discussion on ambulation in Chapter 19 for ambulation procedures and precautions. In the home, it is important to keep the floor free of clutter. The walking space should be adequate and allow freedom of movement. Throw rugs and carpet edges are hazards and can cause serious falls. Place wide masking tape over carpet edges to prevent tripping. Throw rugs must be secured or picked up. Electrical cords, children's toys, shoes, socks, and any loose items on the floor must be removed to ensure safe ambulation. Clients who have been in bed for a long period may be weak. When they are allowed to be out of bed, it helps to have another health care worker assist you until the client shows adequate strength. Ask your supervisor to help you make the appropriate decisions.

Special Procedures

Nonsterile Dressings

Dressings are used to protect an open area on the skin from infection, to absorb drainage, or to keep medicines that aid healing on the open area. The licensed nurse changes sterile dressings (dressings that are free of all living microorganisms). If your patient has a sterile dressing in place and drainage is showing through, tape a sterile dressing over the wet dressing. Make absolutely certain that you do not touch the area of the dressing that contacts the wet dressing. Notify your supervisor as soon as possible. You may be asked to replace a dressing that is clean (but not sterile).

Assisting With Medication

Each state has guidelines that outline who can and cannot give medications. As a home health aide (including certified home health aide), you are *not* licensed to give medications. If you choose to give medications to a client, you may be fined or held liable for your actions. The agency you work for is also liable for your actions. It is important that you remember this when assisting with medications. There is a legal difference between administration and assisting. The licensed nurse coordinator tells you what medication your client needs and the time it should be taken.

PROCEDURE 16.1

DRESSINGS: CLEAN, NONSTERILE

RATIONALE

Correct handling of dressings prevents the increased risk for serious infections in an open wound.

ALERT: Follow Standard Precautions.

1. Wash hands.
2. Assemble equipment.
   a. Clean dressings
   b. Tape
   c. Cleansing solution
   d. Paper or plastic bag
   e. Medication to be applied by patient
   f. Disposable nonsterile gloves
3. Identify patient/client.
4. Explain what you are going to do.
5. Position patient comfortably.
6. Open paper bag.
7. Open clean dressings. *Do not touch center of bandage.*
8. Put on gloves.
9. Remove old dressing and
   a. Check amount of drainage.
   b. Check color, consistency, odor.
   c. Check skin around wound.
   d. Note size of wound.
10. To cleanse wound:
    a. Use circular motions.
    b. Clean from center of wound to skin.
11. Assist client with application of medication, if ordered.
12. Apply clean dressing.
    a. Hold dressing by corner.
    b. Tape bandage securely in place.

13. Discard bandages according to agency procedures.
    a. Close bag with soiled bandages inside.
    b. Tape bag closed.
    c. Discard in covered container.
14. Remove gloves and discard according to agency procedures.
15. Clean equipment and put away.
16. Wash hands.
17. Chart the following:
    a. Time and date
    b. Any observation made:

       (1) Drainage (amount, color, odor)
       (2) Size of wound
       (3) Surrounding skin condition

    c. Type of bandage applied
    d. How procedure was tolerated

9/19/03   0900

15 cm of clear slightly pink
drainage on dressing
Skin condition around wound
in good condition
New dressing applied
Tolerated procedure well
_____ S. Jones CMA

When assisting your client with medications, always check the six "rights."

The Rights of Medication

- The right client   Is the medication order for the correct person?
- The right medication   Is this the correct medication?
- The right time   Is this the prescribed time to take it?
- The right route   How to take it? By mouth, apply to the skin, swallow it, suck on it?

PROCEDURE 16.2

ASSISTING WITH MEDICATION IN THE HOME

RATIONALE

Medication errors can cause serious side effects and add to the patient's medical problems. Following each step every time you assist the patient with medication prevents medication errors.

Always follow the six rights of medication.

1. Wash hands.
2. Assemble supplies.
   a. Glass of water or juice
   b. Appropriate medication
   c. Spoon or measuring device, if needed
3. Remind patient when it is time to take medication.
4. Read label on medication.
5. Read physician's order for medication.
6. Read label on medication again.
7. Steady or guide client's hand if necessary.
8. Assist with pouring correct amount of medication into a container. (Pills are to be counted and placed in a container; liquids are measured.)
9. Close medicine container and read label again.
10. Assist patient in taking medication.
11. Record on patient care notes: time, type, route, amount of medication taken.
12. Wipe up spills and replace soiled linen or client's clothing, if necessary.
13. Replace medication in proper storage place.
14. Wash hands.

10/05/03   0900

Assisted with Keflex 50mg po

Tolerated well

_____ G. Jones CHHA

■ The right amount   Is this the prescribed quantity?

■ Document the right way   Are rights documented in the patient record?

Medication Guidelines

There are some basic guidelines to follow when assisting with medications:

■ Always throw old medications in the toilet where they cannot be taken by others. Old medication loses its strength and does not produce the effect it was prescribed for. It can also become toxic and cause illness. Many medications are dated. Do not use after the expiration date.

■ Never allow a client to take medication from an unlabeled container.

■ Keep medications out of reach of children and **disoriented** clients.

■ Always discuss the placement of medications. Clients may take medication by its placement on a shelf rather than by reading the directions (especially when the client is vision-impaired).

disoriented

Being confused about time, place, or identity of persons and objects.

Deep-Breathing Exercises

Deep breathing is an important procedure to remember when working with clients. We normally take a deep breath every few minutes during the day. This deep breath is called a sigh. When we are sleeping or inactive, we do not sigh or deep breathe. Without the sigh, mucus and fluid begin to develop in the lowest part of the lungs. This extra fluid may cause the client to feel short of breath and cause pneumonia. Pneumonia is still a leading complication in most illnesses. You can help prevent this from occurring by encouraging your clients to take a few slow, deep breaths every hour. This simple procedure helps remove mucus and fluid from the lungs. Another way to encourage clients to take a deep breath is to have them cough. The cough helps to force fluid and mucus up the bronchial tree and out of the lungs. This keeps the lungs clear.

Sitting the Patient/Client on the Bedside

When getting a client out of bed, it is a good idea to take a few minutes and have the client sit on the side of the bed (dangling his or her legs) and take a few slow, deep breaths. By allowing the client this time and encouraging slow, deep breaths, your client takes oxygen into the lungs, and the blood pressure is able to equalize. (Have you ever felt dizzy after standing up too fast? If so, this probably happened because it took a few seconds for the blood to reach your brain. You do not want this to happen with your client.) Review the discussion on syncope in Chapter 15.

STERILIZATION IN THE HOME

It may be necessary to use sterilized articles in the process of caring for your client. Remember that sterilization means that all living microorganisms are dead. Just being clean does not mean that an item is sterile. Many agencies purchase disposable items that are used once and then discarded. It is important to remember that sterile disposable supplies are contaminated when they have been used. Do not try to save money by reusing supplies that are used or opened. Microorganisms are too small to see, so even though an article looks clean, it may be contaminated. You may find it necessary to sterilize items in the home. This can be done in two different ways. The method you use depends on the item to be sterilized. Articles that can tolerate moisture and high heat are sterilized by using wet heat (Figure 16.1). Articles that cannot tolerate moisture are sterilized in a dry heat process (Figure 16.2). When working with clients, always remember the aseptic techniques you learned in Chapter 12. It is essential to practice good technique at all times. This protects your client, the family, and yourself! Follow the procedure your agency recommends for sterilizing.

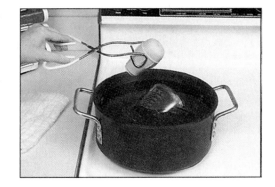

Figure 16.1

Wet heat sterilization.

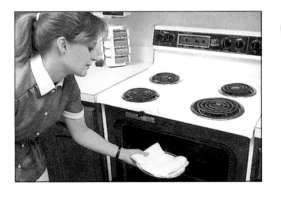

Figure 16.2

Dry heat sterilization.

MAINTAINING A CLEAN ENVIRONMENT

As a home health aide, you may be expected to do some basic cleaning, cooking, and shopping for the client. Your supervisor will establish the jobs that are required to promote the client's progress toward improved health. Your primary responsibility is to the client's health needs. If the environment is not clean, the client may be in jeopardy. The bathroom and kitchen require frequent cleaning to help prevent the spread of microorganisms. You will be expected to keep the bathroom and kitchen clean. It is important for you to understand the client's values concerning cleanliness. Dust on the furniture may be tolerable to the client, but messy cabinets may be intolerable. Things that you are not concerned about may concern the client. To establish a good working relationship, try to discover these details early in your assignment. It usually works best to involve all family members in a plan to maintain a clean environment. A good plan can be organized by deciding what jobs need to be completed each week. Then determine which tasks have to be completed on certain days. Balance the week by assigning tasks to all days so that one day is not extremely busy and another light. When you or your supervisor can encourage the family members to volunteer for some of the tasks, the plan becomes a working agreement.

Housecleaning Method

Try to use the products that are available in the home. If new items are needed, discuss your preferred items, but be flexible and adjust to the products the client prefers. There are a few basic rules to remember when using cleaning products.

abrasive

Compound used to rub away or scrape away another substance.

- Never mix cleaning products. They may cause a harmful reaction to occur (e.g., fumes that irritate eyes or lungs, a corrosive effect on the surface being cleaned).

- Never use cleansers or **abrasive** agents (cleaners with a gritty feel) until you have checked with the client or family. Some newer finishes can easily be scratched.

- Always read instructions thoroughly and follow them exactly.

- When using a tub or container of cleaning solution, change the solution before it becomes dirty. Trying to clean with a dirty solution is impossible.

- Never store cleaning products or tools near food.

- Discard any bottles that are not labeled.

- Remember that most cleaners are toxic, so keep them away from children and disoriented clients.

PROCEDURE 16.3 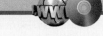 ESTABLISHING A WORK PLAN

RATIONALE
A schedule helps with organization and helps stay in control of household responsibilities.

1. Evaluate the need for basic household duties to be performed.
2. Make a list of the duties you decide must be routinely completed.
3. Ask the family to make a list of duties they feel must be routinely completed.
4. Plan a meeting with family members to discuss routine duties to be completed.
5. Discuss and agree upon the basic duties that will be done by each member of the family.
6. See sample work plan and use it or develop your own.

Sample Work Plan

Day	Duty	Responsible Person
Monday		
Tuesday		
Wednesday		
Thursday		
Friday		
Saturday		
Sunday		

Remember that bacteria cannot move from place to place on their own. They can move only when carried. The most common carriers of bacteria are dust, insects, pests, and people. Proper cleaning reduces dust and discourages insects and pests. People can reduce the chance of spreading bacteria by remembering the importance of washing their hands after going to the bathroom and before handling food for themselves or others.

◯ SAFETY IN THE HOME

The units on safety in Chapter 13 are appropriate for safety in the home. There are additional concerns in the home environment, however, that you need to be aware of.

- Proper lighting must be available at all times.
- Floors and walking areas must be free from clutter, and adequate walking space must be available.
- Stairways need to be blocked by doors or railings to prevent falls.
- Throw rugs are a hazard and may cause clients to fall. Pick them up to provide a safe walkway.
- Use wide masking tape on loose carpet edges.
- Stay with clients while they are smoking, especially if they are sleepy or disoriented.
- Keep ashtrays clean and free of litter so they do not create a fire hazard.
- Be alert about how your client and visitors extinguish cigarettes. Watch furniture for smoke or smoldering.
- The use of extension cords or multiple-socket adapters can create a fire hazard. It is always better to unplug something rather than to overload the electrical system.
- See that a nonskid pad or decals are placed in showers and tubs to prevent slipping.
- Safety rails or bars can be installed around the tub and toilet, if necessary, to provide support for an unstable client.
- Keep all poisons away from food and locked in a cabinet whose use is only for poisons.
- Be sure that all combustible items are kept away from heat and stored in a cool place.
- Remember: *No smoking* must be enforced if the client is using oxygen. A No Smoking sign should be displayed.
- Turn off oxygen before putting a plug in the wall or removing a plug from the wall. The spark that occurs at this time could cause an explosion.
- A client with portable oxygen must not go into an area where there is an open flame (e.g., gas stove with pilot, water heater with pilot).

The kitchen can be especially hazardous. Keep in mind the following precautions when the client and others are in the kitchen.

- A fire extinguisher should be available.
- Keep all handles turned toward the center of the stove when cooking so that they are less likely to be knocked off and so that children cannot pull them off.
- Do not use towels or aprons to lift hot items. The edges can easily catch fire. Use only potholders that provide adequate protection.
- Never reach over an open flame. Turn off the flame before reaching.
- Clients with pacemakers must be kept away from a microwave oven.
- Check the water heater and house heater area for proper circulation of air. These areas should not be used to store other things. If they are cluttered, they are a fire hazard.

Fire is always unexpected. Taking the proper fire precautions will save lives. Take the time to make an escape plan with the family. Only well-thought-out plans can be implemented with assured success. Don't be caught unprepared. Your plan should include the following:

- An operational smoke detector, properly mounted in an appropriate location
- Various routes of escape
- Properly placed equipment (e.g., drop ladder or a slide for a second story)
- Method to remove the client in a safe manner
- An assigned meeting place outside the house

REMINDER   Escape is most important, not valuables. Valuables can be replaced. Family members cannot.

SHOPPING AND PLANNING FOR MEALS

Review Chapter 10 on nutrition. As a home health aide, you may be responsible for planning, shopping, and preparing meals for your client. It is very important for you to follow the diet ordered by the physician. If the client is on a regular diet, it is important for you to discuss the menus with the client. You also want to know the client's preference for between-meal snacks. When planning menus, keep in mind that the meals should be well balanced over a 24-hour period. Each of the food groups should be included in the proper proportions. For some clients, mealtime is the best time of day. For others, meals are unenjoyable. Every person needs healthy, well-balanced meals to maintain or regain good health. The following are things to keep in mind when planning meals:

- Prepare nutritionally balanced meals.
- Do not serve foods that are the same texture.
- Always plan for a variety of foods.
- Serve meals in an attractive manner (e.g., a variety of colors present, not all the same color).
- Keep the cost moderate or within the family budget. Once the menu is decided upon, develop a grocery list.
- Check the household grocery supply for amounts of food on hand.
- Be certain that there are enough of the foods used daily.
- Check other household supplies, such as toilet paper, paper towels, toothpaste, and laundry soap. It saves time if you plan a week's shopping. This keeps you or others from having to return to the store.

When purchasing food, always check the labels of packaged foods. The ingredients are important for people on special diets. The ingredients are listed according to the amount of each item in the package (see Table 16.1). If your client is on a restricted diet, you must carefully select food that meets the diet's **specifications.** If you are unsure, do not buy it. Check with the doctor or your supervisor first.

specifications
Exact way something should be done.

Storing Food

Proper storage of food is essential. If food is not properly stored, nutrients are lost, and foods may spoil before they are used. Proper storage also prevents the growth of bacteria. Only use foods that are fresh. Discard the following:

- All food with an expired date
- Foods that have a strange smell
- Foods that are moldy

Table 16.1 ■ Hot Cocoa Mix Ingredients
sugar
sweet dairy whey
cocoa
corn syrup
solids
nonfat dry milk
hydrogenated vegetable oil
vanilla flavoring

Sugar is the largest amount. Vanilla flavoring is the smallest amount. You might not realize how much sugar is in cocoa mix unless you read the ingredients.

The following are basic guidelines for food storage:

■ Use meat within 48 hours of placing in the refrigerator.

■ Defrost frozen meat in the refrigerator, not on a counter in the kitchen.

■ Fish spoils rapidly. Prepare it as soon as possible after purchase.

■ Fruits and vegetables remain fresh longer if they are kept in the refrigerator. Fruits that are not ripe will ripen faster if placed at room temperature.

■ Breads can be frozen if wrapped carefully or kept in an airtight container. In humid climates, bread will develop mold faster than it will in dry climates.

■ Milk should be refrigerated. Nonfat milk will last longer than whole milk or lowfat milk because there is no fat to sour.

■ Canned foods should be stored in a cool, dark place.

■ Frozen foods can be stored for long periods if they remain frozen. Once they have started to thaw, they should be cooked, and then they can be refrozen. A cookbook will provide guidelines for the safe freezing periods of most foods.

Preparing Food

Food preparation varies from person to person. Discuss with clients their food preferences. Try to please them by preparing foods as close to their desires as possible. If they express a desire to try a special food, or if they especially like the way you prepare food, feel free to use your imagination. Your main restrictions are the ordered diet the client must follow.

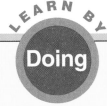

Doing

1. Complete Worksheets 2, 5, 6, and 9 as assigned.

2. Complete Worksheets/Activities 3, 4, 7, and 8 as assigned.

3. Practice all procedures.

4. Prepare responses to each item listed in Chapter Review—Your Link to Success at the end of this chapter.

5. When you are confident that you can meet each objective, ask your instructor for the unit evaluation.

Thinking Critically

1. Time Management Preparing the meals in the Johnston household is a daily crisis because basic food supplies constantly run out. Create a shopping chart for Mr. Johnston that he may keep in the kitchen now that his wife cannot run the house. Explain how you have divided the chart into categories (produce, frozen foods, etc.) so that he may write in items as they run out and have a ready-made shopping list each week.

2. Legal and Ethical Mr. Dimas is very ill. He asks you to arrange for his priest to visit. You belong to a different religion and do not approve of his. You wonder if it is a good idea to call your minister to see him. What should you do, and why?

3. Patient Education Write down instructions you would give to a patient or the patient's family explaining what to do when a sterile dressing becomes saturated with drainage.

4. Medical Math In the home where you are working, all containers are marked in ounces, pints, and quarts. The agency you work for requires that you chart all intake in cubic centimeters (cc's). Choose three examples of containers marked in ounces and convert the measurements to cc's.

5. Safety Alert Mrs. Gonzales's pretty home is filled with scatter rugs and decorative items. Now that she cannot ambulate independently, helping with her shower is a challenge. Make a list of safety changes you would recommend for the bedroom and bathroom and think how you could present these to her.

Portfolio Connection

Once you attain competence as a home health aide, ask for permission to copy your documentation. (Remove all patient identifiers.) Place this copy in your portfolio as evidence of your skills. Place a copy of your on-site trainer's evaluation in your portfolio.

Write a paper describing your doubts and realizations and the barriers that you were able to overcome during the home health aide experience. For example, were you afraid that you couldn't learn to use the equipment? Describe the ways you plan to use the skills, information, and insights that you gained about people and about this job. This assignment must be in standard report format. Participate in job shadowing to help determine your interest in being a home health aide.

Portfolio Tip

Try to balance medically appropriate care with respect for a client's home and its organization.

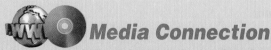

Remember! Media Connection

Use the Companion Website **www.prenhall.com/badasch** and the CD-ROM for additional interactive learning activities.

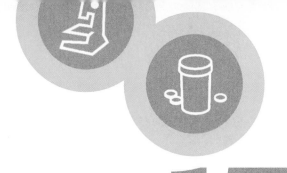

Chapter 17

Electro-cardiogram Technician

STEPS TO SUCCESS

1. Read this chapter.
2. Complete the Learn by Doing assignment at the end of this chapter.

OBJECTIVES

When you have completed this chapter, you will be able to do the following:

✔ Complete all objectives in Part One of this book.

✔ Match vocabulary words with their correct meanings.

✔ List two reasons why the doctor orders an EKG/ECG.*

✔ List four conditions that are determined by an EKG/ECG.

✔ Label a diagram of an EKG/ECG machine and describe the function of each part.

✔ Label a normal EKG/ECG complex.

✔ List three waves recorded on the EKG/ECG cycle, and relate them to the activity of the heart.

✔ List the 12 leads recorded on an EKG/ECG.

✔ Identify the leads according to color and correct placement.

✔ List three common sources of artifacts.

✔ Identify eight common causes of artifacts and their remedies.

✔ Perform an EKG.

✔ Mount EKG/ECG readings.

✔ Compare and contrast normal EKG/ECG readings with abnormal readings.

✔ Attach a Holter monitor to a patient and give clear instructions to the patient.

✔ Explain what a Holter monitor records and why it is used for diagnostic purposes.

✔ Demonstrate the following skills:

- From Chapter 15:
  Pivot transfer from bed to wheelchair and back
  Sliding from bed to gurney and back
  Moving a patient/client in a wheelchair
  Moving a patient/client on a gurney

- From Chapter 22:
  List five filing systems.
  Demonstrate alpha and numeric filing.

*EKG and ECG are both used to indicate an electrocardiogram. Either is correct.

RESPONSIBILITIES OF AN EKG/ECG TECHNICIAN

EKG/ECG

Graphic record of the electrical currents produced by the heart.

irregularities

Different than normal.

heart block

Interference with the conduction of the electrical impulses of the heart that is either partial or complete.

An **ECG** technician works in a general hospital or clinic, or for a physician in private practice. ECG technicians operate equipment that makes a record of the electrical changes that occur during a heartbeat. These recordings help physicians diagnose **irregularities** or changes in the patient's/client's heart. These tests are done routinely after a client reaches a certain age, before surgery, and as a diagnostic tool to detect heart disease and dysfunctions, such as

- Previous heart attack
- **Heart block**
- Enlarged heart muscle
- Rhythm disturbances

As an EKG technician, you are required to do the following tasks:

- Prepare patients/clients for testing.
- Operate the EKG machine and record 12-lead EKG rhythm strips.
- Mount EKG strips.
- File paperwork.
- Maintain equipment and order supplies.
- Prepare copies of EKGs.
- Notify your supervisor immediately of deviations from normal on EKG strips.
- Transport patient/client.

ELECTROCARDIOGRAPH

electrocardiograph

Instrument that records electric currents produced by the heart.

An EKG/ECG is taken with an **electrocardiograph.** An ECG shows the path of the electrical stimulation to the heart.

ECG Functions

See Figure 17.1.

- *Electrodes* are small pieces of metal that pick up the electrical activity of the heart.

Figure 17.1

ECG technician performing an ECG on a client.

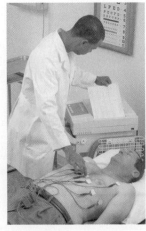

(a)

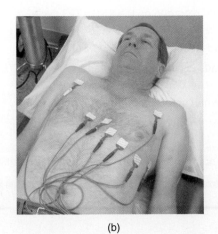

(b)

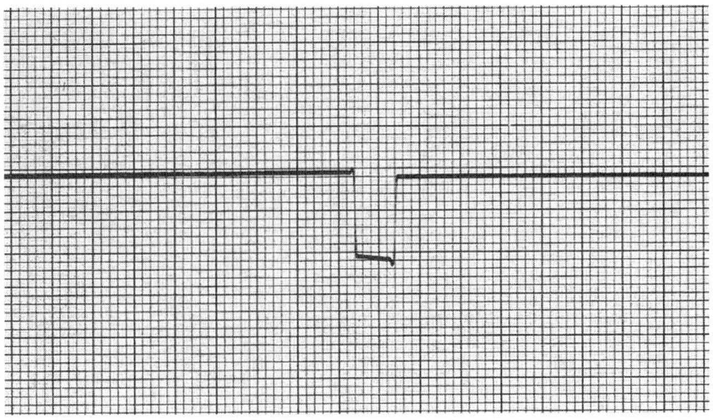

- *Leads* are wires carrying impulses from the electrodes on the patient's skin to the machine.

- *Lead indicator switches* (on old machines) tell the machine which lead to read.

- The *stylus* records the heart's electrical activity on graph paper.

- *Amplifiers* **magnify** the electrical signal the heart generates so that it can be recorded.

- *Speed switches* regulate the speed at which the graph paper runs through the machine.

- *Standardization buttons* (on old machines) are like a ruler. They are a guide to the physician reading the ECG. If you forget to use the standardization button, the ECG may be read incorrectly (see Figure 17.2 for a strip standardization indicator).

- The *sensitivity switch* changes the height of the standard measurement.

- EKG/ECG machines record single leads (Figure 17.3) or multichannel lead strips (Figure 17.4).

ECG/EKG Paper

The ECG/EKG paper is graph paper with small squares that measure the time it takes for each heartbeat (see Figure 17.5 on page 454). ECG paper is heat and

Figure 17.2

Standardization markings.

magnify
Enlarge.

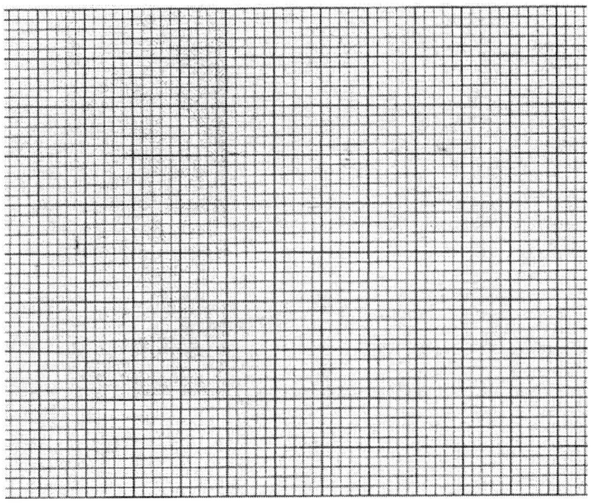

Figure 17.3

Single-channel paper prints one lead at a time.

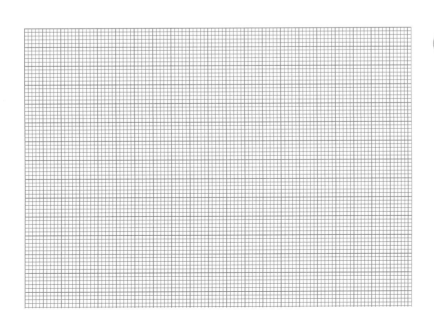

Figure 17.4

Multichannel paper allows all twelve leads to be printed on a full sheet of paper (reduced 20%).

Figure 17.5

ECG graph paper measures electrical activity of the heart and the time it takes to complete each part of that activity.

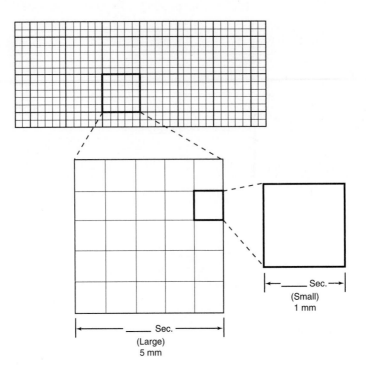

Sec.
(Small)
1 mm

Sec.
(Large)
5 mm

pressure sensitive. The stylus makes an imprint as it moves over the paper. It is important to handle the paper carefully, as it marks easily.

The marks made during an ECG are labeled "PQRST" waves. Each letter identifies an activity in the heart (see Figure 17.6). Each PQRST equals one heartbeat.

EKG/ECG Leads

The standard 12-lead electrocardiogram records electrical activity from 12 different angles of the heart. Recognizing a normal recording from each lead is important. Each angle is identified by a lead name or number (see Figures 17.7 to 17.18). The last six leads are the chest leads. Chest leads (see Figure 17.19) read from the ventral to the dorsal surface (see Figures 17.13 to 17.18). They are called V leads and are placed in very exact places on the chest. To obtain correct readings, EKG technicians must place all leads correctly. Technicians are responsible for reporting abnormal recordings immediately.

Figure 17.6

ECG rhythm strip.

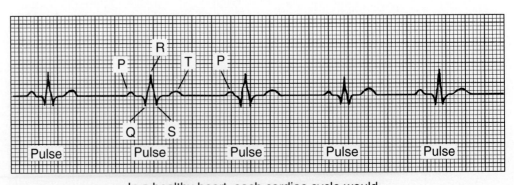

In a healthy heart, each cardiac cycle would be expected to correlate with the patient's individual pulse beats.

Leads 1 Through 3

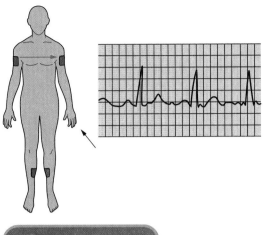

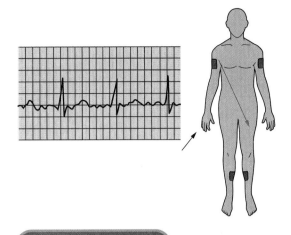

Figure 17.7

Lead 1 reads from the right arm to the left arm and looks similar to this.

Figure 17.8

Lead 2 reads from the right arm to the left leg and looks similar to this.

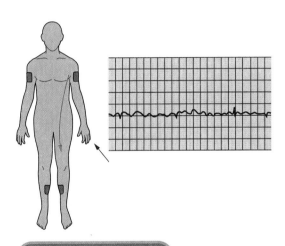

Figure 17.9

Lead 3 reads from the left arm to the left leg and looks similar to this.

Augmented Voltage (Leads)

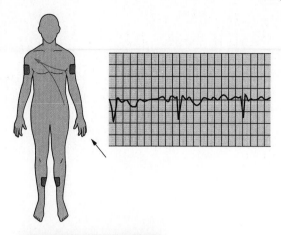

Figure 17.10

Lead AVR reads across the heart to the right shoulder and looks similar to this.

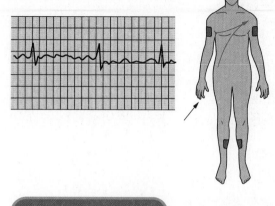

Figure 17.11

Lead AVL reads across the heart to the left shoulder and looks similar to this.

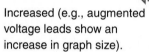

augmented

Increased (e.g., augmented voltage leads show an increase in graph size).

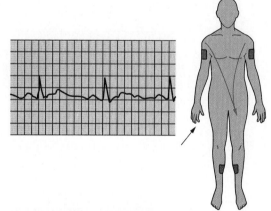

Figure 17.12

Lead AVF reads across the heart toward the feet and looks similar to this.

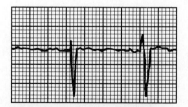

Figure 17.13

Lead V1.

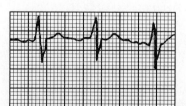

Figure 17.14

Lead V2.

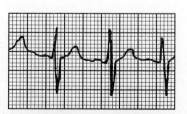

Figure 17.15

Lead V3.

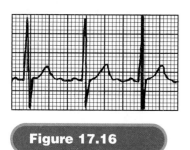

Figure 17.16

Lead V4.

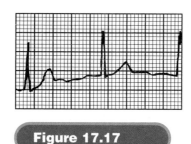

Figure 17.17

Lead V5.

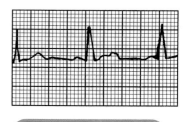

Figure 17.18

Lead V6.

◯ PERFORMING AN EKG/ECG

Placing the Leads on the Patient/Client

Always explain to the patient/client that there is no pain or discomfort during an EKG/ECG. Reassure patients that their privacy is respected and that they are kept covered as much as possible. Tell them the test takes only a few minutes. Reassure patients that there is nothing wrong with them if you have to adjust leads because **artifacts** appear on the strip. Explain that the machine is very sensitive and that it is necessary to hold very still. Talk with patients as you put the leads in place to help them relax and feel more at ease.

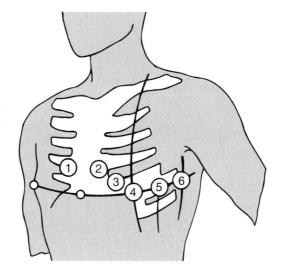

Figure 17.19

Chest or V-lead placement.

artifacts
Unwanted marks on an electrocardiogram.

Correct lead placement is important (see Figures 17.7 through 17.12 and 17.19). The blue squares on Figures 17.7 through 17.12 are placement sites for limb leads. Figure 17.19 shows placement sites for chest or V leads.

EKG/ECG Machines

There are many types of ECG machines. The basic procedure for operating each type of machine may be slightly different. The most common machines are the 12-lead manual EKG machine and the three-channel computerized machine. There is also a single-channel EKG machine. A very high tech machine can interpret the reading and mount the strips automatically. Some patients use a device at home that sends their EKG **impulses** over the telephone for interpretation.

impulses
Measures of electrical activity to the heart tissue recorded on a graph.

Machine Controls

It is important to set each control on the machine so that a correct reading is recorded. Follow all procedures carefully to ensure that you will have an accurate reading.

PROCEDURE 17.1

USING A MULTILEAD ELECTROCARDIOGRAPH (PLACING LEADS ON THE PATIENT/CLIENT, SETTING MACHINE CONTROLS)

RATIONALE

Carefully placing leads and following instructions for operation of equipment ensures a correct EKG reading. Poor technique creates an inaccurate reading and may affect treatment for the patient.

ALERT: Follow Standard Precautions.

Placing Leads on Patient/Client

1. Wash hands.
2. Assemble equipment.
   a. EKG machine with electrodes
   b. Electrode pads
   c. Alcohol wipes or skin cleansing agent
   d. Bath blanket/sheet
   e. Patient gown
3. Identify patient/client.
4. Explain what you are doing and reassure patient that this procedure is painless.
5. Help client change into a patient gown if necessary.
6. Position patient on bed or treatment table in a supine position with arms relaxed beside body.
7. Cover patient with a blanket, leaving arms and legs exposed.
8. Position machine at the side of client.
9. Identify correct location for leg, arm, and chest leads. (Avoid bony areas.)
10. Wipe skin with a cleansing agent to remove oils, scaly skin, or perspiration.
11. Apply electrode patches.
12. Attach leads to snap-on electrode patches. Each lead is color coded to ensure proper placement.
    a. White lead to right arm
    b. Black lead to left arm
    c. Green lead to right leg
    d. Red lead to left leg
    e. Brown leads are chest leads—place each one as indicated:
       (1) V1: fourth intercostal space just to the right of sternum
       (2) V2: fourth intercostal space just to the left of sternum
       (3) V3: midway between position of the fourth and fifth intercostal spaces
       (4) V4: fifth intercostal space

       (5) V5: same level as V4 and just anterior of midaxillary line
       (6) V6: same level as V4 and V5 at midaxillary line

Setting Machine Controls

13. Set machine controls.
    a. Set speed switch to run 25 mm per second. (If there is a severe tachycardia, it may be necessary to set at 50 mm per second.)
    b. Position stylus in center of paper.
    c. Set sensitivity at 1 for normal complexes. If complexes are too small to recognize each wave, set at 2. If complexes are so large that they will not fit on the graph paper, set the sensitivity at ½.
    d. Standardize each lead as instructed by your teacher.
14. Turn on machine.
15. Turn run button on. (Most multichannel EKG machines automatically standardize and record each lead when run button is pushed. See manufacturer's instructions to operate your machine properly.)
16. Turn off machine when all leads are recorded.
17. Remove all leads and electrode patches.
18. Clean remaining gel or paste left from patches.
19. Assist patient in dressing if necessary.
20. Label EKG with patient's name and physician's name.
21. Clean machine so that it is ready for next procedure.
22. Mount EKG and deliver as instructed for interpretation. (See the procedure "Mounting EKGs.")

10/03/03 1000

ECG recorded

Tolerated well

ECG mounted and placed in chart

G. Jones CMA

PROCEDURE 17.2

USING A SINGLE-LEAD ELECTROCARDIOGRAPH (PLACING LEADS ON THE PATIENT/CLIENT, SETTING MACHINE CONTROLS, PERFORMING AN EKG)

RATIONALE

Carefully placing leads and following instructions for operation of equipment ensures correct EKG reading. Poor technique creates an inaccurate reading and may affect treatment for the patient.

ALERT: Follow Standard Precautions.

Placing Leads on Patient/Client

1. Wash hands.
2. Assemble equipment.
   a. EKG machine with electrodes
   b. Conductive gel
   c. Alcohol wipes or skin cleansing agent
   d. Gauze
   e. Rubber electrode straps
   f. Bath blanket/sheet
   g. Patient gown
3. Identify patient/client.
4. Explain what you are doing and reassure client that this procedure is painless.
5. Help patient change into patient gown if necessary.
6. Position patient on bed or treatment table in supine position with arms relaxed beside the body.
7. Cover client, leaving arms and legs exposed.
8. Position machine at the side of patient.
9. Identify correct location for arm and leg leads on fleshy areas. (Avoid bony areas.)
10. Wipe skin with a cleansing agent to remove oils, scaly skin, or perspiration.
11. Apply conductive gel or paste and electrodes. Secure with rubber straps.
12. Connect leads to electrodes. Each lead is color coded to ensure proper placement.
    a. White lead to right arm
    b. Black lead to left arm
    c. Green lead to right leg
    d. Red lead to left leg
    e. Brown lead not attached at this time

Setting Machine Controls

13. Set machine controls. Now that leads are in the proper place, it is important that you set each control on the machine in order to have a correct reading.
    a. Be certain to set speed switch to run 25 mm per second. (If there is a severe tachycardia, it may be necessary to set at 50 mm per second.)
    b. Position stylus in center of paper.
    c. Set sensitivity at 1 for normal complexes. If complexes are too small to recognize each wave, set at 2. If complexes are so large that they will not fit on graph paper, set the sensitivity at ½.
    d. Standardize each lead as instructed by your teacher.
    e. Record 8 to 10 inches for each lead.
14. Turn on machine. A light will come on if the machine is on.
15. Turn lead selector switch to standardization position and quickly press standardization button.
16. Turn lead selector to an off position.
17. Check standardization mark on EKG paper. If machine is operating correctly, this mark will be 10 small blocks high, or 2 large blocks high. Press standardization button as you run each lead.
18. Label each lead if the machine does not automatically.
19. Turn lead selector to lead I and run an 8- to 10-inch strip.
20. Repeat step 19 for leads II and III.
21. Repeat step 19 for AVL, AVR, and AVF, but run only 4- to 6-inch strips.
22. Place brown chest leads in the following locations on the chest wall. After each placement, standardize and run a 4- to 6-inch strip.
    a. V1: fourth intercostal space just to the right of the sternum
    b. V2: fourth intercostal space just to the left of the sternum
    c. V3: midway between position of the fourth and fifth intercostal spaces
    d. V4: fifth intercostal space
    e. V5: same level as V4 and just anterior of midaxillary line
    f. V6: same level as V4 and V5 at midaxillary line
23. Turn off machine.
24. Remove all leads and electrodes.

PROCEDURE 17.2 | USING A SINGLE-LEAD ELECTROCARDIOGRAPH *(Continued)*

25. Clean remaining gel or paste from skin.
26. Assist client in dressing if necessary.
27. Label EKG with patient's name and physician's name.
28. Clean electrodes thoroughly so that machine is ready for the next procedure.
29. Mount EKG and deliver as instructed for interpretation. (See the procedure "Mounting EKGs.")

10/03/03   1000
ECG recorded
Tolerated well
ECG mounted and placed in chart
———— G. Jones CMA

⬤ ARTIFACTS

Artifacts are unwanted marks on the electrocardiogram. These marks are caused not by heart activity but by another source of electrical activity. These unwanted marks make it difficult to read the EKG. There are three common causes:

1. *Alternating-current (AC) interference* occurs when there is an electrical leak from equipment nearby (see Figure 17.20).

Common Causes	**Remedies**
Improper grounding	Check to be certain that equipment is grounded.
Other equipment leaking electricity	Turn off nearby equipment and unplug.
Lead wires crossed and not pointed toward the hands and feet	Adjust the position of the lead wire.
Corroded or dirty electrodes	Clean the electrodes.

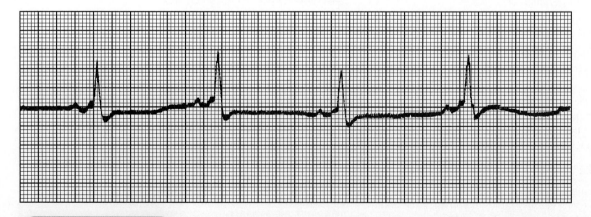

Figure 17.20

AC (60-cycle) interference.

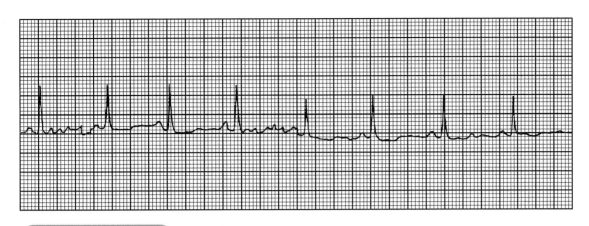

Figure 17.21

Somatic/muscle tremors.

2. *Somatic (body) tremors* can be recognized by a "quivering" baseline (Figure 17.21).

Common Causes	Remedies
Shivering or tense muscles	Warm the patient if cold; reassure if frightened.
Moving or talking	Refrain from moving and talking.
Nervous disorders	Place the patient's hands under the hips to help control tremors.

3. A *wandering baseline* can be recognized because it drifts away from the center of the graph paper (Figure 17.22).

Common Causes	Remedies
Old conductive solution or too little solution	Use fresh solution and apply an adequate amount.

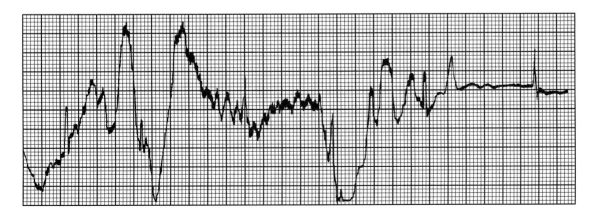

Figure 17.22

Wandering baseline.

Common Causes	Remedies
Improperly applied electrodes	Be certain that the electrodes are not too loose or too tight.
Corroded or dirty electrodes	Keep the electrodes clean.
Lead wires that are pulling on electrodes	Remove tension from the lead wire.
Creams or lotions on the skin under the electrodes	Clean the skin properly.

MOUNTING THE EKG/ECG

Mounting the EKG/ECG strips and submitting them to the physician for interpretation is the final step of the ECG procedures.

PROCEDURE 17.3

MOUNTING EKGS

RATIONALE

Correct mounting of EKG strips ensures that the reading is correct and that the diagnosis is accurate.

There are a variety of standard mount forms used in medicine. Mount the EKG records according to the physician's preference or the standard form used in your facility. Regardless of the form used, there are a few important steps you must follow in mounting every EKG.

1. Neatly trim strips to fit in space provided.
2. Include any unusual-looking complexes in the mounted strip.

3. Fill in the appropriate blanks on the form portion of mount.
4. Sign your name and deliver the completed EKG to the appropriate person for interpretation.

> 10/04/03   1300
> EKG mounted and delivered to Dr.
> Brown's office
> _____ S. Jones CMA

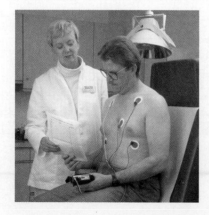

The medical assistant shows the client the diary and gives instructions regarding the Holter monitor before securing it around the patient's waist.

HOLTER MONITORING

Patients who experience occasional chest pain or discomfort without EKG/ECG changes are often tested with a Holter monitor. A Holter monitor is small and easy to carry. The wires are bulky but painless. A small recording device is carried on a strap around the waist or in a shoulder strap (Figure 17.23). Five electrodes are placed on the chest (Figure 17.24). The Holter records all heart activity during the time it is attached to the patient. The patient is instructed to follow routine activities. Instruct the patient that if pain, discomfort, or any symptoms occur, he or she should

1. Push the event button on the monitor.
2. Document in the diary the time of the event and the length of time that the symptoms last.

The physician determines when the client returns to have the monitor and electrodes removed. The recording cassette is removed and placed in a computerized analyzer, where a printout is made from the recording. The printout is analyzed by the physician, who determines treatment or need for additional testing. See the Holter monitor procedure for step-by-step directions in applying the monitor and electrodes.

Being an EKG/ECG technician is an important job on the health care team. You must follow the steps carefully, or the strip that you run will not be accurate and could cause the physician to make a mistake in the diagnosis and treatment. Learn all the steps, and practice until they are very familiar to you. Follow the instructions in the ECG/EKG procedure.

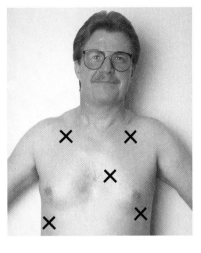

Figure 17.24

Anatomical placement of chest electrodes for Holter monitoring.

PROCEDURE 17.4 | USING THE HOLTER MONITOR

RATIONALE

The Holter monitor records the patient's heart activity. This device is worn by the patient for an extended time. The monitor must be securely placed and programmed to ensure that the reading is correct.

ALERT: Follow Standard Precautions.

1. Wash hands.
2. Assemble equipment.
    a. Prejelled adhesive electrodes
    b. Holter monitor with lead wires
    c. Alcohol wipes
    d. Monitor belt
    e. Razor and shaving cream
    f. Cassette and batteries
    g. Diary for patient records
    h. Nonallergic tape to secure electrodes if needed
    i. Patient's medical record
    j. Pen
    k. Patient gown for women
3. Explain what you are going to do, and show monitor and leads to patient.
4. Ask client to remove clothes from the waist up. Provide a gown for women, instructing them to place the opening in front.
5. Test monitor for proper operation and insert new batteries each time you apply monitor.
6. Shave chest at electrode placement sites if necessary.
7. Rub electrode sites with gauze to prepare skin for good contact.
8. Place electrodes as indicated in Figure 17.24. Follow manufacturer's instructions for details.
9. Place monitor belt with monitor in place around patient's waist or over the shoulder.
10. Instruct client in care of monitor according to manufacturer's instructions.
11. Give patient the diary and instruct him or her to follow a normal routine. If pain, discomfort, or any symptoms should occur, the patient is to
    a. Push event button on monitor.
    b. Document in diary time of event and length of time that symptoms last.
12. Assist client in dressing.
13. Wash hands.

PROCEDURE 17.4 | USING THE HOLTER MONITOR *(Continued)*

14. Record the following in patient medical record:
    a. Date and time monitor was applied
    b. What instructions were given to patient; initial
15. Schedule client for a return visit.

To Remove Monitor:

16. Wash hands.
17. Assist client in removing clothes from the waist up.
18. Remove monitor strap, electrodes, and wires.
19. Clean skin at electrode sites.

20. Assist patient in dressing if necessary.
21. Collect diary from patient.
22. Instruct client according to physician's orders.
23. Wash hands.
24. Place diary in patient's medical record and record time monitor was returned; initial.
25. Place cassette in analyzer for reading.
26. When printout is received from analyzer, attach to medical record, initial, and send or give to physician.

10/04/03   1400
Holter monitor placed and programmed
Instructions given for Holter and diary
Return appointment made
_____ S. Jones CMA

10/05/03   1300
Holter monitor removed and diary placed
in patient chart
Delivered to physician
_____ S. Jones CMA

○ JOBS AND PROFESSIONS

- Assistive personnel
- Nurse assistant
- Clinical medical assistant
- Licensed vocational/practical nurse
- Registered nurse
- Cardiology technician
- Paramedic

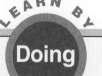

LEARN BY Doing

1. Complete Worksheets 1 and 2 and Worksheet/Activity 3 as assigned.
2. Practice the procedures.
3. Prepare responses to each item in Chapter Review—Your Link to Success at the end of this chapter.
4. When you are confident that you can meet each objective, ask your instructor for the unit evaluation.

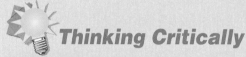 **Thinking Critically**

1. Time Management Describe a patient transfer and set up a plan that will reduce the possibility of a "quivering" baseline when an EKG is given.

2. Cultural Competency Identify cultures that may object to a male technician performing an ECG/EKG on a female. Explain ways to prevent or eliminate alarm or conflict.

3. Patient Education Prepare some diary samples documenting events to show to patients who will be wearing a Holter monitor.

4. Medical Math ECG/EKG graph paper can be run through the EKG machine at different speeds. The standard speed is 25 mm per second. Use Figures 17.5 and 17.6 to determine how fast the pulse rate is in Figure 17.6.

5. Case Study Mrs. Marcolis refuses to allow you to place the electrodes on her chest. She is sure that those "new-fangled machines" will electrocute her. She has been having a lot of chest pain, and the doctor wants to determine if there are changes to her EKG that indicate heart damage. She tells you that this is exactly why she hasn't been to a doctor in 50 years: "The doctors always want to do all these silly tests." You have explained everything about the test very carefully. What can you do to ensure that she allows you to complete the test?

 Portfolio Connection

Once you attain competence as an ECG/EKG technician, ask for permission to copy an electrocardiogram that is mounted and ready for the medical record. (Remove all patient identifiers.) Place this copy in your portfolio as evidence of your skills. Place a copy of your on-site trainer's evaluation in your portfolio.

Write a paper describing your doubts and realizations and the barriers that you were able to overcome during the electrocardiography experience. For example, were you afraid that you couldn't learn to use the equipment? Describe the ways you plan to use the skills, information, and insights that you gained about people and this job. This assignment must be in standard report format.

Participate in a job shadowing to help determine your interest in being an Electrocardiogram technician.

Portfolio Tip

When patients question the need for tests, it often means they are afraid. Always be mentally ready to explain what will happen during a test and to answer questions about the procedure.

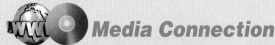

Remember! **Media Connection**

Use the Companion Website **www.prenhall.com/badasch** and the CD-ROM for additional interactive learning activities.

Chapter 18

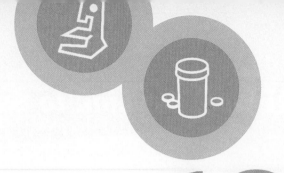

Laboratory Assistant/ Medical Assistant Laboratory Skills; Phlebotomist

MEDIA CONNECTION

Use the Companion Website **www.prenhall.com/badasch** and the CD-ROM for additional interactive learning activities.

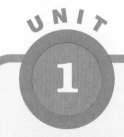

UNIT 1

Laboratory Skills

STEPS TO SUCCESS

1. Complete Vocabulary Worksheet 1 in the Student Workbook.

2. Read this unit.

3. Complete the Learn by Doing assignment at the end of this Unit.

UNIT OBJECTIVES

When you have completed this unit, you will be able to do the following:

✔ Complete all objectives in Part One of this book.

✔ Match vocabulary words with their correct meanings.

✔ Follow 12 general laboratory guidelines.

✔ Practice laboratory safety.

✔ Practice aseptic technique.

✔ Demonstrate loading and operating an autoclave.

✔ Dispose of hazardous materials according to facility policy.

✔ List six ways that laboratory tests help the physician.

✔ Identify information required on all laboratory slips.

✔ Discuss the importance of advance preparation for laboratory tests.

- ✔ List eight types of specimen studies.
- ✔ Identify general rules for testing specimens.
- ✔ List three methods for testing specimens.
- ✔ Discuss quality control in the laboratory.
- ✔ Label a diagram of a microscope.
- ✔ List five ways to prevent loss of your specimen in a centrifuge.
- ✔ Identify steps to acquire a midstream clean-catch urine specimen for male and female.
- ✔ Define *urinary sediment.*
- ✔ List three infectious diseases that can be diagnosed with a sputum test.
- ✔ Explain the reason for testing stool specimens for occult blood.
- ✔ Demonstrate the following:
  - Obtaining a throat culture
  - Preparing a direct smear
  - Streaking an agar plate
  - Preparing a slide from culture grown in an agar plate
  - Gram staining a slide

- ✔ Identify seven items learned from a CBC.
- ✔ Explain why a hematocrit and hemoglobin test are important.
- ✔ Explain the reason for blood glucose testing.
- ✔ Explain the importance of counting WBCs and RBCs.
- ✔ State reasons for doing a WBC differential.
- ✔ List the four blood types.
- ✔ Explain agglutination.
- ✔ Explain an erythrocyte sedimentation rate.
- ✔ Identify the tests done in blood chemistries.
- ✔ Demonstrate the following:
  - Finger stick
  - Hematocrit test
  - Blood glucose test with a glucose meter
  - Diluting blood cells with an Unopette
  - Preparing a blood smear slide
  - Completing a differential white cell count
  - Typing your blood
  - Determining the erythrocyte sedimentation rate

● RESPONSIBILITIES OF A LABORATORY ASSISTANT/MEDICAL ASSISTANT

Laboratory assistants/medical assistants perform a variety of tests. Some of the tests are highly technical: laboratory assistants/medical assistants run tests that assist in diagnosing an illness or disease. Their duties include the following:

- Cleaning laboratory equipment
- Preparing cleaning solutions
- Drying glassware and instruments using a cloth, hot air dryer, or acetone bath
- Examining clean equipment for cracks or chips
- Operating an autoclave to sterilize equipment
- Preparing stains, solutions, and culture media
- Counting blood cells
- Separating plasma from whole blood using a centrifuge
- Incubating cultures
- Using computerized test equipment to test blood specimens
- Performing venipuncture with a Vacutainer™ and/or a needle and syringe
- Monitoring control tests
- Performing laboratory tests on stool, urine, blood, and sputum
- Preparing specimens for processing
- Giving patients instructions for specimen collection or self-testing

Importance of Laboratory Tests

Laboratory tests are important because they are

- A valuable diagnostic tool
- Used to monitor the amount of medication a patient has in his or her system (therapeutic drug level)
- A measure of the body's chemical balance that compares blood and urine samples with normal test values
- A way to use blood and urine tests to diagnose a certain disease or condition

CLIA (see below) periodically sends tests to labs for reading. Tests are returned to CLIA to confirm the laboratory's readings. This is CLIA's quality control on laboratories.

◯ LABORATORY STANDARDS

Medical laboratories and medical offices that perform lab tests on human specimens are regulated by a federal amendment called the Clinical Laboratory Improvement Amendment of 1988 (or CLIA). CLIA sets standards and regulates all laboratories, physicians' offices, and other labs that use human specimens to diagnose, prevent, or treat disease.

As a laboratory assistant/medical assistant you can perform simple tests allowed by CLIA. The lab or medical office must have a CLIA waiver certificate before you perform these tests. The tests include the following:

- Dipstick or tablet reagent urinalysis for bilirubin, glucose, hemoglobin, ketone, leukocytes, nitrite, pH, protein, urobilinogen, specific gravity
- Ovulation tests: visual color test to tell if human luteinizing hormone is present
- Urine pregnancy tests: visual color comparison test
- Erythrocyte sedimentation rate (nonautomated)
- Hemoglobin copper sulfate (nonautomated)
- Fecal occult blood
- Spun microhematocrit
- Blood glucose by glucose monitoring devices cleared by the Food and Drug Administration for home use

Do not perform these tests unless you know that there is a waiver certificate and you have been trained properly.

uniformity

A state of being all the same; does not vary.

Operating a laboratory with **uniformity** and maintaining standards of measure quality are important. People who work in the laboratory must follow the same guidelines that all laboratory workers follow. These guidelines are as follows:

- Clean and cover microscope daily according to manufacturer's guidelines.
- Maintain all infection control logs.
- Report all defective equipment immediately to your supervisor.
- Maintain and observe quality control logs.
- Follow all directions to ensure accurate results from each test.
  - • Refrigerate promptly. • Transport specimens in racks. • Follow instructions when watching for serum separation. • Instruct patients in proper collection of all specimens. • Use appropriate technique with all specimen collections.
- Check temperatures of appliances daily.
- Learn new techniques for testing new material or equipment changes.

- Check expiration dates of all reagents and testing kits weekly.
- Do quality control checks on all testing materials and equipment following manufacturer's directions and CLIA standards.
- Ask the supervisor for help when in doubt regarding any procedure or result.
- Recognize the importance of correct and accurate test results for doctors.
- Report all "stats" immediately.

The medical laboratory is an environment with hazards. The laboratory assistant/ medical assistant or anyone working with laboratory tests must be aware of possible dangers. In the laboratory, you work with patient specimens that must be treated as **hazardous** materials. You also work with various chemicals that can react when mixed together. Some of these chemicals are harmful to the skin, eyes, and/or the respiratory system. To be safe in the laboratory:

hazardous
Dangerous.

- Learn safety measures and follow them carefully.
- Always follow Standard Precautions (review in Chapter 12).

General Safety Practice Guidelines: Personal Safety
The protective equipment you wear includes the following:

- A nonpermeable lab coat to protect your clothes
- Safety eye goggles/glasses to guard your eyes from splashes
- Gloves to keep you from being contaminated by infectious material
- A rubber apron to protect you from **acids** that can spill or splash
- Metal tongs when working with hot objects

acids
Substances that cause the urine to have an acid pH.

Other safety considerations are as follows:

- Never use your mouth to pipette.
- Do not eat, drink, or apply makeup in the laboratory area.
- Flush eyes first, then report eye contamination immediately to supervisor for eye treatment.
- Dispose of all broken glass, needles, or other sharp objects in a sharps container.
- Do not bend, break, or recap needles.
- Follow Standard Precautions and consider all specimens as highly infectious.
- Disinfect counters, surfaces, and equipment daily.

Fire Prevention
- Locate the fire extinguisher.
- Participate in fire drills.
- Report all potential electrical hazards to the supervisor immediately.
- Use grounded plugs for equipment.

Additional Safety Practice Guidelines
- Clearly label and date all **reagents.**
- Label all waste containers with a biohazard symbol.
- Complete incident reports:
  - • Incident or injury to patients or self • Chemical spills • Electrical or fire hazards
- Keep trash from building up in any area.

reagents
Chemical substances that react to the presence of other substances in the blood and urine.

Figure 18.1

Autoclave.

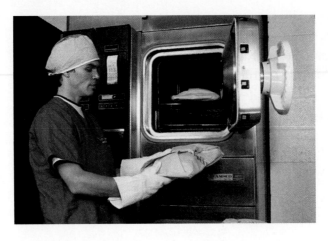

- Keep all posters and decorations away from lights and vents.
- Inspect areas where heating elements are used for possible fire hazards.
- Keep spills wiped up and use a disinfectant when necessary.
- Discard any rag with a flammable substance on it in a metal container with a self-closing lid.

Sterilization

You must sterilize all items in the laboratory that have contact with body tissue or fluids. The most effective way to sterilize equipment is in an autoclave (see Figure 18.1 and Chapter 20). The autoclave produces steam under pressure. The high heat of the steam kills organisms that cause disease. Keep items that you are sterilizing in the autoclave for the specified length of time to ensure that all microorganisms are killed. The autoclave is a heavy piece of equipment with a chamber that withstands high degrees of temperature and a great deal of pressure. Steam under pressure can burn skin, hair, and eyes. Always follow these basic rules when operating an autoclave:

1. Read the directions for the autoclave you are using.
2. Use protective gloves when placing articles in an autoclave or taking them out.
3. Protect yourself if the autoclave is hot from recent use.
4. Do not overload. If you pack material into the autoclave too tightly, the steam cannot circulate and the items will not be sterilized.
5. Allow the temperature and pressure to return to normal before opening the autoclave when sterilization is complete.
6. Clean the autoclave according to the manufacturer's directions. (See Chapter 20 for additional information on sterilization.)

Items that you cannot reuse are not sterilized. Never put body tissue, body fluid, or any article that has been in contact with blood, body fluids, or tissues in the regular trash. Dispose of them in a biohazard container following your facility's policies. All health care workers have the responsibility to protect themselves and others.

The increased concerns over hazardous and/or toxic materials in all areas of work create the need for strict guidelines to protect people. The federal Occupational Safety and Health Administration (OSHA) provides guidelines to help ensure safety. Your laboratory supervisor has these guidelines in a notebook with material safety data sheets (MSDS; see Figure 13.1). The MSDS forms follow OSHA guidelines by explaining how to dispose of and handle hazardous materials safely. The sheets also describe possible physical symptoms of overexposure and proper first-aid treatment if exposed. Ingredients of the hazardous product are also identified on MSDS forms. It is important to follow the general guidelines above and check the MSDS for specific information on each substance.

Contaminated/Hazardous Material

Specimens being analyzed in the laboratory come from patients. The physician often does not know what is causing a client's illness, so you must treat every specimen as though it is contaminated and potentially hazardous. *Always follow Standard Precautions.* When you work in a laboratory or medical office, you must practice good aseptic technique at all times. The most important steps include washing your hands before and after each procedure. Always wear gloves when working with specimens.

Biohazardous Waste Containers

In the medical setting, you must dispose of all contaminated biohazardous materials in biohazardous waste containers. The laboratory containers are lined with red plastic. Put all discarded contaminated/biohazardous materials in the red-lined containers marked "Biohazardous." Empty all containers at the end of each shift or when full. Carefully tie the bag and be certain that it will stay closed. Mark the tied bag "Biohazardous." Reline the container with a new red bag. Place the marked bag in a red sealed container for pickup. Handle all contaminated/hazardous materials according to OSHA guidelines. Never mix them with ordinary trash.

LABORATORY TESTS

Laboratory workers are responsible for testing specimens. The most common specimens include urine, blood, sputum, and stool. The results of these tests provide information about the patient's health. This information helps

- Diagnose the illness
- Determine the cause of the illness
- Confirm a diagnosis
- Evaluate progress
- Regulate treatment
- Establish a baseline for future tests

Guidelines for Laboratory Tests

When you receive a laboratory request, check it for all information. This information includes

- Client's name and address
- Client's age and sex
- Name of test requested
- Time and date of collection
- Physician's name and address
- Method of collection
- Possible diagnosis
- Type and source of specimen
- Medications the patient is taking
- Stat or routine tests

Preparation of Patients/Clients

There are many different kinds of laboratory tests. Some of the tests require very specific preparation. The results of some tests are affected by medication, food, time of day, and type of activity. Know the advance preparation for each test. If you are not certain about preparation, look it up in the procedures manual. Instruct the patient to follow the preparation orders exactly. Advance preparation may include

- **Fasting.** Eating before some tests changes the results of the test (e.g., fasting blood sugar [FBS], glucose tolerance test [GTT], SMA-12 profile). During fasting, patients must not eat or drink fluid (except water). They usually fast for 12 to 14 hours before the test.

■ **Medication restriction.** Many medications can change the chemical and physical qualities of the specimen. The patient needs special instruction if taking medications that can change test results. Medication affects urine specimens more than it affects blood. If the patient can be off the medication without causing injury, the medication is stopped 48 to 72 hours before the tests. The physician makes this decision.

Analyzing Specimens

There are many different studies that help identify and diagnose physical problems.

■ **Urinalysis.** Examines urine chemically, physically, and microscopically.

■ **Hematology.** Examines blood for disease conditions.

■ **Microbiology.** Identifies pathogens in the body.

■ **Histology.** Studies body tissues microscopically to detect diseased tissues.

■ **Cytology.** Examines cells microscopically to discover abnormal cells.

■ **Clinical chemistry.** Examines substances in body fluids, feces, tissues.

■ **Serology and blood banking.** Studies antigen-antibody reactions to discover presence of foreign substance or disease.

■ **Parasitology.** Determines parasite that is causing illness.

General Rules for Testing the Specimen

There are basic steps to follow for testing all specimens.

1. Measure the amount of specimen required for the test carefully. This is very specific.
2. Combine the correct chemical reagent for the test with the specimen.
3. Process the specimen correctly (e.g., centrifuge, heat in a water bath, incubate, heat fix, etc.).
4. Assess the sample by manual or automatic method.
5. Calculate results by hand or machine.
6. Record all the information on the lab report sheet, including
   a. Patient's name, b. Age and sex, c. Time and date, d. Source of specimen, e. Name of test completed, f. Results of test, g. Name of classification

Always follow the approved procedure in your facility.

Methods of Testing Specimens

The *manual method* requires carefully following a series of steps. Some small labs and physicians' offices use manual methods for simple tests (e.g., urinalysis).

Semiautomated analysis is a combination of manual and automated testing (e.g., glucose monitor). To perform a glucose test, you stick the finger to get blood. The glucose monitor measures the glucose in the blood. *Automatic analyzers* can do more than one specimen at a time. These analyzers measure the specimen, add reagent, process the specimen, and give the results.

Quality Control for Specimen Testing

There must be a method for quality control when performing laboratory tests. Performing these test controls tells you that the test is accurate. Quality control helps ensure that the test result is a true picture of the patient's condition. Some tests have the control built in. When the information is reliable, the physician can make a diagnosis. Quality control methods include

- Discarding outdated reagents
- Following the procedure for exact testing
- Routinely verifying that laboratory equipment is reading specimens accurately
- Maintaining equipment by having it serviced routinely

Quality control includes keeping accurate logs. The log includes important information about the test (e.g., expiration date, lot number, date tested, and pass/fail of control). You must initial each test in the log.

⦾ LABORATORY EQUIPMENT

There are many kinds of laboratory equipment. The simple microscope and centrifuge are found in all laboratories. Some equipment is more complicated than others; for example, very advanced computers and analyzers.

Microscope

The microscope is an important tool that magnifies and enlarges objects (see Figure 18.2). You use it to see microorganisms and other components that are too small to see without magnification. The ability to see these components helps find the cause of illnesses. Learning to use the microscope is necessary for laboratory workers.

How to Use a Microscope

There are different types of microscopes. Some microscopes have one eyepiece. These are **monocular** microscopes. Microscopes with two eyepieces are **biocular.**

Basic Parts of the Microscope

- **Base.** Supports the microscope; it keeps the microscope from falling over.
- **Arm.** Supports the eyepiece and is used to carry the microscope.
- **Stage.** Holds slides that are put on the stage after you prepare them.
- **Slide clips.** Hold the prepared slide in place.

monocular
Having one eyepiece.

biocular
Having two eyepieces.

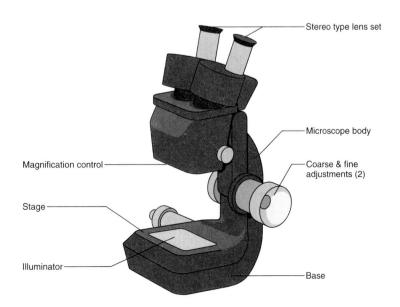

Figure 18.2

Microscope.

Stereo type lens set

Microscope body

Coarse & fine adjustments (2)

Magnification control

Stage

Illuminator

Base

■ **Iris diaphragm.** Adjusts the amount of light that enters the microscope through the opening in the stage.

■ **Mirror or illumination light.** Provides light so that you can see the object on the slide. You control the amount of light with the iris diaphragm. When you use a mirror, you turn the mirror to pick up a light source and *reflect* it into the microscope.

■ **Eyepiece.** Lets you see the object on the slide. Some microscopes have eyepieces that magnify to 10 times (10×), others to 20 times (20×).

■ **Objectives.** Magnify what you have on the slide. Most microscopes have three objectives. The most common objectives are

• High-power objectives that magnify the objects 40 times (40×). • Medium-power objectives that magnify the object 10 times (10×). • Low-power objectives that magnify 4 times (4×). • Oil immersion: the oil immersion objective magnifies 95× to 100×. You put a drop of oil on a specimen that is dark and hard to see. The oil concentrates the light and makes the specimen easier to see.

■ **Body tube.** Connects the eyepiece to the objectives, which are on the revolving nosepiece.

■ **Revolving nosepiece.** The objectives are attached to the revolving nosepiece. You turn it to place the objective over the specimen.

PROCEDURE 18.1

USING A MICROSCOPE

RATIONALE
Proper care and use of the microscope prevents errors.

ALERT: Follow Standard Precautions.

1. Assemble equipment.
   a. Microscope
   b. Lens paper
   c. Slides and slide cover
   d. Specimen
   e. Oil if using oil immersion
2. Wash hands.
3. Place specimen (e.g., hair, scraping from under nails, scraping from tooth) on clean slide (one drop only if liquid specimen).
4. Add required solution.
5. Drop clean slide cover over specimen.
6. Clean eyepiece with lens paper.
7. Clean objectives with lens paper.
8. Turn on illuminating light.
9. Open iris diaphragm.
10. Turn revolving nosepiece to low-power objective.

11. Place slide on stage under slide clips.
12. Turn coarse adjustment knob to move objective close to slide.
13. Look into eyepiece and turn coarse adjustment to move tube upward until you focus specimen.
14. Turn fine-adjustment knob until specimen is clear and focused.
15. Continue steps 12 through 14 using higher objectives until you have best possible focus for specimen.
16. Observe specimen. If setup is for technician or physician, tell that person that slide is ready.
17. Remove slide after it is read.
18. Discard slide according to procedure in your facility.
19. Clean lens and objective with lens paper.
20. Turn off illuminating light.
21. Fill out lab slips according to your facility's policies.

How to Determine Total Magnification of the Specimen

Specimens are very small samples. It is important to know how many times the specimen is magnified. To determine how many times the specimen is magnified, multiply the power of the eyepiece by the power of the objective. For example:

Power of eyepiece 10×
Power of objective 4×
10 × 4 = 40

This means that the specimen is enlarged 40 times its actual size.

NOTE Always remember to record patient's name, account number, date, time, physician's name, type of test, results of test. Always sign with your name and certification.

There are both a coarse adjustment and a fine adjustment on the microscope:

- **Coarse adjustment.** Upper knob on the arm, which moves the objectives up and down. This helps you put the specimen in rough focus.
- **Fine adjustment.** Lower, smaller knob, which moves the objective more slowly. This helps you have a clear image of the specimen (see Figure 18.2).

The microscope must be taken care of. Remember to

- Use special lens paper to clean the eyepiece, or you will scratch the lens.
- Watch the objectives when you move them up and down. This prevents damaging the objectives or breaking the slide.
- Cover the microscope when you are not using it. This keeps out dust.
- Keep the microscope in a safe place where it cannot be knocked to the floor (see the procedure "Using a Microscope").

Centrifuge

The centrifuge is a device that spins at high speed. As the centrifuge spins, it separates heavy or solid components from liquid. The heavy or solid components move to the lower part of the container. This separation allows you to study all components of the specimen. There is one type of centrifuge to process urine and blood in a test tube (Figure 18.3) and another type to process blood in a capillary tube.

Guidelines for Using a Centrifuge

- Counterbalance the tube by placing another tube directly opposite it. This tube must contain a liquid of equal weight. You can usually use water.
- Do not use cracked or scratched tubes. If the tube breaks, the specimen will spill out.
- Turn off centrifuge immediately if a tube breaks.
- Put on rubber gloves and clean the centrifuge.
- Follow the instruction in each procedure for using the centrifuge.

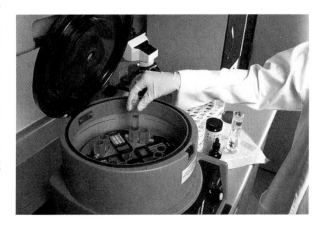

Figure 18.3

Examples of a centrifuge used for blood and for urine.

◉ URINALYSIS

A routine urinalysis provides information about the patient. The urinalysis gives the physician information about the physical, chemical, and microscopic characteristics of the urine. This information tells many different things about the patient's health.

Urine Collection

Proper urine collection is important. The way you collect the urine affects the test. The following are some general guidelines for urine collection:

- Use a clean, dry container.
- A specimen over 32 hours old may give inaccurate test results.
- Refrigerate it and write the collection time on the label if it is necessary to keep a specimen over 2 hours.
- If possible, collect on-site for immediate testing.

Reagent Strips

Your facility may use reagent strips and/or other individual tests. Always follow the procedures of your facility.

Reagent strips have small pads that react to a specific substance. When you dip the strip in a fresh urine sample, there is a chemical reaction. Carefully match the reagent strip with the color chart on the container label. The procedure for using all reagent strips is similar.

Guidelines for Using Reagent Strips

- Check the bottle for an expiration date.
- Keep the bottle in a cool, dry area with the top tightly closed. (Do not refrigerate.)
- Check the strips for a change in color. A tan-to-brown color change indicates deterioration. Do not use the strips.
- Keep the specimen container clean.
- Use freshly voided urine. Urine over 2 hours old gives poor results. Refrigerate if it stands more than 2 hours.
- A clean-catch urine is best for determining leukocytes.
- First urine in the morning is best for determining nitrates.
- Match colors on strips to the color chart on the label. Follow the times on the label carefully.
- Write the type of strips used when recording the type of test.

Microscopic Examination of the Urine

provider 🔊

Physician, physician assistant, nurse practitioner.

Urinary sediment contains the solid materials in the urine. There are many components in the sediment that help the **provider** confirm or determine a diagnosis. The sediment may contain renal or kidney cells, casts, crystals, bacteria, parasites, mucus, or other substances. The sediment settles to the bottom of a centrifuged urine specimen. A small sample of the sediment is placed on a slide for the provider to look at. The provider looks for a cause of illness (e.g., bacteria causing a bladder infection, renal cells indicating renal damage, or red blood cells from irritation). Spinning urine (centrifuging) will be one of your duties.

PROCEDURE 18.2

USING REAGENT STRIPS TO TEST URINE

RATIONALE

Careful testing with reagent strips and accurate reporting of information are essential to reach a correct diagnosis. Al- ways use the proper techniques to prevent contamination of the specimen.

ALERT: Follow Standard Precautions.

1. Wash hands.
2. Assemble equipment.
   a. Reagent strips and bottle
   b. Laboratory report slip
   c. Watch
   d. Urine specimen
   e. Disposable nonsterile gloves
3. Complete laboratory slip.
   a. Name
   b. Sex
   c. Age
   d. Physician
   e. Date
   f. Type of test
4. Put on gloves.
5. Hold specimen to light and observe:
   a. Color (colorless, yellow, light yellow, brown, or- ange, etc.)
   b. Clarity (clear, hazy, cloudy)
6. Write color and clarity on lab slip.
7. Open reagent jar and remove one strip.
   a. Note expiration date. *Do not use if expired.*
   b. Replace jar cover immediately.

8. Hold strip by clear end and immerse in urine.
9. Remove strip immediately by pulling gently over lip of tube to remove excess urine.
10. Hold strip in horizontal position to prevent mixing of chemicals.
11. Hold strip close to color blocks on bottle label and match carefully.
12. Read strip at time indicated and record results.

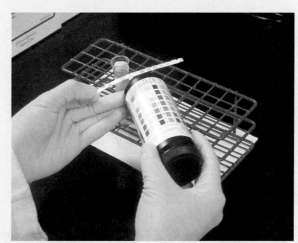

13. Discard reagent strip in biohazard waste.
14. Clean and replace equipment.
15. Remove gloves.
16. Wash hands.
17. Record required information.
18. Report any abnormal results to supervisor immedi- ately.

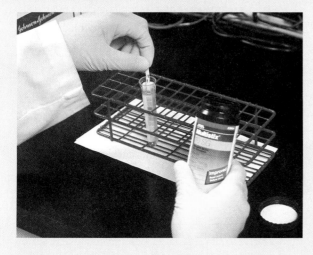

1/03/03	0700
	Reagent strip test, pH 7,
	Protein: Pos., Glucose: 1%, Ketones:
	Tr., Blood: Neg. Positive protein and
	trace blood reported to health care
	provider
	_____ g. Jones Lab Asst.

Special Urine Tests

Measuring Specific Gravity

You can measure specific gravity on a reagent stick. The urinometer is another simple way to check specific gravity. Specific gravity gives the dilution of urine. The normal range for specific gravity of urine is 1.010 to 1.025. An abnormal reading that is not within the range indicates possible problems. High specific gravity is above 1.025. Concentrated (heavy) urine may be caused by dehydration, sugar in the urine from diabetes mellitus, and too many substances in the urine due to kidney disease. Low specific gravity is below 1.010. Diluted urine may be caused by diabetes insipidus, diuretic medications, and kidney disease when unable to concentrate the urine. Specific gravity can also be measured with a refractometer.

Pregnancy Tests

The physician may request a pregnancy test for several reasons, including the following:

- To begin prenatal care early in pregnancy
- To make certain that medication that causes fetal damage is not given
- To prevent the use of procedures that may cause injury to the fetus

A common test for determining pregnancy is a simple urine test. The test is performed on a concentrated urine specimen. The urine is tested for a hormone called hu-

---

PROCEDURE 18.3

MEASURING SPECIFIC GRAVITY WITH URINOMETER

RATIONALE

Careful testing of specific gravity and accurate reporting of information are essential to reach a correct diagnosis. Al-ways use proper techniques to prevent contamination of the specimen.

ALERT: Follow Standard Precautions.

1. Wash hands.
2. Assemble equipment.
   a. Disposable gloves
   b. Glass cylinder (5 inches high)
   c. Urinometer
   d. Fresh urine specimen
3. Put on gloves.
4. Pour urine into cylinder to ¾ mark.
5. Place urinometer in urine.
6. Spin urinometer gently.
7. Place cylinder with lower line of meniscus at eye level.
8. Read specific gravity:
   a. Look at point where lowest part of meniscus crosses urinometer scale.
   b. Read gauge on nearest line.

9. Record reading to enter in computer or on lab slip.
10. Discard urine according to facility's contaminated waste policy.
11. Rinse urinometer with water and dry.
12. Rinse cylinder with water and dry.
13. Remove gloves and discard in contaminated waste.
14. Wash hands.
15. Record specific gravity in computer or on lab list.
16. Document according to facility procedure.

1/01/03	0800
	Sp Gr 1.011
	———— S. Jones MA

PROCEDURE 18.4 MEASURING SPECIFIC GRAVITY WITH REFRACTOMETER

RATIONALE

Careful testing of specific gravity and accurate reporting of information are essential to reach a correct diagnosis. Always use proper techniques to prevent contamination of the specimen.

ALERT: Follow Standard Precautions.

---

1. Wash hands.
2. Assemble equipment
   a. Disposable gloves
   b. Refractometer
   c. Distilled water
   d. Fresh urine sample
3. Put on gloves.
4. Place one drop of distilled water on the glass plate.
5. Close lid.
6. Look through eyepiece to read specific gravity.

NOTE   Make sure it reads 1.000. If reading is not 1.000, follow manufacturer's directions to recalibrate refractometer.

7. Transfer one drop of well-mixed urine onto glass plate of refractometer.

8. Close lid.
9. Look through eyepiece to read specific gravity.
10. Record reading to enter in computer or on lab slip.
11. Discard urine according to facility's contaminated waste policy.
12. Clean refractometer according to manufacturer's directions.
13. Remove gloves and discard in contaminated waste.
14. Wash hands.
15. Record specific gravity in computer or on lab list.

10/10/03   0800
Sp. gravity 1.040, reported to lab tech
_____ S. Jones Lab Asst.

---

man chorionic gonadotropin (HCG). This hormone is produced by the developing fertilized egg. Some of the hormone is secreted into the urine and blood. It is very important to read the manufacturer's instructions carefully before completing a pregnancy test.

To perform an accurate pregnancy test, follow these guidelines:

- Use clean urine containers to collect urine.
- Use the first voided morning specimen for the highest accumulation of HCG.
- Check the specific gravity. If it is less than 1.010, the urine is too dilute.
- Have the urine specimen at room temperature.
- Follow the manufacturer's instructions for storing the reagents.
- Do not use reagents after the expiration date.
- Do not contaminate the specimen.

Testing Urine for Drugs

The collection of urine to determine drug use is becoming more and more common. Some reasons for drug testing:

- Employer requests a preemployment test.
- Department of Transportation requires testing of pilots, truck drivers, and others.
- Employer requests test for employee suspected of using drugs.

There are many strict rules that you *must* adhere to when you collect urine for drug testing. Follow the instructions and proceed step by step. *Be very exact.*

PROCEDURE 18.5

CENTRIFUGING A URINE SPECIMEN

RATIONALE

Careful centrifuging ensures that urine is properly concentrated for testing. Specimens must be properly prepared in order to achieve accurate results.

ALERT: Follow Standard Precautions.

1. Wash hands.
2. Assemble equipment.
   a. Centrifuge
   b. Two centrifuge tubes
   c. Microscope slide (number slide)
   d. Coverslip
   e. Pipette
   f. Disposable nonsterile gloves
   g. Urine specimen
3. Fill in lab slip:
   a. Name
   b. Date
   c. Time
4. Put on gloves.
5. Mix urine to suspend sediment.
6. Pour 10 mL of urine into centrifuge tube.
7. Put tube with urine into centrifuge.
8. Pour 10 mL of water into second centrifuge tube.
9. Place in centrifuge opposite the tube with urine.
10. Secure centrifuge lid.
11. Set centrifuge timer for 4 to 5 minutes. (Allow it to stop on its own.)
12. Remove tube with urine.
13. Carefully invert urine centrifuge tube quickly over sink to pour 9 mL of urine into sink.
14. Turn tube right side up immediately. (About 1.0 cc will remain in tube.)

15. Mix sediment by snapping end of centrifuge tube with finger.
16. Pipette 1 drop of urine on numbered slide.
17. Put on coverslip. (Redo if air bubbles appear under coverslip.)
18. Put slide on microscope stage.
19. Use 10× objective with coarse adjustment to focus on slide.
20. Adjust light source.
21. Follow your facility's policy for reading slide. (If setup is for technician, tell him or her that slide is ready.)
22. Remove slide after it is read.
23. Discard slide according to facility procedure.
24. Clean lens and objective with lens paper.
25. Clean equipment and replace equipment.
26. Remove gloves, and dispose of according to facility policy.
27. Wash hands.
28. Record results if you read the specimen.
29. Document according to facility procedure.

```
1/20/02    0745
   Microscopic Exam: epithelial:
   few/1pf, WBCs: 2-3, /hpf,
   RBCs: few/hpf, casts: neg.,
   crystals: few/hpf
            B Smith MA
```

Clean-Catch Collection

Clean-catch midstream urine collection has a specific procedure. The physician may order a clean-catch urine when he or she suspects that a urinary infection is present or for any urine test. The clean-catch method reduces possible contamination of the specimen. Clean the area around the meatus carefully to remove microorganisms. Collect the urine in a sterile cup using medical aseptic techniques. Pour off part of the specimen for the dipstick test and for spinning down when you

PROCEDURE 18.6

MIDSTREAM CLEAN-CATCH URINE, FEMALE

RATIONALE

Careful instruction of the patient/client helps prevent contaminating the specimen. A clean-catch specimen is essential to accurately diagnose and treat the patient.

ALERT: Follow Standard Precautions.

1. Wash hands.
2. Assemble equipment.
   a. Sterile urine container for clean catch
   b. Label
   c. Disposable antiseptic towelettes
   d. Disposable nonsterile gloves: wear if you handle cup with specimen.
3. Label container.
4. Instruct client to
   a. Wash hands.
   b. Remove container lid and place on counter with inside of lid facing up.
   c. Separate labia to expose meatus.
   d. Take towelette and wipe on side of urinary meatus from front to back.
   e. Dispose of towelette.
   f. Repeat with new towelette on other side.
   g. Wipe directly over meatus with new towelette.
   h. Continue to hold labia open.

   i. Urinate small amount into toilet.
   j. Stop stream.
   k. Place sterile container under meatus and void into container (60 cc).
   l. Stop stream.
   m. Remove container carefully.
   n. Empty bladder.
   o. Carefully replace lid.
   p. Wipe outside of container with paper towel.
   q. Put in designated area.

5. Put on gloves.
6. Finish testing as ordered (e.g., dipstick, set up microscopic exam, drug test).
7. Document procedure according to facility procedure.

10/10/03 0800
Instructed in correct procedure for
collecting clean catch
S. Jones CNA

collect a clean-catch urine. This leaves the urine in the specimen container uncontaminated. If necessary, you can use it for culture and sensitivity testing.

There are other urine specimen tests that may be ordered. Your facility has a procedure manual with instructions for each test that your lab performs. Follow the instructions for collection carefully.

PROCEDURE 18.7

MIDSTREAM CLEAN-CATCH URINE, MALE

RATIONALE

Careful instruction of the patient/client helps prevent contaminating the specimen. A clean-catch specimen is essential to accurately diagnose and treat the patient.

ALERT: Follow Standard Precautions.

PROCEDURE 18.7 | MIDSTREAM CLEAN-CATCH URINE, MALE *(Continued)*

1. Wash hands.
2. Assemble equipment.
   a. Sterile container for clean catch
   b. Label
   c. Disposable antiseptic towelettes
   d. Disposable nonsterile gloves: wear if handling container with specimen
3. Label container.
4. Instruct patient to
   a. Wash hands.
   b. Remove container lid and place on counter with inside of lid facing up.
   c. Cleanse head of penis in a circular motion with towelette. (If uncircumcised, pull back foreskin before cleaning.)
   d. Urinate into toilet. (If uncircumcised, pull back foreskin while urinating.)

   e. Allow stream to begin.
   f. Stop stream and place specimen container to collect midstream.
   g. Remove container before bladder is empty.
   h. Empty bladder into toilet.
   i. Carefully replace lid.
   j. Wipe outside of container with paper towel.
   k. Put in designated area.
5. Put on gloves.
6. Finish testing as ordered (e.g., dip stick, set up microscopic exam, drug test).
7. Document procedure according to facility procedure

> 10/10/03   0800
>
> *Instructed in correct procedure for collecting clean catch*
>
> *S. Jones CNA*

PROCEDURE 18.8 | COLLECTING URINE FROM AN INFANT

RATIONALE

Using the proper technique prevents leakage around the bag and thus prevents contamination of the specimen.

ALERT: Follow Standard Precautions.

1. Wash hands.
2. Assemble equipment.
   a. Specimen container
   b. Disposable urine collector (small plastic bag with opening and sticky area)
   c. Disposable nonsterile gloves
3. Identify patient.
4. Explain to parents what you are going to do.
5. Tell child what you are going to do even if you think that he or she is too young to understand. Children often understand.
6. Put on gloves.
7. Remove diaper.

8. Make certain that skin is clean and dry in genital area.
9. Remove outside cover that is around opening of bag. This has a sticky area that is applied to vulva or around penis. Place over vulva or penis (see figures).

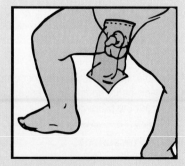

PROCEDURE 18.8 **COLLECTING URINE FROM AN INFANT** *(Continued)*

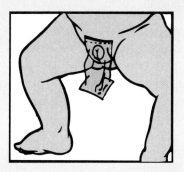

10. Replace diaper.
11. Remove gloves and dispose of according to facility procedure.
12. Check every half hour to see if bag has urine in it.
13. Remove bag when specimen is collected.

14. Rinse, clean, and dry genital area.
15. Replace diaper.
16. Put specimen in specimen container for lab.
17. Label with:
    a. Patient's name
    b. Time of collection
    c. Date
    d. Room number
18. Record collection of specimen.

| 10/25/03 1030 |
| Urine bag applied |
| Specimen successfully collected |
| for testing |
| Sent to lab |
| _____ H. Martinez CNA |

SPUTUM COLLECTION

Sputum is a secretion from the trachea, bronchi, and lungs. It is forced up and out through the mouth by deep coughing. When you collect sputum, make sure that it is not saliva or postnasal drip. Saliva and postnasal drip contaminate a sputum sample. When you collect a sputum sample you must instruct the patient carefully. The doctor orders a sputum specimen to help determine the cause of the illness and whether the patient has an infectious disease. Some of these diseases are

■ Tuberculosis
■ Pneumonia
■ Candidiasis
■ Other fungal infections

Another test is the Papanicolaou stain. This tests for the presence of cancer cells. Collect the sputum for this test in a 95% alcohol solution for a period of 72 hours. Read the procedure for your facility.

PROCEDURE 18.9 **SPUTUM SPECIMEN COLLECTION**

RATIONALE

Careful collection and accurate reporting of information are essential to successfully diagnose and treat the patient.

ALERT: Follow Standard Precautions.

PROCEDURE 18.9 | SPUTUM SPECIMEN COLLECTION *(Continued)*

1. Wash hands.
2. Assemble equipment.
   a. Sputum container
   b. Disposable nonsterile gloves
3. Identify client.
4. Explain what you are going to do.
5. Label container with
   a. Client's name
   b. Date
   c. Time taken
   d. Room number
6. Put on gloves.
7. Help patient rinse mouth if he or she has just eaten.
8. Ask client to take three deep breaths. On the third breath tell resident to cough deep from lungs and try

to bring up thick sputum. (Saliva is not adequate for this test.)

9. The patient may have to try several times to get a good specimen. (You need 1 to 2 tablespoons.)
10. Cover container immediately.
11. Remove gloves and discard according to facility procedure.
12. Wash hands.
13. Record color, amount, odor, and consistency according to facility procedure.

2/03/04   0300

Clear, 0.5cc, thick, stringy

Sent to lab

————— M. Brown MA

STOOL COLLECTION

The patient/client may need to collect a stool specimen. The tests on the stool specimen give the physician information about the patient's digestive system (e.g., blood, bacteria, ova, and parasites in stool). The patient needs to collect the specimen at home. Proper instructions are very important. The following are guidelines for collection of a stool specimen:

■ Feces must not be contaminated with urine.

■ Patient must *not* take a laxative unless instructed to do so.

There are several tests performed on stool samples (see Table 18.1), the most common tests are those for **occult** blood. Screening tests to detect bleeding in the intestinal tract are done routinely. Occult blood may indicate

■ Cancer

■ Polyps

■ Lesions in the colon or rectum

■ Gastrointestinal bleeding

Testing for occult blood is a simple technique that you can do in the office or at home. It consists of three slides. The patient must smear a small amount of stool on slide 1, then slides 2 and 3 for the next three bowel movements. Tell the patient/client that it is important to follow the instructions carefully. When you receive slides from the patient, be sure they are properly labeled.

occult

Hidden, unseen.

Table 18.1 ■ Tests Performed on Stool Specimens

Reason for Test	Type of Specimen
Intestinal amoeba flagellates	Specimen must be at body temperature and checked within 30 minutes.
Ova cystic forms of parasites	Well-formed stool can be taken to lab within a few hours.
Tapeworm	May be examined for ova. If liquid stool, must bring in entire amount. Lab must examine for tapeworm head.

PROCEDURE 18.10

OCCULT BLOOD TEST ON STOOL SPECIMEN

RATIONALE

Careful collection and accurate reporting of information are essential to successfully diagnose and treat the patient. Occult blood in the stool can indicate serious problems.

ALERT: Follow Standard Precautions.

1. Wash hands.
2. Assemble equipment.
   a. Three occult blood slides
   b. Developer per slide manufacturer
   c. Disposable nonsterile gloves
3. Open the back flap of specimen slide.
4. Use the type of liquid developer that coordinates with the type of slide used (i.e., Hemacult developer for Hemacult slides, Serracult developer for Serracult slides).
5. Develop the slides for test results according to manufacturer's directions.
6. Dispose of slides and gloves according to facility's policy.

7. Document the following:
   a. Patient's name
   b. Account number
   c. Date
   d. Time
   e. Physician's name
   f. Type of test
   g. Number of tests
   h. Results e.g. stool sample neg. for occult blood.
   i. Client's diet
   j. Your signature
   k. Your title

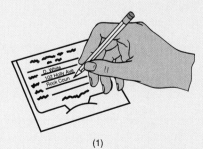

(1)

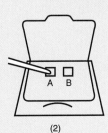

(2)

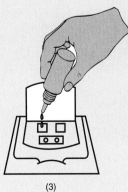

(3)

○ LABORATORY CULTURES

Physicians need a culture of the microorganism that is causing an illness. Knowing what organism is causing the problem helps with the diagnosis and the treatment. Microorganisms that cause strep throat, staph infections, and other illnesses can be treated when they are identified. You need to know how to

■ Obtain a specimen.

■ Place the specimen on the medium, where it can grow and reproduce.

■ Stain a sample of the culture.

Take a specimen for the culture from the affected body sites. These sites include any skin lesion, such as an open, draining sore. Cultures are also taken from any

---

PROCEDURE 18.11 OBTAINING A SPECIMEN FOR CULTURES

RATIONALE

Careful collection and accurate reporting of information are essential to successfully diagnose and treat the patient.

ALERT: Follow Standard Precautions.

1. Wash hands.
2. Assemble equipment.
   a. Sterile swab
   b. Culture medium
   c. Kit for culture
   d. Disposable nonsterile gloves

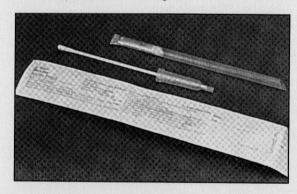

3. Identify patient/client.
4. Put on gloves.
5. Explain what you are going to do.
6. Label culture container from kit.
   a. Patient's name
   b. Date
   c. Physician's name

7. Determine site you are culturing.
8. Remove sterile swab from package.
9. Touch tip of swab to area. *Do not touch anything except area you are culturing.*
10. Rotate tip to cover with specimen.
11. Remove swab from site.
12. Put swab into a sterile container or on culture medium.
13. Be sure that tip is in medium.
14. Prepare as ordered.
15. Dispose of gloves according to contaminated waste policy.
16. Wash hands.
17. Record the following:
    a. Date
    b. Time
    c. Culture site
    d. Where culture is being sent
    e. Signature and classification

5/17/03	1000
Throat culture sent to lab	
S. Yen CNA	

body opening, such as eyes, ears, nose, throat, and vagina. You must be careful when you take a specimen for culturing. Poor technique causes a false test result. You must use a sterile swab to secure the specimen and be careful not to contaminate the sample.

A specimen may be placed on a slide immediately. This is a direct smear. When the technician or doctor reads the smear, he or she can identify the organism. Prepare a direct smear slide following the procedure for using a microscope.

PROCEDURE 18.12 THROAT CULTURES

RATIONALE
Careful collection and accurate reporting of information are essential to successfully diagnose and treat the patient.

ALERT: Follow Standard Precautions

1. Wash hands.
2. Assemble equipment.
   a. Culturette, strep test kit, and so on
   b. Nonsterile disposable gloves
   c. Tongue blade
   d. Pen light
3. Explain procedure to patient/client.
4. Explain that the swab may cause gagging.
5. Have patient in seated position.

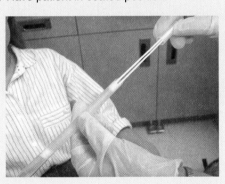

6. Put on gloves.
7. Remove applicator from culture tube.

NOTE Do not contaminate by touching any surface.

8. Ask client to tilt head back.
9. Depress tongue with a tongue blade and illuminate throat with a penlight.
10. Observe for inflamed or purulent area. (Withdraw the tongue blade and tell patient to breathe deeply if patient starts to gag.)
11. Reinsert tongue blade but not as deeply as before.

12. Swab tonsillar area from side to side, including any inflamed or purulent areas. *(Do not touch the tongue, cheeks, or teeth with the swab.)*

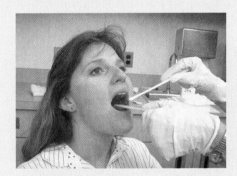

13. Withdraw the swab and tongue blade.
14. Place swab into medium. Do not touch sides.
15. Complete test according to order (e.g., direct smear, manufacturer's test kit, culture, and sensitivity).
16. Label specimen.
17. Clean and replace equipment.
18. Remove gloves and dispose of according to facility policy.
19. Wash hands.
20. Document according to facility procedure.

8/13/03	1500
	Throat culture with culturette,
	strep test kit
	Sent to lab
	_____ G. Nygun CNA

PROCEDURE 18.13

PREPARING A DIRECT SMEAR FOR STAINING

RATIONALE

Following correct procedure ensures that the smear is properly set. Accuracy is essential to successfully diagnose and treat the patient. Following safety precautions helps prevent accidents in the lab.

ALERT: Follow Standard Precautions.

1. Wash hands.
2. Assemble equipment.
   a. Bunsen burner
   b. Saline solution
   c. Clean glass slides
   d. Rubber-tipped slide holder
   e. Wax pencil
   f. Disposable nonsterile gloves
   g. Specimen
3. Put on gloves.
4. Label slide.
5. Light Bunsen burner.
6. Roll swab on slide touching all sides of swab.

7. Allow smear to air dry.
8. Hold slide with smear face up.
9. Attach rubber-tipped slide holder.
10. Pass slide over Bunsen burner flame quickly (slide is warm, not hot).

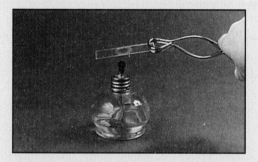

11. Cool slide.
12. Process according to orders.
13. Clean equipment and put away.
14. Remove gloves and dispose of according to facility policy.
15. Wash hands.
16. Document according to facility procedure.

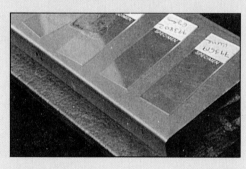

The physician may also request that the microorganism be grown on an *agar plate.* The agar in the plate provides food and moisture. The organisms grow and multiply when you place the agar plate in a warm incubator, at 36 to 37° Celsius (97 to 99° Fahrenheit) for 24 to 36 hours.

A common test is called a culture and sensitivity test. This test identifies the antibiotic that kills the organism. It also identifies the antibiotics to which the organisms are **resistant.** This information helps the physician decide which medication to prescribe. To do a culture and sensitivity test, place paper disks coated with antibiotic on an agar plate streaked with a specimen. If the organism is resistant to the antibiotic, it continues to grow around the disk. If the specimen is sensitive to the antibiotic, the colony around the disk dies. The physician then knows which antibiotic to prescribe for the patient.

resistant

Able to protect itself.

PROCEDURE 18.14

STREAKING AGAR (MEDIA) PLATE FOR CULTURES

RATIONALE

Correctly streaking an agar plate prevents contamination of the specimen. Using the proper technique provides the physician with the information needed for diagnosis and treatment.

ALERT: Follow Standard Precautions.

1. Wash hands.
2. Assemble equipment.
   a. Agar plate with media
   b. Specimen of a direct smear
   c. Pen or marker
   d. Incubator
   e. Disposable nonsterile gloves
3. Label agar plate.
   a. Name of patient
   b. Time
   c. Date
   d. Physician's name
   e. Site of specimen
4. Put on gloves and take swab with specimen from culture tube.
5. Remove lid from agar plate.
6. Place lid on table with inside facing up.
7. Hold plate with agar firmly.
8. Hold swab lightly against agar at top of plate.
9. Roll swab so that all sides touch agar following a side-to-side pattern (see figure p18.11).
10. Continue halfway down agar, being careful not to break into agar.

NOTE Do not go over areas that are already streaked.

11. Roll swab in top-to-bottom pattern in right-hand quarter.
12. Roll swab from side-to-side in left-hand quarter.

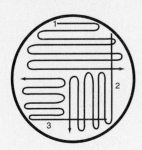

Label lid:
J. White #11333
Wound 1/12/03

NOTE See examples of other patterns. Follow your facility's procedure.

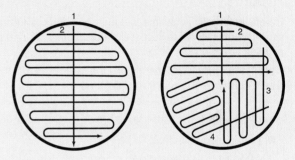

13. Discard swab following facility's contaminated waste policy.
14. Replace cover on plate. Do not touch inside of lid.
15. Place plate with specimen in incubator upside down (agar on top).

NOTE Temperature is 36 to 37° Celsius.

16. Discard gloves according to policy.
17. Wash hands and record the following:
   a. Patient's name
   b. Physician's name
   c. Type of culture (e.g., wound, throat)
   d. Date
18. Clean and replace equipment.
19. Remove gloves and dispose of according to facility policy.
20. Wash hands.
21. Document according to facility procedure.

Gram Stain

Gram staining is a process that dyes and fixes microorganisms. The stain helps make the organism more visible in the microscope. It also helps in identifying the microorganism. The slide can be kept and reviewed if necessary. To prepare a slide from colonies grown in an agar plate for staining, a small colony of organisms is taken from the agar plate. These organisms are placed on a slide and stained.

PROCEDURE 18.15 | **PREPARING A CULTURE SMEAR FROM A GROWTH MEDIUM**

RATIONALE

Careful preparation prevents contamination and provides the information essential to successfully diagnose and treat the patient.

ALERT: Follow Standard Precautions.

1. Wash hands.
2. Assemble equipment.
   a. Culture medium with growth
   b. Slide
   c. Saline solution
   d. Inoculating loop
   e. Disposable nonsterile gloves
3. Put on gloves.
4. Light Bunsen burner.
5. Hold inoculating loop in flame until red hot. (This sterilizes the loop.)
6. Air-cool loop for several minutes. *Do not contaminate.*
7. Remove lid from agar plate.
8. Place lid on table with inside facing up.
9. Carefully touch cool loop to colony.
10. Gently move loop over organisms.
11. Replace lid on plate to prevent contaminating culture.
12. Put small drop of normal saline on slide.
13. Mix specimen on loop with saline on slide.
14. Follow policy in your facility for slide preparation.
15. Allow slide to air dry.
16. Hold loop in flame to destroy microorganisms.
17. Heat-fix smear.
    a. Attach rubber-tipped clamps to slide.
    b. Hold slide with smear face up.
    c. Pass slide over Bunsen burner flame quickly.

18. Label slide.
    a. Name
    b. Date
    c. Physician's name
19. Clean equipment and put away.
20. Remove gloves and dispose of according to facility policy.
21. Wash hands.
22. Document according to facility procedure.

Slide may be prepared:

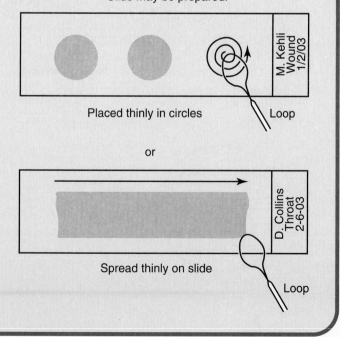

Placed thinly in circles   Loop

or

Spread thinly on slide   Loop

PROCEDURE 18.16

STAINING A SMEAR WITH GRAM STAIN

RATIONALE

Gram staining is a precise series of steps. Following the steps carefully and accurately reporting the information are essential to successfully diagnose and treat the patient.

ALERT: Follow Standard Precautions.

1. Wash hands.
2. Assemble equipment.
   a. Staining rack
   b. Crystal violet
   c. Gram's iodine
   d. 95% ethyl alcohol
   e. Safranine
   f. Wash bottle with distilled water
   g. Slide with fixed smear
   h. Timer or watch
   i. Absorbent paper
   j. Disposable nonsterile gloves
   k. Face shield (check your facility's policy)
   l. Nonpermeable gown (check your facility's policy)
3. Put on
   a. Gloves
   b. Face shield
   c. Gown
4. Put slide face up on staining rack. Do not touch specimen.
5. Flood slide with crystal violet. Time for 30 seconds to 1 minute.

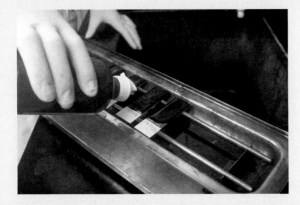

6. Wash off dye with stream from water wash.

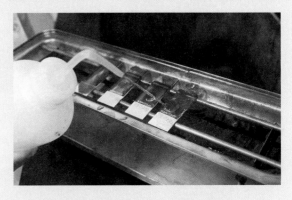

7. Use forceps to tip slide to remove water.
8. Replace slide on stain rack.
9. Flood slide with Gram's iodine and tip to allow runoff.
10. Flood slide again with Gram's iodine. Time for 1 to 2 minutes.

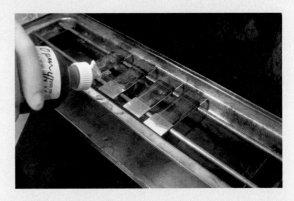

11. Wash off dye with stream from water wash.

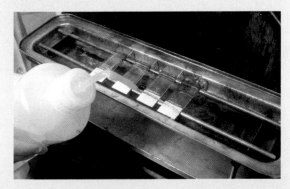

PROCEDURE 18.16 | STAINING A SMEAR WITH GRAM STAIN *(Continued)*

12. Use forceps to tip slide to remove water.
13. Wash slide with 95% ethyl alcohol for 30 to 60 seconds until smear no longer gives off dye.

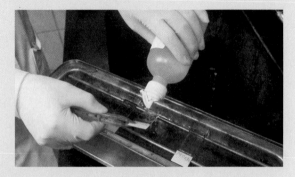

NOTE This step removes stain from gram-negative organisms, which helps identify organism on smear.

14. Replace on rack and rinse with distilled water.

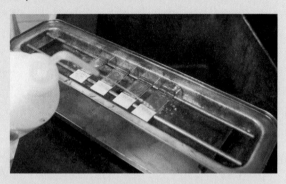

15. Flood slide with Safranine. Time for 30 to 60 seconds.

NOTE This will stain red everything that decolorized.

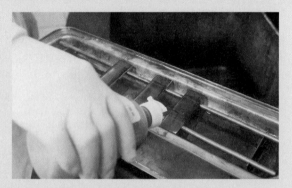

16. Wash slide with distilled water.

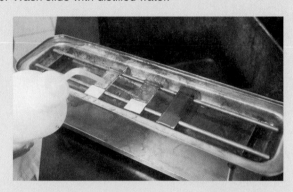

17. Wipe underside of slide (away from smear) with alcohol to remove any stain.
18. Blot slide dry with absorbent paper.

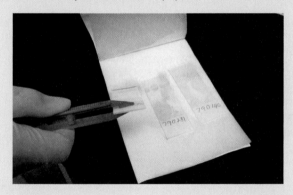

19. Clean work area.
20. Discard gloves according to facility's contaminated waste policy.
21. Remove face shield and gown.
22. Wash hands.
23. Document according to facility procedure.

⦿ BLOOD, BLOOD COMPOSITION, AND BLOOD TESTING

Components of Blood

Whole blood has many formed elements that are suspended in a clear yellow liquid called *plasma*. Plasma makes up 55% of the whole blood. The other 45% has the formed elements. These elements are

- **Erythrocytes.** RBC (carry O_2 to cells, carry away CO_2)
- **Leukocytes.** WBC (protect against infection and disease)
- **Thrombocytes.** Platelets (start the clotting process)

The average adult has 6 to 8 quarts of blood.

Blood Tests

Physicians order blood tests for routine checkups and to help diagnose an illness. There are many blood tests available. This chapter covers the blood tests that the physician orders frequently. (See Table 18.2, which gives you the important reasons for the tests you are doing.) Refer back to the table before you practice a blood test procedure.

The laboratory most often uses capillary/peripheral blood and venous blood. You usually obtain capillary blood from the finger and sometimes from the earlobe. You use a heel stick for infants. The amount of blood is limited to a few drops. This is enough blood to do the following:

- Complete blood count (CBC)
- Hematocrit/microhematocrit
- Some bleeding and coagulation times
- Some chemical and **agglutination** tests

agglutination 🔊
Clumping together (e.g., red blood cells clump together).

When you need a larger amount of blood, you draw venous blood from the veins with a Vacutainer™ or syringe and needle. Some states and schools do not allow students to perform blood tests. Your teacher will tell you what you can do. *Never* practice these tests without training.

Complete Blood Count

The laboratory worker performs many different types of blood tests. The most frequently ordered test is a complete blood count. The complete blood count (CBC) gives a lot of information about the patient's condition. It includes the following:

- RBC (red blood cell) count
- WBC (white blood cell) count
- Hemoglobin determination
- Hematocrit determination
- Differential white blood cell count
- Estimate of the number of platelets
- RBC morphology (size and shape)

Hematocrit/Microhematocrit

A hematocrit measures the volume of packed red blood cells in the blood. When you do this test you separate cell elements from the plasma. You perform this test with

Table 18.2 ■ Common Blood Tests

Test	Abbreviation	Normal Range	Examples of Possible Diagnosis	
			Increase	**Decrease**
White blood cell count	WBC	5000–10,000 mm^3	Acute infection, leukemia, mononucleosis	Viral infections, bone marrow depression
Red blood cell count	RBC	Female: 4–5 million/mm^3 Male: 5–6 million/mm^3	Polycythemia, poisoning, pulmonary fibrosis	Anemia, multiple myeloma, lupus erythemia
Differential white blood cell count	Diff	Neutrophils 50–70%	*Neutrophilia:* acute bacterial infections, parasitic infections, liver disease	*Neutropenia:* acute viral infections, blood diseases, hormone diseases
		Eosinophils 1–4%	*Eosinophilia:* allergic conditions, parasitic infections, lung and bone cancer	*Eosinopenia:* infectious mononucleosis, congestive heart failure, aplastic and pernicious anemia
		Basophils 0–1%	*Basophilia:* leukemia, hemolytic anemia, Hodgkin's disease	*Basopenia:* acute allergic reactions, hyperthyroidism, steroid therapy
		Lymphocytes 20–35%	*Lymphocytosis:* acute and chronic infections, carcinoma, hyperthyroidism	*Lymphopenia:* cardiac failure, Cushing's disease, Hodgkin's disease
		Monocytes 3–8%	*Monocytosis:* viral infections, bacterial and parasitic infections, collagen diseases, cirrhosis	*Monocytopenia:* prednisolone treatment, hairy cell leukemia
Hemoglobin	Hgb	Female: 12–16 g/100 mL Male: 14–18 g/100 mL	Congestive heart failure (CHF), chronic obstructive pulmonary disease (COPD), severe burn	Hodgkin's disease, hyperthyroidism, cirrhosis
Hematocrit/ microhematocrit	Hct, HCT	Female: 40–54% Male: 37–47%	Shock, dehydration, burns	Anemia, leukemia, acute blood loss
Prothrombin time	PT	11–16 sec	Anticoagulant therapy, liver disease, biliary obstruction	Diuretics, pulmonary embolism, multiple myeloma
Erythrocyte sedimentation rate	ESR	(According to method used)	Collagen disease, inflammatory disease, rheumatoid arthritis	Sickle cell anemia, CHF, polycythemia
Platelet count		200,000–400,000/mm^3	Cancer, leukemia, splenectomy	Bone-marrow-depressant drug, pneumonia infection

heparinized

Containing heparin, an anticoagulant.

polycythemia

Condition of having too much blood.

a few drops of capillary blood. Collect the blood in a **heparinized** capillary tube from a finger or earlobe stick for adults. In infants collect the blood from a heel stick. Centrifuge the blood to pack the cells. Low hematocrit readings tell the physician that there is a problem (e.g., anemia). High hematocrit readings provide important information (e.g., **polycythemia**) (see Table 18.2).

PROCEDURE 18.17

FINGER STICK WITH REGULAR LANCET

RATIONALE

Careful technique prevents infection and provides an accurate specimen for diagnosis and treatment.

A regular lancet is used for the puncture if there is no spring-loaded instrument or if the patient has very tough skin (older patients, manual laborers, diabetics).

ALERT: Follow Standard Precautions.

1. Wash hands.
2. Assemble equipment.
   a. Test supplies
   b. Cotton sponge
   c. Alcohol sponge
   d. Lancet
   e. Small bandage (e.g., Band-Aid)
   f. Disposable nonsterile gloves and face shield
3. Explain procedure to patient/client.
4. Wash hands.
5. Put on gloves and face shield.
6. Select finger for stick: third or fourth finger on nondominant hand.

NOTE   Do not use finger with sores, scars, thickened skin.

7. Wipe finger with alcohol sponge.
8. Remove lancet from package and hold it between thumb and index finger.
9. Hold patient's finger firmly with your thumb and forefinger.
10. Make a quick, firm, deep puncture.
11. Wipe away first drop of blood with dry cotton sponge.
12. Collect specimen.
13. Give client a dry cotton sponge to apply pressure to wound.

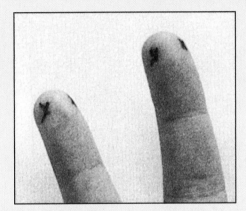

14. Put small bandage on site.
15. Discard lancet into sharps container.
16. Discard all materials according to facility policy.
17. Remove gloves and discard according to facility's contaminated waste policy.
18. Wash hands.
19. Document according to facility procedure.

5/01/04   1300
Finger stick with lancet, on
left third finger
Tolerated well
_____ R. Cese MA

Hemoglobin

Hemoglobin (Hgb) tests measure the oxygen-carrying capacity of the blood. Hemoglobin has the *heme,* which carries iron, and *globin,* which is the protein in the red blood cell. Hemoglobin picks up oxygen in the lungs and transports it to the cells. It also helps carry waste product, CO_2, from the body cells back to the lungs. One way to measure hemoglobin is with a hemoglobinometer.

PROCEDURE 18.18

FINGER STICK WITH SPRING-LOADED PUNCTURE INSTRUMENT

RATIONALE

Careful collection and accurate reporting of information are essential to successfully diagnose and treat the patient.

ALERT: Follow Standard Precautions.

1. Wash hands.

2. Assemble equipment.

    a. Test supplies
    b. Cotton sponges
    c. Alcohol sponge
    d. Spring-loaded puncture instrument
    e. Small bandage (e.g., Band-Aid)
    f. Disposable nonsterile gloves and face shield

3. Explain procedure to patient/client.

4. Wash hands.

5. Put on gloves and face shield.

6. Insert lancet into spring-loaded device and set spring for use. (Follow manufacturer's instructions.)

7. Select the finger.

    a. Small children: use thumb.
    b. Adults/older children: use fourth finger on non-dominant hand.

8. Ask patient to relax hand and dangle it down across the blood-drawing chair or exam table.

9. Wipe finger site with alcohol sponge; allow to dry.

10. Massage finger starting at base of finger and moving to tip of finger.

11. Exert some pressure on fingertip by holding it between your thumb and index finger—"pumping" or "milking" it.

12. Place spring-loaded device against side of fingertip between center pad and outside rim of nail (not dead center) and release according to manufacturer's instructions.

13. Release your hold from finger and wait a few seconds for a drop of blood to begin to form.

14. Wipe away first drop of blood with dry cotton sponge.

15. Collect the following:

    a. Platelet count specimen first
    b. Blood for peripheral smear
    c. Blood for any other test

NOTE   Always wipe away any blood that accumulates between collection of specimens for different tests.

16. Give client a cotton sponge to apply pressure to wound.

17. Apply small bandage.

18. Remove used lancet and place in contaminated sharps container.

19. Discard all materials according to facility policy.

20. Remove gloves and discard in contaminated waste according to facility's policy.

21. Remove face shield.

22. Wash hands.

23. Document according to facility procedure.

5/01/04	1300

Finger stick with spring loaded
puncture instrument on left,
third finger
Tolerated well
_____ R. Cese MA

PROCEDURE 18.19

HEEL PUNCTURE ON AN INFANT

RATIONALE

Following the procedure prevents infection. Careful collection and accurate reporting of information are essential to successfully diagnose and treat the infant.

PROCEDURE 18.19 · HEEL PUNCTURE ON AN INFANT *(Continued)*

ALERT: Follow Standard Precautions.

1. Assemble equipment.
   a. Disposable nonsterile gloves and face shield
   b. Alcohol sponge/iodine wipe
   c. Sterile gauze, 3 × 3
   d. Sterile regular or spring-loaded lancet (2.4 mm)
   e. Test supplies
   f. Small bandage (e.g., Band-Aid)
2. Explain procedure to patient's caregiver.
3. Wash hands.
4. Instruct caregiver to remove baby's lower torso clothing to expose legs and feet. If there is another adult who can hold infant, drape the person's lap with a nonpermeable towel to protect clothing from dropped blood. Infant should be held so that the feet are free and hanging down. If there is no one to hold child, lay the child down on his or her stomach on center of exam table.

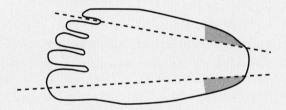

5. Put on gloves and face shield.
6. Examine infant's feet and select heel site.

NOTE   Heel sticks should be performed only on lateral and medial curves of heel (etched areas in figure).

7. Clean bottom of heel with alcohol sponge or iodine wipe. Allow to dry.

8. Take sterile 3 × 3 gauze and wipe area to dry and to increase blood flow to skin.

NOTE   Do not contaminate gauze before using.

9. Open a blue, regular-sized (2.4 mm), sterile lance package.
10. Hold foot tightly and quickly stab site at heel.
11. Withdraw lancet and immediately make a *second* stab perpendicular to first stab, producing T-shaped wound.
12. Release foot for a few seconds.
13. Wipe away first drop of blood with sterile gauze.
14. Hold foot firmly, *avoiding* excessive squeezing, to collect blood. If a capillary tube is used, hold it so that blood flows down.
15. Hold sterile gauze over puncture site until bleeding stops after collection is complete.
16. Put small bandage over site.
17. Discard lancet into sharps container.
18. Discard contaminated material according to facility policy.
19. Remove and discard gloves in contaminated waste.
20. Remove face shield.
21. Wash hands.
22. Document according to facility procedure.

7/01/03	1300
Heel stick with spring loaded puncture instrument on left, lateral heel	
Tolerated well	
	R. Cese MA

PROCEDURE 18.20 · MICROHEMATOCRIT

RATIONALE

Careful collection of capillary blood ensures that the centrifuged specimen is accurate. The results of the specimen reading provide information essential to successfully diagnose and treat the patient.

PROCEDURE 18.20 | MICROHEMATOCRIT *(Continued)*

ALERT: Follow Standard Precautions.

1. Assemble equipment.
   a. Two heparinized microhematocrit tubes
   b. Disposable nonsterile gloves
   c. Face shield
   d. Nonpermeable gown
   e. Lancet
   f. Hematocrit tube clay sealant
   g. Microhematocrit reader card (if not on machine)
   h. Microhematocrit centrifuge
   i. Miscellaneous requisition
   j. Alcohol swab
   k. Dry sponge
   l. Small bandage (e.g., Band-Aid)
2. Explain procedure to patient/client.
3. Wash hands.
4. Select specimen site.
   a. Adult: use fourth finger of nondominant hand.
   b. Child over 3 months: use finger (see the procedures "Finger Stick with Regular Lancet" and "Finger Stick with Spring-Loaded Puncture Instrument").
   c. Young children who are likely to pull away: use thumb.
   d. Infants to 3 months: use heel (see the procedure "Heel Puncture").
5. Put on gloves and face shield.
6. Wipe site with alcohol sponge; allow to dry.
7. Puncture site with lancet.
8. Do not squeeze finger excessively (causes hemolysis and inaccurate results).
9. Gently milk finger.

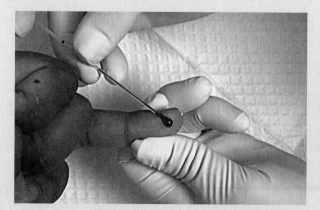

10. Wipe away first drop of blood with a gauze pad. Use second drop of blood.

11. Hold capillary tube to puncture site with marked end away from collection site, tilting in downward direction (allows tube to fill faster). Hold end to puncture site (avoids air bubbles, which cause inaccurate results).
12. Place a finger over end of tube to prevent loss of blood.
13. Fill opposite end of capillary tube with clay sealant. *Do not pack sealant into both ends of tube.*
14. Fill second capillary tube.
15. Put clean gauze over site.
16. Have patient hold firmly.
17. Place both capillary tubes (sealed end to outside) in centrifuge across from each other.
18. Record centrifuge slot numbers on requisition to avoid confusing specimens.
19. Place cover on centrifuge and lock.
20. Close lid and lock.
21. Spin 3 minutes at 10,000 rpm.
22. Apply bandage over puncture site if needed.
23. Wait until centrifuge stops, turning before opening lid. Do not try to stop spinning.
24. Remove capillary tubes and read within 5 minutes.
25. Place tube at right edge of hematocrit scale (top of plasma line at 100% mark).
26. Slide tube left until top of clay sealant is at bottom line, "0."
27. Record point at which top of red cell column crosses line of hematocrit scale. That line is microhematocrit value on the hematocrit scale.
28. Read second tube. Results should agree within 2 percentage points (2%). If more than 3 points, repeat entire process.

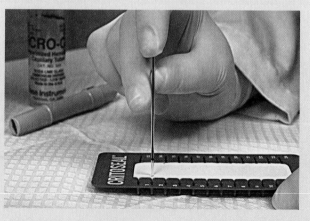

PROCEDURE 18.20 | MICROHEMATOCRIT *(Continued)*

29. Note color of plasma.
    a. Clear or normal
    b. Yellow (may indicate elevated bilirubin; report to the physician)
    c. Pink or red (suggests either hemoglobinemia or poor collection)
30. Discard hematocrit tubes into sharps container.
31. Discard contaminated materials according to facility policy.
32. Remove gloves and place with contaminated waste.
33. Remove face shield.

34. Wash hands.
35. Document on lab slip:
    a. Patient's name
    b. Account number
    c. Date
    d. Site
    e. Results
    f. Physician's name
    g. Signature with classification
36. See reference hematocrit values in Table 18.3.

Table 18.3 ■ Reference Microhematocrit Values

Age	Average Normal (%)	Minimal Normal (%)
Children		
At birth	56.6	51.0
First day	56.1	50.5
End of first week	52.7	47.5
End of second week	49.6	44.7
End of third week	46.6	42.0
End of fourth week	44.6	40.0
End of second month	38.9	35.1
End of fourth month	36.5	32.9
End of sixth month	36.2	32.6
End of eighth month	35.8	32.3
End of tenth month	35.5	32.0
End of first year	35.2	31.7
End of second year	35.5	32.0
End of fourth year	37.1	33.4
End of sixth year	37.9	34.2
End of eighth year	38.9	35.1
End of twelfth year	39.6	35.7
Men		
End of fourteenth year	44	39.6
End of eighteenth year	47	42.3
18–50 years	47	42.3
50–60 years	45	40.5
60–70 years	43	38.7
70–80 years	40	36.0

Table 18.3 ■ Continued

Age	Average Normal (%)	Minimal Normal (%)
Nonpregnant women		
14–50 years	42	36
50–80 years	40	36
Pregnant women		
End of fourth month	42	30
End of fifth month	40	30
End of sixth month	37	30
End of seventh month	37	30
End of eighth month	39	30
End of ninth month	40	30

Source: J. B. Miale, *Laboratory Medicine: Hematology.* St. Louis, Mo.: C. V. Mosby, 1977, p. 426. Reprinted with permission.

PROCEDURE 18.21 USING A HEMOGLOBINOMETER

Accurate measurement with the hemoglobinometer assists in diagnosis and treatment. Hemoglobin carries oxygen to the cells. When it is low, anemia may be a problem. When it is elevated, polycythemia may be indicated.

ALERT: Follow Standard Precautions.

1. Wash hands.
2. Assemble equipment.
   a. Sterile lancet or spring-loaded lance device
   b. Alcohol swab
   c. Cotton balls
   d. Hemoglobinometer
   e. Hemolysis applicator stick
   f. Blood chamber
   g. Lens paper
   h. Small bandage (e.g., Band-Aid)
   i. Disposable nonsterile gloves and face shield
3. Identify patient/client.
4. Explain what you are going to do.
5. Put on gloves and face shield.
6. Clean blood chamber with lens paper.
7. Do finger stick (see the procedure "Finger Stick with Regular Lancet" or "Finger Stick with Spring-Loaded Puncture Instrument").
8. Wipe off first drop of blood with cotton ball.
9. Use second drop of blood to place on clean chamber.
10. Have client hold cotton ball over stick to stop bleeding.
11. Roll hemolysis applicator stick in blood. (This hemolyzes the blood.)

NOTE Blood looks red and cloudy at start. It becomes clear or transparent when it hemolyzes.

12. Cover chamber with coverglass.
13. Push chamber and cover into clip.
14. Look into hemoglobinometer.
15. Slide slide button until the two halves of field are equally light and colors match.
16. Read scale through eyepiece (e.g., 12, 12.5, 13; normal values 12 to 18).
17. Record reading.
   a. Hgb 13 g (example)
   b. Patient's name
   c. Date
   d. Physician's name
18. Place small bandage on patient's finger.
19. Clean and replace equipment according to facility's policy.
20. Remove gloves and face shield.
21. Wash hands.
22. Document according to facility procedure.

Blood Glucose Testing

Diabetic Patient/Client

Diabetes is a disease that affects many people. The diabetic patient does not produce enough insulin. This causes glucose to remain in the blood. Too much glucose in the blood can cause

- Circulatory problems
- Poor healing of lesions on legs and feet
- Changes in the retina (which can lead to blindness)
- Nerve disorders

Some patients with diabetes can successfully control sugar levels in the blood with diet and exercise. Others need medication to control their sugar levels.

The diabetic client controls the disease with diet, exercise, and medication. A clinical study conducted between 1983 and 1993 called the Diabetes Control and Complications Trial (DCCT) showed that controlling glucose levels reduces the risk of eye, kidney, nerve, and cardiovascular disease. New studies confirm the DCCT findings. A laboratory test called Glycosolated Hemoglobin (HbA_1C) provides indications of glucose control. Each number above 7 grams HbA_1C means an increase in the risk of disease for patients with diabetes. Patients who need insulin must check the level of glucose in their blood. The level of glucose tells them how much insulin they need. Patients use a glucose meter to measure the sugar level in their blood before taking insulin.

General Guidelines for Testing Blood for Glucose

1. Read all instructions on the reagents and glucose meter carefully.
2. Store reagent strips according to instructions.
3. Keep the lid on the reagent bottle tightly closed.
4. *Do not touch* the pad on the reagent strip.
5. Use careful technique in obtaining blood specimen.

There are many different glucose meters. Each one is a little different from the others. Learn the steps for the meter that is used in your facility.

Counting Blood Cells

Counting blood cells gives the doctor information about a patient's health. Large laboratories use automated cell counters. In an office or small lab you use a counting chamber. To count blood cells, you must dilute the blood. You use blood diluting pipettes and diluting fluids for this procedure. You count the cells using the diluted blood, a counting chamber called a hemacytometer, a hemacytometer coverslip, and a microscope.

Blood-cell diluting pipettes have three basic parts (see Figure 18.4):

- The calibrated stem is where you aspirate the blood and diluting fluid.
- The bulb is where you mix the contents.
- The short stem is where you attach rubber tubing.

The red-cell diluting pipette mixes RBCs and diluent 1:200. The white-cell diluting pipette is similar except that the dilution is 1:20. The diluent for WBCs destroys RBCs, leaving only WBCs.

An Unopette (Becton-Dickinson) is a disposable blood dilutor. It has a prefilled reservoir, capillary pipette, and a pipette shield. There are Unopettes to dilute WBCs, RBCs, and platelets. Follow the directions for using the Unopette carefully.

Figure 18.4

Blood-cell diluting pipettes.

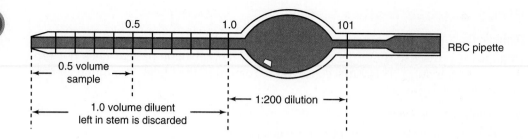

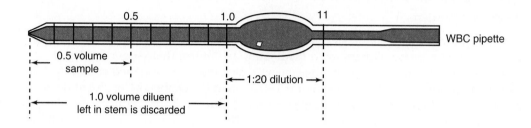

When you use it correctly, it is more accurate than pipettes that require measuring diluents.

You use a hemacytometer to count cells. This is a glass slide. It has two raised areas. There are depressions on three sides. The raised surfaces are marked to help with counting (see Figure 18.5).

Automated Cell Counters

Blood cell counts are often hand counted. There are also many different types of automated equipment that can count cells. The equipment can be simple or very **complex.**

The **automated** cell counter dilutes the blood first. Then the diluted cells are run through a narrow opening. The cells are counted by a laser in some machines. In other machines the cells are counted by an electrical impulse device. Automated cell counting increases the accuracy of the count. Using automated equipment reduces the risks of exposure of lab workers and medical assistants to bloodborne pathogens such as hepatitis B virus and HIV virus (AIDS).

complex

Having two or more related parts.

automated

Method of lab testing that uses equipment to perform a series of steps, as compared to a manual method.

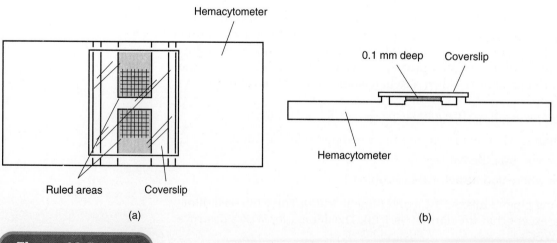

(a)   (b)

Figure 18.5

Hemacytometer: (a) top view; (b) side view.

Blood Smear

A blood smear allows you to see cells in their most natural state. A blood smear is part of the complete blood count (CBC). When you look at a blood smear through the microscope, you see

- Red blood cells
- Thrombocytes
- White blood cells

There are more red blood cells than white blood cells or thrombocytes. The red blood cells

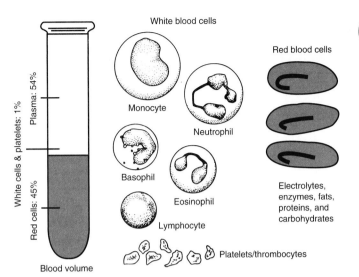

White blood cells

Monocyte

Neutrophil

Basophil

Eosinophil

Lymphocyte

Platelets/thrombocytes

Red blood cells

Electrolytes, enzymes, fats, proteins, and carbohydrates

Plasma: 54%

White cells & platelets: 1%

Red cells: 45%

Blood volume

are **biconcave** disks (see Figure 18.6). They do not have a nucleus. When you stain a red blood cell, the hemoglobin turns reddish brown. The red blood cells should all be the same shape and be filled with hemoglobin. You must report any abnormal appearance.

Thrombocytes (platelets) are the smallest cells. They are round or oval in shape. Thrombocytes do not have a nucleus, and they stain blue (see Figure 18.7). They are small and have irregular shapes.

Figure 18.6

Components of blood.

biconcave

Having a depressed surface on both sides.

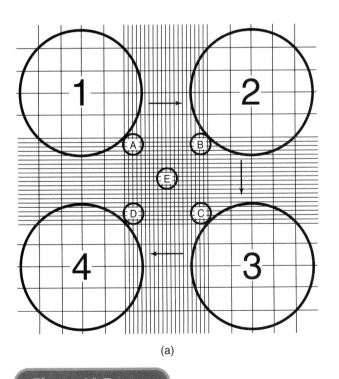

(a)

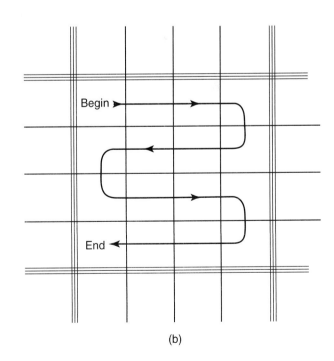

(b)

Figure 18.7

(a) Hemocytometer. Ruled area is the surface of the counting chamber. Count the white cells in the four large outside corner squares (1, 2, 3, 4). Count the red cells in the five smaller squares in the center (A, B, C, D, E). (b) Pattern for counting cells.

PROCEDURE 18.22

DILUTING BLOOD CELLS

RATIONALE

Following the procedure prevents infection. Careful collection of a blood sample will provide information that is essential to successfully diagnose and treat a patient.

ALERT: Follow Standard Precautions.

1. Wash hands.
2. Assemble equipment.
   a. Red and white blood cell diluting pipettes
   b. EDTA anticoagulant
   c. Diluting fluids
      WBC: 27 acetic acid or 0.1 *N* hydrochloric acid
      RBC: normal saline
   d. Gauze pads
   e. Pipette bulb
   f. Pipette shaker
   g. Test tube rack
   h. Nonsterile gloves and face shield
3. Put on gloves and face shield.

NOTE   Blood may be from vial (mix well) or use finger stick method.

4. Hold pipette horizontal to blood source.
5. Put tip of pipette under surface of blood.
6. Use pipette bulb to fill to 0.5 mark.

NOTE   Do not allow air bubbles. Reading is off if there are air bubbles or you are not on 0.5 mark.

7. Wipe outside of pipette with dry gauze pad.

8. Fill diluting fluid container.
9. Put tip of pipette beneath fluid.
10. Hold pipette almost upright.
11. Turn slowly while filling it to 11 mark on WBC pipette or 101 mark on RBC pipette.
12. Put finger over tip of pipette and remove pipette bulb.
13. Rotate pipette to mix sample.
14. Place pipette into tray. (Tray must be labeled with patient's name.)
15. Place pipette on shaker or turn gently to mix.
16. Clean work area.
17. Dispose of materials according to facility's contaminated waste policy.
18. Remove gloves and dispose of according to facility policy.
19. Remove face shield.
20. Wash hands.
21. Document according to facility procedure.

White blood cells are the largest. There are five different types of white blood cells (see Figure 18.6):

Neutrophils	54–62%	
Eosinophils	1–3%	
Basophils	0–1%	Percentage in blood
Lymphocytes	25–33%	
Monocytes	0–9%	

A change in the number of white cells tells the physician that something is happening in the body (e.g., allergic reaction, infection). The white blood cell count is very important when making a diagnosis.

Differential White Cell Count

clumped
Stuck together.

Use a blood smear slide for a differential count. Choose an area on the slide where red blood cells touch but are not **clumped** together. To do a differential count you

PROCEDURE 18.23

COUNTING RED BLOOD CELLS

RATIONALE
Careful collection of this blood sample will provide important data to help the physician determine if the body is making the right amount of red blood cells. Follow procedures carefully to ensure a valid test.

ALERT: Follow Standard Precautions.

1. Wash hands.
2. Assemble equipment.
   a. Disposable nonsterile gloves and face shield
   b. Hemacytometer
   c. Counting chamber with coverglass
   d. Microscope
   e. Diluted blood sample
   f. Watch or timer
3. Put on gloves and face shield.
4. Discard 3 to 5 drops diluted blood from pipette.
5. Center coverglass on counting chamber.
6. Put 1 drop of diluted blood on chamber platform. Drop must touch edge of coverglass.

NOTE Use one drop of blood. If you have air bubbles, repeat steps.

7. Repeat in opposite chamber.
8. Let cells settle for 2 minutes.
9. Put chamber on microscope stage.
10. Use 10× objective to focus on chamber.
11. Bring moat into focus.
12. Move slide to side until indicator arrow appears as a whiter area.

13. Move slide toward you until you see counting area of chamber.
14. Check cells to make sure they are evenly distributed.
15. Find center square of ruled area.
16. Move chamber to center of upper left square of center square.
17. Switch to high power and focus.
18. Count all RBCs in four corner squares.
19. Count all RBCs in center square.
20. Add the five totals together.
21. Multiply by 10,000. This is the RBC count.
22. Repeat on side of chamber. The two counts should be similar.
23. Record number of RBCs.
24. Clean equipment according to facility's procedure.
25. Discard hazardous waste according to policy and remove gloves and face shield.
26. Wash hands.

count and **classify** 100 **consecutive** white blood cells. You must follow a specific winding pattern. This pattern keeps you from counting the same cell twice (see Figure 18.7). You use a differential cell counter to count the cells.

Blood Typing: Antigens and Antibodies
Everyone has a blood type. There are four types: A, B, AB, and O. Blood has both antigens and antibodies. The antigens on the surface of your red blood cells determine your blood type. These antigens are inherited through genes and are on the red blood cells in your body (see Figure 18.8).

- If you have A antigens, you are type A.
- If you have B antigens, you are type B.
- If you have A and B antigens, you are type AB.
- If you have no antigens, you are type O.

classify
To put like items together.

consecutive
Following one after the other.

Figure 18.8

Blood antigens.

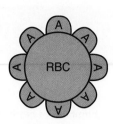

Type A
A antigen is present
(a)

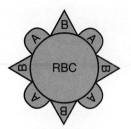

Type B
B antigen is present
(b)

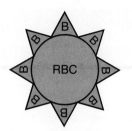

Type AB
A and B antigens
are present
(c)

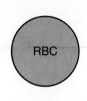

Type O
A or B antigens
are not present
(d)

PROCEDURE 18.24

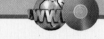

PREPARING A BLOOD SMEAR WITH WRIGHT STAIN

RATIONALE

Follow the procedure carefully to ensure a blood smear that will accept the Wright stain. This will allow evaluation of blood cells leading to an accurate diagnosis.

ALERT: Follow Standard Precautions.

1. Wash hands.
2. Assemble equipment.
   a. Disposable nonsterile gloves and face shield
   b. Clean glass slides
   c. Wright stain
   d. Timer
   e. ECTA anticoagulant blood specimen or capillary blood specimen (wipe off first and use second drop)
3. Put on gloves and face shield.
4. Place a small drop of blood on slide.

NOTE   Center drop on slide about 1/2 inch from end of slide.

5. Hold left side of slide.
6. Put spreader slide in front of drop of blood holding at 30 to 35° angle.
7. Pull spreader slide back into drop of blood.
8. Let blood spread to edges of slide.
9. Push spreader slide forward with a quick smooth motion *(maintain angle)*.

10. Air dry.
11. Label slide.
12. Stain slide.
    a. Put smear slide on staining rack.
    b. Cover slide with Wright stain.

NOTE   Count number of drops used to cover slide. Follow manufacturer's directions.
    c. Time for 1 to 3 minutes.
    d. Add same number of drops of distilled water or buffer to slide.
    e. Blow gently to mix stain and buffer.

NOTE   Mixture is metallic green.
    f. Rinse thoroughly with distilled water.
    g. Drain water from slide.
    h. Dry back of slide.
    i. Let air dry.

13. Clean work area.
14. Dispose of contaminated waste according to facility's policy and remove gloves and face shield.
15. Wash hands.

The antibodies are in the blood plasma. An antibody can combine with an antigen. Our bodies never produce antibodies that can combine with their own blood antigens. For example, if the blood has an A antigen, the plasma does not have an A antibody. The B antibody is in the plasma. The B antibody cannot combine with

PROCEDURE 18.25

PERFORMING A WHITE CELL DIFFERENTIAL

RATIONALE

Follow the procedure carefully to ensure an adequate blood sample. This will allow evaluation of different kinds of white blood cells and an accurate count of cells which will aide in diagnosis and determination of treatment processes.

ALERT: Follow Standard Precautions.

1. Wash hands.
2. Assemble equipment.
   a. Disposable nonsterile gloves
   b. Immersion oil
   c. Lens tissue
   d. Lens cleaner
   e. Differential cell counter
   f. Stained blood smear
3. Clean microscope with lens tissue and put on gloves.
4. Put stained blood smear slide in microscope stage. (Use low-power objective.)
5. Find an area on slide where red blood cells barely touch each other.
6. Add drop of oil.
7. Focus with fine-adjustment knob and increased light.
8. Count 100 consecutive white blood cells in winding pattern (see Figure 18.7).
9. Identify each cell (e.g., lymphocyte, eosinophil).
10. Record each cell in differential cell counter.
11. Record variations in red blood cells:
    a. Size (e.g., macrocytosis, microcytosis)
    b. Shape (e.g., sickle cell, target cells)
    c. Content (e.g., hypochromic)

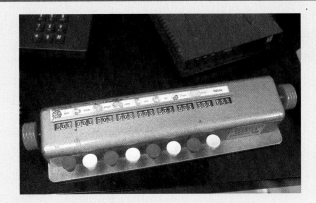

12. Count platelets.

NOTE Take an average; multiply average by 15,000. This gives estimate of platelet count. Normal count is 150,000 to 400,000 per column.

13. Clean microscope with lens tissue.
14. Clean work area.
15. Discard contaminated waste according to facility's policy and remove gloves and face shield.
16. Wash hands.

the A antigen. When an A antigen combines with the A antibody, the reaction is life threatening.

■ Type A blood, B antibody in plasma

■ Type B blood, A antibody in plasma

■ Type AB blood, neither A nor B antibody in plasma

■ Type O blood, A and B antibody in plasma

Another factor in blood typing is the Rh factor. If the Rh factor is present on the red blood cell, you are Rh+. If it is not present, you are Rh−.

Antigen-Antibody Reactions

When a blood antigen combines with the same type of antibody, *agglutination* occurs. The red blood cells clump together. The clumps of cells cannot pass through

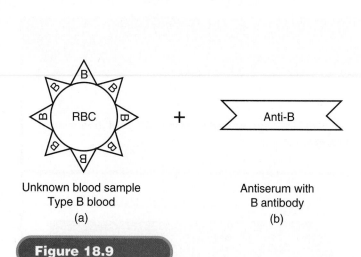

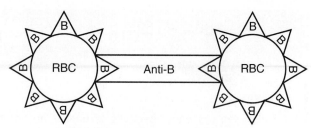

Connecting bridge demonstrates
the antigen-antibody reaction.
The reaction leads to agglutination
of red blood cells. You can see
this reaction without a microscope.
(c)

Unknown blood sample
Type B blood
(a)

Antiserum with
B antibody
(b)

Figure 18.9

the small tubes in the kidney. This can cause kidney failure. The cells also break down and are destroyed (hemolysis). When this happens, oxygen cannot be circulated to the tissues. Carbon dioxide cannot be removed from the tissue, and death results.

Blood Typing and Crossmatching

Blood typing is very important. If the wrong blood is given to a patient, agglutination can occur. To prevent agglutination, you type and crossmatch blood before giving a blood transfusion.

To test blood, you use a manufactured antiserum. The antiserum has antibodies in it. If you use an antiserum with B antibodies on blood with B antigen, you will have clumping. If you use an antiserum with B antibodies on A antigen blood, you will not have clumping (see Figure 18.9).

To crossmatch blood before a transfusion, you perform a series of tests on the patient's blood and the donor's blood. The blood you give the patient must match that of the donor.

Erythrocyte Sedimentation Rate (SR, ESR, Sed. Rate)

The sedimentation rate of blood helps in the diagnosis of some diseases. The speed with which red blood cells fall out of plasma is known as the *sedimentation rate.* An increased sedimentation rate can indicate infection, leukemia, or other problems. When the sedimentation rate decreases it can indicate heart disease, liver disease, or polycythemia.

PROCEDURE 18.26

BLOOD TYPING

RATIONALE

Follow procedure carefully to obtain an accurate blood type. This will help ensure that patients receiving donor blood or products will receive the correct match, therefore receiving appropriate treatment.

ALERT: Follow Standard Precautions.

PROCEDURE 18.26 | BLOOD TYPING *(Continued)*

1. Wash hands.
2. Assemble equipment.
   a. Disposable nonsterile gloves and face shield
   b. Anti-A serum at room temperature
   c. Anti-B serum at room temperature
   d. Anti-Rh serum at room temperature
   e. Two clean slides
   f. Wax pencil
   g. Mixing sticks
   h. Blood specimen
   i. Timer
3. Check expiration date on antiserum.
4. Prepare slides.
   a. Label slides.
   b. Use wax pencil to make two large circles on one slide and one large circle on second slide.

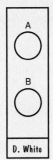 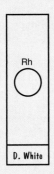

NOTE Make sure that circle is thick enough to prevent blood from crossing it.

5. Put 1 drop of anti-A serum in A circle.
6. Put 1 drop of anti-B serum in B circle.
7. Put 1 drop of anti-Rh serum in Rh circle.
8. Put on gloves and face shield.
9. Put 1 drop of unknown blood specimen *beside* drop of antiserum in each circle.
10. Mix antiserum with blood specimen in each circle.

NOTE Use different mixing stick for each group.

11. Rock slides for 1 minute.
12. Read results before 2 minutes pass.
13. Check slide for agglutination.
14. Record results:

Type of Blood	Anti-A	Anti-B	Anti-Rh or Anti-D
O	Negative	Negative	
A	Positive	Negative	
B	Negative	Positive	
AB	Positive	Positive	
Rh positive			Positive
Rh negative			Negative

15. Clean all equipment.
16. Dispose of contaminated waste according to facility's policy and remove gloves and face shield.
17. Wash hands.

PROCEDURE 18.27 | ERYTHROCYTE SEDIMENTATION RATE USING WINTROBE METHOD

RATIONALE

Carefully follow the procedure to determine how much blood cells drop during a certain time frame. This helps the physician determine if there is an inflammation present in the body.

ALERT: Follow Standard Precautions.

1. Wash hands.
2. Assemble equipment.
   a. Disposable nonsterile gloves and face shield
   b. Calibrated ESR tube—Wintrobe method
   c. Sedimentation rate tubes
   d. Transfer pipettes
   e. Tube holder with level
   f. Venous blood with oxalate/anticoagulant
   g. Timer
3. Check level indicator on tube holder: *must be level.*
4. Put on gloves and face shield.

PROCEDURE 18.27 | **ERYTHROCYTE SEDIMENTATION RATE USING WINTROBE METHOD** *(Continued)*

5. Put sedimentation tube in sed rack with black line in tube at zero on rack.

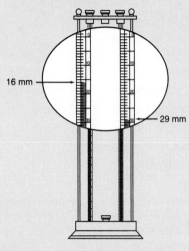

16 mm

29 mm

6. Take tube of specimen blood with anticoagulant and mix gently.

7. Withdraw blood from specimen tube with pipette.

8. Put pipette on bottom of sed tube and release blood slowly as you withdraw pipette.

9. Fill sed tube to zero line. *Note:* If bubbles occur, start over.

10. Recheck rack. It must be level.

11. Follow your facility's procedure for timing fall of red cells.

12. Read at marked line between cells and plasma.

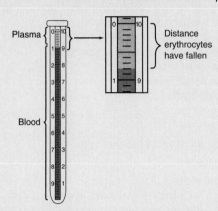

Plasma

Blood

Distance erythrocytes have fallen

13. Record readings (e.g., 20 min, 2 mm). Normal readings: male 0–6.5 mm/hr; female 0–15 mm/hr.

14. Clean equipment.

15. Dispose of contaminated waste according to facility's policy and remove gloves and face shield.

16. Wash hands.

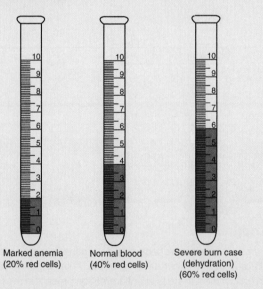

Marked anemia (20% red cells)

Normal blood (40% red cells)

Severe burn case (dehydration) (60% red cells)

Blood Chemistries

The physician uses the results from blood chemistries to help with diagnosis. These chemistries measure chemicals dissolved in the blood. To perform these tests, you need a venous specimen. The phlebotomy unit of this chapter teaches you to draw a venous specimen (see Table 18.4 to familiarize yourself with common blood chemistries). Follow your facility's procedures for tests that you perform.

Table 18.4 ■ Most Common Blood Chemistries and Examples of Disorders They Indicate

Test	Abbreviation	Normal Range	Examples of Possible Diagnosis	
			Results Increased	**Results Decreased**
Alkaline phosphate	ALP	30–115 mU/mL	Liver disease, bone disease, mononucleosis	Malnutrition, hypothyroidism, chronic nephritis
Blood urea nitrogen	BUN	8–25 mg/dL	Kidney disease, dehydration, GI bleeding	Liver failure, malnutrition
Calcium	CA	8.5–10.5 mg/dL	Hypercalcemia, bone metastases, Hodgkin's disease	Hypocalcemia, renal failure, pancreatitis
Chloride	Cl	96–11 mEq/L	Dehydration, eclampsia, anemia	Ulcerative colitis, burns, heat exhaustion
Cholesterol	CHOL	120–200 mg/dL	Atherosclerosis, nephrosis, obstructive jaundice	Malabsorption, liver disease, hyperthyroidism
Creatinine	Creat	0.4–1.5 mg/dL	Chronic nephritis, muscle disease, obstruction of urinary tract	Muscular dystrophy
Globulin	Glob	1.0–3.5 g/dL	Brucellosis, rheumatoid arthritis, hepatic carcinoma	Severe burns
Glucose fasting blood sugar	FBS	70–110 mg/100 mL	Diabetes mellitus	Excess insulin
Two-hour postprandial	2-hr PPBS	< 140 mg/dL	Cushing's syndrome, brain damage	Addison's disease, CA of pancreas
Lactic acid	LDH	100–225 mU/mL	Acute MI, acute leukemia, hepatic disease	
Potassium	K	3.5–5.5 mEq/L	Renal failure, acidosis, cell damage	Malabsorption, severe burn, diarrhea
Serum glutami-coxaloacetic	SGOT	0–41 mU/mL	MI, liver disease, pancreatitis	Uncontrolled diabetes mellitus with acidosis
Serum glutamicpyruvic transaminase	SGPT	0–45 mU/mL	Active cirrhosis, pancreatitis, obstructive jaundice	
Sodium	NA	135–145 mEq/L	Diabetes insipitus, coma, Cushing's syndrome	Severe diarrhea, severe nephritis, vomiting
Free thyroxine	T4	1–2.3 mg/dL	Thyroiditis, hyperthyroidism, Graves' disease	Goiter, myxledema, hypothyroidism
Total bilirubin	TB	0.1–1.2 mg/dL	Liver disease, hemolytic anemia, lupus erythemia	
Triglycerides	TRIG	40–170 mg/dL	Liver disease, atherosclerosis, pancreatitis	Malnutrition
Uric acid	UA	2.2–9.0 mg/dL	Renal failure, gout, leukemia, eclampsia	

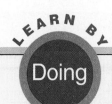

Doing

UNIT 1 ACTIVITY

1. **Complete Worksheets 1 through 7 and Worksheet/Activity 8 as assigned.**
2. **Practice all procedures.**
3. **When you are confident that you can meet each objective, ask your instructor for the unit evaluation.**

UNIT 2

Phlebotomist

STEPS TO SUCCESS

1. Read this unit.
2. Complete the Learn by Doing assignment at the end of this unit.

UNIT OBJECTIVES

When you have completed this unit you will be able to do the following:

✔ Complete all of the objectives in Part One of this book.

✔ List six things the physician can tell from blood samples.

✔ Define vocabulary words.

✔ List three components of blood.

✔ Describe what changes occur in the blood after injury or infection.

✔ List four rules to follow when collecting blood samples.

✔ Match the blood collection tube stopper colors with their content and general use.

✔ Label a diagram of the arm, and identify the veins most often used in venipuncture.

✔ State three ways that blood samples are obtained.

✔ Give two reasons why a syringe and needle are used to draw a blood sample.

✔ Discuss why correct disposal of needles, syringes, and contaminated material is important.

✔ List two serious illnesses spread by contaminated needles and materials.

✔ Demonstrate how to use a Vacutainer™ correctly to withdraw blood.

✔ Demonstrate how to use a needle and syringe correctly to withdraw blood.

✔ Demonstrate how to complete a finger stick correctly.

✔ Apply all procedural techniques with confidence.

RESPONSIBILITIES OF A PHLEBOTOMIST

Phlebotomists may work in an acute care hospital, private laboratory, physician's office, public health agency, or clinic. They draw blood from the veins of patients for testing by the medical laboratory technician or technologist. The phlebotomist can be a laboratory assistant or medical assistant. Phlebotomy is a job title in some facilities. A phlebotomist may only draw blood and not perform other laboratory or medical assistant tasks. Blood is the primary specimen that laboratory workers use for determining the condition of the patient. The results of these tests give the physician information to help in the diagnosis and treatment of patients. The results of blood tests tell the doctor many things about the patient. Some of these relate to

- Anemia
- Infection
- Organ damage
- Change in cell structure
- Liver disease
- Diabetes

The duties of a phlebotomist include the following:

- Screen, record, and direct telephone calls.
- Answer and relay messages.
- Assist in ordering supplies.
- Keep work area clean and properly stocked.
- Keep collection tray clean and stocked.
- Use sterile techniques.
- Identify specialized equipment and supplies.
- Use correct safety precautions.
- Use equipment and supplies for obtaining blood specimens according to facility policy.
- Use proper techniques in collecting and handling specimens.
- Obtain blood specimens from patients (must be certified and have a knowledge of correct anticoagulants).
- Correctly dispose of contaminated materials according to facility policy.

ABOUT BLOOD

Blood is the fluid that flows through the arteries and veins. It carries nutrients and oxygen to the cells and carries away waste products. Blood is composed of *red blood cells, white blood cells,* and **plasma.** A specimen of blood tells a doctor many things about a patient. When the body is injured or ill, blood cells rupture and release chemicals that help doctors diagnose conditions. Vital organs also release substances into the blood that indicate normal or abnormal function within the body. Foreign bodies such as bacteria are also detected from blood specimens. Blood counts determine whether an infection is present (increased number of WBCs) and if there are enough red blood cells.

plasma

Liquid part of the blood, consisting of water, nutrients, wastes, hormones, antibodies, and enzymes.

Patient Considerations

1. Your patient/client may be afraid of a finger stick or **venipuncture.** Remain calm and patient. Explain exactly what you are doing.

venipuncture

Puncture of a vein.

2. The patient may faint and need you to protect him or her from injury. Review how to treat syncopy in your text.

3. It may be difficult to get into the vein.

a. Obese patients have fat layers over the vein. b. Some patients have small, delicate veins, especially the elderly. c. Veins may be injured from past or recent IVs or blood draws. d. Veins may roll and be difficult to access.

If you have a problem entering the vein, call your supervisor to help.
Never stick a patient more than two times.

PREPARING TO DRAW BLOOD

Venipuncture is an invasive procedure. You break the skin, which is the first line of defense against infection. You must use aseptic technique to protect the patient. Remember to *use Standard Precautions* to protect yourself and your patient.

The following rules help you obtain the specimen you need.

■ Collect enough blood for the test.

■ Obtain the specimen as skillfully and efficiently as possible to prevent a **hematoma** or injury to the patient's vein.

■ Collect the proper specimen.

■ Observe the patient for signs of fainting.

hematoma

Collection of blood beneath the skin.

Important Things for You to Know Before You Draw Blood

There are some basic principles that you must learn before you draw blood. Blood is usually tested in two ways:

■ **Uncoagulated.** Collect the blood in a specimen tube that contains an anticoagulant. This method allows you to test the blood specimen in liquid form with the cells in suspension. The specimen is the same as the blood that circulates through the veins.

■ **Coagulated.** Collect the blood and let it coagulate (clot). As a clot forms, a clear liquid, called serum, leaves the clotted cells. This serum is used in many tests.

Anticoagulants

Many tests require unclotted blood. Learn which anticoagulant to use for each specific test. Blood with an anticoagulant may be suitable for one test or a group of tests. It may not be suitable for other tests. Collection tubes come prepared with the solutions needed for specific tests. The tubes are color coded for each test. Learn the color codes you use for each test before you draw blood (see Table 18.5).

Table 18.5 ■ Selecting the Correct Vacutainer™ Tube for Venipuncture

Color	Contents	General Use
Red-brown	None	Blood chemistry, multipurpose
Blue	Citrate	Coagulation
Violet	EDTA (anticoagulant)	Hematology
Green	Heparin	Blood gas, pH
Gray	Sodium fluoride	Chemistry (glucose) and alcohol
SST/marble	Coagulant activator and separating jell	Chemistry

DRAWING BLOOD

Review the structure of the veins in the arm before you draw blood. This knowledge is essential when you draw blood. Sticking a patient in the wrong place can cause injury. Study Figure 18.10 until you can identify each labeled area and find it on your arm. Review all of the sections in this chapter that are about laboratory safety. Learn the different blood tests and blood chemistries. This helps you understand your job.

Blood can be obtained with a Vacutainer™, syringe and needle, or finger and heel sticks. All three require that you follow the guidelines.

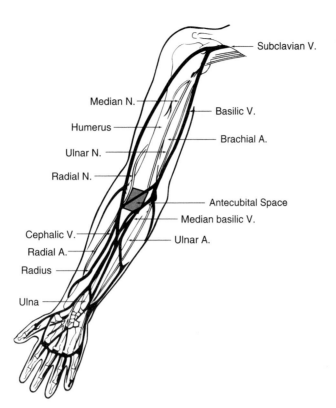

Figure 18.10

Diagram of the arm. A, artery; V, vein; N, nerve.

Guidelines for Blood Withdrawal

1. Select the right collection tube (see Table 18.5 for Vacutainers™).

2. Select the site carefully.

• Never draw blood from an arm with an IV. • Do not use areas that have bruises, a rash, scars, or swelling.

3. Apply a tourniquet above the elbow.

4. Release the tourniquet after 1 minute to prevent bruising and discomfort.

5. Ask the client to open and close the fist to help fill the veins.

6. Cleanse the area for the stick with a sterile swab using a circular motion from the center outward. This removes dirt and bacteria.

7. Hold the skin taut.

8. Use a 15 to 20° angle for entry into the vein.

9. Never press on the vein when removing the needle.

10. *Remember! Do not attempt to draw blood until you are properly instructed in the procedure.*

11. Follow Standard Precautions.

Venipuncture Procedures

Read the following instructions for using a Vacutainer™. Think about each step and why it is important (see Figure 18.11).

Some patients have fragile veins that might be damaged by suction from the Vacutainer™, or have veins that roll. For these patients you can use a syringe and needle. The guidelines are the same as those given in the procedure. The method is different.

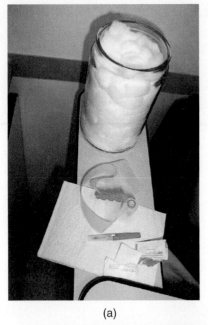

(a)

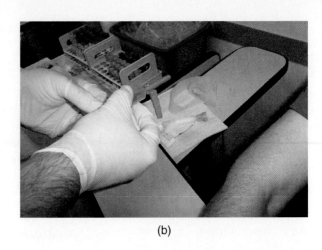

(b)

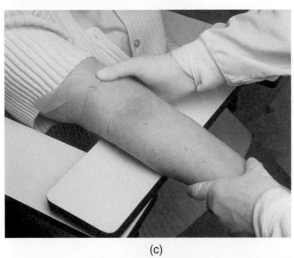

(c)

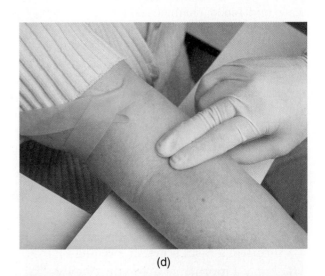

(d)

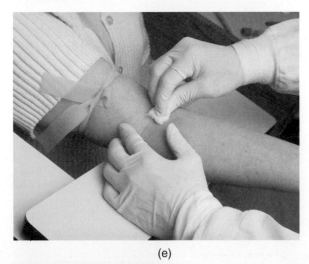

(e)

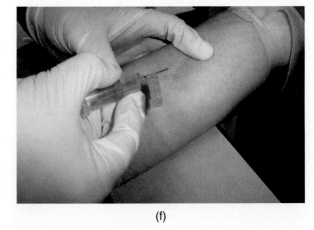

(f)

Figure 18.11

Drawing blood with a Vacutainer™.

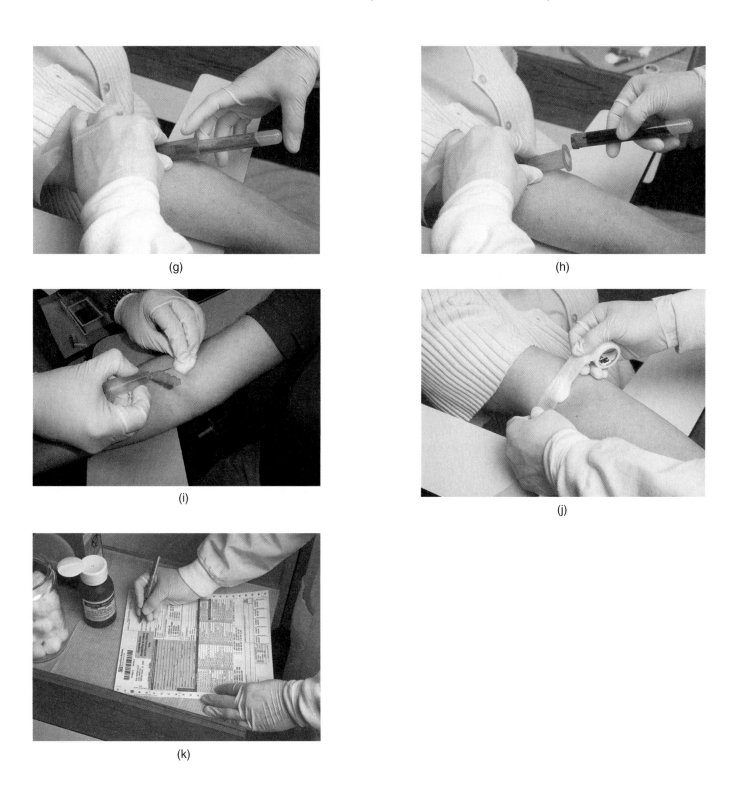

(g)

(h)

(i)

(j)

(k)

Finger or Heel Stick

You use a finger, heel, or earlobe stick (see procedures in Unit 1 of this chapter) when you need a small amount of blood for a test. You obtain a few drops of blood by this method. This is enough for certain tests (for example, PKU on infants, hematocrit, some coagulation tests, and some chemistry tests).

The Collection Tray

Carry a tray with you when you go to the patient/client. If the patient is coming into the laboratory, you have the equipment that you need at your station. If you carry a tray, you must keep it clean and well stocked. Double-check your tray to be certain that you have all the supplies that you need for the test you are doing. The department that you work in has a list of all the supplies that you should carry. Each lab is slightly different. The following is an example of materials that are in a collection tray.

■ Vacutainers™ and syringes
■ Cotton balls and/or sterile gauze
■ Bandages and/or paper tape
■ Tube holders
■ Packaged alcohol swabs
■ Needles (various sizes)
■ Blood culture media
■ Glass slides
■ Lancets
■ Requisitions and marking pen
■ Disposable gloves

How to Dispose of Used Materials

Carefully dispose of used materials (Figure 18.12). Improper disposal causes injury or illness if someone comes in contact with infected materials. It is especially important to be aware of the dangers of contracting hepatitis and AIDS from accidental needle sticks and/or contact with infected body fluids (see the section "Laboratory Standards" in Unit 1).

Always follow these rules:

■ *Never drop a needle into a wastebasket, where it may injure someone.*
■ Place used needles in a sharps container (see Figure 18.12). Follow the laboratory's procedure for safe disposal of the needles.
■ When drawing blood from a patient who is in isolation, take only the materials that you need into the room. Discard the used needles in the disposal container inside the patient's room. Dispose of them according to the facility's policy for contaminated materials. Follow the rules for the removal of specimens from the isolation room.

Figure 18.12

Sharps container.

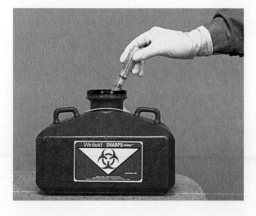

PROCEDURE 18.28

DRAWING BLOOD WITH A VACUTAINER™

RATIONALE

Carefully following the procedure for drawing blood with a Vacutainer™ will help ensure that a viable blood specimen is collected. A viable specimen will help provide accurate results that will aid in diagnosis and monitoring of various conditions.

ALERT: Follow Standard Precautions.

1. Wash hands.
2. Assemble equipment.
   a. Alcohol wipes or 70% alcohol
   b. Sterile cotton wipes
   c. Sterile compresses
   d. Vacutainer™ system with appropriate tube(s), needle, and holder
   e. Small bandage
   f. Disposable nonsterile gloves
   g. Nonpermeable long-sleeved gown
   h. Face shield
3. If going to client's room, check collection tray for materials required.
   a. Vacutainer™ or syringe
   b. Cotton balls or sterile gauze
   c. Bandages or paper tape
   d. Tourniquet
   e. Tube holders
   f. Packaged alcohol swabs
   g. Needles (various sizes)
   h. Blood culture media
   i. Glass slides
   j. Lancets
   k. Requisitions and marking pen
   l. Disposable nonsterile gloves
4. Identify patient/client.
5. Explain procedure to patient.
6. Attach needle to Vacutainer™ (or syringe).
7. Select correct tube for blood sample you are going to draw.
   a. *Red-brown:* blood chemistry, multipurpose
   b. *Blue:* coagulation
   c. *Violet:* hematology
   d. *Green:* blood gas, pH
   e. *Gray:* chemistry (glucose) and alcohol
8. Insert tube into holder and push tube stopper onto needle.
9. Select site for venipuncture by palpating antecubital space:
   a. Carefully examine both arms.
   b. Select suitable site.
10. Put on gloves and face shield.

11. Apply a tourniquet 3 to 4 inches above patient's elbow.
12. Clean venipuncture site with alcohol wipe. *Do not touch area after cleaning.*
13. Remove needle cover.
14. If you are right-handed, use your left hand to pull skin over puncture site tightly. (If left-handed, use right hand.)
15. Carefully insert needle through skin into vein. (This will take practice to do correctly.)
    a. Bevel tip of needle should be up.
    b. Puncture skin and vein in one motion.
16. Place two fingers at end of holder; with your thumb, push Vacutainer™ onto needle to end of holder. (You may need to use more than one tube.)
17. Release tourniquet as soon as blood begins to enter tube, and obtain as many samples as needed.
18. Remove last Vacutainer™ from holder when enough blood has been obtained.
19. Remove needle from vein when blood stops flowing into tube. Place gauze over puncture site.
20. Apply pressure with sterile compress to puncture site and have patient elevate arm for a few minutes.
21. Discard needle in correct disposal container.
22. If tube contains additives, gently invert 8 to 10 times to mix additives with blood. Do not shake.
23. Apply small bandage to puncture site.
24. Clean area of all used material and discard properly according to facility's contaminated waste policy.
25. Label collection tube:
    a. Patient's name
    b. Date
    c. Time
    d. Technician's initials
26. Remove gloves, face shield, and gown.
27. Check to see that bleeding has stopped.
28. Wash hands.
29. Fill out paperwork or forms that are required.
30. Make certain that blood sample is delivered to proper place for testing.

PROCEDURE 18.29

USING A NEEDLE AND SYRINGE TO DRAW BLOOD

RATIONALE

Using a needle and syringe is a gentler method of drawing blood from small, fragile vessels. A small-gauge needle can be used to puncture the vessel and less suction pressure can be exerted with the syringe than a Vacutainer™.

ALERT: Follow Standard Precautions.

1. Wash hands.
2. Assemble equipment.
   a. Sterile compresses
   b. Tourniquet
   c. Sterile disposable needle, usually 1½ or 1¼ inches, 21 gauge
   d. Sterile disposable syringe: 5-, 10-, 20-, or 30-cc size
   e. Test tube(s) with or without additives, depending on tests to be done
   f. Disposable nonsterile gloves
   g. Nonpermeable gown with long sleeves
   h. Face shield
3. If you are going to client's room, check collection tray for materials required.
   a. Syringe
   b. Needles (various sizes)
   c. Cotton balls or sterile gauze
   d. Bandages or paper tape
   e. Tourniquet
   f. Tube holders
   g. Packed alcohol swabs
   h. Blood culture media
   i. Glass slides
   j. Lancets
   k. Requisitions and marking pen
   l. Disposable nonsterile gloves
   m. Nonpermeable gown
   n. Face shield
4. Identify patient/client.
5. Explain procedure to patient.
6. Attach needle to syringe. Leave on needle cover.
7. Select correct tube for blood sample you are going to draw.
   a. *Red-brown:* blood chemistry, multipurpose
   b. *Blue:* coagulation
   c. *Violet:* hematology
   d. *Green:* blood gas, pH
   e. *Gray:* chemistry (glucose) and alcohol
8. Select site for venipuncture by palpating anticubital space.

   a. Carefully examine both arms.
   b. Select suitable site.
9. Put on gloves and face shield.
10. Apply tourniquet 3 to 4 inches above patient's elbow.
11. Clean venipuncture site with alcohol wipe. *Do not touch area after cleaning.*
12. Remove needle cover.
13. If you are right-handed, use your left hand to pull skin over puncture site tightly. (If left-handed, use right hand.)
14. Carefully insert needle through skin into vein. (This will take practice to do correctly.)
    a. Bevel tip of needle should be up.
    b. Puncture skin and vein in one motion.
15. Having entered vein, use your right hand (if you are right-handed) or left hand (if you are left-handed) to pull syringe plunger slowly to withdraw blood. As soon as blood starts to flow into syringe, release tourniquet.
16. When you have drawn required amount of blood, place sterile compress over puncture site and withdraw needle.
17. Apply pressure over puncture site for a few minutes and have patient elevate arm.
18. Remove stopper from Vacutainer™ and fill tube with correct amount of blood.
19. If you are using tubes other than Vacutainers™, cap tubes.
20. Label collection tube with patient's name, date, and time.
21. If tube has an additive, gently invert 8 to 10 times to mix blood and additive. *Do not shake.*
22. Apply small bandage to puncture area.
23. Discard syringe and needle in correct disposal container.
24. Remove gloves, face shield, and gown.
25. Wash hands.

JOBS AND PROFESSIONS

- Assistive personnel
- Clinical medical assistant
- Laboratory assistant
- Nurse assistant
- Licensed vocational/practical nurse
- Registered nurse
- Phlebotomist
- Laboratory technician

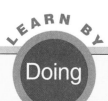

UNIT 2 ACTIVITY

1. Complete Worksheets 1, 3 and 4 and Worksheet/Activity 2 as assigned.

2. Practice all procedures.

3. Prepare responses to each item listed in Chapter Review—Your Link to Success at the end of this chapter.

4. When you are confident that you can meet each objective, ask your instructor for the unit evaluation.

Thinking Critically

1. Medical Terminology Use information in Part One of this text and a medical dictionary to list laboratory tests or medical terms used in the laboratory. Use these terms to write a scenario about a patient who had these tests performed.

2. Legal and Ethical Control tests are important quality indicators in the laboratory. Explain the legal and ethical reasons for their requirements of accuracy and consistency.

3. Communication Role-play with a classmate how to explain to a patient the importance of fasting before some tests. Develop a bulleted list to place in your portfolio of successful techniques and strategies for communicating with patients.

4. Computers Identify at least five laboratory tests that are commonly performed by a computerized analyzer. Describe the primary differences (advantages vs. disadvantages) between the computerized test and the manual test that measures the same thing.

5. Patient Education The daughter of an older, non-English-speaking patient tells you her mother is terrified of giving a blood sample because she believes the procedure puts her at risk of being infected with a fatal disease. Write a list in understanding terms of the Standard Precautions that are taken during the procedure for the daughter to translate. Review your list to be sure it clearly states the protective measures that are required to ensure each patient's safety.

6. Case Study An 8-year-old girl is in the reception area of the laboratory. Her mother warns you that her daughter is frightened of needles and becomes hysterical every time she gets a shot or has blood drawn. Explain how you will approach the child, what you will communicate to her, and what you are going to do to complete the phlebotomy.

Portfolio Connection

When you are competent in all laboratory assistant and phlebotomy skills, ask for permission to copy the results of tests that you completed. (Remove all patient identifiers.) Place these copies in your portfolio as evidence of your skills. Place a copy of your on-site trainer's evaluation in your portfolio.

Write a paper describing your doubts and realizations and the barriers that you were able to overcome during your laboratory experiences. For example, were you afraid that drawing blood might make you faint? Describe the ways you plan to use the skills, information, and insights that you gained about people and about this job. This assignment must be in standard report format.

Portfolio Tip

Remember that lack of information and understanding is often at the heart of a patient's resistance to procedures. Keeping this in mind will help you to realize that the patient's objections are not directed at you personally.

Remember! 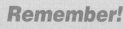 Media Connection

Use the Companion Website **www.prenhall.com/badasch** and the CD-ROM for additional interactive learning activities.

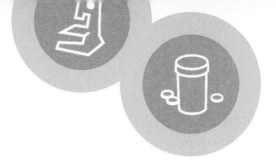

Chapter 19

Physical Therapy Aide

MEDIA CONNECTION

Use the Companion Website
www.prenhall.com/badasch and the CD-ROM
for additional interactive learning activities.

STEPS TO SUCCESS

1. Read this chapter.

2. Complete the Learn by Doing assignment at the end of this chapter.

OBJECTIVES

When you have completed this chapter, you will be able to do the following:

✔ Complete all objectives in Part One of this book.

✔ Describe the responsibilities of a physical therapy aide.

✔ Name four conditions treated with ultraviolet light.

✔ Describe four conditions treated with diathermy.

✔ Explain the physical therapy aide's main responsibility when setting up a patient for a diathermy treatment.

✔ List three conditions commonly treated by ultrasound.

✔ Document the most important question to ask a patient when preparing for an ultrasound treatment.

✔ Identify two kinds of thermotherapy and the conditions they treat.

✔ Identify two ways to give cryotherapy and conditions they treat.

✔ Define *hydrotherapy* and list the three reasons hydrotherapy is used.

✔ Define *guarding technique* and *guarding belt*.

✔ Explain the purpose of range of motion (Chapter 15).

✔ List five commonly used ambulation devices.

✔ List two transporting devices commonly used (Chapter 15).

✔ Demonstrate the following skills:

  • From Chapter 15: Pivot transfer from bed to wheelchair and back
  Sliding from bed to gurney and back
  Moving a patient/client in a wheelchair
  Moving a patient/client on a gurney
  Lifting with a mechanical lift
  Range of motion

  • From Chapter 22: Customer service

✔ Explain the role of physical therapy in the team concept of patient care.

✔ Demonstrate each procedure in this chapter.

THE PHYSICAL THERAPY DEPARTMENT

The physical therapy department is made up of a number of trained people who work as a team to assist and direct patients in the rehabilitation process. Their main goal is to reduce pain, prevent deformity, and promote healing. They also attempt to restore function or assist patients/clients by teaching them new ways to adjust to their disabilities. The entry-level job title for this department is "physical therapy aide." Physical therapy workers may be employed in the following facilities and agencies:

- Acute care facilities
- Long-term care facilities
- Rehabilitation centers
- Schools for disabled persons
- Public health agencies
- Home health care agencies
- Sports medicine centers

RESPONSIBILITIES OF A PHYSICAL THERAPY AIDE

As a physical therapy aide, you are required to do the following tasks:

- Prepare equipment (e.g., hydrotherapy pools)
- Assist patients:
  - With walking and gait training • To dress and undress • To position themselves • To remove and replace braces, splints, and slings
- Change linen on beds and tables
- Fold linen
- Clean equipment and work area
- May inventory materials and supplies

PREPARING PATIENTS/CLIENTS FOR THERAPY

As an aide in the physical therapy department, you assist the therapist and prepare

- The patient
- Supplies
- Equipment

There are various types of therapy, and each requires a slightly different preparation. Some of the most common types of therapy are discussed below.

Ultraviolet-light therapy is used to treat

- Acne
- Pressure sores
- Psoriasis
- Wound infections

This treatment can cause severe burning. For this reason, the patient cannot be left unobserved in the room during a treatment.

NOTE Do not turn on the light before the therapist is ready to start the treatment.

Diathermy is a heat-inducing treatment that increases the circulation in the treated area. It is often used to treat

- Muscle problems
- Arthritis
- Bursitis
- Tendonitis

Metal attracts heat during this procedure, so it is your responsibility to

- Have the patient remove all metal jewelry, belts, hairpins, and so on.
- Ask the patient if they have any metal implants in joints or in other parts of the body. If they do, report it to the therapist right away.

Ultrasound uses high-frequency sound waves to penetrate deep tissues. It is most commonly used to treat

- Pain
- Muscle spasms
- Problems in circulation

Ultrasound is also used to diagnose. However, physical therapy uses it only in a therapeutic mode. Because ultrasound vibrates tissues, caution has to be taken with patients with joint implants. Always ask patients during the preparation if they have any joint implants. If so, report it to the therapist.

Thermotherapy refers to heat treatments. Heat is used to speed up the healing process. Heat causes the blood vessels to expand (dilate). This allows more blood to circulate to the area and helps the healing process. The blood brings oxygen and food needed for healing. If the area is swollen and/or inflamed, the blood helps absorb and carry away the extra fluid. This type of treatment is used to

- Relieve pain
- Promote muscle relaxation
- Reduce muscle spasms
- Reduce inflammation
- Treat skin ulcers
- Treat perineal lacerations
- Reduce swelling
- Promote drainage

There are two kinds of thermotherapy. One type is moist heat. The other type is dry heat. *Moist heat* is applied with

- Hot soaks
- Hot compresses
- Hot packs

Dry heat is applied with

- Heat lamps
- Infrared lights
- Standard electric bulbs
- Heating pads

PROCEDURE 19.1

PREPARING MOIST HOT SOAKS

RATIONALE

Using the correct temperature for the hot moist pads and careful observation of the treated area prevents injury.

ALERT: Follow Standard Precautions.

1. Wash hands.
2. Assemble equipment.
    a. Hydroculator pad
    b. Towel
3. Identify patient/client.
4. Explain what you will be doing and reassure patient that procedure is painless.
5. Cover warm hydroculator pad with towel.
6. Expose site to be treated.
7. Position patient for comfort.
8. Apply covered warm hydroculator pad to appropriate site.

9. Wash hands.
10. Recheck patient frequently; look for
    a. Severely reddened areas
    b. Irritated areas
    c. Painful areas
11. Remove soaks as ordered.
12. Position client for comfort.
13. Wash hands.
14. Report and record patient's tolerance of treatment and any changes in condition you observed.

You need to prepare hot packs so that they are ready when needed. Always check the skin for signs of extreme redness or burning. If patient complains of discomfort, remove the packs immediately.

Cryotherapy means cold therapy. Cold therapy causes the blood vessels to get smaller (contract). This slows the flow of blood to the area. This reduces the amount of fluid and helps reduce pain. Cold application is used to

■ Relieve pain
■ Reduce body temperature
■ Control bleeding
■ Reduce inflammation
■ Prevent edema

Cryotherapy can be given in two ways: dry cold and moist cold. *Dry cold* includes the use of

■ Ice bags
■ Ice collars

Moist cold includes the use of

■ Cold compresses
■ Cold packs
■ Ice massage

Prepare cold packs for cryotherapy (cold, moist, or dry treatments) so that they are ready when needed. Always check the skin for signs of whiteness (blanching) or bluishness. If these occur, stop the treatment immediately.

PROCEDURE 19.2 | MOIST CRYOTHERAPY (COLD) COMPRESSES

RATIONALE

Using correct temperature for moist cryotherapy and careful observation of the treated area prevents injury.

ALERT: Follow Standard Precautions.

1. Wash hands.
2. Assemble equipment
    a. Cool, wet cloth
    b. Plastic cover
    c. Dry towel
3. Apply cool, wet cloth as ordered.

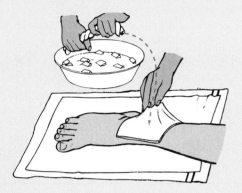

4. Cover wet area with plastic cover.
5. Cover plastic with dry towel.
6. Wash hands.

NOTE Wear gloves if there are broken areas on the skin.

7. Recheck frequently for
    a. Coolness of cloth
    b. Position
    c. Patient's comfort needs (reapply PRN)
8. Remove as ordered.
9. Dry skin.
10. Dispose of supplies and clean area.
11. Wash hands.
12. Report and document effects of treatment.

11/20/03   1100
No skin reddened or irritated areas
Moist, cold towels applied times 15
minutes
Recheck skin at site
No reddened or irritated areas
Patient states: Pain is better
after treatment but returns in
about an hour
—————— A. Cantina student

Hydrotherapy is water therapy. Hydrotherapy is usually given in a whirlpool. The whole body may be treated or just a limb. This treatment is used to

- Apply soothing medication
- Promote relaxation
- Improve circulation and mobility of an injured limb
- Loosen and remove dead skin

This treatment is accomplished in various-sized tubs ranging from small basins to a swimming pool. Your responsibility is to

- Assist the client in disrobing or exposing the area to be treated.
- Ensure that the water temperature is correct (95° F–105° F).
- Secure the client to ensure there is no danger of injury.

PROCEDURE 19.3

DRY CRYOTHERAPY: ICE BAGS/ICE COLLARS

RATIONALE

Using correct temperature for dry cryotherapy and careful observation of the treated area prevents injury.

ALERT: Follow Standard Precautions.

1. Wash hands.
2. Assemble equipment.
   a. Ice bag or commercial cold compress
   b. Ice
   c. Cover for ice bag
3. Fill bag with ice. (Run water over cubes to soften sharp edges.)
4. Remove air from bag by pressing sides together.
5. Close end and check for leaks.
6. Cover bag with cloth. (Never apply bag directly to skin; it may stick, burn, and tear skin when removed.)

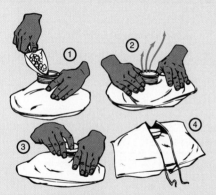

7. Identify patient/client by checking order and name with patient's armband or patient chart.
8. Position ice bag as ordered.

NOTE Wear gloves if there are broken areas on the skin.

9. Secure bag so that it does not move away from affected area.
10. Provide needed comfort measures for patient.
11. Wash hands.
12. Return frequently to check for
    a. Coolness of ice bag
    b. Position of ice bag
    c. Color of skin (remove ice if skin is bluish in color and report)
13. Remove ice bag at ordered time.
14. Wash hands.
15. Recheck skin, and report and document effects of treatment.
16. Wash hands.
17. Empty bag, dry, and return to appropriate area for cleaning.

11/20/03   1100
No skin reddened or irritated areas
Dry cold compress applied times 15
minutes
Recheck skin at site
No reddened or irritated areas
Patient states: Pain is better after
treatment but returns in about an hour
_____ A. Cantina student

- Disinfect and clean the equipment.
- Assist the patient when large areas of the body are to be submerged.
- Clean the tub after each treatment.

⬤ GUARDING TECHNIQUES

Use guarding techniques when moving patients/clients from place to place. These techniques protect the patient while transferring a patient from the bed to a gurney or chair, chair to a chair, chair to a toilet, or commode and back again. You use a variety of techniques to transfer the client.

- **Pivot technique.** You generally use this technique when moving a patient who can bear weight on at least one foot. It works best when moving from a bed or chair to a chair, toilet, or commode and back again.

- **Sliding technique.** You use sliding when a client needs to be moved and cannot get up or bear weight on either foot. It works best when moving from bed to gurney, chair, commode, or toilet and back again. Paraplegic and quadriplegic patients may use a flat boardlike device to slide on. This provides security and decreases the chance of separation between chairs and bed and so on.

- **Lifting technique.** Use this technique when there is ample help and strength to support the client fully while moving him or her from one support to another.

You also use guarding techniques when the patient is ambulating (walking). All patients who can support themselves are encouraged to walk alone or with the assistance of another person. Patients who are uncomfortable usually resist having to move. Your encouragement is needed to keep their body functions as normal as possible. There are a variety of techniques you may use:

- A guarding belt (walking belt) supports and helps the client feel secure.

- You may support the patient by placing an arm around the patient's waist and holding one arm firmly.

- Some patients may need to hold on to you. Just your hand may be enough to steady them in those first few steps after a lengthy stay in bed.

- Some patients may require two people to assist them. One person on each side of the client should hold each arm and hold the person securely around the waist.

- Walking next to a rail is helpful. Patients often feel insecure when they are dependent on another person for support. A solid railing provides the extra security they need.

Safety is very important at all times. The patient may lose his or her balance, feel faint, or the legs can collapse. Prevent injury by helping the resident to the floor. Protect yourself from injury by using good body mechanics. Stay with the patient and call for help. A licensed nurse should evaluate the patient before moving him or her. Ask for help when lifting a patient from the floor.

PROCEDURE 19.4   AMBULATING WITH A WALKING BELT

RATIONALE

Using a gait belt protects the patient from falling when ambulating. It ensures the safety and security of the patient.

ALERT: Follow Standard Precautions.

1. Wash hands.
2. Assemble equipment.
   a. Gait belt/walking belt (correct size)
   b. Patient's robe
   c. Patient's footwear
3. Identify patient.
4. Explain what you are going to do.
5. Assist client to sitting position on side of bed.

PROCEDURE 19.4 | AMBULATING WITH A WALKING BELT *(Continued)*

6. Encourage patient to take a few deep breaths and ask if he or she feels dizzy. (If dizziness is present, let patient sit a while before walking.)

7. Assist patient with robe and slippers.

8. Secure walking belt around patient's waist over clothing.

9. Tighten belt and buckle securely.

NOTE   Belt is too tight if you cannot put two fingers behind it.

10. Stand in front of patient with broad base of support.

11. Instruct patient to put hands on your shoulder.

12. Ease patient to a standing position and hold hand grip securely at back of belt.

13. Ambulate client as ordered.

14. Observe patient for weakness or discomfort.

15. Return client to room and make comfortable.

16. Document and report patient's tolerance of procedure.

17. Return walking belt to storage area so that it will be available for the next procedure.

18. Wash hands.

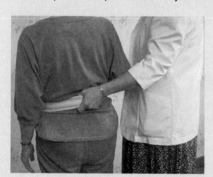

11/08/03   0830
Ambulated with gait belt in
hallway for 10 minutes
Tolerated well
No dizziness or discomfort
Patient states that it "feels good to
be out of bed."
_____ S. Munoz student

EXERCISING

Physical therapy department personnel work with patients to maintain normal functions of all parts of the body. They use range-of-motion exercises to move all joints in the body. This is accomplished through

- **Active ROM.** The client moves the body part without help.
- **Passive ROM.** Someone else moves the body part for the patient. (See the procedure "Range of Motion" in Chapter 15.) The physical therapist directs an exercise program that improves strength and mobility. These exercises may use complicated machines or simple items, such as a rubber ball that can be routinely squeezed. Regardless of the technique you use, it is essential that you are secure with the procedure before you attempt to assist a client.

REHABILITATION EQUIPMENT

Ambulation Devices

Ambulation devices assist patients/clients to walk (see Figure 19.1a–f). Some of the most common devices are described in the next paragraphs.

Canes provide a third base of support for patients who are slightly unstable on their feet. Use a cane when patients are

- Slightly weaker on one side

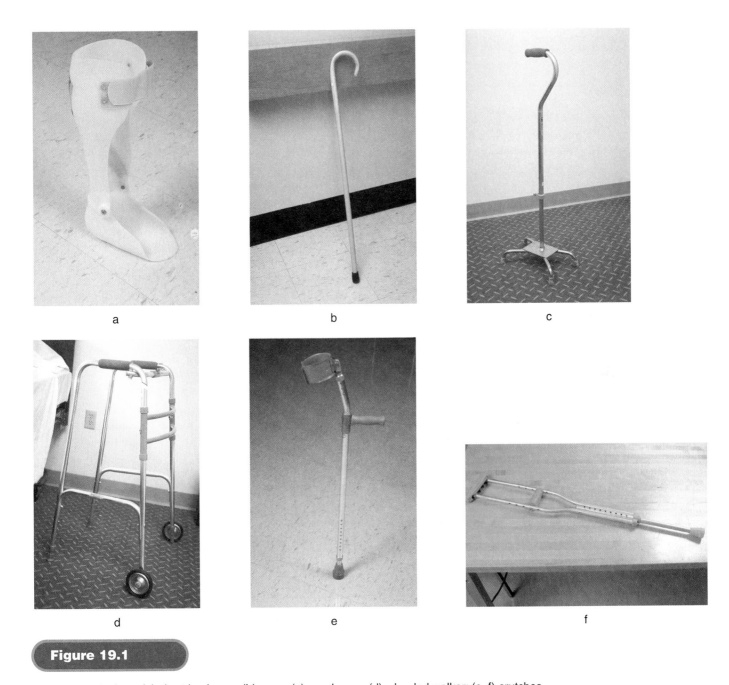

a   b   c

d   e   f

Figure 19.1

Ambulation devices: (a) short leg brace; (b) cane; (c) quad cane; (d) wheeled walker; (e, f) crutches.

■ Easily thrown off balance

■ Insecure walking alone

Special considerations to keep in mind when preparing a cane for use include the following:

■ The patient's height

■ Use of a single-foot cane or multifoot cane

■ Condition of rubber tips

■ Weight and appearance of the cane

PROCEDURE 19.5

WALKING WITH A CANE

RATIONALE

Correctly sized, safe canes and careful safety instruction protects the patient from falls or injuries.

1. Wash hands.
2. Assemble equipment.
   a. Cane in good repair and with rubber tip
   b. Patient's/client's footwear
   c. Patient's/client's robe
3. Identify patient.
4. Assist client with shoes and robe.
5. Explain what you are going to do.
6. Position client in a standing position (have a co-worker help you if necessary).
7. Check height of cane. Top of cane should be at the patient's hip joint.
8. Check arm position at side of body and hold top of cane. Arm should be bent at a 25 to 30° angle.
9. Have patient hold cane in hand on strongest side of body (unaffected side).
10. Assist client as needed while ambulating. Most physicians order a standard gait procedure.
    a. With cane in hand on strongest side, move cane and weakest foot forward.
    b. Place body weight forward on cane and move strongest foot forward. (Patient will have cane's maximum support when this procedure is used when walking on flat surface, hill, or stairs. Remember: Weak leg and cane move together.)
11. When you have completed ordered ambulation, return patient to the starting place.
12. Provide for patient's comfort.
13. Place cane in proper location. If client is capable and physician permits ambulation without assistance, leave cane in a convenient place for patient.
14. Wash hands.
15. Report and document patient's tolerance of procedure.
    a. Date
    b. Time

c. Ambulated with cane (e.g., 15 minutes in hall)
d. How tolerated
e. Signature and classification

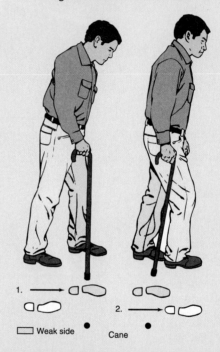

1. →
2. →

☐ Weak side   ● Cane

11/03/03   2100

Height of cane correct
Checked for safety
Instructions given with emphasis
on using the cane on the
affected side
Ambulated without difficulty 15
minutes in hall
Tolerated well
_____ S. Munoz student

Crutches provide support and stability by promoting use of the hands and arms more than the legs. Use them when patients are able to bear weight

■ On one foot or leg

■ Only partially on one leg or on both feet and legs

Special considerations when preparing crutches for use include the following:

■ Adjusting their height for the patient. Keep in mind:
   • Axillary pressure—too much pressure causes injury • Hand level

■ The patient's footwear (slippery soles, open toes, etc.)

■ Condition of rubber tips, hand pads, and axillary pads

■ Securing all joints on the crutches

PROCEDURE 19.6 | WALKING WITH CRUTCHES

RATIONALE

Measuring crutches to fit properly and careful instruction in how to safely use crutches prevents injury.

1. Wash hands.
2. Assemble equipment.
   a. Crutches in good repair with rubber tips
   b. Patient's footwear
   c. Patient's robe, if necessary
3. Identify patient.
4. Explain what you are going to do.
5. Help patient with shoes and robe.
6. Check fit of crutches to patient.
   a. Have client stand with crutches in place. (Ask a co-worker to assist if necessary.)
   b. Position foot of crutches about 4 inches to side of patient's foot and slightly forward of foot.
   c. Check distance between underarm and crutch underarm rest. It should be about 2 inches.
   d. Check angle of patient's arm. When hand is on hand rest bar and crutches are in walking position, arms should be at a 30° angle.
7. Remind patient that the hands support most of the body weight, not the underarms (axilla).
8. Assist client to ambulate following gait method ordered. There are a variety of crutch walking gaits. The following will provide guidelines to the most commonly used:
   a. Three-point gait (beginners)
      (1) One leg is weight-bearing.
      (2) Place both crutches forward along with non-weight-bearing foot. Weight will be supported primarily by weight-bearing foot.

(3) Shift weight to *hands* on crutches and move weight-bearing foot forward.
   b. Four-point gait (beginners) (see figure below)

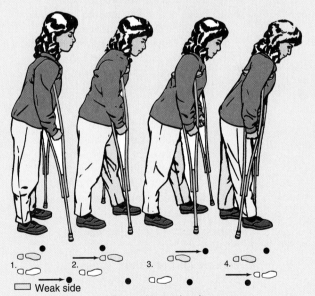

Four-point crutch gait

(1) Both legs are weight-bearing.
(2) Place one crutch forward.
(3) Move foot on opposite side of body forward, parallel with forward crutch.
(4) Place other crutch forward and parallel with first crutch.
(5) Move other foot forward so that it rests next to first foot.

PROCEDURE 19.6 | WALKING WITH CRUTCHES *(Continued)*

c. Two-point gait (advanced) (see figure below)

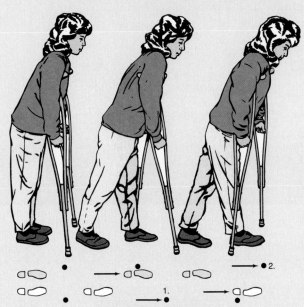

Two-point crutch gait

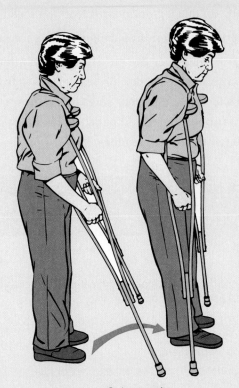

Swing-to gait

(1) Both legs are weight-bearing.
(2) Place one crutch forward and move opposite foot forward with it.
(3) Place other crutch forward and parallel with first crutch. Then move opposite foot forward so that it is even with other foot.

d. Swing-to gait (arm and shoulder strength are needed) (see figure at top right)

(1) One or both legs are weight-bearing.
(2) Balance weight on weight-bearing limb.
(3) Place both crutches forward.
(4) Shift weight to *hands* on crutches.
(5) Swing both feet forward until parallel with crutches.

CAUTION: Placing crutches too far forward can result in a fall!

e. Swing-through gait (advanced: arm and shoulder strength are needed) (see figure at bottom right)

(1) One or both legs are weight-bearing.
(2) Balance weight on weight-bearing limb(s).
(3) Place both crutches forward.
(4) Shift weight to *hands* on crutches.
(5) Swing both feet forward just ahead of crutches.

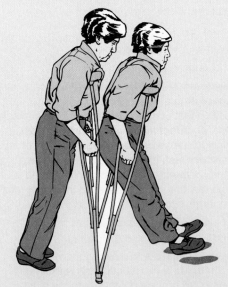

Swing-through gait

9. Return to room.
10. Ensure that client is comfortable.
11. Wash hands.

PROCEDURE 19.6 | WALKING WITH CRUTCHES *(Continued)*

12. Record the following:
    a. Date
    b. Time
    c. Distance ambulated
    d. How tolerated
    e. Signature and classification

12/10/03   2000
Measured crutches for
correct size and safety
Instructed patient in safe
use to prevent additional injury
Ambulated for 15 minutes in hallway
Tolerated well
_____ S. Munoz student

Walkers provide support and stability. Use them when patients are

■ Relearning to walk

■ On limited weight-bearing

■ Unstable on their feet

Special considerations to keep in mind when preparing walkers for patient use include the following:

■ Adjusting the walker to the patient's height

■ The patient's footwear (open toes, slippery soles, etc.)

■ Securing all joints on walker

■ Condition of rubber tips

These devices give the patient additional support and aid in balancing while walking or standing. Patients must be able to use their hands and arms to adapt properly to these devices. Some additional devices that aid in ambulation include the following:

Braces provide specific support for weakened muscle joints or immobilize an injured joint. Patients use them when they have

■ Weakened joints or muscles

■ Injuries that need to be stabilized

Special considerations to keep in mind when preparing braces for a patient include the following:

■ They are custom-made for each patient; they are not meant to be shared.

■ They may require padding to protect the skin.

■ There is only one way to apply a brace; be sure that you know the correct way.

A *prosthesis* is an artificial body part or an aid to a part of the body that minimizes a disability. When a body part is missing, the prosthesis gives a natural appearance and provides maximum usability for the person. The prosthesis most commonly dealt with in physical therapy is the artificial arm or leg. Special

PROCEDURE 19.7 — WALKING WITH A WALKER

RATIONALE

Measuring a walker to fit properly and careful instruction in how to safely use a walker prevents injury.

1. Wash hands.
2. Assemble equipment.
   a. Walker in good condition
   b. Patient's footwear
   c. Patient's robe if necessary
3. Identify client.
4. Tell client what you are going to do.
5. Stand patient up with walker. (Ask a co-worker to help if necessary.)
6. Check to see if walker fits patient properly.
   a. Walker's handgrips should be at top of patient's leg or bend of leg at hip joint.
   b. Arm should be at a 25 to 30° angle.
7. Assist patient to ambulate as ordered. Basic guidelines for walking with a walker are as follows:
   a. Patient begins by standing inside frame of walker.
   b. Patient lifts walker (never slides) and places back legs of walker parallel with toes (never ahead of toes).
   c. Patient shifts weight onto hands and walker (for balance and support).
   d. Patient then walks into walker.
   e. Place yourself just to side and slightly behind client. This position will allow you to observe and be close enough to assist if necessary.
8. When you have completed the ordered ambulation, return patient to his or her starting place.
9. Provide for patient's comfort.
10. Place walker in proper location. If client is capable and physician permits ambulation without assistance, leave walker in a convenient place for patient.
11. Wash hands.
12. Report and document patient's tolerance of procedure.
13. Record the following:
    a. Date
    b. Time
    c. Distance and amount of time ambulated
    d. How tolerated
    e. Signature and classification

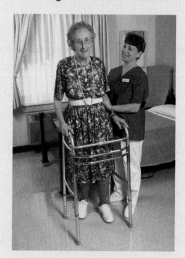

12/04/03   0800

Checked walker for safety measures
Instructed patient in correct use
of walker
Ambulated in hallway for 10 minutes
Patient complained of dizziness
initially
Dangled from bed until dizziness
subsided
Tolerated with some difficulty with
fatigue
Patient stated "I feel really tired
after using the walker."
——————— S. Munoz P.T. Aide

considerations to keep in mind when preparing a prosthesis for a patient include the following:

- You must have the right device.
- The end resting against the patient is padded.
- All straps must be in good condition.
- It is clean and the overall appearance is natural.
- Report tender areas at attachment site.

Transporting Devices

Transport devices include equipment to move patients from one place to another. The most common transporting devices are wheelchairs and gurneys. Gurneys and wheelchairs make it easy to move patients who are unable to walk. You are responsible for a variety of procedures as a physical therapy aide. Be sure that you are knowledgeable and confident about each procedure before you begin work with patients.

Adaptive-Assistive Devices

Adaptive-assistive devices include equipment that helps a person perform daily activities. These devices range from special holders for silverware to devices that help people put on socks or button clothing.

○ JOBS AND PROFESSIONS

- Assistive personnel
- Nurse assistant
- Medical assistant
- Licensed vocational/practical nurse
- Registered nurse
- Physical therapist
- Home health aide

Doing

1. Complete Worksheet 1 as assigned.
2. Complete Worksheet/Activity 2 as assigned.
3. Practice all procedures.
4. Prepare responses to each item listed in Chapter Review—Your Link to Success at the end of this chapter.
5. When you are confident that you can meet each objective, ask your instructor for the unit evaluation.

Thinking Critically

1. Communication Describe what you would say to a patient who was going to have his first hydrotherapy treatment. What special precautions would you take? What would you tell the patient about the possible outcome of his treatment?

2. Medical Terminology Use Part One of this text and a medical dictionary to make a list of 10 medical terms related to the muscular skeletal systems. Use these terms to write a scenario about a patient with a condition affecting the muscles and/or the skeletal system.

3. Legal and Ethical Explain what it means to "know your limitations" as a physical therapy aide working in the physical therapy department.

4. Patient Education Mrs. Watkins has an exercise program designed by her physical therapist to restore full ROM after her complex leg fracture. The exercises cause some discomfort and she wants to stop exercising, insisting that a limited, shuffling gait is good enough. How would you explain to her the importance of her ROM exercises and the restoration of normal functioning? Find a partner and role-play how you would overcome her objections.

5. Safety Alert Review and expand your personal plans for exercise and good body mechanics. You cannot help clients if you are not in fit condition yourself.

Portfolio Connection

When you are competent as a physical therapy aide, ask for permission to copy your documentation of treatment for a patient. (Remove all patient identifiers.) Place this copy in your portfolio to document your skills. Place a copy of your on-site trainer's evaluation in your portfolio.

Write a paper describing your doubts and realizations and the barriers that you were able to overcome during your physical therapy experiences. For example, were you concerned about helping care for patients/clients who are experiencing a lot of pain? Describe the ways you plan to use the skills, information, and insights that you gained about people and about this job. This assignment must be in standard report format.

Portfolio Tip

Encourage all patients/ clients to keep a list of their questions and concerns for the medical staff. This both saves time for the staff and helps patients/clients bring their concerns to the attention of the medical staff.

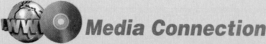
Remember! **Media Connection**

Use the Companion Website **www.prenhall.com/badasch** and the CD-ROM for additional interactive learning activities.

Chapter 20

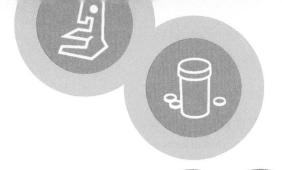

Central Supply/ Central Processing Worker

STEPS TO SUCCESS

1. Complete Vocabulary Worksheet 1 in the Student Workbook.

2. Read this chapter.

3. Complete the Learn by Doing assignment at the end of this chapter.

OBJECTIVES

When you have completed this chapter, you will be able to do the following:

✔ Complete all objectives in Part One of this book.

✔ Complete vocabulary words in the crossword puzzle.

✔ Identify functions of a central supply/central processing department.

✔ Describe the responsibilities of the central supply/central processing department worker.

✔ Describe the subdepartments of central supply/central processing.

✔ Identify six categories of cleaning agents and their specific functions.

✔ List items of appropriate clothing to be worn in the decontamination, preparation, sterilization, and inventory areas.

✔ List three methods of packaging items.

✔ List two types of sterilization and explain two important things to remember about each.

✔ Select items that require special care during sterilization.

✔ Demonstrate proficiency in each procedure pertinent to central supply/central processing.

distribute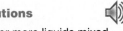
To deliver.

equipment
Instruments, machines, or items used to perform a task.

THE CENTRAL SUPPLY DEPARTMENT

Central supply department workers prepare, store, and **distribute** medical supplies throughout a medical facility. This department is responsible for maintaining a ready inventory of supplies and **equipment** for medical services. This department also monitors cleaning and sterilization of areas and equipment in order to maintain infection control within the medical setting.

RESPONSIBILITIES OF A CENTRAL SUPPLY WORKER

As a central supply worker, you do the following tasks:

instruments
Tools and measuring devices.

- Answer, screen, record, and direct telephone calls.
- Relay and record messages taken from an intercom.
- Record charges and maintain accurate files.
- Clean **instruments,** containers, and equipment.
- Assemble and wrap procedure trays.
- Operate autoclaves to sterilize items.

solutions
Two or more liquids mixed together.

- Use antiseptic **solutions** to sterilize items.
- Circulate inventory according to expiration dates.
- Deliver supplies and equipment as needed.
- Maintain accurate inventory of supplies and equipment.

STANDARD PRECAUTIONS

When working with equipment contaminated with body substances, always follow Standard Precautions. Review the guidelines in Chapter 12.

DECONTAMINATION

There are two main areas in the central supply department that you must be able to recognize. These are clean and dirty areas. They may or may not be marked accordingly. *Clean areas* have items that are unopened or wrapped and dated. *Dirty areas* usually have trash receptacles or unwrapped items that may be clean or soiled. There may also be a hopper (a large toilet-type basin) for washing away contaminated fluids, waste, and so on.

decontamination
Removal of unclean matter and living organisms.

The dirty area is called **decontamination.** All other areas in the department are considered clean areas. Central supply workers wear protective gowns when moving from the decontamination area to a clean area or from clean areas to a dirty area.

The decontamination area receives soiled items that are collected for cleaning and reprocessing. In this area, the workers remove all visible soil on items that are reused. Various types of cleaning agents are used in central supply. Each manufacturer provides directions on how to use each cleaner. Some of the cleaners you use fall under the following categories:

- *Blood solvents* dissolve dried blood or other proteins on instruments. These solvents must be washed away with a neutral detergent before the cleaning process continues.
- *Chlorinated detergents* clean heavily soiled items, and they have a bleaching action.

PROCEDURE 20.1 — DECONTAMINATION AREA

RATIONALE

The decontamination area is a dirty area. Wearing protective equipment prevents self-infection. Following exactly the proper procedure in your facility prevents transmission of infection to staff, patients, and visitors.

ALERT: Follow Standard Precautions.

1. Wear protective equipment.
   a. Head cover
   b. Scrub suit or cover gown
   c. Gloves
   d. Protective eyewear
   e. Mask/shield
   f. Shoe covers (may be required)
2. Determine proper cleaning substance for items to be washed, and dilute according to directions.
3. Unclamp, open, or take apart all items.
4. Soak instruments to loosen dried substances.
5. Scrub instruments under water to decrease the chance of spreading contaminated material through the air.
6. First rinse with tap water and then with distilled or demineralized water to prevent corrosion and mineral deposits on instruments. Wipe large items with a disinfectant and leave to air-dry.
7. Place delicate items into automatic washer baskets and place in washer.
8. Add detergent as directed by manufacturer.
9. Operate automatic washer by following washer directions.
10. Pass items to preparation area.

- *Germicidal detergents* clean large items that cannot be put in a sterilizer. These detergents are allowed to air-dry to maximize the aseptic action.
- *Neutral detergents* clean most instruments, glass, plastic, and rubber items.
- *Soap* washes items that can be damaged by stronger detergents (e.g., silicone items, hands, or skin on other parts of the body).
- *Washing machine detergent* is more **concentrated** than other detergents but has a low sudsing action.

concentrated
Increased strength, strong solution.

NOTE Abrasives are *not* used in central supply, because they make small scratches on instruments that provide a place for pathogens to hide.

Ultrasonic cleaning may be necessary. When it is, it follows the automatic washing step or is in place of the automatic washing step. When hinges or **serrated** areas cannot be cleaned properly by other methods, central supply workers use ultrasonic cleaning. High-frequency sound waves vibrate the detergent solution. This loosens the contaminated material from instruments with hard-to-clean areas.

serrated
Sawlike notches.

When the items are clean, they are transferred to the preparation area through a passageway. In a large central supply area, this passage may be a conveyor belt that leads to another room or a sliding window that allows articles to be placed into the clean area. Large items are passed through a doorway or a short hallway. When transferring items from a dirty area to a clean area, remember what you learned in Unit 1, "The Nature of Microorganisms," in Chapter 12.

Use good technique so that you do not transfer bacteria from the dirty area to the clean area.

PROCEDURE 20.2 — ULTRASONIC CLEANING PROCEDURE

RATIONALE

The decontamination area is a dirty area. Ultrasound is one method of cleaning contaminated equipment. Wearing protective equipment prevents self-infection. Following exactly the proper procedure in your facility prevents transmission of infection to staff, patients, and visitors.

ALERT: Follow Standard Precautions.

1. Wear protective equipment.
   a. Head cover
   b. Scrub suit or cover gown
   c. Protective eyewear
   d. New shoe covers (may be required)
2. Measure detergent and add to water in machine.
3. Follow machine directions for operations.
4. Rinse instruments in tap water.
5. Thoroughly dry each item.
6. Pass items to preparation area.

● PREPARATION AREA

In the preparation area, instruments and supplies are arranged for special procedures on trays or in packages. Items are also checked for damage and for proper working condition.

The preparation area is a clean area. You are required to wear the following:

- Scrub suit
- Head cover
- Shoe covers (in some departments)

This area may be combined with the sterilization area in small facilities. Each area is separate in larger facilities. Learn the procedures for both areas.

PROCEDURE 20.3 — CLEANING EQUIPMENT FROM A TRANSMISSION-BASED PRECAUTION PATIENT

RATIONALE

Transmission-Based Precaution patients usually have more serious infections. Proper precautions in cleaning is essential. Wearing protective equipment, using the correct cleaning method, and carefully following procedure prevents contaminating yourself, staff, patients, and visitors.

ALERT: Follow Standard Precautions.

1. Wear correct clothing.
   a. Head cover
   b. Cover gown
   c. Mask
   d. Gloves
2. Determine proper cleaning substance for items to be washed, and dilute according to directions.
3. Open bag holding items to be cleaned. Remove items from bag.

PROCEDURE 20.3 — CLEANING EQUIPMENT FROM A TRANSMISSION-BASED PRECAUTION PATIENT *(Continued)*

4. Fold bag and place in trash container.

5. Unclamp, open, or take apart all items.

6. Soak instruments to loosen dried substances.

7. Scrub instruments under water to decrease the chance of spreading contaminated material through the air.

8. First rinse with tap water and then with distilled or demineralized water to prevent corrosion and mineral deposits on instruments. Wipe large items with a disinfectant and leave to air-dry.

9. Place delicate items into automatic washer baskets and place in washer.

10. Place all items into automatic washer.

11. Carefully remove gloves by pulling the cuff over hand, causing glove to be inside out when removed. Dispose of in trash container.

12. Remove cover gown, head cover, and mask, and dispose of according to hospital policy.

13. Add detergent as directed by manufacturer.

14. Operate automatic washer by following washer directions.

Items being prepared for sterilization are placed on trays or in packages with other items that are used for specific procedures. These are called *procedure trays* or *packs*. When organizing a tray, always check each item for broken areas, and be certain that it works properly.

Packaging Methods

There are different packaging methods. They include the following:

- Heat-sealed packages that peel open
- Tape-sealed packages that peel open
- Packages wrapped in cloth or special paper for sterilization

PROCEDURE 20.4 — STERILE WRAP, ENVELOPE

RATIONALE

Properly prepared sterile wrap packages prevent contaminating equipment, dressings, and instruments. Improperly contaminated prepared sterile wrap packages can cause serious infection when used on a patient.

1. Select the appropriate size of outer wrap.
   a. Wrapper should be large enough to completely enclose items to be sterilized.
   b. A double thickness is desirable.
   c. Wrapper should not be drawn too tightly, just enough to hold package together.

2. Place items to be wrapped in center of outer wrap. Sides of tray holding items to be sterilized should be aligned with corners of wrapper.

PROCEDURE 20.4 | STERILE WRAP, ENVELOPE (Continued)

3. Fold corner closest to you past center of pack; holding corner, fold it back, making a flap.

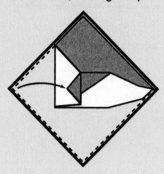

4. Fold left corner of wrap just past center and fold corner back, making a flap.

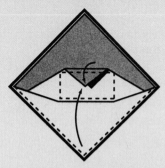

5. Fold right corner of wrap past center (overlap center) and fold back, making a flap.

6. Fold corner farthest from you over package.

7. To provide a double thickness, wrap package again following steps 2 through 6.

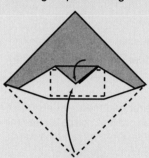

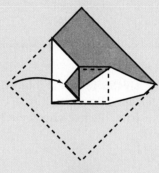

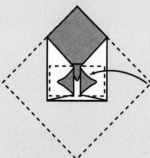

8. Using heat-sensitive tape, secure the edges.

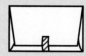

9. Date and label package; follow the procedure "Dating and Labeling Sterile Items."

PROCEDURE 20.5

STERILE SQUARE WRAP FOLD

RATIONALE

Properly prepared sterile wrap packages prevents contaminating equipment, dressings, and instruments. Improperly prepared, contaminated sterile wrap packages can cause serious infection when used on a patient.

1. Select appropriate size of outer wrap.
   a. Wrapper should be large enough to completely enclose the items to be sterilized.
   b. If outer wrap is to be used as a sterile field over a table:
      (1) Wrap should allow at least 6 inches overhang on all four sides of the table.
      (2) A double thickness is desirable.
   c. Wrap should not be drawn too tightly, just enough to hold package together.

2. Place items to be wrapped in center of outer wrap. Corners of tray holding items to be sterilized should be square with corners of wrapper.

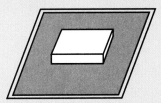

3. Fold edge closest to you past center of pack; continue holding edge and fold back to make a 1-inch band.

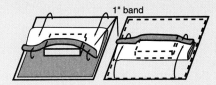

4. Grasp edge farthest from you and pull over items to be sterilized.

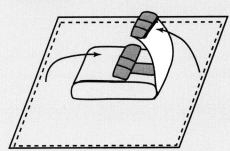

5. Hold the same edge and fold back to make a 1-inch band. (There should be a 2-inch overlap of edges at center of package.)

6. Fold the left edge just past center; holding same edge, fold back to make a band.

7. Fold the right edge just past center; holding same edge, fold back to make a band (overlapping at center).

8. Wrap package again following steps 3 through 7 to provide a double thickness.

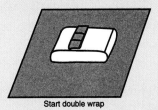

Start double wrap

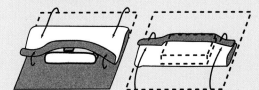

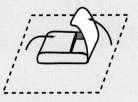

9. Use heat-sensitive tape to secure edges.

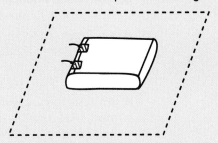

10. Date and label package; follow procedure "Dating and Labeling Sterile Items."

PROCEDURE 20.6 · LINEN PREPARATION

RATIONALE

Correct linen preparation prevents the possibility of transferring microorganisms to a patient. Careful evaluation for tears and defects, correct folding, and carefully following procedure protect patients from transfer of microorganisms from contaminated linen packs.

1. Inspection
   a. Spread linen over an illuminated worktable and look for holes, tears, or other defects.
   b. Circle defects with a pencil and send for repair.
   c. Prepare linen without defects for sterilization.
2. Folding
   a. Fold linen according to department procedure.
   b. Sort and stack linen on shelves according to use.
3. Assembly of linen packages
   a. Packages should not exceed 12 by 12 by 20 inches or weigh more than 20 pounds.
   b. Place last item to be used on bottom and first item to be used on top.
   c. Place gauze sponges in the center of the package so that steam can enter each piece of fabric more easily.
4. Wrapping the linen pack
   a. Select an outer wrapper large enough to enclose the items completely.
   b. Wrap the linen as described in the procedure "Sterile Square Wrap Fold."
      (1) Square fold for large packs
      (2) Envelope fold for small packs
   c. Date and label as described in the procedure "Dating and Labeling Sterile Items."

⬤ STERILIZATION

In the sterilization area, the clean items are placed in an *autoclave*. The environment in the autoclave kills all microorganisms. The items inside the autoclave are exposed to steam or gas and steam under pressure for a specific period of time. Items that may be damaged from steam, pressure, or gas are placed in a chemical disinfectant. There are some basics that you need to remember when sterilizing. The following serves as a reference guide. (See Chapter 18 for small autoclaves.)

Steam Sterilization

- The steam and microorganisms must be in contact for a specific amount of time. The time is determined by the temperature of the steam.
- All items must be completely dry before they are removed from the autoclave. *Remember that pathogens are transported by moisture.*

Gas Sterilization

- The gas, steam, and microorganisms must be in direct contact for a specific period. This time is determined by the concentration of gas and the temperature inside the autoclave.

ethylene oxide

Gas that kills living microorganisms.

- All **ethylene oxide** gas is removed from the sterilized items before they are stored or used.

Sterilizing Plastics, Oils, Powders, and Solutions

- Plastics require ethylene gas sterilization, as heat deteriorates plastics.
- Oils and powders require a dry heat sterilization.
- Solutions require a special steam sterilization method designed just for solutions.

PROCEDURE 20.7 — STERILIZING WITH ETHYLENE OXIDE GAS

RATIONALE

Following the exact procedure for the equipment you are using for sterilization prevents accidental transfer of microorganisms to the patient.

1. Prepare the gas sterilizer.
   a. Place recording chart in monitor.
   b. Add ink to pens if required.
   c. Check for humidity-sensing element in the chamber.
   d. Preheat sterilizer.
2. Snap master switch "on."
3. Check indicators to ensure that adequate gas supply is available.
4. Depress Sterox selector button.
5. Set timer for length of time required for exposure to gas.
6. Set humidity timer for length of humidification period.
7. Load items into sterilizer.
8. Start the sterilization cycle by depressing the lock door cycle button.
9. Monitor indicators showing when the cycle is complete.
10. Unload sterilizer when cycle is complete.
11. Close door of sterilizer; do not engage holding arm.
12. Aerate sterilized items by following department procedure.

PROCEDURE 20.8 — DATING AND LABELING STERILE ITEMS

RATIONALE

Following the exact procedure for dating and labeling equipment and other sterile packages ensures that the packages are rotated according to procedure. Rotation prevents the use of packages that have passed the safety date and become unsterile.

1. Date all packages with the day of sterilization.
2. Label packages with name of pack and a listing of items in package.
3. Initial pack as you wrap it.
4. Mark sterilizer number on each package.
5. Rotate sterilized items by date. Packages that are closest to their expiration date are placed forward on the shelf so that they are used first.

Monitoring the Effectiveness of Sterilization

Each central supply department has procedures for evaluating the effectiveness of the sterilization **cycle.** A permanent record is kept of this monitoring system to ensure infection control. Occasional inspections of the medical facility require inspection of these records. The following gives you an overview of commonly used monitoring devices.

- *Mechanical monitoring* is accomplished by graphing the pressure/vacuum gauge, temperature gauge, and/or **humidity** gauge readings during the sterilization cycle. These records are then filed by date and time.

cycle
Repeating steps (e.g., a wash cycle).

humidity
Wetness, or moisture.

Figure 20.1

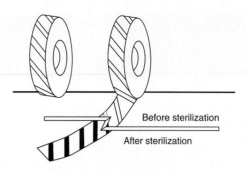

Before sterilization

After sterilization

Autoclave sterilization indicator tape. Before sterilization (top) the tape is a certain color. After sterilization (bottom) the tape changes color. A chemical change during sterilization causes the tape to change color.

■ *Chemical monitoring* is done by using strips of material with a chemical on it that changes color after exposure to enough heat or steam. A tape treated with this chemical secures packages for sterilization. Packages that are sterilized are identified easily by the color change on the tape (see Figure 20.1).

■ *Biological monitoring* is accomplished by placing small containers with live bacteria that are highly resistant in the autoclave during the sterilization cycle. After sterilization, the bacteria are placed in a supportive environment. The bacteria are checked after a specified time. If any bacteria have survived or reproduced, sterilization did not occur.

INVENTORY AND DISTRIBUTION

The inventory and distribution area maintains an accurate count of supplies and equipment on hand and delivers items as necessary. This is accomplished by replacing discarded items immediately and seeing that broken equipment is repaired in a timely manner. All supplies and sterile equipment are rotated on the shelves to ensure that sterility of items does not expire. Items must be resterilized before use if they are not frequently used and the sterilization time expires.

There are various types of delivery systems in the medical facility. Most medical systems use volunteers to pick up and deliver equipment to departments. Some use the central supply/central processing staff to do these duties. Other facilities use a pneumatic tube system that carries small items from place to place and a dumbwaiter elevator for larger items. Most facilities use freight elevators rather than passenger elevators to deliver very large items. The use of freight elevators keeps medical supplies separate from the general public and lowers the possibility of contamination. It is also better if the visitors are not exposed to equipment.

JOBS AND PROFESSIONS

■ Assistive personnel

■ Clinical medical assistant

■ Home health aide

■ Licensed vocational/practical nurse

■ Nurse assistant

■ Registered nurse

■ Surgical assistant

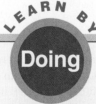

LEARN BY Doing

1. **Complete Worksheets 1 through 3 and Worksheets/Activities 4 and 5 as assigned.**
2. **Practice all procedures.**
3. **Prepare responses to each item listed in Chapter Review—Your Link to Success at the end of this chapter.**
4. **When you are confident that you can meet each objective, ask your instructor for the unit evaluation.**

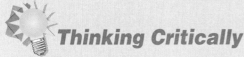
 ## Thinking Critically

1. **Time Management** Always work through your inventory checklist in an organized way. If you are interrupted, mark where you were working before you stopped and evaluate your priorities when you get back.

2. **Communications** Using your daily inventory checklist for central supply, create a plan for how you will explain the system to the volunteers who help you.

3. **Legal and Ethical** One way to prevent the spread of infection is to use the various sterilization processes found in the central supply/central processing area. Describe these processes and how they are monitored for effective sterilization.

4. **Medical Math** You may handle drainage bottles of different sizes. Determine how many ounces are in containers that measure 250 cc, 2,500 cc, and 1,000 cc.

5. **Case Study** Samual Witt is your co-worker. He likes to work quickly so that he can be done with his work early. You notice that he neglects to wear all of the necessary protective equipment. Sometimes he walks from the decontamination area into the clean area without removing his gown and other protective wear. Describe a way to respond to this observation that would serve to protect Samuel and other co-workers. Explain the possible negative and positive outcomes of your actions.

Portfolio Connection

Once you attain competence as a central supply/central processing worker, ask for permission to photocopy sterilization test strip results. Place copies in your portfolio to demonstrate your understanding of the sterilization process.

Write a paper describing your doubts and realizations and the barriers that you were able to overcome during your central supply/central processing experience. For example, what frightened you, and what moved you beyond your fear? Describe the ways you plan to use the skills, information, and insights that you gained about the people you worked with and about this job. This report must be in standard report format.

Portfolio Tip

Take time to organize and plan your work and it will go more smoothly and efficiently. Put copies of any work plans you create in your portfolio.

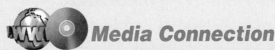 **Remember!** **Media Connection**

Use the Companion Website **www.prenhall.com/badasch** and the CD-ROM for additional interactive learning activities.

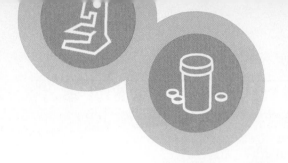

Chapter 21

Environmental Services Technician/ Housekeeper

MEDIA CONNECTION

Use the Companion Website **www.prenhall.com/badasch** and the CD-ROM for additional interactive learning activities.

STEPS TO SUCCESS

1. Read this chapter.

2. Complete the Learn by Doing assignment at the end of this chapter.

OBJECTIVES

When you have completed this chapter, you will be able to do the following:

✔ Complete all objectives in Part One of this book.

✔ Define new vocabulary words.

✔ Describe the responsibilities of an EVS/housekeeper.

✔ Match department names with their abbreviations.

✔ List seven supplies and types of equipment found on a service cart.

✔ Give two reasons why a service cart is important.

✔ Define *germicidal solution.*

✔ List 14 guidelines to use in the EVS/housekeeping department.

✔ List five areas to check that are not usually found in your home.

✔ Describe HAI and explain how to prevent it.

✔ List seven general rules to follow when you clean a patient's room.

✔ Explain the cleaning process for preparing a room for a new patient.

✔ List seven specialized departments in the hospital.

✔ Identify the area within a specialized department that requires aseptic cleaning.

✔ Explain why it is important to keep all public areas clean and attractive.

✔ List duties required in the linen area.

✔ Differentiate between general cleaning, cleaning special areas, and cleaning sterile areas.

✔ Demonstrate each procedure pertinent to an EVS/housekeeper.

◯ RESPONSIBILITIES OF AN EVS/HOUSEKEEPER

EVS/housekeeper workers are responsible for the cleanliness of the environment. Cleanliness helps prevent the spread of infection and creates a more pleasant environment for patients, employees, and visitors. An EVS/housekeeping employee is an important member of the health care team because he or she provides a therapeutic environment for the delivery of care. The information in this chapter discusses the hospital environment; however, you can transfer these skills to any health care setting, including clinics, medical-professional offices, and private health care agencies.

As a housekeeper, you are required to do the following tasks:

- Load a service cart with appropriate supplies and materials.
- Clean assigned areas (for example, room, offices, laboratories):
    - Wash floors, furniture, and equipment. • Dust. • Vacuum. • Clean blinds.
    - Empty ashtrays. • Empty trash. • Scour sinks, tubs, and mirrors.
    - Disinfect bedsprings and unit equipment. • Wash walls, ceilings, and windows as needed.
- Replenish soap and towels.
- Replace cubicle curtains.
- Replace soiled draperies.
- Provide daily cleaning of sterile areas.
- Report malfunctioning equipment.
- Keep utility and storage rooms orderly.
- Move furniture, equipment, and supplies.
- Sweep, mop, wet-wash, and vacuum floors.
- Polish using a buffing machine.
- Clean light fixtures.
- Turn and change mattresses.
- Hang draperies and blinds.
- Collect soiled linens and transport them to the laundry.
- Provide an odor-free environment.

◯ ABBREVIATIONS

EVS workers work in many areas of the hospital. They must know the abbreviations that are used for the different departments. They must also be aware of each department's overall responsibilities. As you read the abbreviations for the departments, refer back to Unit 2 of Chapter 2, which discusses the different areas and lists the responsibilities of the workers. Following is a list of many of the departments in the hospital and abbreviations that might be used.

Emergency room	ER
Electrocardiology	EKG/ECG
Environmental services	EVS
Laboratory	LAB
Radiology	X-Ray
Orthopedics	Ortho
Obstetric	OB

Medical-surgical	MED-SURG
Food service	Dietary
Physical therapy	PT
Occupational therapy	OT
Central supply	CS
Neurology	Neuro
Rehabilitation	Rehab
Gynecology	GYN

Other areas are usually not abbreviated:

Respiratory
Pharmacy
Linen room
Billing
Admitting
Medical records
Volunteers
Pulmonary lab
Dialysis
Chapel

● CARE AND CLEANING OF EQUIPMENT

Use a service cart to keep supplies and equipment where they are easily available as you clean. The carts save many trips to other areas for supplies. They help you be more efficient and save time. Each facility has an equipment list of the things to include on the cart. Not all carts require exactly the same things. Set up your cart according to your assignment. You are also responsible for cleaning your cart at least once a week and as needed. Some standard equipment might include the following:

■ Cleaning brushes
■ Cleaning cloths
■ Dust mop and dustpan
■ Toilet bowl brushes
■ Cleaners such as **germicidals**
■ Deodorizing solutions
■ Wet mop
■ Paper goods
   • Toilet paper • Paper towels and paper towel dispenser key • Tissues
   • Wastebasket liners
■ Gloves (wear gloves according to facility policy)

germicidals
Solutions that kill most bacteria.

After you complete your duties for the day, clean your cart and the equipment. Dispose of all trash, and leave the cart ready for the next day's work.

You must keep the equipment clean and in good repair. When equipment is in good repair, your work is much easier. It must also be clean so as to prevent the spread of microorganisms. Review Chapter 12, "Controlling Infection." The patients and other workers *depend on you* to protect them from the spread of disease and infection.

PROCEDURE 21.1

STOCKING THE SERVICE CART

RATIONALE

A properly stocked cart saves time and ensures that you have all of the supplies and equipment that you need. Using the right supplies helps prevent the spread of infection to patients, staff, and visitors.

1. Check your service cart to make sure that
   a. Wheels are working.
   b. Storage areas are clean.
   c. Shelves are sturdy.
   d. There are no broken areas.
2. Gather supplies.
   a. Gloves
   b. Mopping bucket
   c. Germicidal solution
   d. Spray bottle with germicidal solution
   e. Paper towel dispenser key
   f. Plastic bags:
      (1) Trash containers (small and large)
      (2) Sanitary napkin containers
      (3) Laundry containers
   g. Mop wringer
   h. Dust mop that has been specially treated
   i. Dustpan
   j. Dust mop with long handle
   k. Cleaning brushes
   l. Cleaning cloths
   m. Toilet bowl cleaner
   n. Toilet paper
   o. Paper towels
   p. Hand soap
   q. Putty knife
   r. Deodorizing solutions
3. Restock your cart at the end of your shift so that it is ready for the next day.
4. Wash hands.

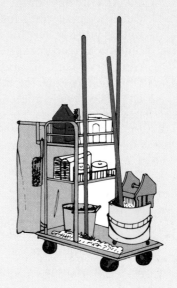

There are some general guidelines that you follow:

- Always use Standard Precautions.
- Follow the manufacturer's instructions for operating and maintaining equipment.
- Store equipment properly.
- Report any defect or problem.
- Clean, rinse, and wring out a wet mop after use. This helps it last longer and prevents odor and mildew.
- Never store brooms and brushes on the straw or bristles because they bend out of shape.
- Keep cleaning cloths separate from linen to prevent contamination.
- Empty dust, trash, vacuum bags, and so on every day.
- Do not shake dust mops, cleaning cloths, or linen as this causes the spread of microorganisms.

■ Wipe down all equipment after use, including

• Caution signs • Scraping knives • Ladders • Hoses • Sweepers, vacuums • Measuring cups • Buckets and pails and their wringers

■ Do not leave solutions in buckets when they are not in use.

■ Do not leave cleaning solutions where a child or confused patient can reach them.

■ Label all containers to prevent mistakes.

■ Do not pull plugs from the socket by the cord.

⬤ GENERAL CLEANING DUTIES

Everything in the environment must be kept clean, odor free, and safe. Dust and microorganisms are always in the air around us, and it is a daily battle to keep them controlled. It is a very large task to keep everything clean. Areas in a health care facility must be cleaned more frequently than those in the home. The health care environment has many more microorganisms that cause illness and disease. Cleanliness requires following procedure, being aware of all areas around you, and taking pride in keeping everything clean and in tip-top order. Part of your responsibility is to recognize the need to clean an area, change dirty filters, and use detergent, odor-control, and germicidal solutions appropriately. Remember from Part One that a germicide kills bacteria, but a bacteriostatic only slows growth. Odor is controlled by cleanliness, nonaerosol sprays, solutions added to buckets, and small bottles with wicks. The scent must be very light or odorless. You need to be watchful and aware of areas that you might not be as concerned with or need to clean as often in your home. Some of these are as follows:

■ Closets and lockers

■ Cubicle curtains

■ Radiators

■ Heating and cooling ducts

■ Air conditioners

■ Light fixtures

■ Screens

■ Windows

■ Refrigerators

■ Drinking fountains

■ Transportable equipment such as wheelchairs, gurneys, and commodes

■ Venetian blinds

■ Corridors

■ Stairways

■ Sprinkler heads

PROCEDURE 21.2 CLEANING CLOSETS AND LOCKERS

RATIONALE

Closets and lockers become dirty from an accumulation of dust and dirt over a period of time. You are responsible for cleaning staff and patient closets to help prevent the spread of infection to patients, staff, and visitors.

PROCEDURE 21.2 | CLEANING CLOSETS AND LOCKERS *(Continued)*

1. Gather equipment.

   a. Bucket
   b. Cleaning solution
   c. Two cleaning cloths
   d. Treated dust mop
   e. Stepstool or ladder
   f. Vacuum
   g. Putty knife
   h. Screwdriver
   i. Spray bottle
   j. Water
   k. Gloves
   l. Deodorizing solution

2. Put on gloves.

3. Prepare cleaning solution.

4. Vacuum and damp-dust inside and outside of closet or locker. (Don't forget the top.)

5. Submerge cloth in cleaning solution.

6. Wring solution out of cloth.

7. Wipe all outside surfaces with cloth. (Wash out cloth frequently to remove dirt; if you don't do this, you will be spreading around the dirt.)

8. Wipe all surfaces with a dry cloth to remove extra solution and water spots.

9. Wipe all inside surfaces with moistened cleaning cloth.

10. Wipe all inside surfaces with a dry cloth.

11. Remove gloves.

12. Wash hands.

PROCEDURE 21.3 | CLEANING STAIRWAYS

RATIONALE

Stairways can be a hazard by causing slips and falls. Following all steps in the procedure helps prevent accidents. Keeping the stairway well cared for helps prevent the spread of infection to patients, staff, and visitors.

1. Gather equipment.

   a. Wet mop
   b. Bucket
   c. Dusting: mop, pan, brush, and cloth
   d. "Caution" sign
   e. Strong cleaning agent
   f. Germicidal solution
   g. Glass cleaner
   h. Hand buffing pad
   i. Gloves
   j. Deodorizing solution

2. Put on gloves.

3. Clean all fixtures around stairway.

   a. Lights
   b. Signs
   c. Windows
   d. Pictures

4. Dust all railings and ledges. (It may be necessary to use extension poles with dusting equipment to reach high places.)

5. Clean all spots on walls and base plates.

6. Dust-mop stairs; start at top using a side-to-side motion. Continue to platform or bottom of stairs, whichever comes first.

7. Pick up dust and dirt with a dustpan and brush.

8. Clean area around doors.

   a. Hinges
   b. Knobs
   c. Jambs and ledges
   d. Polish all metal

9. Place "Caution" signs appropriately; rope off half of stairway. (Leave an adequate walkway.)

10. Damp-mop area enclosed by rope.

PROCEDURE 21.3 | CLEANING STAIRWAYS *(Continued)*

11. Refinish/wax stairs.

12. Dust-mop again.

13. Move rope and "Caution" sign to other side of stairway and repeat the procedure. (Never remove "Caution" signs before the floor is completely dry.)

14. Recheck area before leaving for missed spots.

15. Clean equipment and return it to its storage area.

16. Remove gloves.

17. Wash hands.

PROCEDURE 21.4 | WASHING WINDOWS

RATIONALE

Clean windows create a feeling of openness and cleanliness. This gives patients, staff, and visitors a sense of security about the cleanliness of other parts of the facility.

1. Gather equipment.
   a. Vacuum with attachments
   b. Ladder
   c. Double bucket
   d. Cleaning cloth or sponge
   e. Squeegee
   f. Gloves
   g. Lint-free cloth
   h. Paper towel
   i. Window cleaner
   j. Germicidal solution

2. Put on gloves.

3. Remove all objects from window.
   a. Curtains (tie back or take down)
   b. Items on ledge
   c. Blinds (cleaned and pulled up or taken down)
   d. Screens—remove and clean

4. Vacuum ledge, window grooves, and corners.

5. Wash window frame and ledge with germicidal solution.

6. Rinse and dry frame and ledge.

7. Apply window cleaner with spray bottle, brush, or sponge. Be sure to get into corners.
   a. Use a side-to-side movement.
   b. Overlap slightly with each stroke.

8. Rinse if necessary, using the same technique.

9. Remove water with squeegee by doing the following:
   a. Place the rubber edge of the squeegee flat against the window in an upper corner.
   b. Move the squeegee across the window in a sweeping motion to the opposite side.
   c. Wipe rubber edge of squeegee with a cloth.
   d. Repeat this motion across the window until all sections have been wiped.
   e. Wipe bottom edge of window with a cloth.
   f. Wipe all water drops from ledge or floor.

10. Wipe any streaks with a lint-free cloth.

11. Replace all items removed from the window:
    a. Curtains or drapes
    b. Blinds
    c. Decorations, etc.

12. Recheck window for missed spots.

13. Clean equipment and return it to its storage area.

14. Remove gloves.

15. Wash hands.

PROCEDURE 21.5 | CLEANING CORRIDORS

RATIONALE

Dirty mops and equipment pick up microorganisms and transfer them to other areas. Clean corridors give the facility a feeling of openness and cleanliness and prevent transmission of infection to patients, staff, and visitors.

1. Gather equipment.
   a. Bucket
   b. Disposable gloves
   c. Wet mop
   d. Dusting: mop, pan, and brush
   e. Vacuum
   f. Germicidal solution with deodorizing solution
   g. Stainless steel polish
   h. "Caution" signs
   i. Cleaning cloths
   j. Ladder or stepstool
2. Put on gloves.
3. Clean all fixtures. (Check to see if all fixtures are working properly.)
   a. Lights
   b. Vents
   c. Signs
   d. Drinking fountains
   e. Telephones
   f. Pictures
   g. Window blinds
   h. Mirrors
   i. Drapes or curtains
   j. Ashtrays (if there is an area set aside for smoking)
4. Empty and wash all trash containers in assigned area.
5. Clean windows or glass partitions.
6. Clean marks or spots from walls/wall guards.
7. Clean all ledges.

8. Clean area around door:
   a. Hinges
   b. Polish all metal
   c. Knobs
   d. Door jambs and ledges
9. Place "Caution" signs appropriately in corridor; rope off half of the corridor. (Always leave adequate walking space.)
10. Dust-mop the floor.
11. Damp-mop or use a floor washing machine.
12. Refinish/wax and buff floors.
13. Dust-mop again.
14. Move rope and "Caution" signs to other side of corridor and repeat procedure. (Never remove "Caution" signs before floor is completely dry.)
15. When finished, check area for missed spots.
16. Clean equipment and return it to its storage area.
17. Remove gloves.
18. Wash hands.

PROCEDURE 21.6 | CLEANING DRINKING FOUNTAINS

RATIONALE

Drinking fountains are a problem area if not kept clean. Sputum and nasal spray can be accumulated in the fountains. Keeping the fountains clean prevents transmission of infection to patients, staff, and visitors.

PROCEDURE 21.6 | CLEANING DRINKING FOUNTAINS *(Continued)*

1. Gather equipment.
   a. Cleaning cloth
   b. Cleaning solution
   c. Metal polish
   d. Gloves
2. Put on gloves.
3. Discard any trash from fountain.
4. Submerge cloth in cleaning solution or use spray bottle with cleaning solution.
5. Wring cloth.

6. Wipe all surfaces on fountain. (Be sure to remove stains or marks of any kind.)
7. Polish all metal parts with a metal polish and soft, dry cloth.
8. Wipe up any splashes or spills.
9. Report any fountains that are not working properly.
10. Return all equipment to its storage area.
11. Remove gloves.
12. Wash hands.

● CLEANING ROOMS THAT ARE OCCUPIED BY PATIENTS

It is difficult to be a patient in a hospital. The patient is in an unfamiliar environment. Patients are sick, and they may have many worries. It is important to make their surroundings as pleasant as possible. It is also very important for you to be pleasant. You must also protect them from further illness or complications caused by a *hospital-acquired infection* (HAI). *HAI* is a common term used in health care facilities to describe infections that patients acquire in the hospital—they did not have the infection or illness when they were admitted. It is usually caused by a breakdown in asepsis. If you do not clean correctly, the patients' safety is in danger. You have a major responsibility to help prevent HAI. When you clean the patient's room, there are some rules to follow:

■ Follow Standard Precautions.

■ Work quietly, efficiently, and quickly.

■ Be careful around equipment such as IVs, suction machines, and tubing.

■ Do not put one patient's belongings with another patient's things. This causes cross-contamination.

When you clean the room, be sure to do the following:

■ Empty the wastebasket and replace the bedside bag.

■ Pick up any litter that is on the floor.

■ Wipe off the furniture.

■ Clean the phone, call bell, and TV control.

■ Remove spots from around light switches, on walls, and so on.

■ Mop or vacuum the floor.

■ Dust ledges and check light fixtures, vents, and so on.

■ Notice the cubicle curtains. Are there any spots or spills on them? Are they hanging correctly?

■ Clean the bathroom:

• Empty the wastebasket and pick up any litter. • Clean the basin and faucets and polish the mirror. • Clean the shower or tub and the faucets. • Wipe fixtures with an odor-control solution. • Check the shower curtain for mildew or tears. • Wipe down ledges, wall switches, spots on walls, and so on. • Replace soap, toilet paper, and paper towels. • Clean the toilets and exposed pipes.

■ Replace things just as you found them. Be certain that the telephone, water pitcher, call bell, TV control, tissues, and reading materials are within the patient's reach.

■ Check the overall appearance of the room before you leave, and report any problems or repairs.

■ Notify the nurse if the patient needs anything.

PROCEDURE 21.7 | CLEANING THE OCCUPIED PATIENT ROOM

RATIONALE

Providing the patient with a clean, safe room gives a sense of security. A clean environment helps prevent the spread of infection and prevents reinfection of the patients from their own organisms. It also protects other patients, staff, and visitors.

ALERT: Follow Standard Precautions.

1. Gather equipment.
    a. Cleaning cart with standard supplies
    b. Vacuum
    c. Gloves
2. Put on gloves.
3. Dispose of all loose trash and the bedside bag in trash container.
4. Pull plastic over trash in container and tie off. Place in larger trash container to be removed from the area. Repeat process with all trash containers in room.
5. Wipe out the inside of each trash container with cloth dampened in cleaning solution.
6. Place clean plastic liner in all emptied trash containers. Secure top of plastic over edge of container.
7. Use a cloth dampened in germicidal solution to wipe off and dry:
    a. Bedside table
    b. Bed rails
    c. Chairs
    d. Cabinets
    e. Any spots on walls, door jambs, and light switches (Don't forget to rinse your cleaning cloth frequently so that you are not spreading dirt.)
8. Place a clean bedside bag at bedside.
9. Clean floors:
Uncarpeted floors—dust mop
    a. Use a treated dry mop.
    b. Start in the corners.

    c. Move mop from left to right.
    d. Work your way toward the door. (Pick up or move light objects and dust under them.)
    e. Dampen wet mop with germicidal solution.
    f. Remop room.
Carpeted floors—vacuum
NOTE Start in the corner and work your way toward the door. (Pick up or move light objects and vacuum under them.)
10. Wipe all ledges, vents, sprinkler heads, and lights with cloth dampened in germicidal solution.
11. Wipe all ledges, vents, sprinkler heads, and lights with dry cloth to remove cleaning solution and water spots.
12. Clean bathroom.
    a. Use separate rags and brushes.
    b. Clean toilet according to facility policy.
    c. Clean mirrors.
    d. Polish porcelain.
    e. Wipe tiles and walls.
    f. Clean floor.
    g. Check to be certain that there are soap, toilet paper, and paper towels.
13. Check room for additional needs before leaving.
14. Report any broken items in the room.
15. Return all equipment to its storage area.
16. Remove gloves.
17. Wash hands.

● CLEANING UNOCCUPIED ROOMS

When patients are admitted to the hospital, their room is their home (see Figure 21.1). Regardless of the reason for their admission, there is cause for some anxiety. The environment is very important for both their feeling of comfort and their protection against infection.

There are specific procedures that must be completed before the room is ready for a new patient.

■ Your supervisor will inspect the room with you and help determine what needs to be done.

■ In some hospitals, the walls and ceilings are washed after each patient is discharged. In other hospitals, this is done according to a rotation schedule. Follow the policy of your facility.

■ Follow the directions for cleaning an unoccupied room. In addition, you will wash the bed and make the bed.

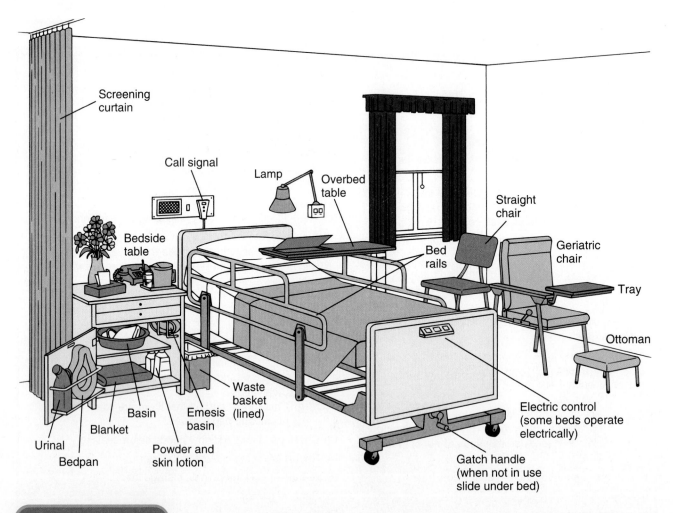

Figure 21.1

Typical patient unit.

PROCEDURE 21.8 — CLEANING THE UNOCCUPIED PATIENT ROOM

RATIONALE

Patients' rooms have many areas where microorganisms can hide. Careful cleaning and disinfecting protect new patients from becoming infected with microorganisms from previous patients. Hospital-acquired infection is a major problem that can be prevented by following facility procedure.

ALERT: Follow Standard Precautions.

1. Gather equipment.
    a. Service cart with standard supplies
    b. Vacuum with attachments
    c. Gloves
2. Put on gloves.
3. Evaluate the condition of the room with your supervisor.
4. Clean all furniture thoroughly.
5. Remove furniture from room.
6. Remove curtains and drapes if necessary.
7. In room and bathroom, wash ceiling and walls with germicidal solution, being sure to clean:
    a. Vents
    b. Lights
    c. Sprinkler heads
    d. Television
    e. Doors
    f. Metal protection plates
    g. Curtain rods or tracks
8. Clean windows and window frames.
9. Thoroughly clean floors following the procedure decided upon when the room was evaluated before cleaning.
10. Replace all furniture.
11. Make beds.
12. Replace drapes and curtains if necessary.
13. Inspect room before leaving area.
14. Return all equipment to its storage area.
15. Remove gloves.
16. Wash hands.

PROCEDURE 21.9 — DUSTING

RATIONALE

Proper dusting picks up dust and prevents flying dust particles. Dust contains microorganisms that cause infection. Carefully following facility procedures helps prevent dust with microorganisms from becoming airborne and infecting other patients, staff, and visitors.

1. Gather equipment.
    a. Dust cloth
    b. Extension for high places
    c. Spray cleaner/wax
    d. Gloves (according to facility policy)
2. Fold dusting cloth in half several times until it is about the size of your hand.

Fold dusting cloth

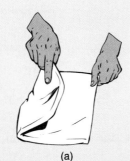
(a)

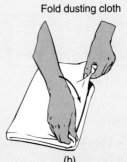
(b)

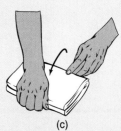
(c)

PROCEDURE 21.9 | DUSTING *(Continued)*

3. Begin dusting at the highest point near the entrance of a room. Move systematically around the room until you reach the entrance again. (Dust all surfaces in a room.)

4. Use long, straight strokes from side to side or up and down.

5. Use a spray cleaner/wax or liquid on wood surfaces. Follow manufacturer's directions.

6. Complete all dusting in an area before moving to another area. Conserve your motions by planning.

7. Check the room before leaving for missed areas.

8. Return all equipment to its storage area.

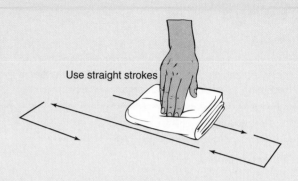

Use straight strokes

PROCEDURE 21.10 | CLEANING FURNITURE

RATIONALE

Proper dusting picks up dust and prevents flying dust particles. Dust contains microorganisms that cause infection. Carefully following facility procedures helps prevent dust with microorganisms from becoming airborne and infecting other patients, staff, and visitors.

1. Gather equipment.
   a. Cleaning solution
   b. Gloves
   c. Two cloths
   d. Bucket or spray bottle
   e. Vinyl cleaner
   f. Vacuum with appropriate attachments
   g. Furniture polish

2. Put on gloves.

3. Dust furniture.
   a. Wood furniture—use a dry cloth, then furniture polish.
   b. Vinyl and fabric furniture—use a vacuum. Be sure to vacuum in all crevices with a narrow attachment. Use a short bristle brush over surface of fabric.

4. Scrub vinyl with vinyl cleaner.
   a. Spray vinyl cleaner evenly on vinyl.
   b. Let it stand a few minutes (do not allow it to dry).
   c. Scrub very soiled areas with a soft brush.
   d. Wipe vinyl until clean.

5. Rinse vinyl with water-dampened cloth.

6. Wipe vinyl dry with clean dry cloth.

7. Return furniture to its original position.

8. Return all equipment to its storage area.

9. Remove gloves.

10. Wash hands.

NOTE Soiled fabric-covered furniture may require professional cleaning or recovering. Some cleaning solutions cause fabric to spot. Ask your supervisor before applying solutions to fabric.

PROCEDURE 21.11

CLEANING THE BED

RATIONALE

The hospital bed has many areas where microorganisms can hide. Following cleaning procedures is essential for prevent- ing the spread of infection. Proper cleaning helps provide a safe environment for patients, staff, and visitors.

1. Gather equipment.
   a. Bucket
   b. Vacuum with crevice attachment
   c. Cleaning solution
   d. Two cleaning cloths
   e. Cleaning brush
   f. Gloves
2. Put on gloves.
3. Discard all loose trash.
4. Vacuum bed, being sure to clean in all crevices. Use a brush to loosen lint or dust.
5. Remove all tape or stickers from bed. (Use tape remover supplied by your facility.)

6. Dampen a cloth with germicidal solution and wipe:
   a. Pillows
   b. Mattress, both sides
   c. Bedsprings
   d. Side rails
   e. Head- and footboards
   f. Controls
   g. Legs
7. Make a closed bed. (See the procedure "Making a Closed Bed" in Chapter 15.)
8. Remove gloves.
9. Wash hands.

PROCEDURE 21.12

VACUUMING CURTAINS/DRAPES

RATIONALE

Everything in the environment has a potential to carry dan- gerous microorganisms that cause infection. Following clean- ing procedures is essential for preventing the spread of infection. Proper cleaning helps provide a safe environment for patients, staff, and visitors.

1. Assemble equipment.
   a. Vacuum
   b. Ladder
   c. Gloves
2. Put on gloves.
3. Spread out curtains/drapes so that more surface area is showing.
4. Place ladder at one end of curtain.
5. Place short bristle brush attachment on vacuum.
6. Vacuum curtains from top to bottom. (Give special care around pleats and valances.)

7. When all surface area of drape has been vacuumed on one side, move to the other side of curtain.
8. Repeat procedure.
9. Return curtains to their original position when cleaning is completed.
10. Return all equipment to its storage area.
11. Remove gloves.
12. Wash hands.

PROCEDURE 21.13 — REPLACING PRIVACY CURTAIN AND DRAPES

RATIONALE

Everything in the environment has a potential to carry dangerous microorganisms that cause infection. Following cleaning procedures is essential for preventing the spread of infection. Proper cleaning helps provide a safe environment for patients, staff, and visitors.

1. Gather equipment.
   a. Vacuum
   b. Ladder
   c. Cleaning solution
   d. Two cleaning cloths
   e. Gloves (according to facility policy)
2. Vacuum curtains to remove excess dust. (This will prevent dust and bacteria from being flipped into the air.)
3. Unhook drapes/curtains, being careful not to shake them.
4. Remove hooks from drapes/curtains.
5. Place them in a laundry basket.
6. Wipe curtain track with cleaning solution on a dampened cloth.
7. Wipe track with a dry cloth to remove excess solution and water spots.
8. Place hooks in replacement curtains.
9. Attach hooked curtains/drapes to track.
10. Return equipment to its storage area.
11. Deliver soiled curtains/drapes to the appropriate place for cleaning.

CLEANING SPECIALIZED AREAS

Specialized areas in the hospital include the following:

- Surgery department
- Labor and delivery
- Nursery
- Catheterization laboratory (cath lab)
- Emergency department
- Central supply
- Medical laboratory

Although some of these are associated with sterile areas, they do not need to be as aseptic as rooms where sterile procedures are done. Always follow facility procedures for cleaning these areas. You follow many of the procedures you have already learned.

- Remove all trash, litter, and linen. Remember to double-bag in labor and delivery, the emergency room, surgery, and the cath lab.
- Damp-wipe telephones, furniture, equipment, shelves, ledges, and so on.
- Clean all sinks, restrooms, utility rooms, and hoppers.
- Spot-clean where necessary.
- Clean the floor.
- Clean isolettes and basinettes.
- Clean the interiors of autoclaves.

CLEANING STERILE AREAS

You have already learned that *sterile* means that there are *no* living microorganisms. The following are sterile areas:

■ Surgery suites

■ Labor and delivery

■ Cath lab

Each area is cleaned daily. You must be very careful when you work around equipment. If you notice anything unusual about the equipment or if you accidentally unplug it or move something, *report it immediately*. Equipment that has been moved or altered in any way can be life threatening. Follow the policy of the facility you work for. However, there are some basic rules for you to learn and follow.

Cleaning After Each Case

Clean sterile areas after each case, and then more thoroughly when the suites are empty and not scheduled for immediate use. Always follow Standard Precautions.

■ All trash and linen that is removed must be bagged according to facility policy.

■ Remove all trash and clean the containers.

■ Clean the linen hampers after you have removed the linen.

PROCEDURE 21.14

CLEANING STERILE AREAS

RATIONALE

Sterile areas are especially important in infection control. Microorganisms in surgery, nurseries, and cath labs can cause serious illness and even death. Procedures must be followed carefully to protect patients whose resistance is compromised from serious infections.

ALERT: Follow Standard Precautions.

NOTE Daily cleaning using this procedure is necessary in the following areas:

Surgery
Labor and delivery
Catheterization laboratory

1. Gather equipment.
    a. Service cart
    b. Glass cleaner
    c. Gloves
2. Put on gloves.
3. Remove all trash from the area.
4. Replace plastic liners in each trash container.
5. Remove soiled linen from hampers.

6. Using a cloth dampened with a germicidal solution, wipe down the linen hamper inside and outside, including wheels.
7. Clean treatment tables.
    a. Remove all parts and clean thoroughly.
    b. Wipe down all visible areas on the table.
    c. Replace mattress pad.
    d. Cover with sheet.
8. Wipe all furniture and equipment in the room, including wheels, etc.
9. Wipe any spots on walls, ledges, doors, etc.
10. Damp-mop floors with clean germicidal solution.
11. Remove gloves.
12. Wash hands.

Figure 21.2

Kick bucket.

Mayo stands

Adjustable, wheeled, small metal stands that hold equipment and supplies for many procedures.

kick buckets

Metal buckets on wheels that can be kicked out of the way.

IV poles

Poles that raise and lower. IV solutions are hung on these poles.

- Damp-wipe all soiled surfaces, including the operating table, back table, and the **Mayo stands.**
- Spot-check walls and lights.
- Damp-mop the floor around the operating table.
- Remake the operating table.
- You are not expected to clean instruments. This is the responsibility of the operating room personnel.

Additional Daily Cleaning

- You are expected to clean equipment and furniture:
  - All stools • **Kick buckets** and their holders (Figure 21.2) • Operating table • Flat surfaces, counters, cabinets, and so on • **IV poles,** suction units (outside only)
- Spot-clean lights, walls, vents, and so on.
- Damp-mop floors.
- Floor-flooding technique may be required.

CLEANING PUBLIC AREAS

Patients are cared for in hospitals and health care facilities. There are also visitors, health care workers, and a variety of individuals coming and going. The way the environment looks makes a major impression. A safe, clean, odor-free environment is important because it promotes comfort and a sense of confidence. Patients and families feel encouraged and confident that the staff are caring and competent caregivers.

Every area of the facility is visited by someone each day. It is a major task to keep everything clean and pleasant, especially in facilities that never close.

Your assignment may be in the public areas of the hospital. These areas include the following:

- Reception area
- Waiting rooms
- Offices
- Nurses' stations
- Lounges for the staff
- Public restrooms
- Stairways, elevators, and corridors
- Classrooms, meeting rooms, and conference centers

All these areas must be kept clean. Remember that if you do not do a good job, it is obvious to everyone. You have a great responsibility. Take it seriously, and be proud of the appearance of your facility.

MAINTAINING THE LINEN AREA

Not all facilities have a separate linen department. Some have all the linens sent out. If your facility has a linen department, you may be assigned to this area. Health care workers in this area have the responsibility to

- Handle all linen as contaminated; follow Standard Precautions.
- Maintain the clean linen room and the washer/dryer room.

- Count linens from the contract laundry, if your facility uses one.
- Keep the linen carts clean and neat (Figure 21.3).
- Replenish stock in all clean linen storage areas.
- Take linens to areas with special requests.
- Operate the washer and dryer.
- Sort, inspect, and fold linens.
- Maintain inventory of linen.
- Store linen carts out of passageways to prevent congestion.
- Remove excess lint from area.

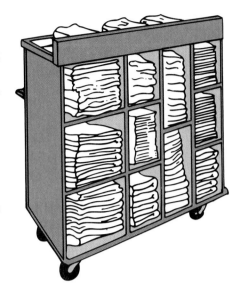

Figure 21.3

Linen cart.

PROCEDURE 21.15 CLEANING LINEN CARTS

RATIONALE

Linen carts are taken from the linen room to patient floors and returned from the floors to the linen room. Carts must be carefully cleaned to prevent transporting microorganisms and contaminating linen.

ALERT: Follow Standard Precautions.

1. Gather supplies:
   a. Clean cloths
   b. Germicidal/detergent solution
   c. Disposable gloves
2. Put on gloves.
3. Wash all racks and bars of cart with germicidal/detergent solution.
4. Wipe with clean cloth.
5. Spray cover of cart on inside and outside with germicidal/detergent solution.
6. Wipe with dry cloth.
7. Wipe wheels and bumpers with cleaning solution and clean cloth.
8. Inspect covers and carts for condition.
9. Remove gloves.
10. Report items needing repair.
11. Store linen carts out of passageways to prevent congestion.

PROCEDURE 21.16 MAINTAINING WASHER/DRYER ROOM

RATIONALE

Laundry may contain fluids, sputum, drainage, and other sources of microorganisms. Correct handling of linens and keeping a clean washer/dryer and laundry room help prevent the spread of infection.

PROCEDURE 21.16 | MAINTAINING WASHER/DRYER ROOM *(Continued)*

1. Gather supplies:
   a. Laundry soap
   b. Additives according to facility policy
   c. Disposable gloves
2. Put on gloves.
3. Separate colors and whites.
4. Place in separate piles.
5. Separate linens in piles by weight (all towels together, all sheets together, etc.).
6. Use manufacturer's operating instructions for washer and dryer.

7. Wash and dry linen according to facility policy.
8. Fold laundry according to facility policy.
9. Inspect laundry for tears or stains (handle according to facility policy).
10. Wipe inside and outside of dryer and washer daily with germicidal solution.
11. Remove gloves.
12. Wash hands.

JOBS AND PROFESSIONS

■ Assistive personnel
■ Clinical medical assistant
■ Licensed vocational/practical nurse
■ Registered nurse

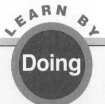

LEARN BY Doing

1. Complete Worksheets 2 and 3 as assigned.
2. Complete Worksheets/Activities 4 through 6.
3. Practice all procedures.
4. Prepare responses to each item listed in Chapter Review—Your Link to Success at the end of this chapter.
5. When you are confident that you can meet each objective, ask your instructor for the unit evaluation.

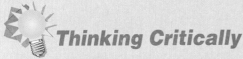

Thinking Critically

1. **Communication** There is an overhead page for you to come immediately to the labor and delivery area. You just started to wet-mop a hallway. Answer the following questions and justify your responses: (1) Whom will you talk to? (2) What will you say? (3) What will you do?

2. **Legal and Ethical** Describe the possible legal results of your leaving a wet floor without signs or a barrier to warn people walking through the area.

3. **Computers** Research and identify ways that computers are used in the environmental services department.

4. **Case Study** Mrs. Summers is a pleasant elderly woman who enjoys talking with you while you are working in her rooms. Today she asks you to do her a favor. She gives you some money to buy her a candy bar from the gift shop.

Describe how you will respond to her, and explain your reasoning.

5. **Patient Education** Mr. Wick is one of the less cheerful patients/clients in the areas you service. Today he tells you that your cleaning is disturbing him and is not necessary for his health. How would you respond to his comments?

6. **Cultural Competency** An elderly patient with limited English language skills is getting more abrupt and demanding every day. Today she wants you to stamp and mail letters for her. When you explain to her that you are not permitted to do some of the chores she is requesting, she becomes angry. The one word you understand that she repeats over and over is "servant." How do you handle this situation? Do you involve other members of the health care team?

Portfolio Connection

Once you attain competency as an environmental services technician/housekeeper, ask for permission to take pictures of areas you cleaned. Be sure that your photos do not show patients or their guests. Place pictures, along with a description of the area, in your portfolio as evidence of your work. Place a copy of your on-site trainer's evaluation in your portfolio.

Write a paper describing your doubts and realizations and the barriers that you were able to overcome during your environmental services/housekeeping experience. For example, did you have fears about going into the surgery area or the morgue? Describe the ways you plan to use the skills, information, and insights that you gained about the people you worked with and about this job. This assignment must be in standard report format.

Portfolio Tip

Don't forget that what is only a small part of your work area is the patient's whole world: leave all patient areas as attractive as you can make them.

Remember! **Media Connection**

Use the Companion Website **www.prenhall.com/badasch** and the CD-ROM for additional interactive learning activities.

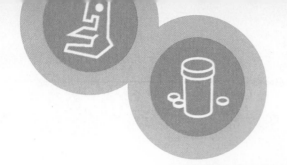

Chapter 22

Health Information Technician

MEDIA CONNECTION

Use the Companion Website
www.prenhall.com/badasch and the CD-ROM
for additional interactive learning activities.

STEPS TO SUCCESS

1. Complete Vocabulary Worksheet 1 in the Student Workbook.

2. Read this chapter.

3. Complete the Learn by Doing assignment at the end of this chapter.

OBJECTIVES

When you have completed this chapter, you will be able to do the following:

✔ Complete all objectives from Part One of this book.

✔ Explain why customer service is important.

✔ Differentiate between a positive and negative personal appearance.

✔ Discuss the importance of office appearance.

✔ List nine guidelines when scheduling clients/patients for appointments.

✔ Describe a tickler file.

✔ Discuss two purposes for writing a letter.

✔ Explain how a letter is a legal document.

✔ Discuss the information that is necessary for a medical history form.

✔ List five filing systems.

✔ List two kinds of registration forms.

✔ Explain how to reach the fair dollar amount for determining fees.

✔ Define *professional courtesy.*

✔ Define *insurance assignment.*

✔ Define *managed care.*

✔ Differentiate between an HMO, a PPO, and an EPO.

✔ Define *CPT codes.*

✔ Define *ICD-9 codes.*

✔ Define *HCPCS codes.*

✔ List three types of bookkeeping systems.

✔ List four items to look for when you receive a check from a patient/client.

✔ Define *W-4* and *W-2 forms.*

✔ Match six items that appear on a paycheck.

✔ Explain how to use a petty cash fund.

✔ Recognize the difference between medical and administrative supplies.

✔ Predict what problems might occur if there were no supply ordering procedure.

✔ Identify the questions to ask regarding business equipment.

✔ Demonstrate the following:
  • Looking professional
  • Scheduling appointments
  • Scheduling a new client/patient: first-time visit
  • Scheduling an outpatient diagnostic test
  • Using a pegboard for charges and services
  • Keeping track of petty cash
  • Writing a letter in three styles

○ RESPONSIBILITIES OF A HEALTH INFORMATION TECHNICIAN

Health information technicians facilitate the efficient operation of a provider's (physician, nurse practitioner, physician's assistant) office. They may also work in clinics or other health care facilities and have varied duties in the front office of physician's offices, clinics, and health maintenance organizations (HMOs).

Duties of the health information technician include the following:

- Answering phones
- Greeting clients/patients
- Processing mail
- Scheduling hospital admissions
- Scheduling laboratory services
- Making appointments
- Preparing insurance forms for Medicare, Medicaid, and workers' compensation
- Typing medical reports
- Maintaining client/patient files
- Handling billing and receipts (in some offices)
- Preparing payroll for office staff (in some offices)
- Typing correspondence

○ CUSTOMER SERVICE

Good customer service has different meanings for different businesses. In a department store or bookstore, it means treating the customer politely and having the items the customer needs. What does it mean in a medical office? The definitions are as varied as the number of patients/clients your office sees. In a medical office, good customer service includes the following:

- Your professional appearance
- The professional appearance of the office
- How you answer a phone call
- The ease in scheduling appointments with the provider
- The way you make patients/clients feel when they walk into the office
- How quickly questions are answered
- How easily billing is done

Be a Professional

The way you are perceived by patients, their family, and other professionals sets the tone for the office. As a health information technician you are responsible for setting a positive tone and image for your employer.

Remember to treat clients/patients the way you expect to be treated when you go to a medical office. Listen to what patients/clients say with their words as well as with their nonverbal communication, and respond paying close attention to your words and nonverbal communication. Review Chapter 5, Unit 1, to reinforce your positive communication skills.

Office Appearance

Office appearance is as important as your appearance. Clients/patients make judgments based on what they see. Patients/clients see the office as a reflection of

PROCEDURE 22.1

LOOKING PROFESSIONAL

RATIONALE

A professional appearance makes a statement about the medical facility. A well-groomed and well-dressed staff says everyone in the facility is interested in the well-being of the pa- tient. Appearance sends a message that the staff is efficient and will take every effort to provide professional service.

1. Dress according to your facility's dress code.
2. Keep jewelry to a minimum (e.g., watch, stud earrings, and a ring).
3. Wear your name badge every day, in view of patients/clients.
4. Wear clean and polished shoes every day.
5. Keep your hair clean.
6. Wear your hair up and off your collar.
7. Use unscented deodorant.
8. Follow rules of good hygiene.
    a. Brush your teeth at least once a day.
    b. Floss daily.
    c. Use mouthwash or breath mints.
    d. Bathe daily.
9. Keep your nails short and clean. (Use light-colored nail polish, and repair chips.)

Female
10. Keep makeup conservative (e.g., no dark, heavy makeup).
11. Do not use perfume or cologne.
12. Wear full-length hose without runs.

Male
13. Do not use cologne or strong aftershave.
14. Keep beard or mustache neatly trimmed.
15. Shave daily. No stubble!

PROCEDURE 22.2

NONVERBAL/BODY LANGUAGE

RATIONALE

Every move that we make sends a message. Positive mes- sages come from good eye contact, smiling, and paying close attention to the person we are interacting with. Nega- tive messages cause the person that we interact with to doubt the efficiency of the staff responsible for patient care.

1. Make eye contact with clients/patients as they enter the office.
2. **Maintain** eye contact as you **converse** with patients/clients.
3. Smile.
4. Keep an open **stance**. (Crossed arms or hands indicates an unwillingness or a barrier in communication.)
5. Give your full attention to one client/patient at a time, even when you have multiple tasks (e.g., telephone, other patients).
6. Keep your hands away from your mouth when speak- ing.

maintain   Keep up.

converse   Talk, have a conversation.

stance   The way you stand.

the quality of care they will receive. Make sure that the office is always clean and orderly. Verify the following:

- Furniture is in its place and in good repair.
- Magazines are neatly arranged in racks or on tables.
- Exam rooms are clean and ready for the next patient. (For example, the table sheet is clean and equipment is clean and ready.)
- Rooms and hallways are well lit.
- Toys are in only one area of the waiting room.
- There is a trash can available for clients/patients.

Letter Writing

Writing is an important tool of communication between you and your clients/patients. When you write to a client/patient you must communicate clearly, factually, and **concisely.** A letter has many purposes. The two most common are

- To give information
- To ask for information

concisely
Brief; to the point.

A letter to a patient/client is a legal record. Always use the following guidelines when preparing a letter:

- Gather all information you need before writing a letter.
- Determine if the letter needs to be formal or informal.
- Understand the purpose of your letter (for example, asking for payment).
- Ask yourself what results you want from the reader of the letter.
- Be specific.
- Use simple wording (for example, *use* instead of *utilize*).
- Be as brief as possible without omitting any important facts.
- Read the letter carefully.
- Ask yourself, "Will the reader understand what the writer wants them to do?"

Letter Styles

The most common style is the block-style letter (see Figure 22.1). To write a block-style letter, follow this format:

1. **Date line.** Six lines from the top of the page
2. **Inside address.** Three to eight lines from the date
3. **Salutation.** Two lines from inside address
4. **Message.** Two lines below salutation

salutation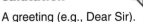
A greeting (e.g., Dear Sir).

   - Single-space between salutation and first paragraph • Double-space between paragraphs
5. **Complimentary closing.**
   - First letter of first word capitalized (for example, *Truly, Sincerely*) • Comma after the complimentary close (for example, *Sincerely yours*)
6. **Writer's typed name.** At least five lines from the complimentary closing
7. **Title of writer.**
   - Typed next to writer's name (for example, *Gus Doors, President*) or • One line below writer's name: *Gus Doors President*
8. If preprinted letterhead is not used, the office name and address follow the writer's title

Figure 22.1

THE BLOCK LETTER

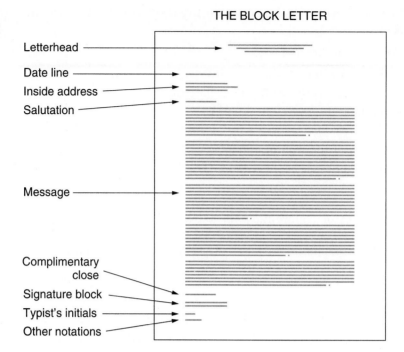

Letterhead

Date line

Inside address

Salutation

Message

Complimentary close

Signature block

Typist's initials

Other notations

9. Identification initials. Two lines below title of writer or office name

- Initials of writer in capital letters followed by a colon and initials of typist in lowercase letters (for example, *GD:mmp*)

10. Enclosure notation. If a letter contains additional paperwork, this notation must be placed one or two lines below the identification initials (for example, *Enclosure;* if more than one, *Enclosures 2, 3,* and so on)

There are other styles of letters that your provider may prefer. See Figures 22.2 and 22.3 for other styles.

Figure 22.2

THE MODIFIED SEMIBLOCK LETTER

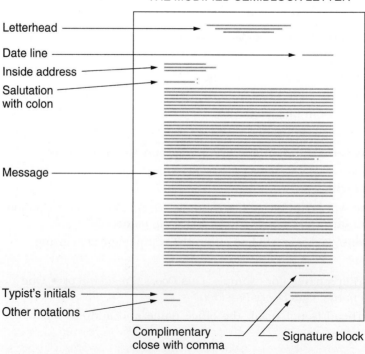

Letterhead

Date line

Inside address

Salutation with colon

Message

Typist's initials

Other notations

Complimentary close with comma

Signature block

THE SIMPLIFIED LETTER

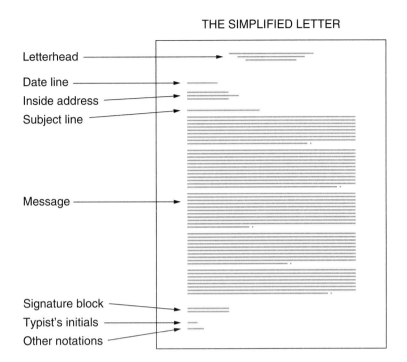

Letterhead

Date line
Inside address
Subject line

Message

Signature block
Typist's initials
Other notations

Figure 22.3

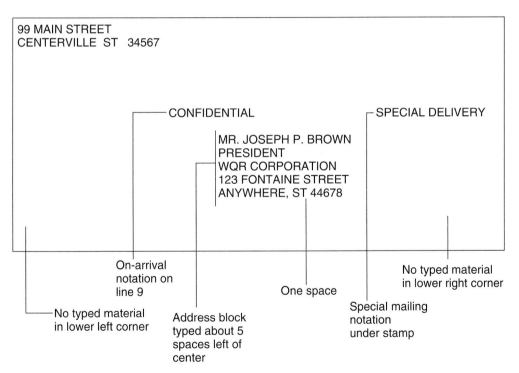

99 MAIN STREET
CENTERVILLE ST   34567

CONFIDENTIAL   SPECIAL DELIVERY

MR. JOSEPH P. BROWN
PRESIDENT
WQR CORPORATION
123 FONTAINE STREET
ANYWHERE, ST 44678

On-arrival
notation on
line 9

No typed material
in lower left corner

Address block
typed about 5
spaces left of
center

One space

Special mailing
notation
under stamp

No typed material
in lower right corner

Figure 22.4

Envelopes

When addressing envelopes, follow the guidelines of the postal service. Remember to put a return address so that the letter can be returned to you if the addressee has moved. Figure 22.4 shows a sample envelope.

● SCHEDULING

For a smooth-running day it is important to know how to schedule clients/patients for office visits, procedures, and surgeries. Scheduling is done in one of two ways: Appointments are written manually in an appointment book, or a computer system maintains appointment schedules.

Scheduling Office Visits

When scheduling visits, follow these guidelines:

1. A patient/client visit is scheduled every 15 minutes, 30 minutes, or hourly, depending on your provider's specialty (see Figures 22.5 and 22.6).

2. Learn to recognize the patients/clients who require more time with the provider.

3. Always ask the purpose of the appointment (for example, checkup, cold) to allocate enough time for the visit.

Figure 22.5

Standard appointment sheet.

Date 1-8-03				
7	30	IAN GALLAGHER		
	45	DEE ANN SHERMAN		
8	00	/////////////////		
	15	MARY KELHI		
	30			
	45			
9	00			
	15			
	30			
	45			
	00			

Figure 22.6

Medical appointment schedule for more than one service at a time.

Month _____

Date _____

Day _____

		Dr. Smith	Dr. Jones	Ultrasound Machine
8:00				
8:15			GREEN, LOIS 412-6190	
8:30			BACK PAIN	DR. JONES: MRS. GREEN
8:45				
9:00				
9:15				
9:30				
9:45				

4. Ask the patient/client what would be the most convenient time for an appointment.

5. If you are not able to schedule the patient/client at the time and date requested, express regret and ask for a second choice.

6. Ask for a phone number where the patient/client can be reached during the day in case a cancellation is necessary.

7. Offer to call the client/patient as cancellations occur if the patient/client desires an earlier appointment. Use a tickler file as a reminder. (See page 579.)

8. Always repeat the appointment time and date to the patient/client to avoid confusion.

9. When a patient/client cancels an appointment, note the date, time, and reason for the cancellation in the chart.

10. Give all patients/clients appointment cards when scheduling a follow-up visit. Put the following information on the appointment card:

   • Provider's name • Provider's address and phone number • Patient's/Client's name • Date and time of next appointment

---

PROCEDURE 22.3

SCHEDULING OFFICE VISITS

RATIONALE

Careful scheduling is essential for a well-run office. Appointments must be scheduled to prevent long waits for patients.

Accommodating the patient as much as possible tells the patient that you are concerned about him or her.

1. Assemble materials.
   a. Pen or pencil
   b. Appointment book
   c. Appointment reminder cards for tickler file
   d. Appointment cards
   e. Calendar
   f. Procedure list with approximate time allotments for each procedure
   g. Written instructions for patient/client preparation prior to visit

2. Prepare provider schedules for at least three months.
   a. Mark out vacation or holiday times.
   b. Schedule monthly, weekly, or daily meetings.
   c. Mark schedule to identify hours for patient/client appointments.

3. Follow the correct procedure for the type of appointment system in your office.

4. Write clearly and neatly so that names and procedures are easy to read.

5. Schedule appointments.
   a. By phone:
      (1) Clarify reason for appointment.
      (2) Discuss most convenient time for client/patient (e.g., A.M., P.M.).
      (3) Offer various times.
      (4) Ask for proper spelling of first and last names once a time is chosen.
      (5) Ask for information, such as birthday or Social Security number, if name is common (e.g., Smith, Jones).
      (6) Write patient's/client's telephone number and where he or she can be reached during the day of appointment.
      (7) Allocate **sufficient** time for the visit when scheduling a procedure.
   b. In person:
      (1) Follow steps 1 to 5 of procedure above.
      (2) Give patient/client an appointment card with date and time of appointment.
   c. For appointments more than three months in the future:
      (1) Ask patient/client to address an appointment reminder card.
      (2) Fill in month patient is to return.
      (3) Instruct patient/client that a card will be sent as a reminder to call and make an appointment.
   d. Place appointment reminder card in tickler file so that it is sent at the correct time.

---

sufficient   Enough.   🔊

Scheduling Surgeries/Procedures

Learn how your provider wants to schedule surgery and procedures in the hospital or office. Use the following guidelines to help you with this scheduling:

- Determine how long each procedure takes.

- Learn how to schedule patients/clients around these procedures.

- Establish what days and times your provider prefers to do surgeries (for example, Monday, Tuesday, all day, just in the morning).

- Learn the admitting procedure for the hospital where your provider performs surgery.

- Provide the patient/client with the following information:

  - Surgery time • Time patient/client needs to arrive at the office or hospital • Registration instructions (admitting forms) if going to the hospital • The hospital's address, telephone, and directions • Written instructions to follow prior to surgery (for example, *NPO after midnight*)

- Give the client/patient verbal and written instruction because the person may be nervous or apprehensive and forget what you said.

- Maintain good lines of communication with the office personnel of all referring providers and assisting providers.

Learning how your office functions allows you to schedule a smooth-running day.

PROCEDURE 22.4 SCHEDULING A NEW PATIENT/CLIENT: FIRST-TIME VISIT

RATIONALE

Gathering essential information from each new patient provides the information needed for patient care and timely billing for services rendered. The patient feels secure when everything is taken care of efficiently.

1. Assemble materials.

   a. Appointment book
   b. Scheduling guidelines
   c. Telephone
   d. Pencil

2. Ask patient/client for the following:

   a. First, last, and middle names
   b. Birth date
   c. Home address
   d. Telephone number

3. Ask patient/client if this is a referral. If yes:

   a. Determine information you need from the referring provider.
   b. Add this information to the medical chart. (Your provider needs to send a consultation report to the referring provider.)

4. Ask what the chief complaint is and when it started.

5. Find the first appointment that allows the appropriate amount of time.

6. Offer a choice of days and times.

7. Enter the following:

   a. Patient's/client's name (*NP* next to name indicating new patient)
   b. Time and date of appointment
   c. Patient's/Client's day telephone number

8. Explain payment procedure (e.g., patient/client must pay for visit, your office will bill).

9. Give directions to the office.

10. Explain parking arrangements.

11. Repeat day, date, and time the appointment is scheduled.

Scheduling Diagnostic Tests

Diagnostic procedures are frequently scheduled to be performed in other facilities. The following is basic information necessary to schedule an appointment:

- Patient's/Client's name
- Age or date of birth
- Reason for the diagnostic test

Give the client/patient the appointment information and instructions to prepare for the test. When scheduled for a test like an upper gastrointestinal series (UGI) give written guidelines that explain how to prepare for the test.

Tickler File

A tickler file reminds you of tasks that need to be done at a certain time (for example, by day, week, or month). When you create a tickler file, arrange 12 file dividers in a file. You need 1 divider for each month and 1 for each day of the month (1 through 31). When a client/patient needs to be seen at a later date:

1. Fill out a reminder card with the patient's/client's name and address.
2. Fill in the blank space with the date of the patient's/client's last visit.
3. Place the card in the file the month prior to the next required visit.
4. Each month, take cards from that month's folder, and mail them to the client/patient.

Check this file routinely. The tickler file tells you what to do and when to do it. The card that is in the file reminds you to notify the client/patient to make an appointment (see Figure 22.7).

PROCEDURE 22.5 SCHEDULING OUTPATIENT DIAGNOSTIC TESTS

RATIONALE

Patients are often fearful about diagnostic tests. Scheduling the diagnostic tests as soon as possible and when it is most convenient for the patients helps give confidence that they are cared for in a timely and caring way.

1. Assemble materials.
   a. Written order from provider
   b. Patient's chart
   c. Test preparation instructions for client/patient
   d. Name, address, and phone number of laboratory
   e. Telephone
2. Read provider's order.
3. Ask patient/client when he or she is available.
4. Call test lab.
   a. Order test
   b. Set up time and date
   c. Give name, age, address, and telephone number of patient/client

   d. Ask if there are special instructions for patient/client prior to the test
5. Provide patient/client with the following:
   a. Name, address, and telephone number of laboratory
   b. Date and time
   c. Instructions (in writing) for preparation prior to test
6. Verify instructions with patient/client.
7. Record test time in patient's/client's chart.
8. Put a reminder in the tickler file or on a calendar to check for results.

Figure 22.7

Appointment reminder card to be placed in a tickler file.

As you requested, Dr. R. C. Smith is reminding you that it has been _____ since your last visit.

Please call (000) 888-0000 to schedule an appointment.

R. C. Smith, M.D.
11372 City Drive
Scottsdale, WA 88888

REGISTRATION

New patients/clients must complete two basic forms when registering:

1. Client/patient information forms
2. Medical history forms

Client/Patient Information Forms

The client/patient information form gives the following information:

- Patient's/client's name, address, and phone number
- Birth date, sex, marital status, Social Security number
- Patient's/client's employer name, address, and phone number
- Insurance company's name, address, and phone number
- Insured's employer name, address, and phone number
- If the patient/client is a minor, name of the responsible party

Medical History Forms

The medical history form gives the provider the necessary information to evaluate the patient's/client's physical condition. The patient/client must give you the following information (see Figure 22.8):

- Previous surgeries
- Allergies
- Chronic illness
- Medications taken
- General medical history
- Childhood diseases

Both forms must be completed accurately to serve the needs of both the client/patient and the provider.

GREEN VALLEY MEDICAL GROUP, INC.
MEDICAL HISTORY

NAME _____

OCCUPATION _____

DATE OF BIRTH _____

MARITAL STATUS: S   M   D   W

ALLERGIES:

Are you allergic to:

Penicillin . . . . Yes _____ No _____

Sulfa . . . . Yes _____ No _____

Aspirin . . . . Yes _____ No _____

Codeine . . . . Yes _____ No _____

Tetanus Injections . . . . Yes _____ No _____

Iodine . . . . Yes _____ No _____

Foods . . . . Yes _____ No _____

Tape . . . . Yes _____ No _____

Other _____

_____

MEDICATIONS:

List all medications, including over the counter, you are currently taking:

_____

_____

_____

_____

_____

HABITS:

Do you:

Smoke?   Yes _____ No _____ How Much _____

Drink Alcohol? Yes _____ No _____ How Much _____

Drink Beverages That Contain Caffeine?

                Yes _____ No _____ How Much _____

Limit Cholesterol   Yes ____ No ____

Use Other Substances   Yes ____ No ____

                What? _____

EXERCISE:

Do you on a regular basis:

Walk . . . . Yes _____ No _____

Run . . . . Yes _____ No _____

Bike . . . . Yes _____ No _____

Swim . . . . Yes _____ No _____

Aerobic Exercise . . . . Yes _____ No _____

Other . . . . Yes _____ No _____

MENSTRUAL HISTORY (FEMALES):

Date of last **PAP** & results_____

Date of last normal period _____

Date of last mammogram & results _____

Length of cycle (days) _____

Usual duration (days) _____

Number of pregnancies_____

Number of children _____

PRESENT COMPLAINTS:

Do you have:

Headaches . . . . Yes _____ No _____

Fever . . . . Yes _____ No _____

Cough . . . . Yes _____ No _____

Chest Pains . . . . Yes _____ No _____

Nausea . . . . Yes _____ No _____

Vomiting . . . . Yes _____ No _____

Diarrhea . . . . Yes _____ No _____

Constipation . . . . Yes _____ No _____

Black Stools . . . . Yes _____ No _____

Bloody Stools . . . . Yes _____ No _____

Painful Urination . . . . Yes _____ No _____

Recent Weight Gain or Loss . . . Yes _____ No _____

Other Complaints _____

_____

PAST ILLNESS:

Have you ever had:

High Blood Pressure . . . . Yes _____ No _____

Heart Trouble . . . . Yes _____ No _____

Pneumonia . . . . Yes _____ No _____

Hepatitis . . . . Yes _____ No _____

Cancer . . . . Yes _____ No _____

Diabetes . . . . Yes _____ No _____

Tuberculosis . . . . Yes _____ No _____

Asthma . . . . Yes _____ No _____

Ulcers . . . . Yes _____ No _____

Seizures . . . . Yes _____ No _____

Sexually Transmitted Disease . . Yes _____ No _____

Blood Disorder . . . . Yes _____ No _____

Other _____

_____

OPERATIONS:

Have you had any surgery:

Appendix . . . . Yes _____ No _____

Tonsils . . . . Yes _____ No _____

Gallbladder . . . . Yes _____ No _____

Stomach . . . . Yes _____ No _____

Hemorrhoids . . . . Yes _____ No _____

Female Organs . . . . Yes _____ No _____

Thyroid . . . . Yes _____ No _____

Hernia . . . . Yes _____ No _____

Heart . . . . Yes _____ No _____

Other _____

_____

_____

Figure 22.8

Medical history form.

⬤ FILING SYSTEMS

Proper filing helps ensure you can find information when you need it. The filing system serves to

- Store information and records safely
- Keep related materials together
- Retrieve files quickly when needed

The following are the five most common systems:

1. Alphabetical
2. Numerical
3. Color coding
4. Chronological
5. Geographic

Each filing system involves the same basic procedures:

- Sorting
- Coding
- Indexing
- Storing or filing

Sorting is the placement of each item according to the particular filing system you are using. Alphabetical sorting requires placing all items with the same letters together. Numerical sorting requires placing all items with the same numbers together. Color sorting requires placing all items with the same colors together. Chronological sorting requires placing all items with the same dates together. Geographical sorting requires placing all items from the same region together.

Coding identifies items that belong to a certain category. For example, surgical files may be assigned a number or letter to identify them as separate from laboratory files.

Indexing organizes items in the order in which they are filed. The American Medical Records Management Association has established rules that provide guidelines for indexing items.

Alphabetical System

The alphabetical system is simple and economical, and it is the most common method for filing records. This system follows the order of the alphabet. If you have not used the alphabet for a long time, take time to review it.

Sorting

To set up an alphabetical filing system, place all charts with the same first letter of the last name together (all *A*'s, all *B*'s, and so on).

- Samuelsen
- Samuelson
- Masters
- Mendoza
- Puertas
- Putnam
- Cruz
- Culver

When there is more than one chart that begins with the same letter, alphabetize by the second, third, fourth letters (or as many as necessary). The boldface letters in the following list determine the files' placement in an alphabetical listing.

- **Cr**uz
- **Cu**lver
- **Ma**sters
- **Me**ndoza
- **Pue**rtas
- **Put**nam
- **Samuelse**n
- **Samuelso**n

Coding

If your files are separated by a code, place all *A*'s with the same code together, all *B*'s with the same code together, and so on. Some systems do not separate coded files. In files that are not separated, the codes identify specific things. For example, an office may have several doctors, and each doctor may be identified by a different color. All charts can be filed together, or they can be separated, depending on the office procedure.

Indexing

Make three columns on a page and label the columns 1, 2, and 3. When filing by name, place the last name in the column labeled 1, the first name in the column labeled 2, and the middle name or initial in the column labeled 3. For example, if the name is Alec Monroe Goldman, it is indexed as

1	**2**	**3**
Goldman	Alec	Monroe

It is important to label charts by this indexing method. This makes placing them in order a simple task.

Charts with initials instead of a first name are placed before spelled-out names. C. Todd Sherman is indexed as

1	**2**	**3**
Sherman	C.	Todd

Names that are hyphenated are considered one name, as if the hyphen were not there. For example, Kellie Bell-White is indexed as

1	**2**	**3**
Bell-White	Kellie	

Apostrophes are ignored when indexing, so Timothy Gallagher O'Bannon is indexed as

1	**2**	**3**
OBannon	Timothy	Gallagher

Last names with prefixes are joined as one name, so Carlos A. De Leon is indexed as

1	**2**	**3**
DeLeon	Carlos	A.

Abbreviated names are indexed as if they were spelled out in full. For example, St. Gustov Edward is indexed as Gustov Saint Edward, or

1	**2**	**3**
Edward	Gustov	(Saint)

If a title precedes one name or a given name and a middle name, the title is the first indexing number. Father Gerald Rahn, Queen Erin, and Princess Monica are indexed as

1	**2**	**3**
Gerald	Rahn	(Father)
Erin	(Queen)	
Monica	(Princess)	

Titles and degrees before or after a complete name are placed in parentheses after the name for identification. For example, Dr. DeeAnn Marie Sherman or DeeAnn Marie Sherman, M.D., is indexed as

1	**2**	**3**
Sherman	DeeAnn	Marie (Dr.)
Sherman	DeeAnn	Marie (M.D.)

Store or File

Place files in alphabetical order for easy retrieval. Place the names in order by looking for the first letter that is different, indicating the sequence. For example, Gallagher, Kevin DeWayne, is filed before Gallagher, Shaun Patrick Michael, because the *K* in Kevin comes before the *S* in Shaun.

Follow the instructions in your Student Workbook to practice sorting, coding, indexing, and filing.

Numerical System

The numerical system is another simple way of maintaining client/patient charts. Use a notebook or computer to record the number assigned to each client/patient. This allows you to find the client/patient name by the assigned number. The assigned number is often referred to as a medical record number or patient/client number.

■ Assigned numbers are placed in numerical order.

■ Assign each new patient/client a number (for example, 001, 002, 003).

accessible

Available to obtain.

Keep a log in a notebook or computer of the client/patient name and number as you assign them. This record must be **accessible** to all staff. For example, assign numbers as follows:

File Number	**Client/Patient Name**
001	Mendoza
002	Samuelsen
003	Putnam
004	Puertas
005	Masters
006	Culver
007	Cruz
008	Samuelson

Terminal Digits

Numbers can indicate many different things. Grouping by **terminal** digits means that you group items according to the last few digits of their assigned number (for example, 432.80, 321.80 or 879.90, 320.90). The terminal digits in these examples are 80 and 90, so all the 80s are filed in order by the first three digits, and all the 90s are filed in the same fashion (for example, 321.80, 432.80 and 320.90, 879.90). Let's pretend that you have items that need to be filed according to their assigned number. First sort these items by grouping all the same number of digits together (for example, all two-digit numbers together, all three-digit numbers together). These are basic rules to follow:

terminal

Last or ending.

- When zeros precede numbers, ignore them. Zeros are often added to numbers because computers call for a specific number of digits in a space. For example, the sequence 0001, 0935, 0087 is filed 0001, 0087, 0935. Because you ignore zeros before numbers when filing, you sort 0001 as a one-digit number, 0087 as having two digits, and 0935 as having three digits.

- Coding is often done by the terminal-digit method. Take the last digits of the assigned numbers and group together all those that are the same. File in ascending order within these groupings. For example, 546.10, 386.30, 957.10, and 752.30 are grouped with all numbers ending with 10 together and all numbers ending with 30 together (546.10, 957.10, 386.30, 752.30).

- Indexing places items in ascending numerical order within their groups. (For example, 546.10 and 957.10 are in one group, and 386.30 and 752.30 form another group.)

- Place files according to their numerical order.

Follow the instructions in your Student Workbook for sorting, coding, indexing, and filing numerically.

Color-Coding System

Color coding helps reduce the chance of filing errors. The following are guidelines for using this method.

1. Assign a color sticker to each letter of the alphabet (for example, blue is *A*, yellow is *B*, green is *C*).
2. Determine how many stickers to apply on a patient's/client's chart (depending on chart size). *Example:* If you use three colors on the chart and the client's/patient's name is Mr. Gates, place the stickers in the order that corresponds to the first three letters of the patient's/client's last name (for example, *G* is yellow, *A* is blue, and *T* is purple).
3. Place the color stickers on the side of the chart that faces out when filed.

Chronological System

Chronological filing arranges files in the order of their occurrence, usually by day. This method is most often used in storing research items. Because each day, month, and year can be referred to by number, it is easy to follow the basic numerical system.

1. Sort by placing all items of the same year together.
2. Code each item as in any filing system.
3. Index by placing all files of the same month and year together.
4. File each item by date within the appropriate month and year grouping.

Geographical System

Geographical filing is done according to location. This method is often used for storing records of research studies in specific geographical areas. File alphabetically according to the name of the state, then alphabetically according to the city. File in the following manner:

- Alphabetically according to the state name
- Alphabetically according to the city name
- Alphabetically according to the names of companies

Whichever filing method you use, follow the basic rules for filing under the appropriate system. The following is an example of filing by company name:

Company Name	City	State
A.G. Corporation	Mills	Illinois
Blosson Inc.	Lakewood	California
Gamble Corporation	Reno	Nevada
General Corporation	Redlands	California
K.G. Inc.	Lakes	Utah
K.M.B. Corp.	Mills	Illinois
M.M. General	Lakewood	California
M.W.G. Corporation	Great Lakes	Florida
Water Inc.	Silverton	Illinois

The following items are alphabetized by state and city:

State	City	Company Name
California	Lakewood	Blosson Inc.
California	Lakewood	M.M. General
California	Redlands	General Corp.
Florida	Great Lakes	M.W.G. Corp.
Illinois	Mills	A.G. Corp.
Illinois	Mills	K.M.B. Corp.
Illinois	Silverton	Water Inc.
Nevada	Reno	Gamble Corp.
Utah	Lakes	K.G. Inc.

● FEES

A fee is a charge for professional services rendered by the provider. The following guidelines help determine how to establish fees:

- All fees must be the same for all patients/clients and insurance companies.
- To arrive at a fair dollar amount, research the following resources:
  - Call other providers and/or office staff who have the same type of practice. (For example, if your provider is a family practice provider, talk with another family practice office.) • Ask various insurance companies to provide you with the average dollar amounts they reimburse for services. • Check the state guidelines on charges allowed.

Professional Courtesy

It is a common practice for providers to extend professional courtesy to other providers and some patients/clients for services rendered. A provider can decide not to charge a patient/client or other provider for services rendered or charge at a discounted rate. Learn the billing policy in your office so that you can deal appropriately with these types of accounts.

⬤ BILLING

Each office needs to establish a billing policy. This policy will provide the following information:

- When to bill a patient/client.
- When to bill the patient's/client's insurance.
- When the patient/client pays for services as they are rendered.
- When to inform the patient/client about your payment policy. (For example, when the patient/client sets up an appointment, tell him: "Mr. Puertas, it's the policy of our office to request payment at the time of service.")
- Whether you will supply patients/clients with a superbill (Figure 22.9) to send to their insurance company.
- Whether you will accept assignment. Accepting assignment means that you accept what the client's/patient's insurance allows. *Example:* Your provider charges $55 for an office visit, but the insurance company will allow a fee of only $35 for an office visit. The insurance company then pays you a percentage of the fee allowed (e.g., 80% of the allowed fee, or $28). The patient is responsible for the difference between $28 and $35. In this case the provider collects $7 from the patient/client. The provider writes off the remaining $20.

Because there are so many different types of insurance and insurance plans, it is important to have a clear understanding of what companies your provider has contracts with and how those contracts work.

Insurance

You may deal with as many different insurance plans as you do clients/patients. Each insurance company has guidelines and regulations detailing what it considers covered and uncovered benefits. The insurance company also indicates what amount it will pay to the provider of service. It is important that the client/patient insurance information is correct and can be verified. Billing must follow the insurance company's guidelines, or it will not pay. Always request that the client/patient bring his or her insurance card (see Figure 22.10) so that a copy can be kept in the person's chart, insurance forms that are completed and signed, and information that explains policy deductibles.

Managed Care

Managed care is defined as a cost-effective way of providing service to the clients/patients. The following managed care plans provide this type of benefit for the patient.

Health Maintenance Organization

A health maintenance organization (HMO) contracts with a medical group or provider to be the primary care provider for its members. The HMO pays the provider or medical group for its services on a monthly basis. The amount, which is **prepaid,**

prepaid

Paid ahead of time.

BRISTOL PARK MEDICAL GROUP, INC.

3160 Redhill Avenue • Costa Mesa, CA 92626

NEW PATIENT
NEW FAMILY **FAMILY PRACTICE**

DATE MO DAY YR	DR	MED REC NO	DOB	LOC	APPT	REASON FOR VISIT	DOCTOR'S USE ONLY

PATIENT NAME	VISIT NO	CO-PAY	
RESPONSIBLE PARTY NAME			Lab charges are subject to change without notice. You will receive a separate bill from Smith Kline Laboratories

MEDICINE 7.50			SMITH KLINE LABORATORY 1.75			INJECTIONS			
LIMITED OV. (ROUTINE)	90050	40.00	CHEMZYME	80019	29.75	DPT	°C	90701	22.00
INTERMED OV.—PELVIC	90060	55.00	CHEMZYME Plus	80019-51	51.00	H.I.B. VACCINE	°C	90749	22.00
EXTENDED OV.	90070	70.00	W/HDL/LDL			M-M-R		90707	30.00
PERIODIC EXAM	90088	70.00	PRENATAL PANEL	80055	90.50	ORAL POLIO		90712	13.00
COMPREHENSIVE H & P	90080	125.00	W/HbsAg P-5			TETANUS TOX (T-D)		90718	13.00
REDUCED OV.	90040	30.00	PAP SMEAR (1 SLIDE)	88150	24.50	T.B. PPD	°C	90749	13.00
INIT. OV. (NEW PATIENT)	90000	50.00	BIOPSY - 1 SPECIMEN	88304	79.75	T.B. TINE		86585	13.00
INIT. TREATMENT PROGR.	90010	55.00	BIOPSY - MULTI SPECIMENS	88305	86.75	ALLERGY		95150	13.00
UNUSUAL HOURS	99050	35.00	(SPECIFY # OF SPECIMENS)			BICILLIN-CR	°C	90749	13.00
HOSPITAL E.R. (INTERM.)	90560	65.00				CORTISONE	°C	90749	14.00
						ESTROGEN	°C	90749	13.00
						FLU VACCINE		90724	13.00
SURGERY 225.00			SPECIMEN HANDLING	99000	12.00	IV SET-UP	°C	99070	28.00
PROCTO-SIGMOIDOSCOPY	45300	90.00	(PAP'S & BIOSPIES ONLY)	—	—	MEASLES MONOVALENT		90705	13.00
FLEXIBLE SIG W/O BIOPSY	45330	190.00	VENIPUNCTURE	90018	7.00				
TENDON INJECTION	20550-58	90.00	**BPMG LABORATORY**						
INCISION & DRAINAGE	10060-58	90.00	BLOOD-OCCULT (STOOL)	89205	15.00	**SUPPLIES**			
CRYOCAUTERY—INITIAL	17340-58	79.00	G C CULTURE °C	87087	15.00	STERILE TRAY		99070	35.00
CRYOCAUTERY—SUBSQ	17340	45.00	GLUCOSE-METER	82948	12.00	STERILE SETUP		99070	25.00
LAC. SIMPLE (2.5cm)	12001-58	90.00	GRAM STAIN	87205	15.00	SURGERY ROOM CHARGES		99200	50.00
LAC. SIMPLE FACE (2.5cm)	12011-58	157.50	HEMATOCRIT	85014	15.00	ELASTIC BANDAGE		99070	
LAC. SIMPLE (2.5 TO 7.5cm)	12002-58	146.25	KOH ONLY	87220	14.00	CAST MAT'L. (PLASTER)		99070	
ELECTROFUL BODY	17100-58	78.75	KOH/SALINE °C	87999	28.00	CAST MAT'L. (LIGHTCAST)		99070	
ELECTROFUL FACE	17000-58	112.50	MONO-SPOT	86300	15.00	CRUTCHES		99070	40.00
POST-OP CARE	99024	00.00	SALINE ONLY	87210	14.00	EYE TRAY		99070	8.00
			STREP SCREEN	87060	12.00	LAVAGE TRAY		99070	12.00
			URICULT	87087	15.00				
SPECIAL PROCEDURES			URINALYSIS	81000	15.00				
AUDIOGRAM, BASIC	92551-52	36.00	UA DIP ONLY	81002	10.00	**BILLING**			
EAR LAVAGE	69210-52	10.00	URINE PREG	84703	15.00	COPAY		99095	
ECG—ROUTINE	93000	60.00	WRIGHT'S STAIN	—	—	ADJUSTMENT			
HOLTER MONITOR	93262	325.00	NASAL OR SPUTUM	89190	15.00	COPAY (SPECIAL)		99098	
IPPB	94650	30.00	STOOL	87205	15.00	INFERTILITY (50%)		99092	
MANIPULATION	96600	45.00				FAMILY PLANNING		99091	
SPIROMETRY	94010	45.00	**X-RAY 13.00**						
			CHEST (2V)	71020	65.00				
NON-COVERED PROCEDURES			CHEST (1V)	71010	50.00				
ALLERGY SERUM	95155	47.00	LUMBOSACRAL SPINE (3V)	72100	65.00	**BUSINESS OFFICE USE**			
DME/ORTHOTICS	99099		SINUSES COMPLETE (3V)	70220	90.00	DISABILITY FROM:		—	—
DRUG SCREENING	82660	35.00	KNEE (2V)	73560	60.00	DISABILITY TO:		—	—
ELECTIVE PHYSICAL	90750		FOOT (3V)	73630	60.00	ADJUSTMENTS: PROF DISCOUNT			
FLU INJECTION	90724	13.00	TOE (3V)	73660	45.00	COURTESY DISCOUNT			
FORM COMPLETION	99080	15.00	WRIST (3V)	73110	65.00	VIP DISCOUNT DO NOT BILL			
			FINGER (3V)	73140	45.00	AUTO ACCIDENT (3RD PARTY)			
			KUB	74000	50.00	PRIME INSURANCE			
						RECALL: YES MONTHS _____			

ICDA-DIAGNOSIS	X	ICDA-DIAGNOSIS	X	ICDA-DIAGNOSIS	X	ICDA-DIAGNOSIS	X	ICDA-DIAGNOSIS	X	ICDA-DIAGNOSIS	X	ICDA-DIAGNOSIS

Document Creations (714) 324-3919

Figure 22.9

Superbill. (Courtesy of Bristol Park Medical Group, Inc.)

capitation

Payment to provide care for a set number of people.

depends on the number of clients/patients that are enrolled with the medical group or physician. The amount that is paid is called **capitation.** For example, Dr. Smith is a primary care provider who has 10 members of an HMO enrolled with her. The HMO pays Dr. Smith $10 per month per client/patient whether or not the client/

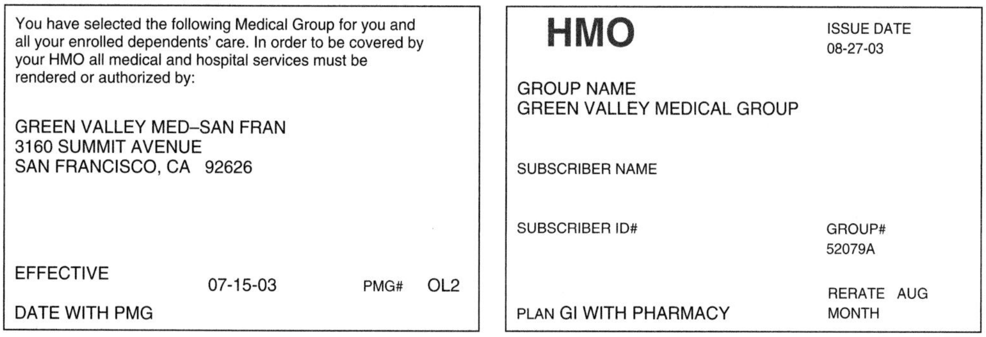

Figure 22.10

Insurance card.

You have selected the following Medical Group for you and all your enrolled dependents' care. In order to be covered by your HMO all medical and hospital services must be rendered or authorized by:

GREEN VALLEY MED–SAN FRAN
3160 SUMMIT AVENUE
SAN FRANCISCO, CA 92626

EFFECTIVE
DATE WITH PMG   07-15-03   PMG#   OL2

HMO   ISSUE DATE
                                       08-27-03

GROUP NAME
GREEN VALLEY MEDICAL GROUP

SUBSCRIBER NAME

SUBSCRIBER ID#   GROUP#
                                       52079A

PLAN GI WITH PHARMACY   RERATE   AUG
                                       MONTH

patient comes to Dr. Smith. If the client/patient comes to see Dr. Smith once or 10 times in one month, the doctor still receives only one $10 payment per month.

The HMO covers most of the costs for procedures except for a copayment that is the responsibility of the client/patient. If the client/patient needs the care of a specialist (for example, an orthopedist), the primary care provider must direct the client/patient to the appropriate specialist by giving the client/patient a referral authorization.

Preferred Provider Organization

A preferred provider organization (PPO) contracts with a provider or medical group that has agreed to provide care at a reduced rate. The PPO often pays 90 to 100% of the cost. The client/patient pays the balance. The client/patient does not have to choose a primary care provider but must see a provider on the contracted list or pay all fees that are higher than the PPO has agreed to pay. There is usually a deductible that the patient/client is responsible for each year.

Exclusive Provider Organization

An exclusive provider organization (EPO) contracts with a medical group or provider to provide services to its members at a reduced cost. The member must see only the providers contracted with the EPO. If the member sees a noncontracted provider, he or she is responsible for all costs.

Always instruct the patient/client to bring the following information to ensure correct billing:

- Insurance card
- Insurance forms that are complete and signed
- All met or paid deductibles

Remember that if you contract with an insurance plan, you need to follow the company's guidelines when billing for any services **rendered.** Appropriate billing results in correct reimbursement.

rendered

Given or provided.

Billing Codes

Procedure and diagnostic codes were developed for billing purposes. These codes are accepted universally by programs such as Medicare and Medicaid. There are three types of codes: the Current Procedural Terminology (CPT) system, the Health Common Procedure Coding System (HCPCS), and the International Classification of Diseases 9th Revision Clinical Modification (ICD-9-CM).

Current Procedural Terminology (CPT)

Use the CPT coding system for reporting medical services and procedures performed by providers and other medical professionals. It is a communication method that is nationally accepted by all health insurance programs.

It is important to use the correct CPT code. The code that you use affects the reimbursement your office receives from the insurance plans you do business with. Improper coding can result in loss of payment. Remember that CPT codes

- Are five-digit numeric
- Describe procedures, services, and supplies used
- Are accepted and required by all insurance carriers, with few exceptions
- Are revised annually, and codes are added, changed, or deleted
- Can make a difference in your reimbursement

Health Common Procedure Coding System (HCPCS)

The HCPCS coding system was developed in 1983 by the Health Care Financing Administration (HCFA) to process bills to Medicare for supplies, materials, and injections. Use it when certain procedures and services are not defined in the CPT. Remember that HCPCS codes

- Are five-digit alphanumeric (the first digit is a letter between *A* and *Z*)
- Describe supplies, material, and services provided by a medical professional
- Are required when billing Medicare and Medicaid
- Are revised annually, and codes are added, changed, or deleted
- Can make a difference in your reimbursement

International Classification of Diseases 9th Revision Clinical Modification (ICD-9-CM)

Use the ICD-9-CM codes to define the diagnosis. Remember that ICD-9 codes

generic
Major group (e.g., heart disease or skin disease).

- Are three- to five-digit numerics (the first three digits represent a **generic** disease; the fourth and fifth digits describe the disease in a more specific manner)
- List the most important diagnosis first if the client/patient has more than one diagnosis

vital
A must, essential.

When you are billing, it is **vital** that all the procedural and diagnosis codes coordinate. Insurance companies return any claims that do not have matching procedural and diagnosis codes. For example, suppose that a patient comes in with chest pain, and the procedure that is marked on your superbill or fee ticket is a foot x-ray instead of a chest x-ray. The insurance company will question the claim and return it for clarification.

● COLLECTIONS

delinquent
Late.

Delinquent accounts are a major problem and need careful handling. One person is usually in charge of delinquent accounts. Outside collection agencies may be hired and paid a set fee or percentage for each account they collect. Ask the following questions regarding the collection policy of your facility:

- When to consider an account delinquent (for example, after 30 or 60 days)
- When to contact a patient/client regarding the outstanding balance on an account
- How and when to inform a client/patient that his or her account will be sent to collections
- What the collection agency's reputation and policies are (some agencies have unusual methods of dealing with clients/patients that may cause problems for your office)

PROCEDURE 22.6   MANAGING DELINQUENT ACCOUNTS

RATIONALE

Delinquent accounts create tension between office staff and patients. Following proper procedure provides a professional approach and eases the tension between the involved parties.

1. Assemble materials.
   a. Delinquent accounts
   b. Office letterhead
   c. Collection letter form
   d. Facility policy for collection of delinquent accounts
2. Sort accounts by number of days delinquent (e.g., 30 days, 60 days, 90 days, and so on).
3. Decide which action to take:

   a. Make phone calls to client/patient as reminders and record response on billing record.
   b. Choose collection letter according to policy.
   c. Prepare collection letter.
   d. Mail collection letter.
   e. Note when letter is sent.
4. Send account information to collection agency according to your facility's policy.

⬤ BOOKKEEPING

Bookkeeping is the method of recording income for services by the provider. You also use bookkeeping to record expenses, such as office supplies, rent, and telephone, that occur during the daily operations of a business. Your office may select a computerized or manual record-keeping system. As a health information technician you may be responsible for keeping the daily records. To maintain accurate records, you must learn the system your office works with. The following are commonly used methods:

- Single-entry
- Double-entry
- Pegboard

Single-Entry Bookkeeping

This is a simple and inexpensive method of accounting. This system requires the following parts:

- **General ledger.** Maintain a logbook with all day sheets.
- **Day sheets.** Record all charges for one day for each patient/client.
- **Accounts receivable ledger.** Record amount the patient/client pays for service.
- **Accounts payable ledger.** Record all fees that you pay for the purchase of equipment, supplies, or services.

Double-Entry Bookkeeping

This system requires recording two entries per financial transaction on a ledger of accounts (see Figure 22.11):

- **Credit entry.** An addition or payment
- **Debit entry.** A deduction or charge

Figure 22.11

Ledger of accounts.

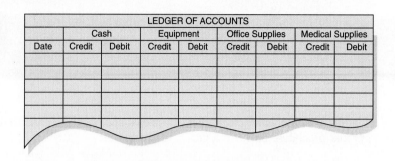

	LEDGER OF ACCOUNTS							
	Cash		Equipment		Office Supplies		Medical Supplies	
Date	Credit	Debit	Credit	Debit	Credit	Debit	Credit	Debit

	LEDGER OF ACCOUNTS					
	Cash		Equipment		Office Supplies	
Date	Credit	Debit	Credit	Debit	Credit	Debit
10/9/03		−400.⁰⁰			+ 400.⁰⁰	

For example, suppose you need to purchase $400 worth of office supplies with cash. Your ledger reflects a debit to Cash of $400 and a credit to Office Supplies of $400 (see Figure 22.11). This provides an automatic check-and-balance system.

Pegboard (One-Write) Bookkeeping

This method allows you to record information on several kinds of forms at the same time. These forms include the following (see Figure 22.12):

- **Day sheet.** A record of all daily financial transactions. One sheet is used per day.
- **Superbill (statement-receipt).** A three-part carbon copy form; copies go to the client/patient, insurance company, and office billing.
- **Ledger cards.** A financial record of the client's/patient's account. You keep the ledger card where it is easily accessible and separate from the client's/patient's chart.
- **Clipboard.** Where the day sheet, superbill, and ledger card are kept for easy record keeping.

PROCEDURE 22.7

USING A PEGBOARD FOR CHARGES AND SERVICES

RATIONALE

The pegboard system provides an easy and efficient way of record keeping and billing. It is important to follow the procedure carefully to prevent errors that are difficult to correct.

1. Assemble materials.
   a. Pegboard
   b. Calculator
   c. Day sheet
   d. Carbon paper (sheets may be NCR sheets; these do not require carbon paper)

   e. Receipts
   f. Ledger cards
   g. Balance sheet from day before
   h. Pen

2. Set up pegboard.
   a. Put on day sheet.

PROCEDURE 22.7 | **USING A PEGBOARD FOR CHARGES AND SERVICES** *(Continued)*

    b. Put carbon over day sheet.

    c. Put receipts over pegs lined up with first open writing line on day sheet.

3. Put in balance from the preceding day.

4. Determine which clients/patients you will see.

5. Pull patient/client ledger cards.

6. Put cards in order of scheduled appointments.

7. Add ledger card to pegboard as clients/patients are seen (one card at a time).

    a. Put card under first receipt.

    b. Align entry line of ledger with carbon on receipt.

8. Enter information on superbill.

    a. Client's/patient's name

    b. Date

    c. Receipt number

    d. Existing balance from ledger card

9. Remove superbill and clip it to patient/client chart.

After the patient/client sees the provider:

10. Ask client/patient for superbill.

11. Enter fee for service (use fee schedule).

    a. Find receipt on pegboard.

    b. Replace client/patient ledger under receipt.

    c. Put service code and fee on receipt.

12. Record amount paid and new balance.

13. Give completed receipt to client/patient.

14. Repeat steps 7 through 13 for each client/ patient.

15. File ledger card at the end of the day or immediately.

At the end of the day:

16. Total all columns on day sheet.

NOTE This system allows you to see errors quickly and is easy to learn and maintain.

CHECKS (PAYABLE/RECEIVABLE)

If you are responsible for writing checks for bills, the office policy tells you the following:

■ When bills are paid (for example, first or last day of the month)

■ What recording system to use

■ How to write checks clearly to prevent misunderstandings

■ Which accounts are paid in full and which are sent partial payments

If you are responsible for receiving checks from clients/patients, look at the check to verify the following information:

■ The check is made out to the right provider or office name.

■ The written amount is the same as the number amount.

■ The address and telephone numbers on the check are current.

■ The check is signed by the person whose name is on the check.

Confirming this information prevents problems with the bank or client/patient later.

PAYROLL

The payroll system is complex. All businesses must follow certain federal and state regulations for payroll. A business may hire an outside agency to prepare its payroll or have an employee complete the payroll. Even if you are not the one responsible for maintaining these records, you must understand the way the payroll

Figure 22.12

Day sheet.

PATIENT NAME	PATIENT NUMBER	DEP#	DATE OF SERVICE	SSN FOR OVER 5 YEARS DOB FOR UNDER 5 YEARS	SERVICE CODE	INFORMATION (CRUTCH RETURNS, NAME ON CHECK)	CODE	INIT. PMT.TYPE	DEBIT AMOUNT	CREDIT AMOUNT

416776

GREEN VALLEY MEDICAL GROUP INC.

Costa Mesa (714) 555-3242	Irvine (714) 555-1090	Santa Ana (714) 555-7100	Mission Viejo (714) 555-1600	San Francisco (714) 555-3199	Mountain Valley (714) 555-3130

Payment type codes:
1 = Cash   3 = Insurance check
2 = Credit Card   4 = Check

Service codes:
#901 Co-payment   #998 PMT check
#997 PMT Insurance   #999 PMT Cash

GREEN VALLEY MEDICAL GROUP INC.

Facility name _____

Date _____

	PATIENT NAME	PATIENT NUMBER	DEP#	DATE OF SERVICE	SSN FOR OVER 5 YEARS DOB FOR UNDER 5 YEARS	SERVICE CODE	INFORMATION (CRUTCH RETURNS, NAME ON CHECK)	PMT.TYPE CODE	INIT.	DEBIT AMOUNT	CREDIT AMOUNT
	Sally Morton	346-72	08	11-22-03	555-55-5555	901		1	DC	15⁰⁰	15⁰⁰
1											
2											
3											
4											
5											
6											
7											
8											
9											
10											
11											
12											
13											
14											
15											
16											
17											
18											
19											
20											
21											
22											
23											
24											
25											

Payment type codes:
1 = Cash   3 = Insurance check
2 = Credit Card   4 = Check

Service codes:
#901 Co-payment   #998 PMT check
#997 PMT Insurance   #999 PMT Cash

Cash total	
Check total	
Grand total	

X _____

Balanced by

---

system works. Employers must maintain clear records of their payroll system. Every employer must keep the following information for each employee:

1. **W-4 form.** This form gives the number of exemptions the employee claims. It tells the employer how much to withhold from the payroll check for taxes and affects the employee's take-home pay (see Figure 22.13).

2. **Time card.** This is a record of the employee's actual work time (see Figure 22.14). The employee's earnings for the pay period are determined from the person's time card.

3. **Payroll register.** This includes the following information (see Figure 22.15):

   a. Information copied from the time card b. Employee's name c. Number of exemptions (from W-4) d. Hourly rate and hours worked e. **Gross pay** plus overtime f. Taxable earnings for **FICA** g. Unemployment insurance h. Other deductions (for example, savings bonds, insurance) i. **Net pay** j. Check numbers

gross pay

Money earned before deductions are removed.

FICA

Federal Insurance Contribution Act.

net pay

Money earned after deductions are removed.

Fom W-4 (2003)

Purpose. Complete Form W-4 so that your employer can withhold the correct Federal income tax from your pay. Because your tax situation may change, you may want to refigure your withholding each year.

Exemption from withholding. If you are exempt, complete only lines 1, 2, 3, 4, and 7 and sign the form to validate it. Your exemption for 2003 expires February 16, 2004. See **Pub. 505,** Tax Withholding and Estimated Tax.

Note: *You cannot claim exemption from withholding if: (a) your income exceeds $750 and includes more than $250 of unearned income (e.g., interest and dividends) and (b) another person can claim you as a dependent on their tax return.*

Basic instructions. If you are not exempt, complete the **Personal Allowances Worksheet** below. The worksheets on page 2 adjust your withholding allowances based on itemized deductions, certain credits, adjustments to income, or two-earner/two-job situations. Complete all worksheets that apply. **However, you may claim fewer (or zero) allowances.**

Head of household. Generally, you may claim head of household filing status on your tax return only if you are unmarried and pay more than 50% of the costs of keeping up a home for yourself and your dependent(s) or other qualifying individuals. See line **E** below.

Tax credits. You can take projected tax credits into account in figuring your allowable number of withholding allowances. Credits for child or dependent care expenses and the child tax credit may be claimed using the **Personal Allowances Worksheet** below. See **Pub. 919,** How Do I Adjust My Tax Withholding? for information on converting your other credits into withholding allowances.

Nonwage income. If you have a large amount of nonwage income, such as interest or dividends, consider making estimated tax payments using **Form 1040-ES,** Estimated Tax for Individuals. Otherwise, you may owe additional tax.

Two earners/two jobs. If you have a working spouse or more than one job, figure the total number of allowances you are entitled to claim on all jobs using worksheets from only one Form W-4. Your withholding usually will be most accurate when all allowances are claimed on the Form W-4 for the highest paying job and zero allowances are claimed on the others.

Nonresident alien. If you are a nonresident alien, see the **Instructions for Form 8233** before completing this Form W-4.

Check your withholding. After your Form W-4 takes effect, use Pub. 919 to see how the dollar amount you are having withheld compares to your projected total tax for 2003. See Pub. 919, especially if your earnings exceed $125,000 (Single) or $175,000 (Married).

Recent name change? If your name on line 1 differs from that shown on your social security card, call 1-800-772-1213 for a new social security card.

Personal Allowances Worksheet (Keep for your records.)

A	Enter "1" for **yourself** if no one else can claim you as a dependent	**A** _____
	You are single and have only one job; or	
B	Enter "1" if: You are married, have only one job, and your spouse does not work; or .	**B** _____
	Your wages from a second job or your spouse's wages (or the total of both) are $1,000 or less.	
C	Enter "1" for your **spouse.** But, you may choose to enter "-0-" if you are married and have either a working spouse or more than one job. (Entering "-0-" may help you avoid having too little tax withheld.)	**C** _____
D	Enter number of **dependents** (other than your spouse or yourself) you will claim on your tax return	**D** _____
E	Enter "1" if you will file as **head of household** on your tax return (see conditions under **Head of household** above) .	**E** _____
F	Enter "1" if you have at least $1,500 of **child or dependent care expenses** for which you plan to claim a credit .	**F** _____
	(**Note:** *Do not* include child support payments. See **Pub. 503,** Child and Dependent Care Expenses, for details.)	
G	**Child Tax Credit** (including additional child tax credit):	
	If your total income will be between $15,000 and $42,000 ($20,000 and $65,000 if married), enter "1" for each eligible child plus **1 additional** if you have three to five eligible children or **2 additional** if you have six or more eligible children.	
	If your total income will be between $42,000 and $80,000 ($65,000 and $115,000 if married), enter "1" if you have one or two eligible children, "2" if you have three eligible children, "3" if you have four eligible children, or "4" if you have five or more eligible children.	**G** _____
H	Add lines A through G and enter total here. **Note:** *This may be different from the number of exemptions you claim on your tax return.*	**H** _____

For accuracy, complete all worksheets that apply.	If you plan to **itemize or claim adjustments to income** and want to reduce your withholding, see the **Deductions and Adjustments Worksheet** on page 2.	
	If you have **more than one job** or are **married and you and your spouse both work** and the combined earnings from all jobs exceed $35,000, see the **Two-Earner/Two-Job Worksheet** on page 2 to avoid having too little tax withheld.	
	If **neither** of the above situations applies, **stop here** and enter the number from line H on line 5 of Form W-4 below.	

- **Cut here and give Form W-4 to your employer. Keep the top part for your records.** - - - - - - - - - - - - - - - - -

Form **W-4**	**Employee's Withholding Allowance Certificate**	OMB No. 1545-0010
Department of the Treasury Internal Revenue Service	**For Privacy Act and Paperwork Reduction Act Notice, see page 2.**	**2003**

1 Type or print your first name and middle initial	Last name		2 Your social security number

Home address (number and street or rural route)	3 ☐ Single ☐ Married ☐ Married, but withhold at higher Single rate.
City or town, state, and ZIP code	**Note:** *If married, but legally separated, or spouse is a nonresident alien, check the "Single" box.*
	4 If your last name differs from that shown on your social security card, check here. You must call 1-800-772-1213 for a new card. ☐

5	Total number of allowances you are claiming (from line **H** above **or** from the applicable worksheet on page 2)	**5**
6	Additional amount, if any, you want withheld from each paycheck	**6** $
7	I claim exemption from withholding for 2003, and I certify that I meet **both** of the following conditions for exemption:	
	Last year I had a right to a refund of **all** Federal income tax withheld because I had **no** tax liability **and**	
	This year I expect a refund of **all** Federal income tax withheld because I expect to have **no** tax liability.	
	If you meet both conditions, write "Exempt" here	**7**

Under penalties of perjury, I certify that I am entitled to the number of withholding allowances claimed on this certificate, or I am entitled to claim exempt status.

Employee's signature
(Form is not valid unless you sign it.) ► _____ **Date** ►

8 Employer's name and address (Employer: Complete lines 8 and 10 only if sending to the IRS.)	9 Office code (optional)	10 Employer identification number

Cat. No. 10220Q

Figure 22.13

W-4 Form.

Figure 22.14

Example time card. A time card has 31 days.

			Verified by	
# _____ Loc_____	Dept_____	Super_____		

Name _____

Period Ending _____

Scheduled Hours _____ 4–10's _____ Night Shift _____

DO NOT WRITE IN THIS SPACE

Reg Hours _____	Vac Hours _____
OT Hours _____	Sick Hours _____
Dbit Hours _____	SDiff Hours _____
Hol Hours _____	Other Hours _____
Persl _____	Acctg _____

	Morning In	Noon Out	Noon In	Night Out	Extra In	Extra Out
8						
1						
9						
2						
10						
3						
11						
4						
12						
5						
13						
6						
14						
7						
15						

The balance shown above is correct, and receipt is acknowledged.

Signature _____

calculated

Figured out.

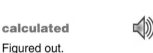

4. Employee earnings record. This record contains the following information (see Figure 22.16):

a. Employee's name and address b. Social Security number c. Number of exemptions claimed d. Date of birth and marital status e. Rate of pay and hours worked f. Earnings, deductions, and net pay g. Check numbers h. Year-to-date earnings

The amount of employee tax withheld is decided by federal and state regulations. A certain amount of money is withheld from the employee's paycheck to pay federal and state taxes on each paycheck. The following are the taxes withheld (see Figure 22.17):

1. Federal income tax. See Table 22.1.

2. Federal Insurance Contribution Act (FICA). This is commonly known as the Social Security tax. The amount of the deduction is **calculated** from the FICA tax tables. The employer must match (also pay) the same amount that is deducted from the employee's gross income.

3. State income tax. Like the federal tax, the state tax is withheld from the employee's paycheck for deposit toward the employee's annual taxes. Employers have tax tables to help them determine the amount to withhold.

4. State disability insurance (SDI). States establish this fund for persons who are temporarily unable to work. Contributions to this fund are made by the employee.

				EARNINGS			TAXABLE EARNINGS		DEDUCTIONS				
NAME	No. Exemp.	Hrly. Rate	Hours Wkd.	Reg.	Over-time	Total	FICA	Unemp. Ins.	FICA	FWT	Total	Net Pay	Chk. No.
Bart, Gwen	2	5.60	40	224.00	—	224.00	224.00	224.00	15.01	40.00	55.01	168.99	65
Evans, Sid	1	7.40	42	296.00	22.20	318.20	318.20	318.20	21.32	80.00	101.32	216.88	66
Murray, June	3	10.00	44	400.00	60.00	460.00	460.00	460.00	30.82	69.00	99.82	360.18	67
Sokol, Larry	2	8.00	36	288.00	—	288.00	288.00	288.00	19.16	24.00	43.16	244.84	68
				1208.00	82.20	1290.20	1290.20	1290.20	86.31	213.00	299.31	990.89	

PAYROLL PERIOD January 8–14,20--

Figure 22.15

Payroll register.

NAME	_Bart, Gwen_		SOCIAL SECURITY NO. _046 12 1930_
ADDRESS	_14 Pawling Avenue_		DATE OF BIRTH _June 5, 19--_
	Troy, New York 12180		MARITAL STATUS _Married_
NO. OF EXEMPTIONS _2_			HOURLY RATE _$5.60_

Line No.	Week Ended	Hours Wkd.	EARNINGS Reg.	Over-time	Total	DEDUCTIONS FICA	FWT	Total	Net Pay	Check No.	Year-to-Date
1	1/7	41	229.60	2.80	232.40	13.60	41.00	54.60	177.80	22	232.40
2	1/14	40	224.00	—	224.00	13.10	40.00	53.10	170.90	65	456.40

Figure 22.16

Employee earnings record.

BRISTOL PARK MEDICAL GROUP, INC.
3160 REDHILL AVE
COSTA MESA CA   92626   1 - 55

PAYROLL PERIOD FROM	TO	DATE
10-01-03	10-14-03	10-18-03

CONTROL NO.	EMPLOYEE NO.	DEPT.	EMPLOYEE NAME	SOCIAL SECURITY NUMBER	EXEMPTIONS FED.	STATE	OTHER	MAR. STA.

EARNINGS					TAXES		
TYPE	DESCRIPTION	RATE	UNITS	AMOUNT	TYPE	WITHHELD	YEAR-TO-DATE
12	REGULAR		40.00	520.00	FIT	71.81	71.81
21	OVERTIME		.25	4.88	FICA	40.15	40.15
					SIT	8.94	8.94
					DI	4.72	4.72

DEDUCTIONS NO.	DESCRIPTION	AMOUNT	PERIOD-TO-DATE	DEDUCTIONS NO.	DESCRIPTION	AMOUNT	PERIOD-TO-DATE

TOTALS						CHECK NUMBER
Y-T-D GROSS	Y-T-D TAXES	CURRENT GROSS	CURRENT TAXES	DEDUCTIONS	NET CHECK	
524.88	125.62	524.88	125.62		399.26	8018735

Figure 22.17

Employee pay stub.

5. **Unemployment insurance.** The amounts paid and who pays into such funds vary from state to state. This fund is for workers who have lost their jobs.

6. **Other deductions.** Employees can request that other deductions be withheld from their paychecks, such as

   a. Health insurance b. Loan repayments c. Credit union payments or deposits d. Christmas club e. Pension funds f. Charitable contributions

The employer must keep an individual record for each employee. The Federal Wages and Hour Law requires the employer to send a wage and tax statement (W-2 form; see Figure 22.18) to the employee no later than January 31 of each year. It contains some of the following information:

■ Preceding year's gross earnings

■ Federal income tax withholdings

Table 22.1 ■ Example of a Wage Withholding Table

Biweekly Payroll Period—Single Person for Wages Paid After December 2003												
And the wages are—		And the number of withholding allowances claimed is—										
At least	But less than	0	1	2	3	4	5	6	7	8	9	10
		The amount of income tax to be withheld shall be—										
$ 580	$ 600	$ 81	$ 68	$ 54	$ 41	$ 28	$15	$ 1	$ 0	$ 0	$ 0	$ 0
600	620	84	71	57	44	31	18	4	0	0	0	0
620	640	87	74	60	47	34	21	7	0	0	0	0
640	660	90	77	63	50	37	24	10	0	0	0	0
660	680	93	80	66	53	40	27	13	0	0	0	0
680	700	96	83	69	56	43	30	16	3	0	0	0
700	720	99	86	72	59	46	33	19	6	0	0	0
720	740	102	89	75	62	49	36	22	9	0	0	0
740	760	105	92	78	65	52	39	25	12	0	0	0
760	780	108	95	81	68	55	42	28	15	2	0	0
780	800	111	98	84	71	58	45	31	18	5	0	0
800	820	114	101	87	74	61	48	34	21	8	0	0
820	840	117	104	90	77	64	51	37	24	11	0	0
840	860	120	107	93	80	67	54	40	27	14	1	0
860	880	123	110	96	83	70	57	43	30	17	4	0
880	900	128	113	99	86	73	60	46	33	20	7	0
900	920	134	116	102	89	76	63	49	36	23	10	0
920	940	139	119	105	92	79	66	52	39	26	13	0
940	960	145	122	108	95	82	69	55	42	29	16	2
960	980	150	126	111	98	85	72	58	45	32	19	5
980	1,000	156	131	114	101	88	75	61	48	35	22	8
1,000	1,020	162	137	117	104	91	78	64	51	38	25	11
1,020	1,040	167	142	120	107	94	81	67	54	41	28	14
1,040	1,060	173	148	123	110	97	84	70	57	44	31	17
1,060	1,080	178	154	129	113	100	87	73	60	47	34	20

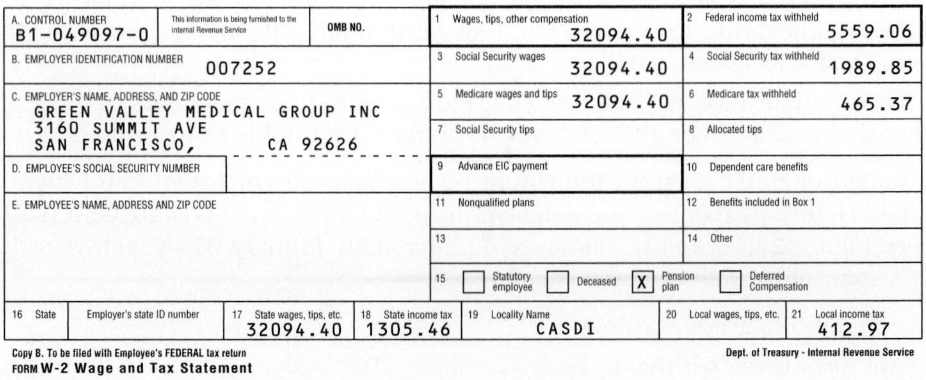
A. CONTROL NUMBER B1-049097-0
This information is being furnished to the Internal Revenue Service
OMB NO.
1 Wages, tips, other compensation 32094.40
2 Federal income tax withheld 5559.06
B. EMPLOYER IDENTIFICATION NUMBER 007252
3 Social Security wages 32094.40
4 Social Security tax withheld 1989.85
C. EMPLOYER'S NAME, ADDRESS, AND ZIP CODE
GREEN VALLEY MEDICAL GROUP INC
3160 SUMMIT AVE
SAN FRANCISCO, CA 92626
5 Medicare wages and tips 32094.40
6 Medicare tax withheld 465.37
7 Social Security tips
8 Allocated tips
D. EMPLOYEE'S SOCIAL SECURITY NUMBER
9 Advance EIC payment
10 Dependent care benefits
E. EMPLOYEE'S NAME, ADDRESS AND ZIP CODE
11 Nonqualified plans
12 Benefits included in Box 1
13
14 Other
15 Statutory employee | Deceased | X Pension plan | Deferred Compensation
16 State | Employer's state ID number | 17 State wages, tips, etc. 32094.40 | 18 State income tax 1305.46 | 19 Locality Name CASDI | 20 Local wages, tips, etc. | 21 Local income tax 412.97
Copy B. To be filed with Employee's FEDERAL tax return
FORM W-2 Wage and Tax Statement
Dept. of Treasury - Internal Revenue Service

Figure 22.18

Example of one type of W-2 form.

- FICA taxes withheld
- Total FICA wages paid
- Contributions to a retirement plan

If employees terminate employment during the year, a W-2 must be sent to them within 30 days of the last payment of wages.

⦿ PETTY CASH FUND

Petty cash is an amount of money set aside for the purchase of small items for the office (for example, postage stamps, office supplies). It is important to keep an accurate record of this account. Use the following guidelines for maintaining a petty cash account.

1. **Designate** an amount to keep in petty cash (for example, $75).

2. Only one person in the office is responsible for handling the petty cash.

3. Design a **disbursement** form (see Figure 22.19) with the following information:

   a. Today's date b. Amount given c. Paid to d. Signature of person receiving the cash e. Signature of the person who authorized the expense f. Expense (for example, stamps, copy paper)

designate

To appoint or determine.

disbursement

Payment.

Figure 22.19

Example of one type of disbursement form.

PETTY CASH DISBURSEMENT	No. _22_
Date _1-8-03_	_$24.20_
	Amount
Paid To _Tom Gates_	
Expense _Car Fare_	
Authorized by _Petty Cash_	
	Signature
Cash received by _____	
	Signature

PROCEDURE 22.8 — KEEPING TRACK OF PETTY CASH

RATIONALE

Petty cash provides money that is needed for daily expenses. Careful record keeping ensures that petty cash will balance and provide necessary cash as needed.

1. Assemble materials.
   a. Petty cash record form
   b. Disbursement forms
   c. Disbursement journal
   d. Checks as needed
   e. List of petty cash expenditures
2. Decide amount of money to keep for petty cash.
3. Write check to set up fund.
4. Cash check.
5. Write amount of cash in balance column in journal.
6. Write amount to Miscellaneous in disbursement.
7. Use petty cash disbursement form each time a withdrawal is made.

8. Record amount in disbursement journal.
9. Enter new balance.

To replenish petty cash:

10. Write check. (Amount spent plus balance must equal beginning balance.)
11. Total the expense column and put charges in correct disbursement column.
12. Record amount added to fund.
13. Record new balance in petty cash fund.

auditing

Formal checking for correctness.

replenish

Refill or build up again.

4. Attach a receipt to the disbursement form for **auditing** purposes.

5. Replenish the fund when necessary by writing a check for the total amount of receipts/disbursement slips. This restores the petty cash account to the starting amount (for example, receipts total $73.25, check written for $73.25 for reimbursement to petty cash fund).

SUPPLIES

It is impossible to operate a medical practice without the proper supplies. Keeping supplies stocked is an important responsibility. Following are the two types of supplies and some examples of each type:

- Medical supplies
  - Disposable products (for example, gowns, specimen containers, needles, gloves) • Medications • Cleaning and disinfectant solutions
- Administrative supplies
  - Expendable items (for example, stationery, pens, registration forms) • Facial tissue, toilet tissue • Paper drinking cups

Your office policy for ordering supplies indicates the following:

- When to order supplies
- Names of companies that supplies are purchased from (when placing order, keep in mind the delivery time)
- What record keeping is done for ordering supplies

BUSINESS EQUIPMENT

Your office will have office equipment to help run the medical practice smoothly. Always follow manufacturers' directions when using equipment.

Copier

Identify the following:

- Where the on/off button is
- Whether you need to turn off the copier daily or at the end of the week
- What features the copier has:
  - To enlarge and reduce copies • To sort/group copies • To do back-to-back copying • To staple copies • To produce copies in different colors
- The maximum number of copies that can be made at one time
- Where the paper tray is
- How you put the paper in the copier
- Where the copying paper is kept
- How a paper jam is cleared
- Where and how you change ink cartridges
- The name and phone number of the maintenance/repair company

Facsimile (Fax)

Identify the following:

- Where the on/off button is
- All the functions, such as automatic dial, and redial

- Whether you place the pages to be faxed facing up or down
- How you dial:
  - Whether you need to request an outside line • Listening for a tone before dialing the fax number • Which key is pressed to start the fax operation
- Where a list of the most frequent numbers faxed is
- How you put paper in the fax
- Where the fax paper is kept
- How you clear a paper jam
- The name and phone number of the maintenance/repair company

Telephone

Identify the following:

- How many incoming lines there are
- What all the features are:
  - Transfer • Hold • Speaker • Redial • Phone number memory • Conference calls
- Whether there are public lines and private lines

Your learning and practicing all the operational guidelines of your office assists in providing good-quality service for your clients/patients. Doing so also makes you an important and valuable part of your office.

1. Complete Worksheets 2 through 4 as directed by your instructor.

2. Ask your instructor for directions to complete Worksheet 5.

3. Complete Worksheets 6 through 8 and Worksheet/Activity 9 as directed by your instructor.

4. Practice all procedures.

5. Prepare responses to each item listed in Chapter Review—Your Link to Success at the end of this chapter.

6. When you are confident that you can meet each objective ask your instructor for the unit evaluation.

Thinking Critically

1. Communication Describe how you would explain office policy on professional courtesy discounts to a patient who is insistent on getting a reduced rate.

2. Legal and Ethical Mrs. Smith's husband calls and asks you why his wife has an appointment with the doctor. Write an example of how you would respond to him.

3. Patient Education Mr. Morgan is calling to make an appointment with a physician. When you ask what the appointment is for, he does not want to tell you. Write a paper about how you would explain to Mr. Morgan why you must know the reason for the appointment. Write the explanation just as you would say it to the patient.

4. Computers List the ways computers are used in the health care information department.

5. Medical Math Create a spreadsheet to show charges, receipts, and balance due.

6. Case Study A patient is upset because he doesn't understand what kind of insurance he has. Write an explanation of the benefit coverage of HMOs and PPOs to help the patient determine what kind of insurance he has. Write the explanation just as you would say it to the patient.

7. Time Management The office manager has established strict rules for the amount of time to be spent on each office task such as billing, correspondence, and so on. However, time needs are changing. Describe the kind of documentation you would collect to show her that you need to change the time allocations to handle the workflow efficiently.

Portfolio Connection

Once you attain competence as a health information technician, ask for permission to copy a letter, a spreadsheet, and other forms and documents that you have completed. (Remove all patient identifiers.) Place these copies in your portfolio as evidence of your skills. Place a copy of your on-site trainer's evaluation in your portfolio.

Write a paper describing your doubts and realizations and the barriers that you were able to overcome during your health information technician experience. For example, were you afraid that you couldn't learn to use the equipment? Describe the ways you plan to use the skills, information, and insights that you gained about the people you worked with and about this job. This assignment must be in standard report format.

Portfolio Tip

Always keep patient confidentiality in mind, particularly when working in areas to which clients have access. We are all trained to keep sensitive documents confidential. Remember that this applies to computer screens also. If you have to leave your computer, exit or reduce any screen that might be displaying confidential computer records.

Remember! 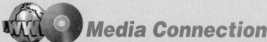 **Media Connection**

Use the Companion Website **www.prenhall.com/badasch** and the CD-ROM for additional interactive learning activities.

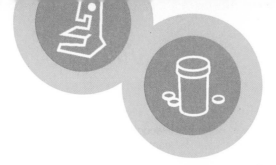

Chapter **23**

Clinical Medical Assistant

MEDIA CONNECTION
Use the Companion Website
www.prenhall.com/badasch and the CD-ROM
for additional interactive learning activities.

STEPS TO SUCCESS

1. Complete Vocabulary Worksheet 1 in the Student Workbook.

2. Read this chapter.

3. Complete the Learn by Doing assignment at the end of this unit.

OBJECTIVES

When you have completed this chapter, you will be able to do the following:

✔ Complete all objectives from Part One of this book.

✔ Match vocabulary words with their correct meanings.

✔ Measure and record height and weight of an adult, child, and infant.

✔ Summarize the importance of measuring the circumference of an infant's head.

✔ Explain what a drastic change in growth patterns may indicate.

✔ Explain how to read a visual acuity test and the importance of the results.

✔ Compare and identify examination positions by name.

✔ List four basic examination techniques and explain their purposes.

✔ Compare similarities and differences between a general physical examination and a limited examination to rule out a condition.

✔ Identify symptoms of 12 physical conditions and state the appropriate patient education for each.

✔ Explain two types of pediatric appointments.

✔ List 13 guidelines to follow when preparing for a surgical procedure.

✔ Reread Chapter 20, "Central Supply/Central Processing Worker":
  • Decontamination
  • Preparation area
  • Sterile wraps
  • Sterilization
  • Monitoring effectiveness of sterilization

✔ Name five public health issues that require an official report with a public agency.

✔ Match common prescription abbreviations with their meanings.

✔ Match controlled substances with their assigned schedule level.

✔ Name four drug reference books.

✔ Describe methods to ensure safekeeping of medication.

✔ Write a formula for calculating medication dosage.

✔ Match metric measures with their equivalent standard measure.

✔ Name the six "rights" of medication administration.

- ✔ Recognize the guidelines for preparing and administering medications.
- ✔ Explain why it is important to observe liquid medication, and describe what to observe.
- ✔ Match the route of administration with its description.
- ✔ Explain why injections are given instead of other methods of medication administration.
- ✔ Describe areas where it is not appropriate to give an injection.
- ✔ Describe syringe- and needle-handling techniques that prevent accidental needle sticks.

- ✔ Recognize different types of parenteral medication containers.
- ✔ Name medications commonly administered by the Z-track method.
- ✔ Differentiate between intradermal, subcutaneous, intramuscular, and Z-track injections.
- ✔ Name and explain the purpose of common immunizations.
- ✔ Demonstrate all procedures in this chapter.
- ✔ Apply all procedural techniques with confidence.

● RESPONSIBILITIES OF A MEDICAL ASSISTANT

Medical assistants (MAs) help health care providers examine and treat patients. They perform the tasks that keep a medical office or clinic running smoothly. Some MAs perform both *clinical* and **administrative** tasks. Other MAs are trained in only one of these areas. Some offices require a clinical medical assistant and an administrative medical assistant and do not expect one person to do tasks in both areas.

administrative

Pertaining to processing, such as handling of paperwork, that assists in patient care and supports the physician.

Clinical duties most commonly include the following:

- ■ Measuring and recording vital signs
- ■ Interviewing patients to obtain medical history
- ■ Explaining medical treatment to patients
- ■ Preparing patients for examinations
- ■ Assisting the doctor
- ■ Disposing of contaminated supplies
- ■ Collecting and preparing specimens for shipment to medical laboratories
- ■ Practicing aseptic techniques
- ■ Disinfecting medical instruments
- ■ Instructing patients in self-care and child care, including medication, diet, and treatments
- ■ Drawing blood
- ■ Calling patients and pharmacies as directed by the health care provider
- ■ Preparing patients for x-ray
- ■ Performing electrocardiograms (EKGs)
- ■ Applying dressings and assisting with treatments
- ■ Cleaning consulting and examination rooms and work areas
- ■ Performing simple laboratory tests

MAs are an important part of a medical practice. They work in ambulatory care offices as well as those of physicians, chiropractors, optometrists, and podiatrists. The MA position was first recognized in the 1930s, and the position continues to change with advances in medicine. There is a national association that certifies MAs when they meet specific criteria (see Chapter 2).

TAKING MEASUREMENTS

To determine a healthy body weight, compare the client's bone size and height. Bone size is identified as small, medium, or large.

Weighing the Patient: Adult and Child Over 3 Years of Age

Height and weight are recorded during the patient's/client's first visit. Weight is measured in pounds and ounces or in kilograms. The **initial** measurements are a baseline for future visits. Body weight indicates a person's nutritional status. A drastic weight loss or gain can indicate an illness. Patients with edema may need to be weighed daily to help the provider determine the amount of fluid the patient is retaining. Height and weight are also used to determine medication dosage. When weights are closely monitored, always do the following:

initial
First.

- Use the same scale.
- Weigh the patient at the same time of day.
- Determine changes in clothing weight.

Use a scale to measure weight. Measuring accurately is important; always balance the scale at zero before weighing. Two common types of scales are the digital scale, which displays the weight in numbers, and the balance scale.

When weighing a patient/client, guard the person as he or she steps on and off the scale to prevent tripping and falling. Do not allow patients/clients to lean on or hold onto anything while you weigh them, because you cannot get an accurate weight if they do.

PROCEDURE 23.1 | MEASURING WEIGHT ON A STANDING BALANCE SCALE

RATIONALE

Accurate measuring of weight requires an understanding of exactly how to use the balance scale. Correct weight is an important indicator of patient health.

1. Wash hands.
2. Assemble materials.
   a. Paper/medical record
   b. Pen
3. Balance scale at zero. (Balance-bar pointer must stay steady in center of balance area. If pointer does not center, scale will read weight incorrectly. With the weights on zero, turn balance screw until pointer remains centered.)
4. Ask patient/client to step onto scale.
5. Pointer should rise to top of balance bar.
6. Move large weight on balance bar to estimated patient/client weight. Pointer must continue to rest against top of balance bar.

7. Move small weight to right until pointer hangs free at center of balance bar.
8. Read patient/client weight by:
   a. Reading number next to notch on which biggest weight is resting (e.g., 150).
   b. Add number on upper bar to which smallest weight is pointing (e.g., 21).
   c. Sum of these two numbers is patient's/client's weight (171).
9. Write weight in patient's/client's medical record.

10/01/03   1000
Weighed 124 lb. on balance scale
_____ M. Gonzales CMA

NOTE Always remember to record date, time, personal care or treatment given, any complaints, problems reported to the team leader/head nurse, and any other required information. Always sign with your name and certification.

Measuring Height: Adult and Child Over 3 years

Height is measured in feet and inches or in centimeters. Most balance scales have a measuring bar to determine height. Compare the size of the bone structure and the height in Table 23.1 to determine a healthy weight range.

Measuring Height, Weight, and Head Circumference: Infants and Toddlers (Under 3 Years of Age)

Infant and toddler growth is rapid and requires frequent monitoring. Infants are usually seen every 2 months to monitor growth and development patterns. Careful measuring and graphing of these patterns can help detect early changes that are important.

Measuring Head Circumference

Measuring head circumference screens infants and toddlers for abnormal head size. Watching head size can alert the provider if a problem such as hydroencephaly is present. Always place the measuring tape over the occipital bone on the back of the head and wrap forward just above the ears to center of forehead.

Table 23.1 ▪ Height and Weight Table for Adults

Men						Women			
	Bone Structure						**Bone Structure**		
Height		**Small**	**Medium**	**Large**	**Height**		**Small**	**Medium**	**Large**
feet & inches	**in.**				**feet & inches**	**in.**			
5' 2"	62	128–134	131–141	138–150	4' 10"	58	102–111	109–121	118–131
5' 3"	63	130–136	133–143	140–153	4' 11"	59	103–113	111–123	120–134
5' 4"	64	132–138	135–145	142–156	5' 0"	60	104–115	113–126	122–137
5' 5"	65	134–140	137–148	144–160	5' 1"	61	106–118	115–129	125–140
5' 6"	66	136–142	139–151	146–164	5' 2"	62	108–121	118–132	128–143
5' 7"	67	138–146	142–154	149–168	5' 3"	63	111–124	121–135	131–147
5' 8"	68	140–148	145–157	152–172	5' 4"	64	114–127	124–138	134–151
5' 9"	69	142–151	148–160	155–176	5' 5"	65	117–130	127–141	137–155
5' 10"	70	144–154	151–163	158–180	5' 6"	66	120–133	130–144	140–159
5' 11"	71	146–157	154–166	161–184	5' 7"	67	123–136	133–147	143–163
6' 0"	72	149–160	157–170	164–188	5' 8"	68	126–139	136–150	146–167
6' 1"	73	152–164	160–174	168–192	5' 9"	69	129–142	139–153	149–170
6' 2"	74	155–168	164–178	172–197	5' 10"	70	132–146	142–156	152–173
6' 3"	75	158–172	167–182	176–202	5' 11"	71	135–148	145–159	155–176
6' 4"	76	162–176	171–187	181–207	6' 0"	72	138–151	148–162	158–179

PROCEDURE 23.2 | MEASURING HEIGHT OF ADULT/CHILD (OVER 3 YEARS OF AGE)

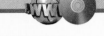

RATIONALE

Height measurement is an indicator of normal or abnormal growth and development. Accurate measurement helps determine whether the child is developing normally.

1. Wash hands.
2. Raise height-measuring rod on back of scale so that tip of height-measuring rod is above patient's/client's head.
3. Instruct patient/client to remove shoes.
4. Ask patient/client to step onto scale and turn around to face away from balance bar.
5. Instruct patient/client to place heels against back of scale and stand straight.
6. Lift up measuring rod so that it points out above patient's/client's head.
7. Lower rod gently until it rests on patient's/ client's head.
8. Instruct patient/client to step off scale.
9. Read numbers just above edge of hollow bar of rod at back of scale.
10. Record height on medical record in feet and inches, centimeters, or inches only, according to your provider's policy.

10/02/03	1500
	Height 33 in.
	____ M. Gonzales CMA
	or
10/02/03	1500
	Height 82.5 cm.
	____ M. Gonzales CMA

PROCEDURE 23.3 | MEASURING THE HEAD CIRCUMFERENCE OF AN INFANT/TODDLER (UNDER 3 YEARS OF AGE)

RATIONALE

Head circumference is an indicator of normal or abnormal growth development. Accurate measurement helps determine whether the infant/toddler is developing normally.

1. Wash hands.
2. Obtain measuring tape.
3. Identify the patient.
4. Explain procedure to parent.
5. Place infant in supine position.
6. Position measuring tape over occipital bone and wrap toward forehead. Bring tape just above ears to the center of the forehead.

10/04/03	1000
	Head circumference measures 15 in.
	____ M. Gonzales CMA
	or
10/04/03	1000
	Head circumference measures 37.5 cm
	____ M. Gonzales CMA

PROCEDURE 23.4

MEASURING THE HEIGHT OF AN INFANT/TODDLER

RATIONALE

Height is an indicator of normal or abnormal growth development. Accurate measurement helps determine whether the infant/toddler is developing normally.

1. Wash hands.
2. Obtain tape measure or measuring bar.
3. Place infant on flat surface.
4. Place zero mark of tape or measuring bar level with top of infant's head.
5. Ask parent or co-worker to hold top of head gently at zero mark.
6. Gently straighten legs.
7. Read measurement that is level with infant's heel.
8. Wash hands.

10/04/03	1000
	Height 21 in.
	_____ M. Gonzales CMA
	or
10/04/03	1000
	Height 52.5 cm
	_____ M. Gonzales CMA

Measuring Infant and Toddler Height

Infant and toddler heights indicate normal or abnormal growth patterns. Always use the same technique to measure their height and weight. Never estimate height. Use a tape measure or the ruler on the scale or tabletop.

Measuring Weight: Infant/Toddler

Infant and toddler weights are an important measure of growth patterns. Weight in an infant can change very quickly during an illness. Weight loss is an important indicator of dehydration. *Do not* change from weighing with clothes during one visit to weighing without clothes the next visit. Be consistent.

The growth chart in Figure 23.1 is a method of graphing growth patterns. The curved lines flowing across the chart indicate normal growth. Slightly differing levels of growth are normal. A large difference in the expected growth pattern may indicate a problem (for example, glandular imbalance or nutritional deficiency).

PROCEDURE 23.5

MEASURING THE WEIGHT OF AN INFANT/TODDLER

RATIONALE

Infant weight is an indicator of normal or abnormal growth development. Accurate measurement helps determine whether the infant/toddler is developing normally.

PROCEDURE 23.5 MEASURING THE WEIGHT OF AN INFANT/TODDLER *(Continued)*

1. Wash hands.
2. Assemble equipment.
    a. Infant balance scale
    b. Towel
    c. Growth chart
3. Ask parent to remove infant's clothing.
4. Place clean towel on scale cradle to decrease shock of cold metal against infant.
5. Balance the scale at zero with towel in place.
6. Place infant face up on scale. Keep diaper or towel over infant's genital area in case of elimination.

7. Place one hand over infant (almost touching) to give a sense of security.
8. Slide weight easily until scale balances.
9. Read scale in pounds and ounces or in kilograms.
10. Return infant to parent.
11. Balance the scale at zero mark.
12. Record weight on growth chart and in patient's chart.

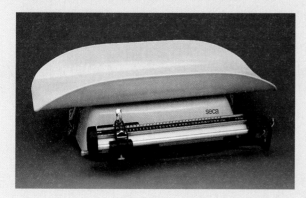

```
10/05/03   0800
                Measured on balance scale, wt. 25 lb.
                _____ M. Gonzales CMA
          or
10/05/03   0800
                Weighed mother and then mother
                and child to determine weight
                Infant too distressed to weigh
                on infant balance scale
                Wt. 25 lb.
                _____ M. Gonzales CMA
```

Testing Visual Acuity

Vision acuity (clearness) testing helps the provider detect eye disease or injury. Vision acuity tests are usually part of a physical examination. A provider always does a vision acuity test when the patient complains of eye pain, itching, tenderness, or injury. The provider can identify changes and evaluate the treatment more effectively when there is a **baseline** acuity test.

To read the result of the visual acuity test on a Snellen chart (Figure 23.2), find the fraction to the left of the line the patient is able to read. For example, if the patient reads all the letters in the line marked 20/20 and is unable to read line 20/15, the patient's vision is 20/20. The top number means that the patient is 20 feet from the chart. The bottom number is the distance at which a patient with normal vision can read that row of letters. If line 20/50 is the last line read, the patient's vision is 20/50. This means that the patient is able to read at 20 feet what a person with normal vision sees at 50 feet. The chart in Figure 23.3 is read the same way.

baseline

A number, graph, or indication to use as a guideline. A measurement taken at a later time may differ from the baseline, indicating a possible cause for concern.

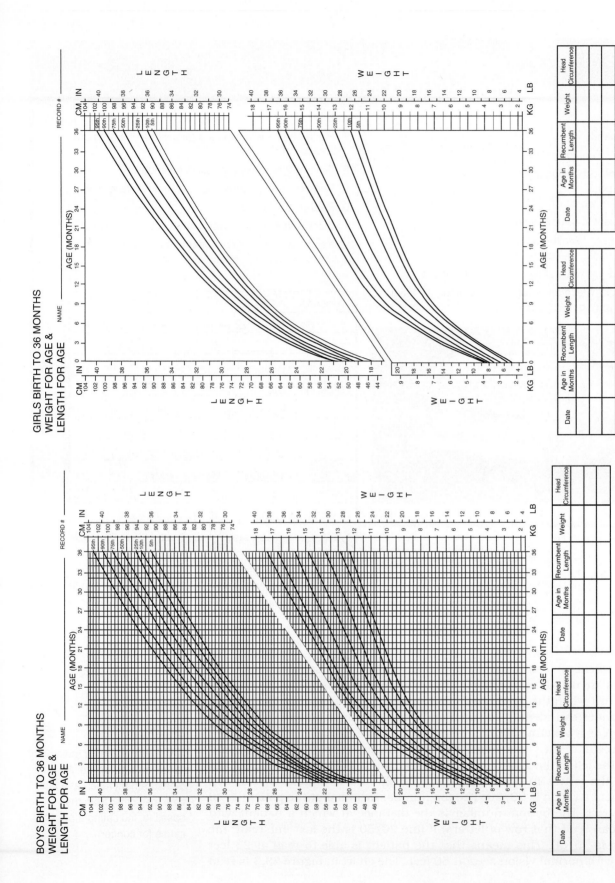

Figure 23.1

Growth charts for girls and boys from birth to 36 months.

PROCEDURE 23.6

TESTING VISUAL ACUITY: SNELLEN CHART

RATIONALE

Vision affects all activities of daily living. Correct measurement of visual acuity is essential to determine whether patient has normal or abnormal eyesight.

1. Explain procedure to patient.
2. Position patient 20 feet (6 meters) from Snellen chart.
3. Ask patient to cover left eye and read smallest line of letters that he or she can see.
4. Record the distance patient is from the chart compared to the size of letters patient can see clearly (e.g., 20/20, 20/30, 20/40).
5. Record results with minus number if patient makes an error on a line:
   a. 20/40: with one error = 20/40 − 1
   b. 20/40: with two errors = 20/40 − 2

6. Record results with plus number if patient reads 20/40 line and two symbols in the 20/30 line = 20/40 + 2.
7. Repeat test with right eye covered.
8. Repeat test, allowing patient to use both eyes.
9. Repeat each test with patient wearing glasses (if he or she has prescription lenses).

> 12/18/03 1400
>
> Snellen chart, 20/40 both eyes
>
> M. Gonzales CMA

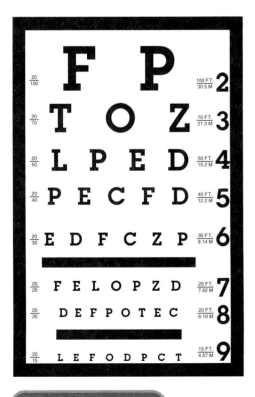

Figure 23.2

Snellen eye chart for English readers.

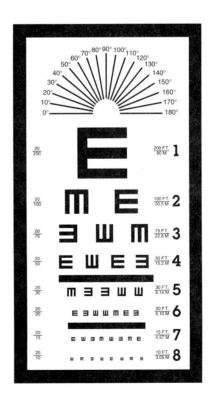

Figure 23.3

Snellen eye chart for non-English readers and children. Have young children and non-English-speaking clients use their fingers to indicate directions of the *E*.

● STANDARD PRECAUTIONS

When working with patients it is important *always* to follow Standard Precautions to protect yourself when contact with blood or body fluids is possible. Review Chapter 12 and read Tables 23.2 and 23.3.

Table 23.2 ▪ Standard Precautions With Risk Categorization

Infection-control guidelines exist to protect employees and patients against infectious viruses and bacteria. The Standard Precautions you take depend on the (1) potential for contact with blood, (2) potential for contact with any body fluids, and (3) tasks (procedures) that you perform. This table tells you what to wear when you are doing various tasks. Follow these guidelines to protect yourself and others from infection.

Category	Task Requires:	Protect Yourself By:	Have Available:

I: High risk	Direct contact with blood or other body fluids	Washing hands:
		  If you touch blood/body fluids
		  After removing gloves
		Wearing:
		  Gloves
		  Apron or gown
		  Eye protection
		  Face mask
		Never recapping needles or bending/breaking them
		Placing used needles in a sharps container
		Cleaning off blood/body fluids immediately
		Disposing of waste materials
		Being vaccinated for hepatitis B	

II: Low risk	When you have close contact with patients but are not likely to come in contact with blood/body fluids	Washing hands	Mask Eye protection Gloves
III: No risk	Your routine work requires no contact with blood/body fluid	Washing hands, as a general rule	

Table 23.3 ▪ Standard Precautions: Examples of Tasks and Use of Protective Equipment

Task	Gloves	Gown	Mask	Protective Eyewear
Controlling spurting blood	Yes	Yes	Yes	Yes
Controlling minimal bleeding	Yes	No	No	No
Blood drawing	Yes	Yes	Yes	Yes
Oral or nasal suction	Yes	No	Yes	Yes
Handling/cleaning contaminated instruments	Yes	Yes	Yes	Yes
Measuring blood pressure	No	No	No	No

⊙ ASSISTING WITH EXAMINATIONS

Patients/clients need reassurance during a physical examination. The patient/client may not know what to expect and may feel anxious. To help put him or her at ease, be friendly and efficient.

Equipment

Set up equipment according to the provider's request and check all equipment to be sure it works properly. Equipment varies depending on the body areas to be examined. Learn to anticipate each provider's needs and have equipment and supplies ready before he or she asks for them. Basic equipment includes the following:

■ Blood pressure cuff and sphygmomanometer

■ Stethoscope

■ Opthalmoscope (Figure 23.4)

■ Otoscope (Figure 23.5)

■ Percussion hammer (Figure 23.6)

■ Disposable gloves

■ Basin/pan

■ Tape measure (Figure 23.7)

■ Tongue blade (Figure 23.8)

You may need to set up additional equipment. The type of examination determines which equipment the provider will need.

Examination Positions

There are specific positions for each procedure. Putting the patient/client in the correct position makes the examination easier. Always protect the patient's/client's privacy by positioning and draping according to the directions in each procedure.

■ **Horizontal recumbent (supine) position.** Use this position for examination, treatment, and surgical procedures of the ventral (anterior) part of the body (for example, for abdominal pain, removal of stitches in chest).

■ **Fowler's position.** This position relieves patients who are having trouble breathing (for

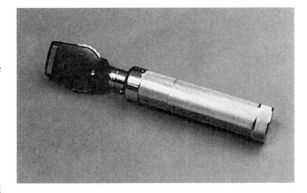

Figure 23.4

Ophthalmoscope.

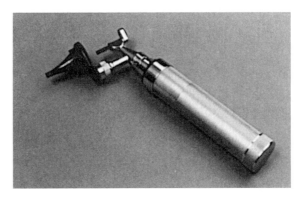
Figure 23.5

Otoscope.

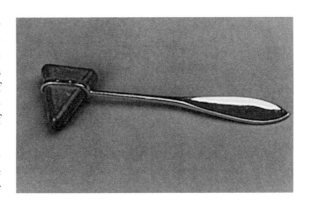
Figure 23.6

Taylor percussion hammer.

Figure 23.7

Tape measure.

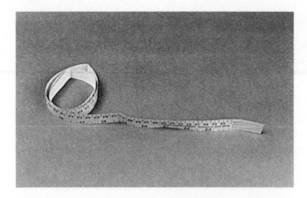

Figure 23.8

Tongue blade.

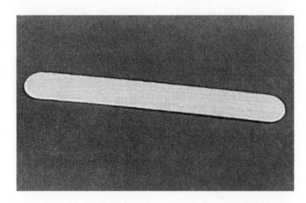

example, asthma, chest pain). This position allows examination of the anterior and posterior chest (for example, listening to heart and lung sounds).

■ **Trendelenburg position.** This position helps restore blood flow to the brain when the body experiences shock. This position also helps promote drainage of congested lungs.

■ **Dorsal lithotomy position.** Use this position to examine or perform surgical procedures on the peritoneal and rectal areas (for example, vaginal exam, cystoscopy).

■ **Prone position.** Use this position for examination, treatment, or surgical procedures of the dorsal (back) part of the body.

■ **Left lateral position and left Sims' position.** Use this position for minor rectal examinations and treatments.

■ **Knee-chest position.** Use this position for rectal examinations and surgical procedures. Some examination tables adjust to support the patient's abdomen and chest.

PROCEDURE 23.7 HORIZONTAL RECUMBENT (SUPINE) POSITION

RATIONALE

Placing the patient in the correct position for treatment, examinations, and for comfort measures is essential for safe and accurate care of the patient.

1. Wash hands.
2. Explain to client what you are going to do.
3. Assist patient to a position lying flat on his or her back in good alignment, with a small pillow under the head.

4. Drape cover so that he or she is not exposed, leaving all edges of drape loose.

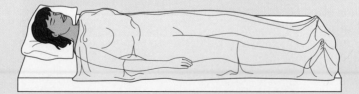

PROCEDURE 23.8

FOWLER'S POSITION

RATIONALE

Placing the patient in the correct position for treatment, examinations, and for comfort measures is essential for safe and accurate care of the patient.

1. Wash hands.
2. Explain to patient what you are going to do.
3. Assist client to a position lying flat on his or her back in good alignment.
4. Keep patient covered so that he or she is not exposed.
5. Knees may bend slightly.
6. Adjust backrest to one of the following positions according to patient's or physician's needs.

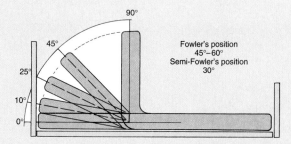

Fowler's position
45°–60°
Semi-Fowler's position
30°

7. Drape cover so that patient is not exposed, leaving all edges of drape free.

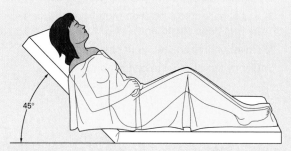

PROCEDURE 23.9

TRENDELENBURG POSITION

RATIONALE

Placing the patient in the correct position for treatment, examinations, and for comfort measures is essential for safe and accurate care of the patient.

1. Wash hands.
2. Explain to patient what you are going to do.
3. Assist client to a position lying flat on his or her back in good alignment.
4. Drape cover so that he or she is not exposed, leaving all edges of drape loose.
5. Lower the head of the table until the body is at a 45° angle. Legs may be bent or extended.
6. Reassure patient that he or she will not slide off table.

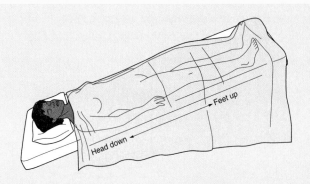

PROCEDURE 23.10 DORSAL LITHOTOMY POSITION

RATIONALE

Placing the patient in the correct position for treatment, examinations, and for comfort measures is essential for safe and accurate care of the patient.

1. Wash hands.
2. Explain to client what you are going to do.
3. Assist patient to a position lying flat on his or her back in good alignment.
4. Cover patient so that he or she is not exposed.
5. Gently assist client to bend knees.

6. Separate legs by placing each foot flat on bed about 2 feet apart or in stirrups attached to examination table.
7. Move patient's hips to edge of end of table when stirrups are available.
8. Drape with half-size sheet positioned with one corner toward head and opposite corners between legs. Secure side corner around legs.

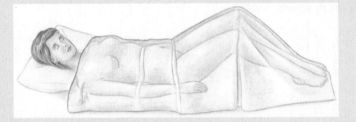

PROCEDURE 23.11 PRONE POSITION

RATIONALE

Placing the patient in the correct position for treatment, examinations, and for comfort measures is essential for safe and accurate care of the patient.

1. Wash hands.
2. Explain to client what you are going to do.
3. Assist patient to a position lying flat on his or her back.

4. Cover client so that he or she is not exposed.
5. Assist patient to turn onto stomach, keeping him or her covered.

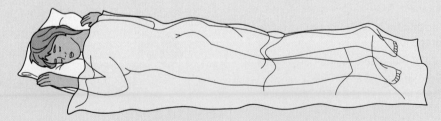

PROCEDURE 23.12

LEFT LATERAL POSITION AND LEFT SIMS' POSITION

RATIONALE

Placing the patient in the correct position for treatment, examinations, and for comfort measures is essential for safe and accurate care of the patient.

1. Wash hands.
2. Explain to client what you are going to do.
3. Assist patient to a position lying flat on his or her back.
4. Cover client so that he or she is not exposed.
5. Assist patient to turn onto left side.

6. Position patient's left arm slightly behind him or her on bed.
7. Gently bend both knees.
8. Place right leg slightly forward of left leg for lateral position.
9. Bend right knee toward chest for Sims' position.

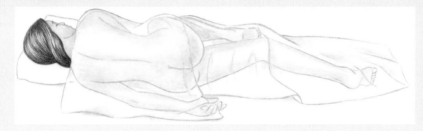

PROCEDURE 23.13

KNEE-CHEST POSITION

RATIONALE

Placing the patient in the correct position for treatment, examinations, and for comfort measures is essential for safe and accurate care of the patient.

1. Wash hands.
2. Explain to client what you are going to do.
3. Assist patient to a position lying flat on his or her back.
4. Cover patient so that he or she is not exposed.
5. Assist patient to turn onto his or her stomach, keeping client covered.
6. Instruct patient to raise hips upward by kneeling on both knees.

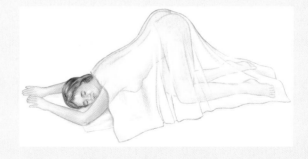

PROCEDURE 23.13 | **KNEE-CHEST POSITION** *(Continued)*

7. Rest patient's head and shoulders on a pillow.

8. Extend arms above head on bed.

9. Drape with a large sheet, allowing edges to hang free.

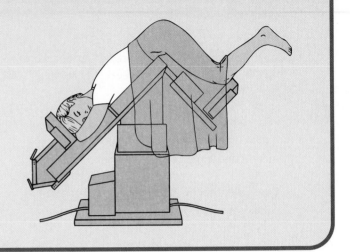

Examination and Diagnostic Techniques

Examinations require four basic techniques.

1. **Observation/Inspection.** Here the provider looks at the patient/client for normal and abnormal appearance. Skin, eyes, hair, nails, movements, or actions that look unusual may be important in determining an illness (see Figure 23.9a).

2. **Palpation.** In this procedure, the provider feels parts of the body for unusual or abnormal conditions. Feeling and applying pressure also allow the provider to locate tender or painful areas (see Figure 23.9b).

3. **Percussion.** Providers use their fingers to tap over areas of the body. The sounds the provider hears during percussion indicate the fullness, emptiness, and size of internal organs (see Figure 23.9c).

4. **Auscultation.** The provider listens to body sounds through a stethoscope. Sounds of the heart and lungs, bowel sounds, and even the flow of blood through arteries can be heard (see Figure 23.9d).

These four techniques give a provider clues about how the body is working. For example, if a patient complains of a chest cold, the provider listens to the chest with a stethoscope. Gurgling sounds or very little airflow in the lungs tell the provider that the lungs are congested with fluid. A chest x-ray confirms what **auscultation** indicated.

When a patient/client complains of pain or other problems, the provider uses the four basic examination techniques. Prepare each patient/client for observation, palpation, percussion, and auscultation. Tell patients/clients what you want them to do. Remember that patients/clients are often nervous. Show patience and understanding.

To determine a final **diagnosis** the physician looks for clues from the following sources:

■ Patient/client history

■ Physical examination findings

■ Vital signs

■ Laboratory results

auscultation

Listening for sounds within the body.

diagnosis

Identification of a disease or condition.

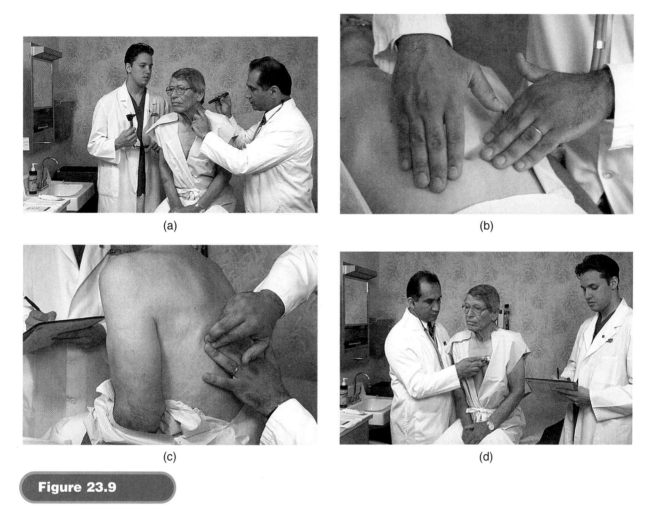

(a) (b)

(c) (d)

Figure 23.9

Methods of physical examinations: (a) inspection; (b) palpation; (c) percussion; (d) auscultation.

- Diagnostic test results
- Symptoms described by the patient

If there is more than one possible diagnosis, the provider needs to rule out each possible condition before determining a final diagnosis. For example, a patient complaining of abdominal pain may need additional tests to

- Rule out (R/O) appendicitis
- Rule out (R/O) gastroenteritis
- Rule out (R/O) pelvic inflammatory disease (PID)

The provider makes a final diagnosis when tests rule out possible conditions and provide evidence of a specific disease.

General Physical Examination

Regular, routine examinations help identify early signs of illness or conditions that can develop into a disease or illness. The health questionnaire (see Figure 23.10) is a very important part of the routine physical. It provides information about the client's lifestyle. It also gives a history to alert the provider of possible problems. To prepare a patient/client and the exam room, follow the steps in the procedure.

Figure 23.10

Patient/client questionnaire.
(Courtesy of Bristol Park
Medical Group, Inc.)

MEDICAL
HEALTH QUESTIONNAIRE

NAME _____ AGE _____ DATE _____

HISTORY OF PAST ILLNESS/INJURIES (HAVE YOU HAD?):   MEDICAL RECORD # _____

	YES	NO	UNSURE
MEASLES	☐	☐	☐
MUMPS	☐	☐	☐
CHICKEN POX	☐	☐	☐
DIABETES	☐	☐	☐
STROKES	☐	☐	☐
CANCER	☐	☐	☐
RHEUMATIC FEVER OR HEART DISEASE	☐	☐	☐
TUBERCULOSIS	☐	☐	☐
SEXUALLY TRANSMITTED DISEASE	☐	☐	☐
CONGENITAL ABNORMALITIES	☐	☐	☐
OTHER SERIOUS DISEASES	☐	☐	☐

LIST _____

	YES	NO
HAVE YOU EVER BEEN HOSPITALIZED OR BEEN UNDER MEDICAL CARE FOR VERY LONG?	☐	☐
IF YES, FOR WHAT REASON? _____		
HAVE YOU HAD ANY HEAD INJURIES?	☐	☐
HAVE YOU EVER BEEN KNOCKED UNCONSCIOUS?	☐	☐
OPERATIONS:		
HAVE YOU HAD ANY SURGERY?	☐	☐
PLEASE DESCRIBE _____		

FAMILY HISTORY	IF LIVING:		IF DECEASED:		HAS ANY BLOOD RELATIVE EVER HAD?	YES	NO
	AGE	HEALTH	AGE	CAUSE			
FATHER					CANCER		
MOTHER					TUBERCULOSIS		
BROTHER / SISTER					DIABETES		
					HEART TROUBLE		
					HIGH BLOOD PRESSURE		
HUSBAND / WIFE					STROKE		
SON / DAUGHTER					CONVULSIONS		
					SUICIDE OR SEVERE DEPRESSION		
					MENTAL ILLNESS		
					BLEEDING TENDENCY		
					GOUT OR OTHER ARTHRITIS		
					ALCOHOL OR DRUG PROBLEMS		

SOCIAL HISTORY: ☐ SINGLE ☐ MARRIED ☐ SEPARATED ☐ DIVORCED ☐ WIDOWED

	YES	NO
DO YOU LIVE ALONE?	☐	☐
DO YOU HAVE DEPENDENTS AT HOME?	☐	☐
DO YOU EXERCISE REGULARLY?	☐	☐
DO YOU SMOKE?	☐	☐
HOW MUCH?		
HAVE YOU *EVER* SMOKED?	☐	☐
HAVE YOU EVER FELT YOU SHOULD CUT DOWN ON YOUR DRINKING?	☐	☐

	YES	NO
HAVE PEOPLE EVER ANNOYED YOU BY CRITICIZING YOUR DRINKING?	☐	☐

ARE YOU CURRENTLY EMPLOYED?
☐ FULL TIME ☐ PART TIME ☐ NOT EMPLOYED
WHAT IS YOUR JOB? _____
YEARS OF EDUCATION COMPLETED:? _____
HOW MUCH *WORK TIME* HAVE YOU LOST DUE TO YOUR HEALTH?
PAST SIX MONTHS: _____
PAST ONE YEAR: _____
PAST FIVE YEARS: _____

SYSTEMIC REVIEW (DO YOU CURRENTLY HAVE ANY OF THE FOLLOWING?):

GENERAL	YES	NO
RECENT WEIGHT CHANGE	☐	☐
SKIN:	YES	NO
JAUNDICE	☐	☐
HIVES, ECZEMA OR RASH	☐	☐
FREQUENT INFECTION OR BOILS	☐	☐
ABNORMAL PIGMENTATION	☐	☐
HEAD-EYES-EARS-NOSE-THROAT:	YES	NO
EYE DISEASE OR INJURY	☐	☐
DO YOU WEAR GLASSES/CONTACTS?	☐	☐
DOUBLE VISION	☐	☐
HEADACHES	☐	☐
GLAUCOMA	☐	☐

HEAD-EYES-NOSE-THROAT (cont'd):	YES	NO
SNEEZING OR RUNNY NOSE	☐	☐
NOSE BLEEDS	☐	☐
CHRONIC SINUS TROUBLE	☐	☐
EAR DISEASE	☐	☐
IMPAIRED HEARING	☐	☐
ITCHING EYES OR NOSE	☐	☐
TRANSIENT EPISODES OF UNCONSCIOUSNESS	☐	☐
DIZZINESS	☐	☐
NECK:	YES	NO
STIFFNESS	☐	☐
THYROID TROUBLE	☐	☐
ENLARGED GLANDS	☐	☐

REC-0100 2/95   (OVER PLEASE)

Patient/client teaching is an important part of a medical assistant's responsibilities. Encourage patients to adopt good health habits. Provide written material when the examination is complete. This helps patients/clients understand their role in their care. Following are some examples of patient/client education topics:

- Self-care
- Medication
- Awareness of special condition
- Self-examination
- Breast exam
- Blood pressure
- Lifestyle changes that promote good health
- Dietary habits
- Balancing work, family, and private time

SYSTEMIC REVIEW: (Cont'd)

RESPIRATORY:	YES	NO
SPITTING UP BLOOD..	☐	☐
CHRONIC OR FREQUENT COUGH	☐	☐
ASTHMA/WHEEZING OR DIFFICULTY BREATHING.............	☐	☐
PLEURISY OR PNEUMONIA................................	☐	☐

CARDIOVASCULAR:	YES	NO
CHEST PAIN/ANGINA PECTORIS OR HEART ATTACK		
SHORTNESS OF BREATH WALKING OR LYING DOWN ......☐		☐
HIGH BLOOD PRESSURE................................☐		☐
SWELLING OF HANDS, FEET OR ANKLES ....☐		☐
AWAKENING IN THE NIGHT SMOTHERING.........☐		☐
HEART MURMUR/PALPITATIONS......................☐		☐

GASTROINTESTINAL:	YES	NO
PEPTIC ULCER (STOMACH/DUODENAL)............☐		☐
HEARTBURN/INDIGESTION.............................☐		☐
VOMITING BLOOD OR FOOD ....☐		☐
GALLBLADDER DISEASE ....☐		☐
LIVER TROUBLE/HEPATITIS ....☐		☐
PAINFUL/BLOODY BOWEL MOVEMENTS ....☐		☐
HEMORRHOIDS/PILES OR BLACK STOOLS.......☐		☐
CHANGE IN BOWEL HABITS (DIARRHEA, ETC.).............☐		☐
CRAMPING OR PAIN IN THE ABDOMEN ....☐		☐
DOES FOOD STICK IN THROAT? ....☐		☐

GYNECOLOGICAL: (FEMALE ONLY)
AGE PERIODS STARTED _____
HOW LONG PERIODS LAST _____ DAYS
FREQUENCY OF PERIODS _____ DAYS
NUMBER OF PREGNANCIES _____
NUMBER OF MISCARRIAGES/ABORTIONS _____
DATE OF LAST PAP SMEAR _____ RESULTS_____
DATE OF LAST MAMMOGRAM _____ RESULTS _____

GENITOURINARY:	YES	NO
LOSS OF URINE ....☐		☐
FREQUENT URINATION (DAY OR NIGHT).............☐		☐
BURNING OR PAINFUL URINATION ....☐		☐
BLOOD IN URINE ....☐		☐
KIDNEY TROUBLE (STONES, ETC.) ....☐		☐

LOCOMOTOR-MUSCULOSKELETAL:	YES	NO
VARICOSE VEINS...☐		☐
ANY DIFFICULTY IN WALKING.......................☐		☐
ANY PAIN IN CALVES OR BUTTOCKS ON WALKING,		
RELIEVED BY REST ....☐		☐

NEUROLOGIC:	YES	NO
HAVE YOU HAD FAINTING SPELLS..................☐		☐
CONVULSIONS ....☐		☐
PARALYSIS ....☐		☐

HEMATOLOGIC:	YES	NO
ARE YOU SLOW TO HEAL AFTER CUTS ....☐		☐
BLOOD DISEASE ....☐		☐
ANEMIA...☐		☐
PHLEBITIS ....☐		☐
EXCESSIVE BLEEDING OR ABNORMAL BRUISING.............☐		☐

ENDOCRINE:	YES	NO
THYROID DISEASE..☐		☐
HORMONE THERAPY.....................................☐		☐
ANY CHANGE IN HAT OR GLOVE SIZE ....☐		☐
ANY CHANGE IN HAIR GROWTH....................☐		☐
HAVE YOU BECOME COLDER THAN BEFORE,		
OR HAS SKIN BECOME DRIER ....☐		☐

PSYCHIATRY:	YES	NO
HAVE YOU EVER BEEN ADVISED TO SEEK		
OR HAVE YOU SOUGHT TREATMENT FOR:		
DEPRESSION..☐		☐
ANXIETY AND/OR PANIC................................☐		☐
SEVERE STRESS ....☐		☐
ALCOHOL AND/OR DRUG ABUSE ....☐		☐

PLEASE LIST ALL KNOWN ALLERGIES (DRUGS, FOOD, ANIMALS, ETC.):

_____   _____
_____   _____
_____   _____

HEALTH RISKS:

I HAVE RECEIVED A HANDOUT COVERING THE FOLLOWING SUBJECTS:

☐ SUBSTANCE USAGE   ☐ PHYSICAL ACTIVITY HABITS   ☐ SAFE SEX PRACTICES
☐ HEALTHY DIETARY HABITS   ☐ STRESS CONTROL   ☐ PERSONAL SAFETY
☐ SELF EXAMINATION (BREAST/TESTICLES)

I UNDERSTAND I CAN ADDRESS ANY CONCERN/QUESTIONS CONCERNING THE ABOVE INFORMATION WITH MY MEDICAL PROVIDER.

SIGNATURE OF PERSON ACQUIRING THIS INFORMATION:_____

SIGNATURE OF PATIENT: _____ DATE _____

QUESTIONNAIRE REVIEWED BY: _____ DATE _____
(MEDICAL PROVIDER)

Figure 23.10

Continued.

PROCEDURE 23.14

GENERAL PHYSICAL EXAMINATION

RATIONALE

Your assistance in gathering accurate information prior to the physician's examination helps facilitate the examination process. Your assisting at various intervals during the exami- nation to help position the patient, hand the physician sup- plies and instruments, or respond to the patient's requests helps provide a smooth, well-organized process.

ALERT: Follow Standard Precautions.

1. Wash hands.
2. Take patient/client to scale; measure weight and height; document.

3. Take patient/client to examination room. If patient is new, review patient questionnaire and clarify unclear information. (Some providers prefer that the MA complete the patient questionnaire.) See example of patient questionnaire in Figure 23.10.

PROCEDURE 23.14 — GENERAL PHYSICAL EXAMINATION *(Continued)*

4. Interview patient and document the following:
   a. Date and time.
   b. Principal complaint or purpose of visit. Document verbatim the patient's description of the injury.

   NOTE If injury occurred at work or may be work related, special authorization is required prior to treatment.

   c. Age.
   d. Any known allergies.
   e. Current medications.
   f. Medications recently stopped.
   g. Date of last rectal exam.
   h. Female's date of last.
      (1) Normal menstrual period
      (2) Mammogram
      (3) Pap smear

5. Measure body temperature and blood pressure; document.

6. Count pulse and respiratory rate; document.

7. Note any visible symptoms.

8. Instruct patient/client to have a seat while waiting for physician.

9. Notify or signal provider that patient is ready for conference.

10. Prepare patient for examination when provider indicates.

11. Instruct patient/client to
    a. Remove all clothes. (Offer to assist patients.)
    b. Put on gown with opening in back. (Some providers prefer opening in front when doing breast examination.)
    c. Have a seat while waiting for physician.

12. Check room and have the following equipment and supplies ready:
    a. Opthalmoscope
    b. Otoscope with ear shields
    c. Percussion hammer
    d. Disposable gloves
    e. Basin/pan
    f. Tape measure
    g. Tongue blade
    h. Lubricant
    i. Anal scope
    j. Vaginal speculum for women

13. After the examination:
    a. Give medication or treatment if ordered.
    b. Instruct patient to dress. (Offer to help patients.)
    c. Remove instruments and tray to cleaning area.

14. Wash hands.

15. When patient/client is dressed:
    a. Complete patient teaching as necessary.
    b. Direct client according to provider's order (for example, to laboratory for lab work, to radiology department for x-ray, to receptionist to make next appointment and payment arrangements).

16. Document treatments, procedures, and medication given.

17. Clean examination room for next patient/client.

18. Wash hands.

- Exercise
- Smoking cessation

A patient may complain of symptoms that require an examination other than his or her general physical examination visits. The following information guides you in preparing for the most common types of examinations.

Eye, Ear, Nose, and Throat Examinations

Eye, ear, nose, and throat examinations are known as EENT examinations. This type of examination may be routine or may be done when a patient complains of the following:

- Decreased hearing
- Congested nose
- Sore throat

PROCEDURE 23.15   LIMITED EXAMINATION

RATIONALE

Your assistance in gathering accurate information prior to the physician's doing a limited examination helps facilitate the examination process. Your assisting at various intervals during the examination to help position the patient, hand the physician supplies or instruments, or respond to the patient's requests helps provide a smooth, well-organized process.

ALERT: Follow Standard Precautions.

1. Wash hands.
2. Take patient/client to scale; weigh and document.
3. Take patient/client to examination room and instruct him or her to have a seat.
4. Interview the patient/client and document the following:
    a. Date and time
    b. Principal complaint
    c. Age
    d. Allergies
    e. Current medication
5. Measure body temperature; document.
6. Count pulse and respiration; document.
7. Measure blood pressure; document.

- Red and irritated eyes
- Runny nose
- Earache
- Head and facial pain

The physician examines the eyes, ears, nose, and throat and may also examine the chest if these symptoms occur.

The eye may need a light eye patch to prevent further damage from trauma. After surgery, instillation of a local anesthetic may be needed for therapeutic use. A pressure eye patch is used for corneal abrasions, to control postoperative edema and hemorrhage from trauma.

During an EENT examination, the provider may decide to culture drainage in the throat. The culture helps identify the specific bacteria causing an ear or throat infection. Use good technique when obtaining a specimen for culture. If a specimen is contaminated, the test results will be incorrect. Review the procedure "Obtaining a Specimen for Culture" in Chapter 18. See Table 23.4 for common EENT conditions, possible treatments, and patient teaching. The following procedures may be necessary to treat or diagnose various eye, ear, nose, and throat conditions.

Table 23.4 ■ Common EENT Conditions, Possible Treatments, and Patient Education

Condition	Possible Treatments	Patient Education
Cataracts	Surgery	1. Encourage patient. 2. Provide patients and family with written information as to pre- and postoperative expectations.
Conjunctivitus	Medication Eye irrigation (wash) Warm compresses Allergy testing	1. Teach ways to prevent reinfection and cross infection. 2. Teach need for good lighting. 3. Teach to rest eyes periodically. 4. Teach application of medication.

Table 23.4 ■ Continued

Condition	Possible Treatments	Patient Education
Glaucoma	Medication Surgery Close observation	1. Instruct patient not to lift heavy objects. 2. Teach stress-reduction techniques. 3. Teach importance of taking prescribed medication.
Sty	Warm compress Incision and drainage Medication	1. Teach application of warm compress. 2. Instruct to reduce reading or straining of eye. 3. Instruct to keep out of direct sunlight. 4. Instruct not to rub eyes. 5. Teach ways to keep eye clean.
Otitis	Medication Heat Removal of fluid from behind the membrane Surgery (myringotomy)	1. Teach recognition of symptoms. 2. Teach use of vaporizers and decongestants.
Otosclerosis	Surgery (stapedectomy)	1. Encourage patient. 2. Provide written postoperative care instructions.
Deviated nasal septum	Surgery	1. Encourage patient. 2. Provide written postoperative care instructions.
Nasal polyps	Surgery	1. Encourage patient. 2. Provide written postoperative care instructions.
Laryngitis	Vaporized cool mist medication Reduction of irritants	1. Teach use of vaporizer. 2. Teach medication administration. 3. Teach need for environment free of smoke or irritants.

PROCEDURE 23.16

EYE IRRIGATION (CONTINUOUS)

RATIONALE

A continuous eye irrigation washes the eye of irritants and can help to prevent eye damage. Your quick, efficient action following this procedure helps ensure the best outcome for the patient.

ALERT: Follow Standard Precautions.

1. Wash hands.
2. Explain what you are going to do.
3. Assemble equipment.

   a. Sterile towel
   b. Sterile basin
   c. IV tubing
   d. IV pole
   e. 1,000 cc IV normal saline
   f. Cotton balls
   g. Litmus/pH paper for chemical burn
   h. Topical anesthetic
   i. Plastic trash bag
   j. Disposable gloves

4. Perform a visual acuity test unless severity of situation or physician's order contraindicates.
5. Wash hands thoroughly.
6. Place client in supine position.
7. Put on gloves.
8. Turn client's head to side affected to prevent solution flowing over nose and into other eye.
9. Place towel under patient's head and/or place basin beneath eye.
10. Use litmus paper to determine if irritant is acid or alkaline.

PROCEDURE 23.16 | EYE IRRIGATION (CONTINUOUS) *(Continued)*

11. Spike 1,000 cc IV bag with IV tubing (chemical burn: use at least 1,000 cc of normal saline to dilute and wash out harsh chemical).
12. Close clamp.
13. Invert IV bag on IV pole.
    Instill topical anesthetic to eye according to policy and/or physician's orders.
14. Separate patient's eyelid with thumb and index finger on nondominant hand.
15. Open clamp on IV tubing and begin irrigation.
16. Hold tubing at 45° angle.
17. Ask patient to rotate eye clockwise.
18. Direct stream at inner canthus so that the normal saline solution flows across the cornea to the outer canthus.
19. Stop the flow of solution periodically and ask patient to close eye. (This will move secretions from upper to lower conjunctival sac.)
20. Dry eyelid with cotton balls.
21. Wipe from inner to outer canthus.
22. Use new cotton ball for each wipe.
23. Remove gloves.
24. Wash hands thoroughly.

25. Perform visual acuity test on physician's direction.
26. Document the following on client's chart:
    a. Date
    b. Time
    c. Duration of irrigation
    d. Type of solution
    e. Amount of solution
    f. Visual acuity test before and after irrigation
    g. Patient's tolerance of procedure
    h. All instructions given patient
    i. Signature and certification

1/01/03	1400

Visual acuity test prior to irrigation
bilaterally 20/20
Topical anesthetic applied to OS
Irrigated OS with 250 cc normal
saline for 30 minutes
Tolerated well
Visual acuity test post irrigation
20/20 biaterally
———— M. Gonzales CMA

PROCEDURE 23.17 | FLUORESCEIN STAINING OF THE EYE

RATIONALE

A fluorescein strip test identifies any foreign body or injury to the eye. Once a foreign body or injury is identified, the proper action can be taken to restore the eye. Your quick, efficient action following this procedure helps ensure the best outcome for the patient.

ALERT: Follow Standard Precautions.

1. Wash hands.
2. Assemble equipment and supplies.
   a. Normal saline solution
   b. Fluorescein strip
   c. Tissues
   d. Cobalt blue light
   e. Cotton balls
   f. Disposable gloves

3. Explain procedure to patient/client.
4. Place patient flat on examination table or in a semi-Fowler's position.
5. Tilt patient's head toward affected side.
6. Provide patient with tissue.
7. Put on gloves.
8. Remove fluorescein strip from sterile package.

PROCEDURE 23.17   FLUORESCEIN STAINING OF THE EYE *(Continued)*

9. Moisten tip of fluorescein strip with drop of sterile solution.

10. Hold strip in one hand. *Do not contaminate tip.*

11. Gently evert patient's lower eyelid with other hand.

12. Touch lower conjunctival sac gently with tip of fluorescein strip.

13. Instruct patient to blink eyes gently. This will spread dye over corneal and conjunctival surfaces.

14. Assist physician with examination.

    a. Hand cobalt blue light to physician.

    b. Irrigate eye after examination to prevent chemical conjunctivitis from fluorescein.

    c. Dry eye with cotton ball.

    d. Apply eye patch if ordered by physician.

15. Remove gloves.

16. Wash hands and document the following on client's chart:

    a. Date

    b. Time

    c. Vital signs

    d. Fluorescein strip test result

    e. Irrigation solution used

    f. Amount of irrigation

    g. All instructions given patient

    h. Patient's condition on discharge

    i. Medications given

    j. Signature and certification

> 1/01/03   1700
>
> Complained of an irritation in OS
>
> Vital signs normal
>
> Fluorescein strip identified foreign object
>
> Removed by Dr. Smith
>
> Irrigated with 60 cc normal saline and eye patch applied to OS
>
> Instructed in self-care
>
> ———— S. Kim CMA

PROCEDURE 23.18   LIGHT EYE PATCH APPLICATION

RATIONALE

Applying a light eye patch protects the eye from further damage and irritation from light.

ALERT: Follow Standard Precautions.

1. Wash hands.

2. Assemble supplies.

    a. Gauze, 4 × 4

    b. Tape

    c. Plastic or metal eye shield

    d. Gauze eye patch

    e. Disposable gloves

3. Explain what you are going to do.

4. Place client flat or in semi-Fowler's position on exam table.

5. Wash hands thoroughly.

6. Put on gloves.

7. Instruct patient to close eye.

8. Gently apply gauze eye patch over patient's closed eye.

9. Secure gauze patch with two pieces of tape.

10. Apply a metal or plastic shield over eye patch per physician's order.

11. Remove gloves, wash hands.

12. Instruct patient that monocular (one eye) vision alters

    a. Depth perception

    b. Field of vision

PROCEDURE 23.18 | LIGHT EYE PATCH APPLICATION *(Continued)*

13. Tell patient
    a. Not to drive
    b. Not to operate machinery
14. Document the following on patient's chart:
    a. Date
    b. Time
    c. Type of patch applied

    d. All instructions given patient
    e. Patient's condition on discharge
    f. Signature and certification

1/01/03   1300
light eye patch applied to OS
Instructed in self-care techniques
_____ S. Cash CMA

PROCEDURE 23.19 | AUDIOMETRIC (HEARING) EXAMINATION

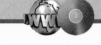

RATIONALE

Audiometric testing provides diagnostic information about hearing acuity. Loss of acuity may indicate nerve damage, the presence of a tumor, or other problems.

1. Wash hands.
2. Assemble and prepare equipment.
    a. Acoustically shielded booth
    b. Earphones and cushions (clean before using)
    c. Audiometric report form
    d. Otoscope
    e. Manual audiometer
3. Take client to examination room.
4. Check both ears with otoscope to ensure clearness of ear canals. (Eardrum should be visible.)
5. Seat patient in acoustically shielded booth so that he or she cannot see manipulation of dials of audiometer.
6. Begin test with better ear, if patient can hear better with one ear than the other.
7. Instruct client prior to putting on earphones:
    a. He or she will hear a series of tones of various sound levels.
    b. First one ear will be tested and then the other.
    c. He or she is to raise a finger each time he or she hears a tone.
    d. Client should keep his or her finger up for as long as he or she hears tone, *no matter how faint it is.*
    e. Instruct patient to lower finger *only* when he or she no longer hears sound.

    f. Instruct patient to push button on response terminal (in place of raising finger) if booth is used.
8. Place earphones over patient's ears. Make sure that each earphone is centered over ear canal and that cushions fit snugly.
9. Place blue earphone over left ear.
10. Place red earphone over right ear.
11. Do not allow patient to handle earphones.
12. Close door to audiometric test booth.
13. Present one or two tones of different frequencies at easily heard levels so that patient becomes familiar with procedure.
14. Set frequency dial at 500 Hz, hearing dial at 30 dB.
15. Decrease dB level by 10 until patient responds by lowering his or her finger or depressing response terminal. For example, 500 Hz

    30 dB
    20 dB
    10 dB
    0 dB
    − 10 dB
    − 20 dB

PROCEDURE 23.19 — AUDIOMETRIC (HEARING) EXAMINATION *(Continued)*

16. When there is no response from patient, increase dB level by 5 until patient responds by raising his or her finger or depressing response terminal. For example, 500 Hz

    0 dB
    5 dB
    10 dB
    15 dB
    20 dB
    25 dB
    30 dB
    35 dB
    40 dB

17. *Interrupt tone; present at same level to confirm that patient has heard sound.* Follow preceding instructions for dB. Increase Hz value to

    1,000
    2,000
    3,000
    4,000
    6,000
    8,000

18. Do *not* set up rhythm in turning tone off and on. Patients may respond based on rhythm anticipation and not on "true" hearing levels.

19. Do *not* prolong test unnecessarily. If responses become inconsistent beyond reasonable expectation, terminate test and repeat at later date.

20. Document results on graph (blue ink for left ear and red ink for right ear), fill in all areas, and sign and date side 2 of the audiometric form.

TESTER COMPLETES

PURPOSE OF TEST		PLACE WHERE TESTED		TEST RELIABILITY	
BASELINE	☐	MOBILE UNIT	☐	GOOD	☐
PRE-EMPLOY	☒	OFFICE	☒	FAIR	☒
BASELINE/PRE-EMPLOYMENT	☐	PLANT	☐	POOR	☐
MONITOR	☐				

TESTER SIGNED __Nurse__ DATE ____

CALIBRATED __2-15-03__   AUDIOMETER NUMBER __10 C 344__

Left Ear   Right Ear

500	1000	2000	3000	4000	5000	6000	500	1000	2000	3000	4000	5000	6000
0	0	5	0	5	0	10	0	5	15	0	0	5	20

Otoscopy: Left _____   Right _____

DATE ENTERED: __4-1-03__
SIGNATURE __S. Fraga__

1/01/03   1300

Testing indicates some hearing loss

Dr. Iso notified

Test results in chart

_____ I. Eu Min CMA

PROCEDURE 23.20 — EAR IRRIGATION

RATIONALE

Wax can build in the outer ear canal, diminishing hearing. Irrigating the ear helps remove excess ear wax or foreign matter, which can help restore hearing. Remember that irrigating the ear can cause dizziness initially and nausea following the procedure.

ALERT: Follow Standard Precautions.

1. Wash hands.
2. Assemble equipment and supplies.

    a. Irrigation syringe
    b. Basin
    c. Waterproof drape
    d. Towels (two)
    e. Container for solution
    f. Irrigating solution

PROCEDURE 23.20 | **EAR IRRIGATION** *(Continued)*

g. Cotton-tip applicators
h. Otoscope
i. Debrox (if ordered)
j. Disposable gloves

3. Take allergy history. (If known or possible allergies to irrigation solution exist, notify physician.)

4. Check with patient/client for the following:

   a. History of eardrum perforation
   b. Complications from previous ear irrigations

5. Explain procedure to patient.

6. Position patient in one of two ways:

   a. Sitting with head tilted slightly forward and toward affected side
   b. Lying on examination table with head tilted toward affected side

7. Check auditory canal with otoscope.

8. Wash hands thoroughly.

9. Put on gloves.

10. Instill ear wax softener according to physician's order.

11. Prepare solution as specified by physician.

12. Place emesis basin close to patient's head, under ear.

13. Ask patient to hold basin.

14. Test irrigating solution. (Temperature of solution should be between 95° and 105° F.)

15. Gently pull outer ear to straighten ear canal.

16. Draw solution into syringe.

17. Insert tip of irrigating syringe at opening of auditory canal.

18. *Do not occlude (block) opening.*

19. Point tip of syringe upward and toward posterior end of ear canal.

20. Gently instill solution against canal wall.

21. Observe return flow for debris.

22. Observe patient for

   a. Pain
   b. Dizziness

NOTE Discontinue procedure immediately if symptoms occur.

23. Continue irrigation until return flow is clear, or 500 cc of solution is used.

24. Inspect ear canal with otoscope for cleanliness.

25. Remove basin.

26. Dry ear and neck with towel.

27. Turn patient on affected side to facilitate drainage of residual debris.

28. Measure and record amount of solution returned.

29. Remove gloves, wash hands.

30. Document the following on client's chart:

   a. Date
   b. Time
   c. Which ear irrigated
   d. Volume of solution
   e. Temperature of solution
   f. Appearance of canal before and after irrigation
   g. Appearance of return flow
   h. Patient's tolerance of procedure
   i. Instructions given patient
   j. Condition on discharge
   k. Signature and certification

10/10/03   0900

Right ear irrigated with 500 cc 97°
degree irrigating solution
A 2 mm ear wax plug removed
Patient tolerated procedure well
No dizziness, nausea, or pain
_____ R. Tlilayatza CMA

Respiratory Tract Examination

Respiratory tract examinations include the ears, nose, throat, and chest. Prepare the room with an otoscope, nasal speculum, tongue blade, penlight, and stethoscope. The upper respiratory system is usually examined when the patient experiences the following symptoms:

■ Fever

■ Chest pain

■ Cough

Table 23.5 ■ Common Respiratory Conditions, Possible Treatments, and Patient Education

Condition	Possible Treatments	Patient Education
Rhinitis	Medication to relieve symptoms	1. Instruct patient to gently blow nose. 2. Inform patient of complication of closing nostrils when blowing nose (sinus drainage is forced into eustachian tube). 3. Instruct patient to call physician if nasal drainage is yellow or greenish, or puslike (purulent).
Pharyngitis (sore throat)	Medication to relieve symptoms and to kill bacteria if present	1. Perform throat culture if bacteria is suspected cause.
Tonsilitis	Medication Possible surgery	1. Provide pre- and postoperative instruction. 2. Provide instructions for medications.
Laryngitis	Inhalation of steam or medicated cool mist Antibiotics Warm gargle	1. Explain need for steam and/or cool medicated mist. 2. Instruct patient to rest voice.
Bronchitis	Medication	1. Instruct patients who smoke to stop. 2. Explain that bronchi in lungs are irritated.
Pneumonia	Inhalation of steam or medicated cool mist Hospitalization may be necessary Bedrest Medication to relieve symptoms Antibiotics if bacterial pneumonia	1. Obtain sputum for culture and sensitivity. 2. Explain need for sputum specimen. 3. Instruct patient to cough into tissue.
Emphysema	Medication Postural drainage Breathing treatments	1. Stress importance of balanced diet and reduced dairy product intake. 2. Recommend exercise program. 3. Encourage patient to stop smoking.

- Discharge from nose or ears
- Difficult breathing
- Headache
- Tiredness
- Nasal congestion
- Watery eyes

See Table 23.5 for common respiratory conditions, possible treatments, and patient teaching.

Cardiovascular Examinations

Cardiovascular examinations focus on the heart and blood vessels of the body. The provider checks the cardiovascular system during a routine physical. He or she also examines this system when a patient complains of the following:

- Headaches
- Nervousness
- Dizziness
- Chest pain or a squeezing feeling in the chest
- Pain in neck, jaw, and arms

- Fatigue (feeling very tired)
- Shortness of breath
- Enlarged (distended) neck veins
- Rapid heartbeat (palpitations)
- Cold extremities
- Numbness in the extremities
- Hot, reddened area on legs
- Varicose veins

The provider may order an electrocardiogram (EKG/ECG) to measure the heart's activity. Follow the procedure "Mounting EKGs" in Chapter 17. The provider orders an echocardiogram if he or she suspects heart structure damage or disease. The echocardiogram allows the provider to see the inner structure and motion of the heart. The echocardiogram is usually performed in radiology.

The provider may also order tests of the patient's/client's blood. The following blood tests tell the most about the cardiac (heart) muscle:

- Lactic dehydrogenase (LDH)
- Creatine phosphokinase (CPK)

When the EKG/ECG indicates changes and the LDH/CPK are abnormal, the provider assumes heart muscle damage is present. If you are certified and are required to draw blood, refer to Chapter 18 and follow the procedure "Drawing Blood With a Vacutainer™" or "Using a Needle and Syringe to Draw Blood." Process the blood sample according to laboratory guidelines. Remember: Always follow Standard Precautions when drawing blood. See Table 23.6 for common cardiovascular conditions, possible treatments, and patient teaching.

Digestive System Examination

The digestive system examination focuses on the mouth, teeth, tongue, pharynx, esophagus, stomach, and the small and large intestine. The pancreas, liver, and gallbladder are the accessory organs that help digest food. When examining the digestive system, the provider also examines the accessory organs. The provider examines this system during a routine physical or when a patient/client complains of the following:

- Heartburn (burning sensation around and below the location of the heart)
- Abdominal pain
- Abdominal cramps
- Fever
- Vomiting
- Nausea
- Bloating
- Frequent loose stools (diarrhea)
- Constipation
- Hernias
- Blood in the stool
- Pain or burning with bowel movement

To prepare a patient/client and room for the digestive system examination, follow the procedure "Limited Examination." The initial examination may indicate the

Table 23.6 ■ Common Cardiovascular Conditions, Possible Treatments, and Patient Education

Condition	Possible Treatments	Patient Education
Coronary artery disease (narrowing of arteries of the heart)	Medication Surgery Diet	1. Explain importance of low-salt, low-fat diet; weight control; prescribed exercise program. 2. Reduce stress factors. 3. Stress importance of taking prescribed medication. 4. Provide written information on condition.
Myocardial infarction (MI, heart attack)	Medication Rehabilitation	1. Encourage patient to follow prescribed diet, medication program, and exercise program. 2. Provide written instructions and information about condition.
Congestive heart failure (CHF), (tissues of heart and lungs are edematous)	Medication Rest Diet Antiembolism stocking	1. Encourage patient to follow prescribed diet and medication program. 2. Provide written instructions and information about condition.
Hypertension (blood pressure above 140/90)	Medication Diet therapy Exercise program	1. Warn patient not to stop medication without seeing physician. 2. Stress importance of diet and exercise. 3. Explain why blood pressure increases with weight gain and poor dietary habits.
Varicose veins (veins that allow blood to pool and not return to the heart)	Ace bandages Warm soaks Surgery	1. Explain importance of changing position frequently (sitting, standing). 2. Explain application of elastic wrap or elastic stockings and their purpose. 3. Stress importance of elevating legs. 4. Stress importance of loose clothing so that circulation is not impaired.
Thrombophlebitis	Medication Surgery Warm compresses	1. Instruct in application of warm compresses. 2. Instruct in elevation of legs. 3. Teach to watch for danger signs.
Cerebral vascular accident (CVA, stroke)	Hospitalization Physical therapy Occupational therapy Speech therapy Medication	1. Encourage patient to reach highest potential. 2. Teach awareness of adaptive devices and assist in selection.

need for further examinations and tests. The results of a hematocrit and hemoglobin test tell the provider if there is a significant blood loss. Refer to Chapter 18 and follow the procedures "Microhematocrit" and "Using a Hemoglobinometer."

Endoscopy procedures allow the provider to see the inside of the digestive system. The provider uses an endoscope for this examination. The inside of an endoscope is lined with special mirrors and a light. These scopes are fragile and require special care. There are several types of endoscopes. The following procedures are used to view different areas of the digestive system with endoscopes:

■ **Gastroscopy.** Views the pharynx, esophagus, stomach using an endoscope inserted through the mouth.

■ **Colonoscopy.** Views the inside of colon and intestines using an endoscope inserted through the rectum.

■ **Sigmoidoscopy.** Views the lower colon using a sigmoidoscope inserted through the rectum.

The following are common x-ray procedures to help diagnose digestive system disorders:

- **Upper gastrointestinal series (UGI).** Allows fluoroscope viewing of the esophagus, stomach, duodenum, and small intestine. The patient swallows barium, a **radiopaque** liquid. The barium shows the shape and size of the inside of each organ it moves through. If a growth or ulcer is present, the UGI allows the radiologist to see it.

- **Lower gastrointestinal series (LGI)–barium enema (BE).** Views the entire large intestine. Barium is administered as an enema. The radiopaque barium shows tumors, **polyps**, ulcers, **diverticulitis**, changes in **mucosa**, and other changes.

- **Sonograms.** XDisplays on a monitor the movement and shapes of organs inside the body. High-frequency sound waves from the ultrasound equipment reflect these movements and shapes. The radiologist can determine if growths are present or if normal movement or function is absent.

Each radiology procedure requires special patient preparation before the test. Instruct patients in writing and verbally to ensure that they understand. When directing patients, always follow the radiology department guidelines for each test. See Table 23.7 for digestive system conditions, possible treatments, and patient teaching.

radiopaque

Shows as a white material when a fluoroscope x-ray is taken.

polyps

Small tumorlike growths.

diverticulitis

Inflammation of the small sacs in the wall of the colon.

mucosa

Thin lining on the inside of the intestines.

Table 23.7 ■ Common Digestive System Conditions, Possible Treatments, and Patient Education

Condition	Possible Treatments	Patient Education
Gastroesophageal reflux (burping gastric juices into esophagus)	Antacids Frequent small meals Surgery	1. Instruct patient to sit up during and after eating. 2. Teach to elevate head when sleeping.
Hiatal hernia	Medication Alteration of diet and eating patterns Surgery	1. Teach diet modifications. 2. Teach need for frequent small meals. 3. Teach weight control. 4. Teach to elevate head when sleeping.
Peptic ulcer	Medication Stress reduction Stopping smoking Alteration of diet	1. Teach diet modification. 2. Instruct patient to watch for bloody or tarry stools.
Appendicitis	Surgery	1. Provide pre- and postoperative instruction.
Colitis	Medication Diet therapy Psychotherapy to relieve anxiety Surgery	1. Encourage patient to follow diet. 2. Teach importance of reducing stress. 3. Provide pre- and postoperative instruction.
Abdominal hernia	Surgery	1. Instruct in signs of strangulated hernia. 2. Provide pre- and postoperative instruction. 3. Provide written material about condition.
Hemorrhoids	Diet therapy Surgery	1. Instruct in diet restrictions. 2. Provide written material about condition.

Urinary System Examination

The urinary system examination focuses on the kidneys, ureters, urinary bladder, and urethra. In the male the prostate, vas deferens, testes, scrotum, and penis are also examined. This system is examined once a year during a general physical and when a patient complains of the following:

- Frequent urination with a feeling of urgency, burning sensation, small amounts of urine
- Pain in kidney area
- Blood in the urine
- Swelling (edema) around eyes and in the feet

Most patients complaining of urinary system disorders require a urinalysis. To collect a routine urine specimen or a clean-catch specimen, follow the procedures in Chapter 18. Remember to use Standard Precautions when handling body fluids. The provider may require blood chemistries to see if waste products are being filtered out of the blood. If you are certified and are required to draw blood chemistries, follow the procedure "Drawing Blood With a Vacutainer™" or "Using a Needle and Syringe to Draw Blood" in Chapter 18. Remember to observe Standard Precautions when handling blood. See Table 23.8 for urinary system conditions, possible treatments, and patient teaching.

Male Reproductive System Examination

The male reproductive system examination focuses on the penis, scrotum, urethra, prostate, epididymis, vas deferens, and testes. This system is examined once a year and when a male patient complains of the following:

- Frequent and urgent urination
- Pain or swelling in the scrotum
- Painful or difficult urination
- Discoloration of the scrotum
- Enlargement of the scrotum
- Urethral discharge
- Genital sores, rash, blistering, or warts

Table 23.8 ■ Common Urinary System Conditions, Possible Treatments, and Patient Education

Condition	Possible Treatments	Patient Education
Cystitis	Medication Increase in water intake	1. Instruct in importance of drinking enough water to dilute bacteria (unless physician restricts fluids). 2. Instruct women always to wipe themselves from front of perineum to back.
Pyelonephritis	Medication Increase of fluids	1. Encourage large intake of water.
Nephrolithiasis	Diet therapy Medication Increase in fluid intake Heat application Surgery	1. Instruct patient to strain all urine and inspect for stones. 2. Provide list of low-calcium foods. 3. Provide pre- and postoperative instruction.

Table 23.9 ■ Male and Female Reproductive System Conditions, Possible Treatments, and Patient Education

Condition	Possible Treatments	Patient Education
Epididymitis	Bedrest Ice application Medication Increase in fluid intake	1. Provide instruction in ice application. 2. Provide written material explaining condition. 3. Encourage increased fluid intake.
Prostatitis	Medication Increase of fluids	1. Provide written material about the condition and surgical considerations.
Gonorrhea	Medication	1. Instruct patient to reveal condition to all sex partners and arrange for medical care. 2. Instruct patient to abstain from sexual activity. 3. Provide written material about condition that promotes responsible sexual habits.
Syphilis	Medication	1. Instruct patient to reveal condition to all sex partners and arrange for medical care. 2. Instruct patient to abstain from sexual activity. 3. Provide written material about condition that promotes responsible sexual habits.
Chlamydia	Medication	1. Instruct patient to reveal condition to all sex partners and arrange for medical care. 2. Instruct patient to abstain from sexual activity. 3. Provide written material about condition that promotes responsible sexual habits.
Genital warts	Medication Surgery	1. Provide written material about condition that promotes responsible sexual habits.
AIDS	Medication to relieve symptoms Incurable	1. Provide emotional support and information about local support groups. 2. Provide written material about condition that promotes responsible sexual habits. 3. Instruct in Standard Precautions to prevent infection of others.

Prepare the patient for a limited examination. Provide gloves, lubricant, and a small light for the doctor. The provider may order a culture, routine urinalysis, or a clean-catch specimen. See Table 23.9 for reproductive system conditions, possible treatments, and patient teaching.

Female Reproductive System Examination

The female reproductive system examination focuses on the perineum, vagina, uterus, cervix, clitoris, ovaries, fallopian tubes, and breasts. The female reproductive system is examined once a year and when the patient complains of the following:

■ Vaginal itching or discharge
■ Swollen, painful breasts
■ Lump or mass felt in breast
■ Pelvic pain
■ Abnormal uterine bleeding
 • Heavy bleeding • Scant menstrual flow • Spotting between periods
■ Absence of regular menstrual flow
■ Inability to become pregnant

Figure 23.11

Equipment for a pelvic examination and Pap smear.

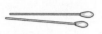
Cotton applicators

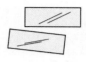
Wooden tongue blade

Microscope slides

Pap smear fixative

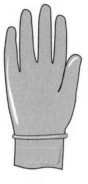
Glove

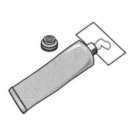
Lubricant

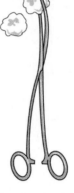
Uterine dressing forceps

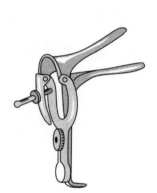
Vaginal speculum

cervix

Neck (e.g., the cervix of the uterus is the neck of the uterus).

Women should have a pelvic (vaginal) examination and Papanicolaou test (Pap test) yearly. General practitioners, internists, gynecologists, and obstetricians routinely perform pelvic exams and Pap tests to identify tissue abnormalities. A Pap smear can help identify unusual cells (for example, cancer cells) on the **cervix.**

The Pap smear requires gentle scraping of the cervix during the pelvic exam. Tissue scraped from the cervix is smeared on a slide. Later the slide is examined under a microscope. Tissue cells and fluids help detect early signs of cancer. Pap smear results are reported using the Bethesda System. For additional information about cervical cancer see the National Cancer Institute's Cancer Information Web site at www.cancernet.nci.nih.gov. For information about the reporting of Pap smear results using the Bethesda System go to www.lhncbc.nlm.nih.gov/apdb/CERVCAN9/ CCMM.HTM.

Equipment for a pelvic examination and Pap smear is shown in Figure 23.11. Prepare the patient and room for a pelvic examination according to the procedure on page 615.

PROCEDURE 23.21 **PELVIC EXAMINATION AND PAPANICOLAOU (PAP) TEST**

RATIONALE

Your assistance in gathering accurate information prior to the pelvic examination helps facilitate the examination process. Your assisting at various intervals during the examination to help position the patient, hand the physician supplies and instruments, or respond to the patient's requests helps provide a smooth, well-organized process. Proper processing of a Pap slide provides a viable specimen that will indicate the presence of healthy or diseased tissue.

ALERT: Follow Standard Precautions.

PROCEDURE 23.21 | PELVIC EXAMINATION AND PAPANICOLAOU (PAP) TEST
(Continued)

1. Wash hands.
2. Take patient/client to scale; weigh and document.
3. Take patient to examination room.
4. Interview patient/client and document the following:
   a. Date
   b. Time
   c. Principal complaint/reason for visit
   d. Age
   e. Allergies
   f. Current medication
   g. Last normal menstrual period
   h. Date of last Pap smear
5. Instruct patient to
   a. Void (empty bladder).
   b. Disrobe from waist down.
   c. Put drape over knees.
6. Assemble equipment and supplies.
   a. Exam gloves
   b. Physician's gown
   c. Eye protection
   d. Vaginal speculum
   e. Light source
   f. Lubricant
   g. Cotton-tip applicators
   h. Cervical scraper
   i. Glass slides
   j. Fixative solution
   k. Slide container
   l. Lab requisition
7. Explain procedure to patient to promote cooperation and lessen anxiety.
8. Assist patient into dorsal recumbent position with buttocks extended slightly beyond end of table, feet in stirrups (see the procedure "Dorsal Lithotomy Position").
9. Tell provider when patient is ready.
10. Put on exam gloves.
11. Hold slides for proper placement of specimens. Prepare slides when exam is completed:
    a. Spray with fixative.
    b. Write patient's/client's name on frosted end of slide.
12. Remove gloves, wash hands.
13. Complete lab requisition with all necessary information.
14. Assist patient/client to sitting position after examination.
15. Instruct patient/client that she will be notified about test results.
16. Send slide and requisition to lab.
17. Document the following:
    a. Pap test, sent to lab
    b. Patient notified that test results will be sent to her
18. Clean room for next patient.

10/10/04   0800
Pap specimen sent to lab
Self-care instruction given
_____ R. Meyer CMA

Breast Exam

When the provider is going to perform a breast exam, it is necessary to instruct the patient/client to remove all clothes above the waist and put on the examination gown with the opening in the front. Take a minute to instruct the patient/client in the simple breast self-examination. Reinforce the fact that just a few minutes each month can save her life. Tell the patient/client to follow the steps in Figure 23.12 once a month about a week after the menstrual cycle ends. Patients/clients who have experienced menopause should perform the check the first day of each month.

See Table 23.10 for female reproductive system conditions, possible treatments, and patient teaching.

Figure 23.12

Visual inspection.

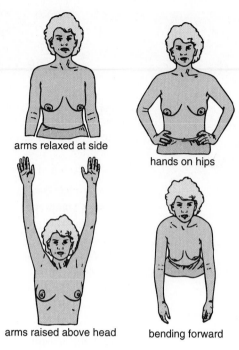

arms relaxed at side

hands on hips

arms raised above head

bending forward

Table 23.10 ■ Conditions of the Female Reproductive System, Possible Treatments, and Patient Education

Condition	Possible Treatments	Patient Education
Vaginitis	Medication Vaginal irrigation	1. Instruct patient in use of vaginal creams, suppositories, or irrigation. 2. Encourage patient to wear cotton underwear.
Pelvic inflammatory disease (PID)	Medication Heat application Vaginal irrigation Surgery	1. Instruct about general hygiene. 2. Provide written material and explanation of condition, and promote responsible sexual habits.
Mastitis	Medication Hot and cold applications	1. Provide information on diet modification (e.g., decrease caffeine and chocolate intake). 2. Instruct patient in use of hot and cold compresses.
Endometriosis	Medication Surgery	1. Instruct patient in use of medication. 2. Provide written information about condition. 3. Provide pre- and postoperative instruction.
Premenstrual syndrome (PMS)	Medication	1. Instruct in diet modification (salt restriction; avoidance of alcohol and caffeine). 2. Instruct to reduce stress.
Breast cancer	Medication Surgery Radiation Radiation Implants	1. Provide written information on condition. 2. Provide pre- and postoperative instruction. 3. Inform about local support groups.

⦾ BREAST SELF-EXAMINATION: A NEW APPROACH

All women over 20 should practice monthly breast self-examination (BSE). Regular and complete BSE can help you find changes in your breasts that occur between clinical breast examinations (by a health professional) and mammograms.

Women should examine their breasts when they are least tender, usually seven days after the start of the menstrual period. Women who have entered menopause, are pregnant or breast-feeding, or who have silicone implants should continue to examine their breasts once a month. Breast-feeding mothers should examine their breasts when all milk has been expressed.

If a woman discovers a lump or detects any changes, she should seek medical attention. Nine out of 10 women will not develop breast cancer, and most breast changes are not cancerous.

BSE: Breast Self-Examination

- BSE is done monthly
- Seven to 10 days from the first day of period
- Same day every month if you are not menstruating (e.g., 1st or 15th of the month)

Look

1. Stand in front of a mirror and look at each breast separately. Note the size, shape, color, contour, and direction of your breasts and nipples.
2. Raise your arms over your head and look at your breasts, as you turn slowly from side to side.
3. Press your hands on your hips and push your shoulders forward. Look at each breast separately.

Feel

Stand in front of a mirror and start BSE just below the collar bone.

1. Use your left hand to examine the right breast. Moisten the pads of your three middle fingertips with body lotion. Apply firm pressure and make small circles as you go back and forth (up and down, circular or spoke style) in a pattern covering all the breast area including the nipple. Extend the examination to the breast tissue in the underarm area.
2. Use your right hand and repeat BSE on the left breast as indicated in step 1.
3. Lie down and raise your right arm above your head. Examine the right breast as before, omitting the underarm area.
4. Still lying down, raise your left arm and repeat the BSE on the left breast, omitting the underarm area.

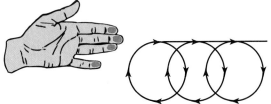

light
medium
deep

Breast Cancer Warning Signs

Most changes that you may find while doing a breast self-examination are benign, but to be sure, have any

> **Figure 23.13**
>
> Palpation with pads of the fingers.

unusual changes or irregularities checked by a physician promptly. Irregularities may include

- Lump or thickening (breast, underarm)
- Red or hot skin
- Orange peel skin
- Dimpling or puckering
- Unusual pain
- Itch or rash, especially in nipple area
- Retracted nipple
- Change in direction of nipple axis
- Bloody or spontaneous discharge from nipple
- A sore on the breast that does not heal

Orthopedic Examination

Orthopedic examinations may require examination of any bony area of the body. All bones of the body are covered with skin and other tissue. X-rays allow the provider to see bones. When injury to a bone occurs, the muscle, tendons, and soft tissue around the injury also require treatment. See Chapter 19 regarding physical therapy for various treatments. See Table 23.11 for conditions affecting bones, possible treatments, and patient education.

Table 23.11 ■ Conditions Affecting Bones, Possible Treatments, and Patient Education

Condition	Possible Treatments	Patient Education
Arthritis	Medication Heat Rest, sometimes Therapy Surgery	1. Provide written information on activities of daily living, medication, exercise, diet, and treatments. 2. Promote a lifestyle that encourages patient's highest physical potential.
Fracture	Medication Bedrest Heat or cold applications	1. Teach cast care. 2. Teach safe movement while wearing a cast. 3. Teach signs of circulation changes. 4. Teach importance of good nutrition.
Scoliosis	Brace Exercise Surgery	1. Teach importance of routine exercise. 2. Encourage the wearing of brace if ordered.
Herniated vertebral disk	Bedrest Traction Therapy Medication Surgery	1. Instruct in use of traction. 2. Provide pre- and postoperative instructions.
Bursitis	Medication Removal of joint fluid Sling Heat Therapy	1. Instruct in application of sling. 2. Instruct in application of heat packs. 3. Provide written instructions on how to prevent bursitis.
Gout	Medication Rest Increased fluid for weight reduction in obese	1. Provide information on medication. 2. Provide instruction in proper diet and provide handout.

⬤ PEDIATRICS

Pediatrics pertains to providing care for children. A pediatrician is a medical doctor specializing in the care of children and infants. Family practice providers also provide medical services for children and infants as well as their parents. There are two types of pediatric appointments:

1. Well-child appointment

2. Sick-child appointment

The well child is checked routinely to evaluate growth and development patterns. Early identification of abnormal development allows quick, effective treatment. Children also receive immunizations at regular intervals. Immunizations prevent many life-threatening diseases.

Education of parents is important with each well check. Giving parents child development information can make your job easier. Parents who are informed about normal development and growth patterns are more relaxed and require less direction. Routine well-child appointments are usually scheduled at the following ages:

- 1 month
- 2 months
- 4 months
- 6 months
- 9 months
- 12 months
- 15 months
- 18 months
- 24 months, and yearly thereafter

The sick child shows signs of infection or disease. Often, sick children wait in a separate waiting room away from well children. This separation helps prevent the spread of infection and disease.

When possible, take the time to show children instruments and other items and to explain how they are used in their care. Children's knowledge and sense of safety make your job more interesting and rewarding.

Childproof your examination and waiting rooms so that they are safe. Never leave a small child alone on an examination table. When weighing infants or giving care, *always* keep one hand on the child to secure its position. When infants or children need treatment that requires them to be absolutely still, restraining procedures are needed. Proper restraint is important to protect the infant/child and ensure accuracy of the procedure.

The parent of a sick child is usually distressed. Take time to explain what you are doing and why you are doing it. Provide the parent with handouts about care and answer questions. Refer a question to the provider if it is out of your scope of training. Your active listening and patience will help calm the parent.

Review Chapter 9 to better understand normal development and birth defects. Review Figure 23.1 for an example of growth charts.

⬤ MINOR SURGICAL PROCEDURES

Surgeries that do not require a general anesthetic or complicated equipment are often considered minor. The following are common minor surgical procedures:

- Suturing lacerations—sewing cuts or separated tissue

■ Incision and drainage (I & D) procedures—opening an abscess (infected area) or cyst (pocket of fluid) and allowing it to drain

■ Removal of foreign bodies from subcutaneous tissue

■ Removal of warts, moles, and skin tags

■ Biopsy—taking small pieces of tissue for microscopic examination

■ Cauterization—burning of small areas of tissue to remove tissue or stop bleeding

Guidelines to Follow When Preparing for Surgical Procedures in the Office

1. Reinforce all instructions given patient by physician/surgeon.
2. Explain all procedures simply, clearly, and calmly.
3. Obtain witnessed informed operative consent for all surgical procedures.
4. Patients having surgical procedures that require IV push, preoperative medication, and local anesthesia must have someone to drive them home following the procedure.
5. Assess the patient's stress level. Note symptoms, address them appropriately, and document them.
6. Assess vital signs every 15 minutes during surgery.
7. Follow Standard Precautions.
8. Complete surgical skin preparation following the physician's order.
9. Have emergency equipment available.
10. Maintain sterile technique during procedures.
11. Apply sterile dressings according to the physician's order.
12. Monitor patients for ½ hour following procedure or until stable for discharge.
13. Discharge all patients from surgery by wheelchair or according to facility policy.

Familiarize yourself with the most common surgical instruments. Give special attention to details. You are responsible for quick, easy identification of instruments when assisting a physician (see pictures of surgical instruments in your Student Workbook).

Suture material and needles are a part of most surgical trays. Familiarize yourself with needle types (see Figure 23.14) and various suture materials (cotton, silk, nylon, catgut, and wire are a few). The size or gauge of sutures is labeled in 0s. A suture label reading 0 contains a thick suture material; a package label that reads 00,000 (5-0) contains a thin suture material. Most suture materials are measured in 0s ranging from 0 to 0,000,000,000 (10-0). Suture packages indicate the type and size of suture needle in the package; if no needle is included, the picture of the needle is absent.

Prepare a patient and surgical room as described on page 643.

Following surgery it is important to clean up and process equipment and used supplies. Always remember to follow Standard Precautions and dispose of hazardous materials according to facility procedures.

Figure 23.14

Types of suture material.

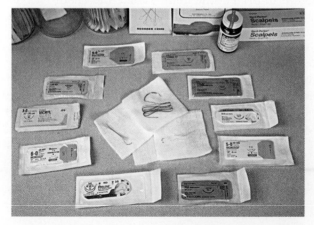

PROCEDURE 23.22

SURGICAL SETUP

RATIONALE

A sterile surgical setup provides a sterile field and sterile supplies and equipment for invasive procedures. Following the procedure is essential to prevent contamination. Con-tamination allows bacteria to enter the body and may cause infection.

1. Wash hands.

2. Assemble equipment and supplies.
   a. Mayo stand or surgical table
   b. Sterile items:
      Fenestrated drape
      Nonfenestrated drape
      Medicine glass for anesthesia
      Sponges, 4 × 4
      5-cc syringe or control syringe
      Needles: 18 gauge–1 inch, 25 gauge–½ or
        1½ inch (or size physician prefers)
      Cautery (physician preference—electric or
        battery)
      Suture material (physician preference)
      Instruments
      Gloves
      Gowns (physician preference)
      Specimen containers
   c. Mask
   d. Cap
   e. Goggles and/or face shield
   f. Lab requisitions
   g. Anesthetic (physician preference)

3. Take patient/client to surgical area.

4. Explain the procedure and check to see if informed consent is signed.

5. Reassure patient.

6. Instruct patient to remove clothing and put on exam gown.

7. Wash hands.

8. Open a sterile drape or towel and place on Mayo stand, or place largest package on a flat surface and open. The outer wrap will serve as a barrier between table and sterile items. This creates a sterile field to work on.

NOTE Be sure Mayo stand is dry. A wet drape allows microorganisms to enter sterile field.

9. Position package so that first edge unfolded will be pulled away from you. (By opening away from you with first motion, you will not have to reach across area again.)
   a. Remove tape.
   b. Loosen corner tucked in at taped edge.
   c. Open by pulling away from you and placing open edges straight across from you.

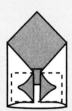

d. Slowly pull corners at right and left of package, opening sides. This exposes inside of package.

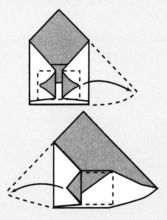

e. Carefully pull back on corner pointing toward you.

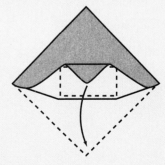

10. Open all supplies and equipment and drop onto sterile field.

11. Cover sterile field with a sterile drape.

12. Position patient at physician's request.

13. Assist as physician requests.

NOTE If you need to handle sterile items, follow next procedure for putting on sterile gloves and removing gloves.

PROCEDURE 23.23 PUTTING ON STERILE GLOVES AND REMOVING GLOVES

RATIONALE

Sterile gloves cover the hands and allow treatment of open skin areas. Following the procedure is essential to prevent contamination of the gloves. Contamination allows bacteria to enter the treatment area and may cause infection.

1. Wash hands.
2. Pick up wrapped gloves.
3. Check to be certain that they are sterile.
   a. Package intact
   b. Seal of sterility
4. Place on clean, flat surface.
5. Open wrapper by handling only the outside. (Figures a and b).

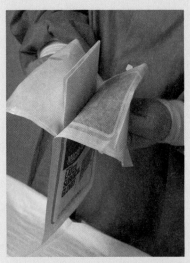

a

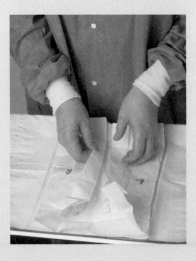

b

6. Use your left hand to pick up the right-handed glove at folded cuff edge, touching only the inside of glove (Figure c).

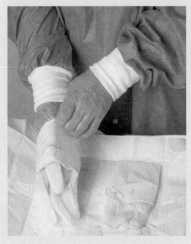

c

7. Put glove on right hand (Figure d).

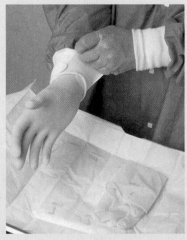

d

8. Use gloved right hand to pick up left-handed glove (Figures e–f).
   a. Place finger of gloved right hand under cuff of left-handed glove.

PROCEDURE 23.23 | PUTTING ON STERILE GLOVES AND REMOVING GLOVES
(Continued)

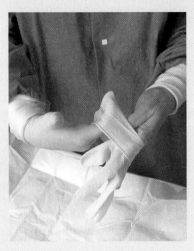

e

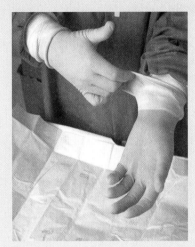

f

b. Lift glove up and away from wrapper to pull onto left hand.

c. Continue pulling left glove under wrist. (Be certain that gloved right thumb does not touch skin or clothing.)

9. Place fingers under cuff of right glove and pull cuff up over right wrist with gloved left hand.

10. Adjust fingers of gloves as necessary.

If either glove tears, remove and discard. Begin with new gloves!

11. Turn gloves inside out as you remove them; dispose of with hazardous materials.

PROCEDURE 23.24 | TAKING DOWN A SURGICAL SETUP

RATIONALE

Instruments are contaminated with blood and body fluids. Correctly breaking down a surgical setup after surgery prevents injury and possible infection to the health care workers.

ALERT: Follow Standard Precautions.

1. Assemble supplies.
   a. Exam gloves
   b. Sharps container
   c. Double red bags in red container
   d. Double red bags
   e. Laundry hamper
   f. Basins
   g. Gown and mask
   h. Detergent
   i. Bacteriocidal
   j. Nonpermeable gloves
   k. Face shield/eye goggle and nose/mouth shield
   l. Nonpermeable gown

2. Wash hands thoroughly.

3. Put on nonpermeable disposable gloves, gown, and face shield.

PROCEDURE 23.24   TAKING DOWN A SURGICAL SETUP *(Continued)*

4. Check Mayo stand to ensure that specimen has been placed in properly labeled specimen container.

5. Place container on counter with lab requisition.

6. Using a Kelly clamp or long-handle forceps, remove all items from tray. Place

    a. Syringes and needles in sharps container

    b. Suture needles in sharps container

    c. Scalpel blade and handle in sharps container

    d. Cautery blade (if it is disposable) in sharps container

    e. Used sponges in biohazardous waste

    f. All instruments in basins with cleaning/disinfecting solutions

    g. All paper material (drapes, towels, etc.) in biohazardous waste

    h. Bloody linens (cloth towels and/or drapes), if used, in double red bag in laundry hamper

7. Remove and discard exam gloves in biohazardous waste.

8. Wash hands thoroughly.

9. Put on disposable gloves.

10. Spray surgical table and Mayo stand with germicide.

11. Discard disposable suction tip (if used) in biohazardous waste.

12. Empty suction bottle (if used) in hopper or toilet.

13. Thoroughly rinse suction tubing and bottle with clear water.

14. Soak suction bottle and tubing (if used) in cleaning agent for 10 minutes, then rinse with water.

15. Discard gloves in biohazardous waste.

16. Put on nonpermeable gloves.

17. Soak suction bottle and tubing (if used) in bacteriocidal for 10 minutes.

18. Rinse suction bottle and tubing (if used) with water.

19. Wash instruments according to facility procedure.

20. Remove gloves.

21. Wash hands thoroughly.

22. Take specimen to lab with completed requisition.

NOTE   Carefully follow facility policies and procedures when working with hazardous material.

PROCEDURE 23.25   CHANGING A STERILE DRESSING

RATIONALE

Proper technique in changing a sterile dressing prevents wound infection and contamination to the health care worker.

ALERT: Follow Standard Precautions.

1. Wash hands.

2. Assemble supplies.

    a. Pair of nonsterile examination gloves

    b. Pair of sterile examination gloves

    c. Sterile dressing material

    d. Tape

    e. Biohazardous waste container

3. Explain procedure to patient.

4. Position patient/client.

5. Put on nonsterile gloves.

6. Remove soiled dressing and examination gloves.

7. Discard in biohazardous waste container.

8. Wash hands.

9. Set up sterile tray.

    a. Place sterile drape on Mayo stand.

    b. Open and place all sterile dressing supplies on sterile field.

    c. Pour wound-cleaning solution or antiseptic into sterile container.

10. Put on sterile gloves.

11. Medicate wound as directed by physician.

12. Apply a double layer of gauze to wound or incision.

NOTE   If moderate to heavy drainage is expected, reinforce dressing. If drainage seeps through to outer layer, wound will be contaminated.

PROCEDURE 23.25 | CHANGING A STERILE DRESSING *(Continued)*

13. Remove gloves and place in biohazardous waste container.
14. Wash hands.
15. Secure dressing with tape.
16. Document the following:

   a. Date
   b. Time
   c. Type of dressing applied
   d. Appearance of wound
   e. Your name and certification

> 12/10/04   1300
>
> Telfa dressing to open wound on
> left, lower abdominal quadrant
> following sterile procedure
> No redness or heat around wound
> Tolerated well with no complaints of
> pain
>
> ———— T. Hoen CMA

PUBLIC HEALTH REPORTING

Some conditions require filing an official report. These reports concern public health issues.

1. Communicable, reportable diseases are identified by the local health agency.
2. Animal bites and scratches are usually reportable to the local public health agency or animal control authority.
3. Real or suspected child abuse is reported to local authorities according to your facility's policy. Child abuse is defined as abuse to a person under the age of 18. The following are examples of abuse:

   a. A physical injury that is inflicted on a child by other than accidental means b. Sexual assault of a child c. Sexual **exploitation** of a child d. Willful cruelty or unjustifiable punishment of a child e. **Corporal** punishment or injury f. **Neglect** g. Abuse in out-of-home care
4. Real or suspected elder abuse or abuse of a dependent adult is reported to local authorities according to your facility's policy.
5. Disorders characterized by a lapse of consciousness are usually reported to the department of motor vehicles or a local health agency.

Reporting conditions such as those listed above protect others from disease or injury. Each state's requirements differ. Learn what reports your state or county requires to protect public health.

exploitation
To use another person for profit or enjoyment.

corporal
Bodily. For example, corporal punishment involves hitting or harming the body.

neglect
To ignore or not provide for.

PHARMACOLOGY AND MEDICATION ADMINISTRATION

Working with medication and administering medication are serious responsibilities. As a medical assistant you are responsible for the following:

- Administering medication
- Being aware of side effects
- Interpreting prescriptions
- Reinforcing the provider's instructions
- Recognizing adverse effects of medications

■ Reporting accurate observations

■ Using references to obtain directions

Common Prescription Abbreviations

Special abbreviations and symbols are used when working with medication. To understand and communicate about medication use the following abbreviations:

cap(s)	capsule(s)
dil	dilute
dr	dram
D/W	dextrose in water
fl or fld	fluid
gal	gallon
gt or gtt	drop
IM	intramuscular
IU	international units
IV	intravenous
kg	kilogram
L	liter
liq	liquid
m or min	minim
mcg	microgram
mEq	milliequivalent
mg	milligram
ml	milliliter
NS	normal saline
OD	right eye
oint	ointment
OS	left eye
OU	both eyes
oz	ounce
pt	pint or patient
pulv	powder
sc or subc or subq	subcutaneous
tinc or tr or tinct	tincture

Legal Issues

There are federal guidelines regulating the manufacture, distribution, dispensing, and sale of medication. Federal regulations are monitored by the Drug Enforcement Agency (DEA) of the Department of Justice. Federal legislation controls the distribution of drugs. State regulations are monitored by the State Department of Health and Human Services.

The medical assistant assists the provider by

■ Monitoring expiration dates of the physician's DEA registration.

■ Keeping records and inventory that are legally acceptable.

- Controlling access to all drugs, controlled substances, and prescription pads.
- Destroying medication when expired. Disposal of controlled substances must be witnessed.

Drugs that can cause addiction and abuse are divided into five groups, called schedules. Each schedule names the drugs and explains their ability to become addicting and/or abused (see Table 23.12).

Table 23.12 ■ Schedule of Controlled Substances

The drugs and drug products that come under the jurisdiction of the Controlled Substances Act are divided into five schedules. Some examples from each schedule are outlined below. For a complete listing of all of the controlled substances, contact any office of the Drug Enforcement Administration or log on to www.DEA.GOV and click on "Drug Scheduling."

SCHEDULE I SUBSTANCES   The substances in this schedule are those that have no accepted medical use in the United States and have a high abuse potential.

acetylmethadol	marijuana	N-ethylamphetamine
dihydromorphine	MDMA (Ecstasy)	peyote
fenethylline	mescaline	psilocybin
heroin	methaqualone	tilidine
LSD		

SCHEDULE II SUBSTANCES   The substances in this schedule have a high abuse potential with severe psychic or physical dependence liability. Schedule II controlled substances consist of certain narcotic, stimulant, and depressant drugs.

amobarbital	meperidine (Demerol)	oxymorphone (Numorphan)
amphetamine (Dexedrine)	methadone	pantopon
cocaine	methamphetamine (Desoxyn)	pentobarbital
codeine	methylphenidate (Ritalin)	phenmetrazine (Preludin)
dronabinol	morphine	phenylacetone
etorphine hydrochloride	nabilone	secobarbital
fentanyl (Sublimaze)	opium	sufentanil
hydromorphone (Dilaudid)	oxycodone (Percodan)	

SCHEDULE III SUBSTANCES   The substances in this schedule have an abuse potential less than those in Schedules I and II, and include compounds containing limited quantities of certain narcotic drugs and non-narcotic drugs.

Tylenol with Codeine derivatives of barbituric acid	chlorphentermine	pentobarbital compounds
amobarbital compounds	clortermine	phendimetrazine
benphetamine	nalorphine	secobarbital compounds
	paregoric	

SCHEDULE IV SUBSTANCES   The substances in this schedule have an abuse potential less than those listed in Schedule III.

alprazolam (Xanax)	ethinamate (Valmid)	midazolam (Versed)
barbital	fenfluramine	oxazepam (Serax)
chloral hydrate	flurazepam (Dalmane)	pentazocine (Talwin-NX)
chlordiazepoxide (Librium)	halazepam (Paxipam)	phenobarbital
clonazepam (Clonapin)	lorazepam (Ativan)	phentermine
clorazepate (Tranxene)	mebutamate	prazepam (Verstran)
detropropoxyphene (Darvon)	meprobamate (Equanil, Miltown)	quazepam (Dormalin)
diazepam (Valium)	methohexital	temazepam (Restoril)
diethylpropion	methylphenobarbital	triazolam (Halcion)
ethclorovynol (Placidyl) paraldehyde		

SCHEDULE V SUBSTANCES   The substances in this schedule have an abuse potential less than those listed in Schedule IV and consist primarily of preparations containing limited quantities of certain narcotic and stimulant drugs generally for antitussive, antidiarrheal, and analgesic purposes. Two examples are buprenorphine and propylhexedrine.

Prescriptions

Prescription drugs are medications that require monitoring by a licensed physician. The Federal Drug Administration determines which drugs must be prescribed by a physician. Prescriptions are instructions to a pharmacist to supply the patient with medication in a specified amount. The prescription also provides directions for taking medication. The prescription is a legal document. There are six parts to complete in a prescription:

1. Patient information and superscription
   - Date • Client's name • Client's address • Age, if child • Rx, meaning "recipe" or "take thou"
2. Inscription
   - Name of medication • Amount of medication
3. Subscription
   - Directions to pharmacist
4. Sig or signa
   - Directions to patient
5. Physician's signature and address, registry number, and controlled substances approval number (BNDD)
6. Number of times, if any, the prescription can be refilled

Medication/drugs are described in three ways:

1. A brand name is assigned to a drug by the manufacturer. The brand name is commonly used in advertising a medication.
2. A generic name often describes the chemical makeup or classification of a drug. Generic names are adopted by the U.S. Adopted Name Council (USAN); Pharmacopia (USP), *a database catalog;* or the United States National Formulary (NF), *the dictionary of drug names.*
3. The chemical name reflects the chemicals in the drug and its structure.

The cost of generic medication is usually less than that of brand-name medication. Patients save money if the doctor prescribes the generic form or tells the patient that a generic medication is acceptable.

Drug Reference Books

There are so many medications available that it is difficult to remember all the important information. To determine the best medication for a patient, doctors often refer to reference books. The following paragraphs briefly describe the most frequently used reference books.

The *United States Pharmacopia* (USP)–*National Formulary* (NF) is published every 5 years. The publication lists only official drugs, and it identifies drug standards. The NF chapter explains the ingredients of each drug. Drug information includes the following:

- Description of drug
- Standards for purity
- Strength and composition
- Storage
- Use
- Dosage

American Medical Association Drug Evaluations is a periodically revised book of officially established and recognized drug names and standards.

The *Physicians' Desk Reference* (PDR) is not an official drug reference book but is the most commonly used. It is published annually; periodic (twice yearly) supplements provide information on newest medications. The PDR contains the following information:

■ Partial list of drug manufacturers, including their addresses

■ Emergency telephone number

■ Brand-name drugs (Section 2, pink pages)

■ Drugs listed by category or classification (Section 3, blue pages)

■ Drugs listed by generic and chemical names (Section 4, yellow pages)

■ Locations of poison control centers (following Section 4) (Section 5)

■ Pictures of drugs with their manufacturers

■ Each drug's composition, uses and action, administration, dosage, precautions, contraindications, and side effects, and its common, generic, and chemical names (Section 6, the largest section of white pages)

■ List of manufacturers of diagnostic drugs and the uses of those drugs (Section 7, green pages)

American Hospital Formulary Services (AHFS) provides periodic supplements that maintain current information. This publication gives unbiased drug information. Drugs are listed by generic names according to their therapeutic or pharmacological class.

It is important for MAs to understand how to use reference books. MAs are responsible for giving medication correctly. Drug reference books provide guidelines for responsible administration of prescribed medication. The *Physicians' Desk Reference* is the most available reference.

Using the *Physician's Desk Reference* (PDR)

The PDR can be used in a variety of ways. To demonstrate this we will use the example of a patient who hands you an oval-shaped pill with Wallace 200 stamped on it. You can take that pill to the PDR and compare it with the pictures in Section 5. An exact comparison indicates that Wallace is the manufacturer and 200 is the dose. To become more familiar with the PDR, follow the steps in this procedure.

PROCEDURE 23.26   USING THE *PHYSICIANS' DESK REFERENCE* (PDR)

RATIONALE

It is essential for the health care worker to know details about medications. The PDR is an essential tool that provides information about medications the health care worker gives. Understanding how to use the PDR helps in finding information in a timely manner.

1. Identify the name of the manufacturer by going to Section 5; compare the tablet with pictures to identify the medication.

   a. Wallace is the manufacturer.
   b. Turn to the page where Wallace pills are displayed.
   c. Match the pill with pictures of pills displayed.

   d. A yellow oval pill marked "Wallace 200" matches "Soma Compound with Codeine 200 mg" in the display.

2. Turn to Section 2, the pink pages. Find "Soma Compound with Codeine 200 mg." Two page numbers are listed.

   a. The first page number refers to Section 5, the picture of the medication.

PROCEDURE 23.26   **USING THE *PHYSICIANS' DESK REFERENCE* (PDR)**
(Continued)

b. The second page number refers to Section 6 and provides product information.

3. Turn to the page number indicated in Section 6 to find specific drug information.

   a. Description of drug
   b. Clinical pharmacology
   c. Indications and usage (describes the reasons for using the drug)
   d. Contraindications (reasons not to give this drug)
   e. Warnings
   f. Precautions

g. Dosage and administration
h. How supplied
i. Storage recommendations

4. Go to Section 1 for more information about a drug. Find the manufacturer:

   a. Wallace Laboratories is listed with the *W*'s in the alphabetical list.
   b. Write requests for information using the address supplied.
   c. Call for assistance using the professional services telephone number or night and weekend emergency number if available.

Storage and Handling of Drugs

Medication requires special handling. To ensure the safekeeping of medications, always:

- Keep medications in a locked area away from other supplies.
- Keep medications in original containers.
- Refrigerate medications that require storage at lower than room temperatures.
- Rotate medications so that the oldest are used before expiration dates.
- Destroy expired medications. (Follow office policy when destroying medication.)
- Keep medications requiring darkness out of the light (in a dark cupboard or container).
- Be aware of medications that react with other materials (for example, some medications react with plastic so must be stored in glass).

To organize the storage of drugs, use a simple, logical system. One example of a system is alphabetic arrangement by classification—for example, all **antibiotics** together, **contraceptives** together, **diuretics** together. Within each classification, separate oral, **parenteral, topical,** and other medications. Federal law requires that you place all controlled substances (see Table 23.12) in a locked cabinet safely separated from other medications. Any controlled substances that are lost or stolen must be reported by the physician to the Drug Enforcement Agency.

Drug Dosage

Giving the right medication dosage is an important part of administering medication. Many medications are prepackaged and ready to give. Some medications require dosage calculation. A simple **formula** for calculating dosage is

$$\frac{\text{dosage you want}}{\text{dosage you have}} = \text{dosage you give}$$

Example: The physician orders 200 mg (milligrams) of a medication. You have 100-mg tablets of the medication.

$$\frac{\text{dosage you want}}{\text{dosage you have}} = \frac{200 \text{ mg}}{100\text{-mg tablets}} = \text{you give two tablets}$$

antibiotics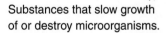
Substances that slow growth of or destroy microorganisms.

contraceptives
Items that serve to prevent pregnancy.

diuretics
Drugs that increase urine output.

parenteral
Not in the digestive system (e.g., injections are parenterally administered).

topical
Surface of the body.

formula
Accepted rule (e.g., a math formula and a baby formula are both guidelines or rules).

Divide 200 mg by 100 mg:

$$100\overline{)200} \atop \underline{200}$$

$$\overset{2}{100\overline{)200}}$$

The patient needs to take two tablets to receive 200 mg of the ordered medicine.

The medication that the doctor orders must be measured in the same terms as the medication you have on hand. For example, if the physician orders a medication in milligrams and you have doses measured in grams, you must convert milligrams to grams. To convert measures, see Table 23.13 or use the following easy steps:

■ To convert grams to grains or grains to grams, you must learn that 1 g = 15 gr.

■ To convert grams to grains, multiply the number of grams × 15. *Example:* 30 g × 15 = 450 gr

■ To convert grains to grams, divide the number of grains by 15. *Example:* 450 gr ÷ 15 = 30 g

■ To convert grams to milligrams, move the decimal three places to the right. *Example:* 1 g = 1,000 mg (1 g = 1,000. mg)

■ To convert milligrams to grams, move the decimal three places to the left. *Example:* 1,000 mg = 1 g (1,000. mg = 1.000 g)

Table 23.13 ▪ Metric Dosage and Apothecary Equivalents

Liquid Measure		Weight	
Metric	**Approximate Apothecary Equivalents**	**Metric**	**Approximate Apothecary Equivalents**
1,000 mL	1 quart = 1 L	30 g	1 ounce
750 mL	1½ pints	15 g	4 drams
500 mL	1 pint	10 g	2½ drams
250 mL	8 fluidounces	7.5 g	2 drams
200 mL	7 fluidounces	6 g	90 grains
100 mL	3½ fluidounces	5 g	75 grains
50 mL	1¾ fluidounces	3 g	45 grains
30 mL	1 fluidounce	2 g	30 grains (½ dram)
15 mL	4 fluidrams	1.5 g	22 grains
10 mL	2½ fluidrams	1 g	15 grains
8 mL	2 fluidrams	0.75 g	12 grains
5 mL	1¼ fluidrams	0.6 g	10 grains
4 mL	1 fluidram	0.5 g	7½ grains
3 mL	45 minims	0.4 g	6 grains
2 mL	30 minims	0.3 g	5 grains
1 mL	15 minims	0.25 g	4 grains
0.75 mL	12 minims	0.2 g	3 grains
0.6 mL	10 minims	0.15 g	2½ grains
0.5 mL	8 minims	0.12 g	2 grains
0.3 mL	5 minims	0.1 g	1½ grains
0.25 mL	4 minims	75 mg	1¼ grains
0.2 mL	3 minims	60 mg	1 grain
0.1 mL	1½ minims	50 mg	¾ grain
0.06 mL	1 minim	40 mg	⅔ grain
0.05 mL	¾ minim	30 mg	½ grain
0.03 mL	½ minim	25 mg	⅜ grain
		20 mg	⅓ grain
		15 mg	¼ grain
		12 mg	⅕ grain
		10 mg	⅙ grain

Table 23.13 ▪ Continued

Liquid Measure		Weight	
Metric	**Approximate Apothecary Equivalents**	**Metric**	**Approximate Apothecary Equivalents**
		8 mg	⅛ grain
		6 mg	1/10 grain
		5 mg	1/12 grain
		4 mg	1/15 grain
		3 mg	1/20 grain
		2 mg	1/30 grain
		1.5 mg	1/40 grain
		1.2 mg	1/50 grain
		1 mg	1/60 grain
		0.8 mg	1/80 grain
		0.6 mg	1/100 grain
		0.5 mg	1/120 grain
		0.4 mg	1/150 grain
		0.3 mg	1/200 grain
		0.25 mg	1/250 grain
		0.2 mg	1/300 grain
		0.15 mg	1/400 grain
		0.12 mg	1/500 grain
		0.1 mg	1/600 grain

Some measurements and equivalents* for pouring medicines (to be memorized):

04 mL (4–5 mL)	=	1 teaspoon	or	1 dram	or	60 drops (gtt)
01 mL	=	¼ teaspoon	or	¼ dram	or	15–16 drops (gtt)
02 mL	=	½ teaspoon	or	½ dram	or	30–32 drops (gtt)
15 mL	=	3 teaspoons	or	4 drams	or	½ ounce (oz)
30 mL	=	6 teaspoons	or	8 drams	or	1 ounce (oz)
1 tablespoon	=	3 teaspoons	or	15 mL	or	½ ounce (oz)
2 tablespoons	=	6 teaspoons	or	30 mL	or	1 ounce (oz)
6 fluidounces	=	1 teacupful	or	150–180 mL		
8 fluidounces	=	1 glassful	or	240–250 mL		
2 pints	=	1 quart	or	1,000 mL		
4 quarts	=	1 gallon	or	4,000 mL		

* These equivalents are approximate only. In practice, the cubic centimeter and the milliliter are equal. Actually, the cubic centimeter is less than the milliliter by 0.000028 cc.

Review Chapter 7, Unit 2. This review will help you remember common medical weights and measures. Use the formula in Chapter 7 to review and practice changing or converting the following:

■ Ounces (oz) to cubic centimeters (cc) or milliliters

■ Milliliters (mL) to ounces (oz)

■ Pounds (lb) to kilograms (kg)

■ Kilograms (kg) to pounds (lb)

Administering Medications

To prevent mistakes and injury to the patient, always follow carefully the six "rights" of medication administration:

1. Right drug

2. Right dose

3. Right route of administration

4. Right time

5. Right patient

6. Right documentation

Guidelines for Preparing and Administering Medications

1. Wash hands.

2. Follow only written medication orders.

3. Do not allow yourself to be distracted while preparing medication.

4. Always read the medication label three times:

a. When taking it from the shelf (do not use medication that is not clearly labeled) b. Before measuring the ordered amount c. When returning the container to the shelf or discarding it

5. Know the drug you are giving. Look it up in one of the reference books to confirm the expected action, dosage, and route of administration.

6. Calculate the ordered dosage if necessary. Verify calculations with a co-worker.

7. Measure medications.

a. Measure solid medications such as pills, tablets, or capsules by dropping the medication from the package into a medicine cup. b. Observe liquid medications for

- Color change • Cloudiness • Sedimentation

NOTE If these conditions exist, discard the medication.

c. Always have a second nurse verify order, dose, and measured medication in syringe when giving

- Insulin • Heparin

d. Gently shake emulsions and suspensions to mix ingredients completely. Shaking distributes all of the ingredients equally. This allows you to give accurate amounts of all ingredients. e. When pouring liquids, place the label of the bottle in the palm of your hand to keep liquid from dripping on label.

Table 23.14 ■ Medication Administration Procedures

Administration Route	Type of Medication	Administration Procedure
Buccal	Tablets	Tablet placed between the gums and cheek of the mouth; absorbed as tablet dissolves
Inhalation	Medicated aerosols, mists, sprays, streams	Liquid medication inhaled through nebulizer, respirator, or inhalation device
Irrigation	Solutions	Solution washed through a body cavity or over a membrane
Installation	Solutions	Medication dropped into area requiring treatment, such as ear or eye
Injunction or topical	Liniments, lotions, ointments, powders, solutions, sprays, tinctures	Medication applied to skin (use gloves to apply)
Oral	Capsules, pills, solutions, spansules, tablets	Medication taken by mouth and swallowed
Parenteral	Sterile solutions	Medicated solution injected into body tissue and absorbed
Rectal	Suppositories, solutions	Medicated solution or suppository inserted into rectum
Sublingual	Tablets	Tablet placed under the tongue to dissolve
Vaginal	Creams, foams, liquids, ointments, solutions, suppositories	Medication applied, inserted, or irrigated (douche)

f. Pour the liquid into a medicine cup; hold at eye level to achieve an accurate measure. g. Clean the neck of the medication bottle before capping. h. Never mix two or more medications unless ordered (check compatibility).

ALERT: Follow Standard Precautions.

8. Apply topical medications to the skin, mucous membrane (including vaginal creams and suppositories), or the cornea of the eye. Always follow the specific directions on the medication. Use aseptic technique to prevent contamination of medication.

9. Never leave medication unattended. Prepare medication and administer immediately. Watch the patient swallow oral medication.

10. Never administer medication prepared by another person.

11. Always verify the patient's name and the order on the chart to ensure that the right medication is given to the right patient.

12. Check patient allergies before administering medication. Look at allergies listed on patient's chart and ask patient if he or she is allergic to the medication.

NOTE Medication can be given in a rectal suppository if the client/patient cannot take by mouth. Use the following procedure when a suppository is ordered.

PROCEDURE 23.27

ADMINISTERING A RECTAL SUPPOSITORY

RATIONALE

Rectal suppositories are used for many reasons. Your proper administration of a rectal suppository prevents in-jury to the mucous membrane and ensures that medication is absorbed correctly.

ALERT: Follow Standard Precautions.

1. Wash hands.
2. Assemble supplies.
   a. Gloves
   b. Suppository
   c. Lubricant
3. Verify medication with physician's order.
4. Identify patient/client.
5. Confirm known medication allergies with patient.
6. Position patient in left Sims' position (see Procedure 23.12).
7. Put on examination gloves.
8. Remove suppository from wrapper.
9. Lubricate tip of suppository.
10. Separate buttocks with gloved hand.
11. Instruct patient to take a deep breath.
12. Insert suppository, tapered end first, into rectum.
13. Use forefinger to advance suppository along rectal wall toward the umbilicus for approximately 3 inches.
14. Hold patient's buttocks together for several seconds or until urge to defecate subsides.

15. Encourage patient to retain suppository for at least 20 minutes.
16. Clean excess lubricant from anus.
17. Remove gloves and discard in biohazardous waste.
18. Document the following:
    a. Date
    b. Time
    c. Route
    d. Medication
    e. Dose
    f. Expiration date
    g. Lot number
    h. Signature and certification

11/30/03   1330

Compazine suppository (Exp. date 10/11/04, lot #223) inserted into rectum

1415

Patient states nausea decreased and no emesis since 1320

_____ H. Alhusdi CMA

13. Observe the patient for unusual reactions. It is good practice to keep the patient for 15 to 20 minutes after:

a. A first-time dose of antibiotic b. A large dose of antibiotic c. An insulin injection d. Administration of allergy serums

14. Discard unused or refused medications. *Never return medication to original containers.*

15. Notify the physician immediately if medication is refused.

16. Record the following on the correct chart:

a. Date b. Time c. Drug d. Amount given e. Route of administration f. Lot number of medication g. Manufacturer's name h. Expiration date

See Table 23.14 for a description of how medications are given.

Medication Administration by Injection

Injections, shots, and hypodermics are parenteral methods of giving medication. The word *hypodermic* means "under the skin." Hypodermic injections put medication under the skin. The medication and needle size determine the depth of the injection. Medications are given by injection to

- Achieve a fast response
- Ensure that the correct amount is administered
- Provide medication when it cannot be given another way
- Provide anesthesia to a specific part of the body
- Place medication in a specific area, such as a joint

Do not give injections in body areas that are

- Burned
- Cyanotic (bluish color)
- Close to large blood vessels, bones, or nerves
- Swollen
- Bruised, injured, or scarred
- Unusual in skin texture or color, or enlarged (for example, moles or warts)

Syringes

Syringes are measuring devices that allow you to force medication through a needle at the tip of the syringe. See Figure 23.15 to identify the parts of a syringe. Syringe sizes vary from very small to 60 mL. The most commonly used syringe is 3 cc/mL.

Tuberculin Syringe

Special syringes are used for administration of small doses. A tuberculin syringe measures up to 1 cc/mL (see Figure 23.16). Note the very fine calibrations on the syringe. These special syringes allow you to measure as small as 0.1 cc. Use this type of syringe for allergy testing and tuberculin skin testing.

Insulin Syringe

An insulin syringe measures insulin in unit measures (see Figure 23.17). Syringe size is determined by the patient's required dosage. The most commonly used are U50 or U100 syringes.

Needles

Needles that attach to syringes for injection come in different lengths and diameters of needle opening (**lumen**). Length of needles for medication administration ranges

lumen

Opening (e.g., opening in a tube or needle).

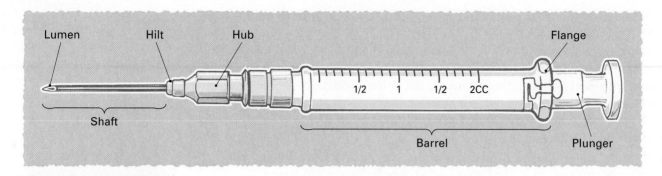

Figure 23.15

A hypodermic needle.

Figure 23.16

Tuberculin syringe.

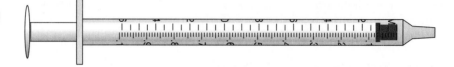

Figure 23.17

Insulin syringes measure in units.

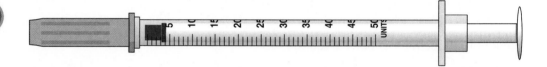

from ½ to 2 inches. You determine needle length according to where you want the medication in the tissue. For example:

- An intradermal injection requires a short, ½- to ⅝-inch needle for medication that goes just under the skin.

- An intramuscular injection requires a needle that is long enough to reach the muscle, usually 1½ to 2 inches.

- A subcutaneous injection requires a ⅝- to 1-inch needle to reach subcutaneous tissue.

Needle diameter, also called needle gauge, describes the size of the opening in the needle. Needle gauges range between 14 and 27. As the number of the gauge increases, the diameter of the needle opening *(lumen)* decreases. For example, a 25-gauge needle has a small opening (lumen). A 16-gauge needle has a large opening (lumen).

Preventing Needle Sticks

Needle sticks injure the skin and introduce infectious agents into the body. Accidental needle sticks that occur after an injection is given can be serious. An accidental needle stick can transfer a disease from one person to another. Transfer of Hepatitis B and AIDS is of greatest concern. (See Tables 23.2 and 23.3 for Standard Precaution task categorization, page 612.) To prevent accidental needle sticks:

1. *Never* recap a needle after giving an injection.
2. *Never* lay down a syringe after giving an injection.

3. Immediately trigger the automatic sharps protective device and place the syringe in a puncture-resistant, leakproof container (a sharps container).

4. Empty sharps containers when they are three-fourths full.

5. Close lid tightly on a sharps container when moving it.

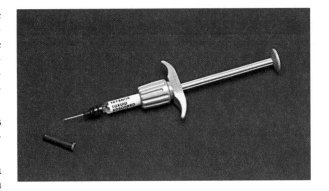

Figure 23.18

Unit-dose cartridge.

Preparing Parenteral Medication

Medication comes in many different types of containers. The following are the most common:

- *Prefilled unit-dose disposable syringes or cartridges* (see Figure 23.18).
- *Ampule.* Small glass container with a narrow neck, allowing for **aspiration** of medication.
- *Vial.* Closed glass container with rubber stopper. Vials are simple unit-dose or multidose containers. Some vials contain powdered medicine and require mixing **(reconstituting)** with a **diluent.** A thin metal flap covers the rubber stopper. Take precautions to prevent cutting your finger when lifting this metal flap.

aspiration

Withdrawal of a fluid.

reconstituting

Adding water to a powdered drug.

diluent

Liquid added to powder that dissolves the powder.

Various Methods of Giving Injections

There are five common methods for giving injections. Each method allows the medication to be absorbed in a different way. The following paragraphs and procedures describe four of these methods. (Medical assistants are not legally approved to use the fifth method, intravenous injection.)

PROCEDURE 23.28 OPENING AN AMPULE AND ASPIRATING MEDICATION

RATIONALE

Checking medication three times prevents giving the patient the wrong medication. Opening ampules according to the procedure prevents glass chips from contaminating medication and possible injury to the health care worker.

1. Wash hands.
2. Assemble supplies.
   a. Alcohol wipe
   b. Medication ampule
   c. Ampule file
   d. Gauze, 2 × 2
3. Check medication label against physician's order when taking ampule from shelf.
4. Tap stem of ampule lightly to empty medication into ampule.
5. Cleanse neck of ampule with alcohol wipe.

6. Place gauze at neck.
7. Hold ampule between fingers at top and bottom.
8. Snap off the top of ampule with quick movement so that glass fragments catch in gauze.
9. File across narrowest part of neck when difficult to break.
10. Discard top of ampule in sharps container.
11. Check medication label against physician's order.

PROCEDURE 23.28 OPENING AN AMPULE AND ASPIRATING MEDICATION
(Continued)

12. Aspirate medication:

    a. Insert tip of needle into ampule below fluid level.

    b. Draw plunger back to pull appropriate amount of medication into syringe.

13. Remove needle from ampule, being careful not to touch edge of container.

14. Check medication label and dosage against physician's order and discard ampule in sharps container.

15. Turn syringe so that needle is pointing up, tap syringe to move air bubble to tip of syringe, then push air through needle if air bubbles are present.

16. Cover needle according to facility policy.

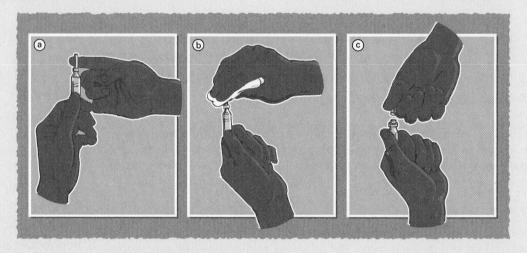

PROCEDURE 23.29 ASPIRATING MEDICATION OR DILUENT FROM A VIAL

RATIONALE

Aspirating medication from a vial requires carefully inserting the needle through the opening of the vial and tipping the vial to ensure that all medication is aspirated into the syringe. It is also important to guard the needle tip from being damaged.

1. Wash hands.

2. Assemble supplies.

    a. Medication vial

    b. Syringe

    c. Alcohol wipe

3. Select the appropriate syringe and needle (attach needle to syringe if necessary).

4. Check medication label against physician's order when taking medication vial from shelf.

5. Remove metal flap from vial and clean top of rubber stopper with alcohol wipe.

6. Carefully remove cap from needle.

7. Draw the same amount of air into syringe as that of medication to be given. (*Example:* Physician's order calls for 1 cc of medication; draw 1 cc of air into syringe.)

8. Check medication label against physician's order before drawing up medication.

9. Puncture rubber stopper on vial top with needle.

10. Push air into medication vial to equalize pressure when medication is aspirated.

11. Aspirate (withdraw) medication into syringe.

12. Remove needle from vial and cover.

13. Check medication label and dosage against physician's order.

14. Return vial to shelf or discard in sharps container.

PROCEDURE 23.30

RECONSTITUTING POWDER DRUGS

RATIONALE

Powdered injectable medication must be diluted with a sterile fluid (dilutant). Your careful measuring of the dilutant helps ensure that a proper dosage is administered.

1. Wash hands.
2. Assemble supplies.
   a. Syringe
   b. Alcohol wipes
   c. Sterile diluent
   d. Medication
3. Check medication label against physician's order when taking vial from shelf.
4. Read reconstitution/dilution instructions on medication vial.
5. Take sterile diluent fluid from shelf and check against medication label.
6. Aspirate diluent (see aspiration procedure).
7. Check medication label against physician's order.
8. Remove metal flap from vial.
9. Clean rubber stopper with alcohol.
10. Select syringe and needle.
11. Remove cap from needle.
12. Puncture rubber stopper of medication vial.
13. Push appropriate amount of diluent into medication vial.
14. Remove needle from vial and dispose of in sharps container.
15. Gently roll medication vial between hands to mix medication powder and diluent.

Intradermal (ID) injections are given just under the surface of the skin (Figure 23.19).

- **Purpose** To administer allergy tests, and some new therapies that stimulate the immune system, tuberculin skin test
- **Amount** Usually between 0.1 and 0.3 mL
- **Sites** Anterior forearm, distal to the antecubital space

Subcutaneous ("sub Q") injections are given in the subcutaneous tissue layer.

- **Purpose** To achieve quick absorption of medication into the bloodstream
- **Amount** No more than 2 mL
- **Sites** Upper outer arm, abdomen, anterior thigh, or scapular portion of the back

Intramuscular (IM) injections are given in muscle tissue.

- **Purpose** Maximum gradual absorption of medication into the bloodstream.
- **Amount** 2 to 5 mL. Doses of 4 to 5 mL should be divided in half and administered in two injections.
- **Sites** Deltoid, dorsal gluteal, vastus lateralis of the thigh, or ventral gluteal.

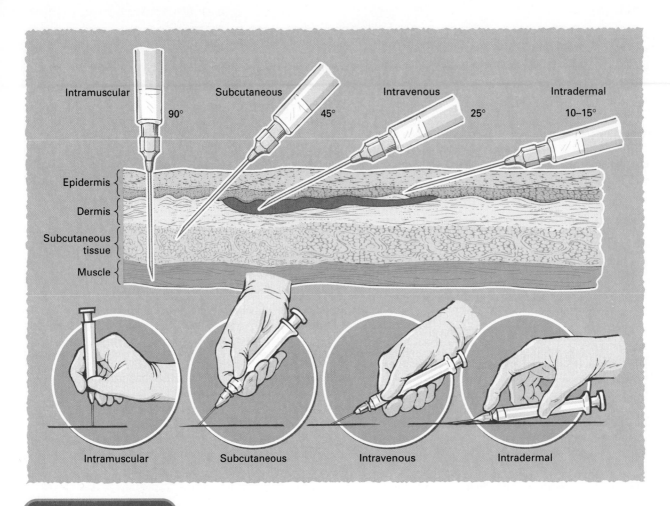

Figure 23.19

Angle of needle insertion for four types of injection.

PROCEDURE 23.31 INTRADERMAL INJECTION

RATIONALE

Intradermal injection technique is important in order to achieve the desired outcome. Your proper technique will help ensure that proper diagnosis and treatment can be determined.

ALERT: Follow Standard Precautions.

1. Wash hands.
2. Assemble supplies and medication.
   a. Tuberculin syringe
   b. Needle, 25- or 26-gauge, ⅜- or ⅝-inch long
   c. Substance for injection
   d. Alcohol wipe
   e. Gloves

3. Verify medication label against physician's order. Put on gloves.
4. Cleanse vial stopper. Draw up medication in a tuberculin syringe.
5. Ask patient/client to identify himself or herself.

PROCEDURE 23.31 | **INTRADERMAL INJECTION** *(Continued)*

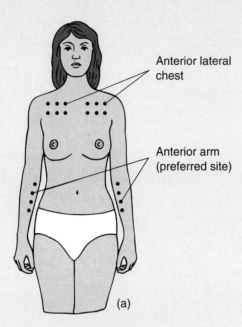

Anterior lateral chest

Anterior arm (preferred site)

(a)

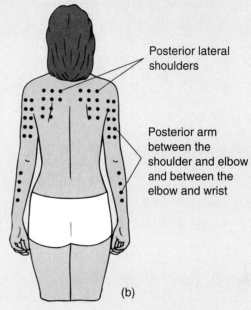

Posterior lateral shoulders

Posterior arm between the shoulder and elbow and between the elbow and wrist

(b)

6. Confirm any known medication allergies. (If known or possible allergies to medication exist, do not administer medication. Report to physician.)

7. Locate injection site: Measure two to three fingers' width distal (toward the wrist) to the antecubital space.

NOTE   If skin at preferred site is burned, irritated, scarred, or highly pigmented, use the following:

    a. Anterior lateral area of chest
    b. Posterior lateral shoulder
    c. Posterior lateral arm between shoulder and elbows or elbow and wrist

8. Put on gloves.

9. Cleanse site with alcohol in a circular motion from center, moving outward.

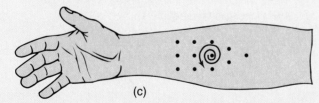

(c)

10. Allow skin to dry completely.

11. Holding patient's forearm in one hand, stretch skin taut.

12. Rotate syringe until bevel of needle is facing up.

13. Position syringe so that the needle is almost flat against patient's skin.

14. Insert needle through epidermis so that point of needle is still visible through skin. (See the figure on the left on page 664.)

15. Advance needle approximately ⅛ inch below skin's surface.

16. Inject medication slowly until a wheal (raised area) appears. (See the figure on the right on page 664.)

17. Remove needle and trigger sharps protective covering and discard in sharps container.

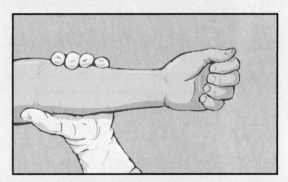

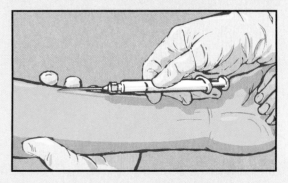

PROCEDURE 23.31 INTRADERMAL INJECTION *(Continued)*

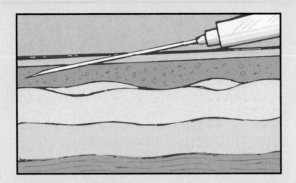

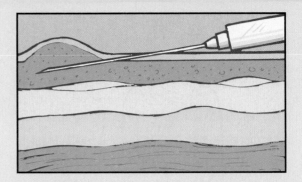

Never massage the area.

18. Apply small bandage if necessary.

19. Remove gloves and dispose of according to facility policy.

20. Wash hands.

21. Document administration in patient's chart.

a. Date
b. Time
c. Route
d. Site
e. Medication
f. Dose
g. Expiration date
h. Lot number
i. Signature and certification

PROCEDURE 23.32 SUBCUTANEOUS INJECTION

RATIONALE

Giving a subcutaneous injection allows quick absorption of medication into the bloodstream. Your careful follow-through of this procedure will help ensure that the prescribed medication is properly absorb.

ALERT: Follow Standard Precautions.

1. Wash hands.

2. Assemble supplies and medication.

   a. Syringe
   b. Needle: 25 gauge, ⅝-inch long
   c. Alcohol wipe
   d. Medication
   e. Disposable gloves

3. Verify medication label against physician's order.

4. Put on gloves.

5. Cleanse top of medication vial.

6. Draw up medication into appropriate syringe.

7. Ask patient/client to identify himself or herself.

8. Confirm any known medication allergies. (If known or possible allergies to medication exist, do not administer medication. Report to physician.)

9. Identify injection site. The preferred sub-Q site to inject insulin is the abdomen.

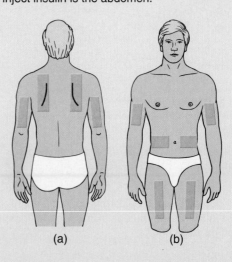

(a)   (b)

PROCEDURE 23.32   SUBCUTANEOUS INJECTION *(Continued)*

10. Cleanse injection site with an alcohol wipe starting at center of site and moving outward with circular motion.

11. Allow skin to dry.

12. Grasp skin firmly between thumb and forefinger to elevate subcutaneous tissue.

13. Smoothly and quickly thrust needle into tissue at 45° angle **except** when giving insulin or heparin; then insert needle at 90° angle.

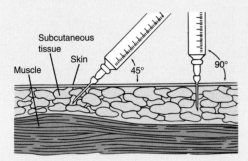

14. After needle is inserted:
    a. Release grasp on skin.
    b. Pull back on plunger to check for blood. (If blood is aspirated, remove needle,

discard needle and syringe, and repeat procedure.)
    c. Slowly inject medication into tissue if no blood is aspirated.

15. Remove needle from tissue quickly and smoothly.

16. Apply pressure over injection site and massage area unless contraindicated due to type of medication given.

17. Dispose of syringe in sharps container.

18. Remove gloves and dispose of according to facility policy.

19. Wash hands.

20. Document administration in patient's chart.
    a. Date
    b. Time
    c. Route
    d. Site
    e. Medication
    f. Dose
    g. Expiration date
    h. Lot number
    i. Signature and certification

PROCEDURE 23.33   IM INJECTION (ADULTS)

RATIONALE

Intramuscular injections allow maximum gradual absorption of medication into the bloodstream. Your careful follow-through of this procedure will help ensure that the prescribed medication is properly absorbed.

ALERT: Follow Standard Precautions.

1. Wash hands.

2. Assemble supplies and medication.
    a. Syringe
    b. Needle: 22 gauge, 1½-inch
    c. Alcohol wipes
    d. Medication
    e. Disposable gloves

3. Verify medication label against physician's order.

4. Put on gloves.

5. Cleanse stopper on vial.

6. Draw up medication into appropriate syringe.

7. Ask patient/client to identify himself or herself.

8. Confirm any known medication allergies. (If known or possible allergies to the medication exist, do not administer medication. Report to physician.)

9. Choose an appropriate site.

10. Cleanse injection site with alcohol wipe starting at the center of site and moving outward with circular motion.

11. Allow skin to dry.

PROCEDURE 23.33 **IM INJECTION (ADULTS)** *(Continued)*

12. Give injection.

    a. Grasp skin firmly.

    b. Hold syringe firmly perpendicular to skin.

    c. Thrust needle into muscle with one quick, smooth motion.

    d. Hold syringe with one hand.

    e. Pull back on plunger with other hand, to aspirate. (If blood appears, remove needle, discard needle and syringe, and repeat procedure.)

    f. Inject the medication slowly, allowing time (10 seconds) for distension of space in muscle to accommodate fluid if no blood appears.

13. Withdraw needle smoothly and quickly.

14. Immediately apply direct pressure to site using alcohol wipe.

15. Massage site unless contraindicated.

16. Discard syringe in sharps container.

17. Remove gloves and dispose of according to facility policy.

18. Document administration in patient's chart.

    a. Date

    b. Time

    c. Route

    d. Site

    e. Medication

    f. Dose

    g. Expiration date

    h. Lot number

    i. Signature and certification

PROCEDURE 23.34 **IM INJECTION (INFANTS AND CHILDREN)**

RATIONALE

Intramuscular injections allow maximum gradual absorption of medication into the bloodstream. Your careful follow-through of this procedure will prevent complications for the child and help ensure that the prescribed medication is properly absorbed.

ALERT: Follow Standard Precautions.

1. Wash hands.

2. Assemble supplies and medication.

    a. Syringe

    b. Alcohol wipes

    c. Needle: 25 gauge, ½- to ⅝-inch

    d. Medication

    e. Disposable gloves

3. Follow steps 3–5 in the procedure "IM Injection (Adults)."

NOTE It is recommended that 1 mL be the maximum volume administered in a single site to small children and infants. The muscles of small infants may not tolerate more than 0.5 mL.

6. Ask child's parent to identify child and confirm known allergies.

7. Select injection site.

    a. Preferred site of IM injection for *infants and toddlers to the age of 3* is lateral thigh (vastus lateralis), using upper outer quadrant. Pinch lateral thigh to raise muscle during injection.

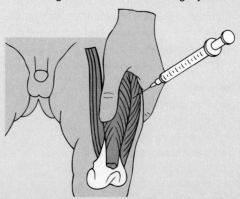

    b. Preferred sites of injection for children over age of 3 are same as for adults. *The dorsogluteal area should not be used until the child has been walking for at least one year.*

PROCEDURE 23.34 | IM INJECTION (INFANTS AND CHILDREN) *(Continued)*

8. Ask a second person (nurse or MA) to help restrain patient.
9. Follow steps 9–18 in "IM Injection (Adults)."

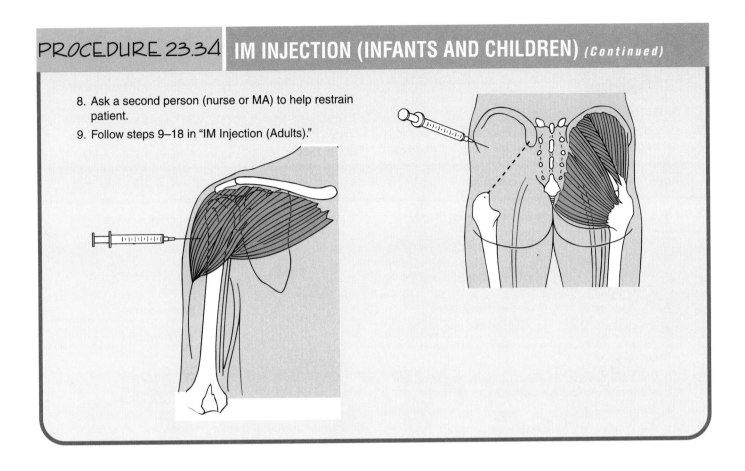

The Z-tract technique is another method of giving an intramuscular injection. Z-tract is recommended when

- Medication is irritating to subcutaneous tissue.
- Medication discolors or stains the tissue.
- Complete absorption of medication in the muscle is important.

The following medications are given by the Z-tract method:

- Immunoglobulin
- Antibiotics
- Vistaril
- Gamma globulin
- Estrogen
- Procaine
- Imferon
- Testosterone
- Narcotics

In the Z-tract technique, the medication is given in the upper outer quadrant of the gluteal muscle of the hips. Pull the tissue laterally away from the injection site. While holding the tissue, give the injection. Remove the needle. Then release the tissue. See the figures in the procedure "IM Z-Track Injection" for a clear view of how the medication is deposited in the muscle.

PROCEDURE 23.35

IM Z-TRACK INJECTION

RATIONALE

Perfecting your Z-track intramuscular injection technique will help prevent staining of subcutaneous tissue, reduce localized irritation, and prevent oozing of medication at the injection site.

ALERT: Follow Standard Precautions.

Follow steps 1–4 of the procedure "IM Injection (Adults)."

5. Draw up medication in appropriate syringe and add 0.3 mL of air to syringe.
6. Tap air bubble to end of syringe so that it is beside tip of plunger.
7. Change needle used to draw up medication.
8. Attach sterile 22-gauge 2-inch needle to syringe.
9. Follow steps 7–8 in the procedure "IM Injection (Adults)."
10. Cleanse injection site with alcohol starting at center of site and working outward with circular motion.
11. Allow skin to dry.
12. Pull skin laterally away from injection site.

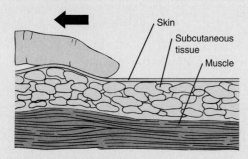

13. Remove needle cap.
14. Insert needle at 90° angle in one swift motion.
15. Pull back on tip of plunger to aspirate. (If blood is aspirated, remove needle, discard needle and syringe, and repeat procedure.)
16. Inject medication slowly, followed by 0.3 mL of air.

17. Wait 10 seconds after completing injection before removing needle.

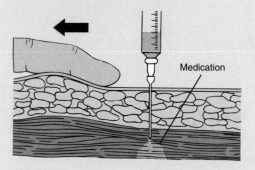

18. Remove needle and allow retracted skin to move back into position. *Do not massage site of injection.*

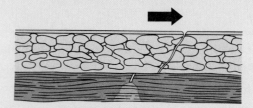

Z-track tissue displacement

19. Document administration in patient's chart.
    a. Date
    b. Time
    c. Medication
    d. Lot number
    e. Expiration date
    f. Route Z-track
    g. Location
    h. Signature and certification

⦿ IMMUNITY AND IMMUNIZATIONS

Immunity is the body's resistance to disease and infection. The body develops immunity in the following ways.

- ▪ The body has a natural resistance to specific viruses, bacteria, or their **toxins**. Natural immunity is present at birth and lasts a lifetime.

- ▪ The body produces antibodies. Antibodies attack foreign substances called antigens, or their toxins. *Example:* When the measles virus enters the body, the patient experiences measles. Antibodies are formed to attack and destroy the virus. If the measles virus enters the body again, the antibodies that destroyed the measles virus before quickly destroy the virus. The patient does not get the measles again. This is called a natural **acquired** immunity.

- ▪ The body receives a **vaccine** of a dead or weakened organism. The body then produces antibodies that destroy the organism. This is called immunization by vaccination.

- ▪ The body receives an **antitoxin** that provides an immediate resistance to toxins formed from an invading organism.

Immunization by Vaccination

Immunization by vaccination is commonly used to prevent the following illnesses:

- ▪ Varicella[8]
- ▪ Whooping cough
- ▪ Diptheria
- ▪ Measles: rubella[7] (3 days, causes birth defects) and rubeola (7 to 14 days) mumps
- ▪ Tetanus
- ▪ Smallpox
- ▪ Hepatitis B[2] and A[9]
- ▪ Haemophilus influenzae type B[4]
- ▪ Inactive polio[5]
- ▪ Pertussis[3]
- ▪ Pneumococcal conjugate[6]

ALERT   If live virus is indicated on vial, always wear eye protection to prevent self-**inoculation** if a splash from syringe-and-needle separation should occur.

The ability to control these diseases has saved many lives. It is important for everyone to be immunized. As a medical assistant, encourage patients to be immunized and to have their children complete each immunization series (see Table 23.15). For additional information about immunizations and the most current updates, see www.aap.org/family/parents/immunize.html or www.cdc.gov/nip. *Important:* Do not immunize ill patients or those who experienced a fever in the previous 24 hours. When giving flu or rubella vaccine, ask patients if they are sensitive to egg protein or feathers. If they are, do not give flu or rubella vaccine. Federal regulations require patients to read specific information and to sign an informed consent *before administration* of DTP, OPV, or MMR.

The following lists briefly describe the diseases for which immunization is routinely provided.

toxins
Poisons.

acquired
Refers to a condition, disease, or characteristic that began after birth.

vaccine
Dead or weakened organisms that stimulate the body to make antibodies.

antitoxin
Substance that provides immunity to a toxin.

inoculation
Instill, to put into the body.

Table 23.15 ■ Recommended Childhood Immunization Schedule United States, 2002

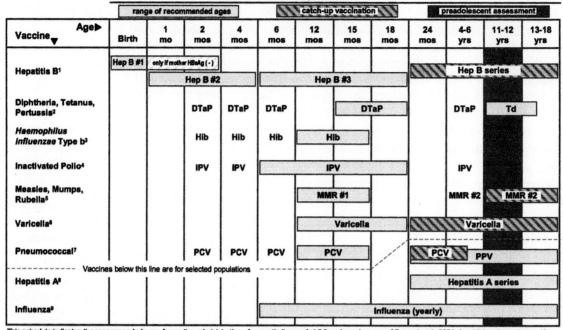

Recommended Childhood Immunization Schedule
United States, 2002

Vaccine ▼	Age ► Birth	1 mo	2 mos	4 mos	6 mos	12 mos	15 mos	18 mos	24 mos	4-6 yrs	11-12 yrs	13-18 yrs
				range of recommended ages			catch-up vaccination			preadolescent assessment		
Hepatitis B[1]	Hep B #1	only if mother HBsAg (-)	Hep B #2			Hep B #3					Hep B series	
Diphtheria, Tetanus, Pertussis[2]			DTaP	DTaP	DTaP		DTaP			DTaP	Td	
Haemophilus influenzae Type b[3]			Hib	Hib	Hib	Hib						
Inactivated Polio[4]			IPV	IPV		IPV				IPV		
Measles, Mumps, Rubella[5]						MMR #1				MMR #2	MMR #2	
Varicella[6]						Varicella				Varicella		
Pneumococcal[7]			PCV	PCV	PCV	PCV				PCV	PPV	
Hepatitis A[8]										Hepatitis A series		
Influenza[9]						Influenza (yearly)						

Vaccines below this line are for selected populations

This schedule indicates the recommended ages for routine administration of currently licensed childhood vaccines, as of December 1, 2001, for children through age 18 years. Any dose not given at the recommended age should be given at any subsequent visit when indicated and feasible. ▨ Indicates age groups that warrant special effort to administer those vaccines not previously given. Additional vaccines may be licensed and recommended during the year. Licensed combination vaccines may be used whenever any components of the combination are indicated and the vaccine's other components are not contraindicated. Providers should consult the manufacturers' package inserts for detailed recommendations.

1. Hepatitis B vaccine (Hep B). All infants should receive the first dose of hepatitis B vaccine soon after birth and before hospital discharge; the first dose may also be given by age 2 months if the infant's mother is HBsAg-negative. Only monovalent hepatitis B vaccine can be used for the birth dose. Monovalent or combination vaccine containing Hep B may be used to complete the series; four doses of vaccine may be administered if combination vaccine is used. The second dose should be given at least 4 weeks after the first dose, except for Hib-containing vaccine which cannot be administered before age 6 weeks. The third dose should be given at least 16 weeks after the first dose and at least 8 weeks after the second dose. The last dose in the vaccination series (third or fourth dose) should not be administered before age 6 months.
 Infants born to HBsAg-positive mothers should receive hepatitis B vaccine and 0.5 mL hepatitis B immune globulin (HBIG) within 12 hours of birth at separate sites. The second dose is recommended at age 1-2 months and the vaccination series should be completed (third or fourth dose) at age 6 months.
 Infants born to mothers whose HBsAg status is unknown should receive the first dose of the hepatitis B vaccine series within 12 hours of birth. Maternal blood should be drawn at the time of delivery to determine the mother's HBsAg status; if the HBsAg test is positive, the infant should receive HBIG as soon as possible (no later than age 1 week).

2. Diphtheria and tetanus toxoids and acellular pertussis vaccine (DTaP). The fourth dose of DTaP may be administered as early as age 12 months, provided 6 months have elapsed since the third dose and the child is unlikely to return at age 15-18 months. Tetanus and diphtheria toxoids (Td) is recommended at age 11-12 years if at least 5 years have elapsed since the last dose of tetanus and diphtheria toxoid-containing vaccine. Subsequent routine Td boosters are recommended every 10 years.

3. Haemophilus influenzae type b (Hib) conjugate vaccine. Three Hib conjugate vaccines are licensed for infant use. If PRP-OMP (PedvaxHIB® or ComVax® [Merck]) is administered at ages 2 and 4 months, a dose at age 6 months is not required. DTaP/Hib combination products should not be used for primary immunization in infants at age 2, 4 or 6 months, but can be used as boosters following any Hib vaccine.

4. Inactivated poliovirus vaccine (IPV). An all-IPV schedule is recommended for routine childhood poliovirus vaccination in the United States. All children should receive four doses of IPV at age 2 months, 4 months, 6-18 months, and 4-6 years.

5. Measles, mumps, and rubella vaccine (MMR). The second dose of MMR is recommended routinely at age 4-6 years but may be administered during any visit, provided at least 4 weeks have elapsed since the first dose and that both doses are administered beginning at or after age 12 months. Those who have not previously received the second dose should complete the schedule by the visit at 11-12 years.

6. Varicella vaccine. Varicella vaccine is recommended at any visit at or after age 12 months for susceptible children (i.e. those who lack a reliable history of chickenpox). Susceptible persons aged ≥13 years should receive two doses, given at least 4 weeks apart.

7. Pneumococcal vaccine. The heptavalent pneumococcal conjugate vaccine (PCV) is recommended for all children aged 2-23 months and for certain children aged 24-59 months. Pneumococcal polysaccharide vaccine (PPV) is recommended in addition to PCV for certain high-risk groups. See *MMWR* 2000;49(RR-9);1-37.

8. Hepatitis A vaccine. Hepatitis A vaccine is recommended for use in selected states and regions, and for certain high-risk groups; consult your local public health authority. See *MMWR* 1999;48(RR-12);1-37.

9. Influenza vaccine. Influenza vaccine is recommended annually for children age ≥ 6 months with certain risk factors (including but not limited to asthma, cardiac disease, sickle cell disease, HIV, and diabetes; see *MMWR* 2001;50(RR-4);1-44), and can be administered to all others wishing to obtain immunity. Children aged ≤12 years should receive vaccine in a dosage appropriate for their age (0.25 mL if age 6-35 months or 0.5 mL if aged ≥ 3 years). Children aged ≤ 8 years who are receiving influenza vaccine for the first time should receive two doses separated by at least 4 weeks.

For additional information about vaccines, vaccine supply, and contraindications for immunization, please visit the National Immunization Program Website at www.cdc.gov/nip or call the National Immunization Hotline at 800-232-2522 (English) or 800-232-0233 (Spanish).

Approved by the Advisory Committee on Immunization Practices (www.cdc.gov/nip/acip), the American Academy of Pediatrics (www.aap.org), and the American Academy of Family Physicians (www.aafp.org).

Pertussis or Whooping Cough

- Highly contagious
- Most prevalent in infants and children under 4 years of age
- Gradual in onset, with sneezing, cough, slight fever, and **listlessness**
- Characterized after 10 to 14 days by a cough that sounds like a whoop (that is, a series of short, quick coughs)
- Treated with antibiotics to help reduce other infections (secondary to pertussis)

Diptheria

- Contagious
- Serious because it produces a false membrane in the throat that makes it difficult to eat, drink, and breathe
- Damaging to the heart and central nervous system
- Often fatal if untreated

Tetanus

- An infection of the central nervous system
- Introduced into the body through any opening in the skin or through the umbilical cord of the newborn
- **Characterized** by headaches, fever, and muscle spasms of the jaw (lockjaw) and throat; eventually all body muscles spasm
- Often fatal

Poliomyelitis

- Caused by one of three polio viruses
- Introduced into the body through the mouth
- Characterized by fever, **malaise,** headache, nausea, vomiting, slight abdominal pain (these symptoms may disappear and recur with pain and **paralysis**)
- Uncommon today, but occurred in **epidemic** proportions before vaccine was discovered

Haemophilus Influenza B

- The main cause of inflammatory diseases in young children
- Very serious, causing diseases from **meningitis** to **septic arthritis**
- Difficult to treat; causes death if treatment is not successful

Measles (Rubeola)

- Contagious
- Caused by virus that affects the skin and respiratory system
- A serious **preventable** childhood infectious disease
- Occasionally complicated by **pneumonia** and/or **encephalitis**
- Preventable by a preparation of human antibodies called **gamma globulin,** which may be given to prevent or modify measles after exposure in individuals who have not received measles vaccine

Mumps

- An infectious disease caused by a virus
- Noticeable when the glands under the ear swell, followed a day or two later by fever, diarrhea, and malaise

listlessness

A state of being without energy.

characterized

Distinguished by; refers to a trait or quality.

malaise

Weakness or discomfort.

paralysis

Loss of sensation and muscle function.

epidemic

Disease that spreads rapidly among people.

meningitis

Inflammation of the membrane covering the brain.

septic arthritis

Bacterial inflammation of the joint caused by bloodborne bacteria carried from another place in the body.

preventable

Able to be kept from happening.

pneumonia

Inflammation of the lungs.

encephalitis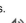

Inflammation of the brain.

gamma globulin

Substance that acts as an antibody to increase immunity.

testicles

Site of production of the male sex cell.

sterility

Absence of living organism or inability to produce offspring.

■ Responsible for swelling and inflammation of the **testicles** or ovaries, in rare cases causing **sterility**

■ Occasionally complicated by meningitis

German Measles (Rubella)

■ Contagious

■ Caused by a virus

■ Characterized by slight fever and swollen glands under the ear, down the neck, and around the back of the neck

■ Known to cause damage to a baby developing in the uterus. (A pregnant woman should be notified immediately if she is exposed to a person with rubella, as she needs to see a physician as quickly as possible.)

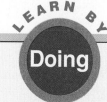

LEARN BY

Doing

1. Complete Worksheets 3, 4, 5, 7, 9, 10, 11, 13, 14, 15 and 16 as directed by your instructor.

2. Complete Worksheets/Activities 2, 6, 8 and 12 as directed by your instructor.

3. Practice all procedures.

4. Prepare responses to each item listed in Chapter Review—Your Link to Success at the end of this chapter.

5. When you are confident that you can meet each objective, ask your instructor for the unit evaluation.

Thinking Critically

1. **Patient Education** Ms. Gonzales has been told that mammograms are acutely painful and she is afraid. List the ways you will reassure her. Include a complete description of the process, what the screening shows the radiologist, and the lifesaving importance of early detection.

2. **Cultural Competency** Research different cultures and identify those that require the husband to be present when the wife is examined by a medical provider.

3. **Communication** When preparing a patient for an examination, always give specific instructions for undressing. For example, remove outer clothes only; remove all clothes; gown to close at the back; gown to close at the front. Patients feel foolish when they do not know what is expected of them. Make a sample list of patient instructions for different examinations.

4. **Computers** Describe ways computers are used in the clinical setting of a medical office.

5. **Medical Math** Describe the equivalencies of millimeters and inches, cubic centimeters and ounces, and pounds and kilograms. Convert 36 inches into millimeters, 4 ounces into cubic centimeters, and 120 pounds into kilograms. Determine the dose to give when 10 grains of a medication are ordered and you have 300-mg tablets available.

6. **Case Study** You are educating a new mother on the importance of immunizing her child. During your explanation she interrupts you and says she has a friend with a child who is mentally impaired. The friend blames early immunizations for her child's impairment. Explain how you will respond to the mother and what you will do.

Portfolio Connection

Once you attain competence as a clinical medical assistant, ask for permission to copy an example of patient charting that you have completed. (Remove all patient identifiers.) Place these copies in your portfolio as evidence of your skills. Place a copy of your on-site trainer's evaluation in your portfolio.

Write a paper describing your doubts and realizations and the barriers that you were able to overcome during your clinical medical assistant experience. For example, were you afraid that you couldn't learn to use the equipment? Describe the ways you plan to use the skills, information, and insights that you gained about the people you worked with and about this job. This assignment must be in standard report format.

Portfolio Tip

When clinical and mathematical details seem overwhelming, focus on the treatments they support and the relief they offer your clients. An extra bonus of this way of thinking is that it gives a procedure rationale to explain to your clients.

Remember! Media Connection

Use the Companion Website **www.prenhall.com/badasch** and the CD-ROM for additional interactive learning activities.

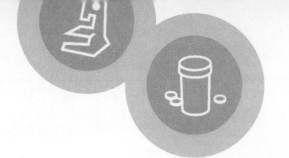

Chapter 24

Dental Assistant

Co-Authored by Vivian Muensterman

STEPS TO SUCCESS

1. Complete Vocabulary Worksheet 1 in the Student Workbook.

2. Read this chapter.

3. Complete the Learn by Doing assignment at the end of this chapter.

OBJECTIVES

When you have completed this chapter, you will be able to do the following:

✔ Complete all objectives in Part One of this book.

✔ Match vocabulary words with their correct meanings.

✔ Describe the responsibilities of a dental assistant.

✔ List eight recognized dental specialties.

✔ Differentiate between posterior and anterior teeth and their functions.

✔ Identify the following:

- Deciduous and permanent teeth by name on a diagram
- Surfaces of a tooth
- Charting symbols and abbreviations
- Dental office equipment by name
- Specific OSHA infection control guidelines for the dental office
- Common dental instruments
- Basic dental tray setups

✔ Apply charting symbols and abbreviations to indicate conditions of teeth on a dental chart.

✔ Label the following:

- Parts of the oral cavity on a diagram
- Teeth on a diagram using the universal method
- Anatomical structures of a tooth on a diagram

✔ Explain the following:

- How to position a patient for a dental procedure
- The importance of observing patients before, during, and after procedures

✔ Describe the following:

- Admitting and seating a patient for a dental procedure
- The dental assistant's position related to the patient and the dentist during a procedure
- Oral evacuation, rinsing, and drying techniques
- Steps for cleaning the treatment room following procedures and between patients

✔ Teach the following:

- How to use disclosing tablets/solution

- The Bass toothbrushing technique
- Dental flossing techniques

✔ Demonstrate the following:

- Basic instrument transfer techniques
- Preparation and transfer of an anesthetic syringe
- Procedure for completion of treatment and dismissing a patient

- How to make a study model
- Assisting techniques during basic restorative procedures

✔ Prepare impression materials.

✔ Mount a full-mouth and bite-wing x-ray series.

✔ Apply all procedural techniques with confidence.

RESPONSIBILITIES OF A DENTAL ASSISTANT

Dental assistants are valued members of the dental health care team. Their primary duty is chairside assisting during oral care procedures. Their basic duty is to maintain **visibility** in the mouth. They also provide instruments and materials as the dentist needs them to complete the dental treatment. Constant observance and consideration of the patient's/client's comfort level and health status are important in the role of a dental assistant. The responsibilities of a dental assistant include the following:

visibility
Ability to see.

- Working directly with the dentist in the treatment room
- Preparing and cleaning dental treatment rooms following infection control guidelines
- Preparing necessary equipment and instrumentation for dental procedures
- Processing and mounting dental x-rays
- Caring for and maintaining dental equipment
- Teaching patients oral hygiene methods
- Taking and pouring study models (may be an expanded role in your state)
- Possibly performing some front office duties
- Exposing x-rays (radiographs) (requires completion of a state-approved radiology course or examination)

DENTAL SPECIALTIES

The dental profession has eight recognized specialties. A dental assistant requires specialized training to work in these areas. Specialized training may occur through on-the-job training in the dental office, through study courses given by the dental societies, or at a school certified by the **ADA.** Dental assistants need to know what the specialties are when their dentist refers patients to the specialist. The following are the eight specialties:

ADA
American Dental Association.

periapical
Around the apex (e.g., of the tooth).

- **Endodontist.** Diagnoses and treats diseases of the dental pulp and **periapical** tissues
- **Oral pathologist.** Studies causes, processes, and effects of diseases of the mouth
- **Oral surgeon.** Performs oral surgery
- **Orthodontist.** Treats and prevents irregularities of the teeth and dental arches
- **Pedodontist.** Cares for teeth and oral conditions of children
- **Periodontist.** Treats and prevents disease of the bone and soft tissues surrounding the teeth

■ **Prosthodontist.** Replaces missing teeth or oral tissues by artificial means, such as crowns, bridges, dentures, and implants

■ **Public health dentistry.** Concerned with the dental health of the population

General dentists may have training in some specialized areas; however, they may choose to refer to a specialist when they feel it is better for the patient.

INTRODUCTION TO DENTISTRY

The oral cavity and the teeth are very important in the total health of the body. The mouth is related directly to eating, physical health, and a sense of well-being. A healthy mouth allows the digestive system to function properly. The mouth allows communication through speaking. When we think our teeth do not look nice, we may hide our mouth with our hand while talking. This makes it hard for others to understand what we are saying. The physical appearance of teeth plays a major role in personal relationships. If we feel unattractive, we may withdraw from social events. Unpleasant breath odor causes others to avoid getting close. Physical appearance of the mouth also affects mental attitudes about ourselves. Poor self-image causes us to lose our self-confidence. As a dental assistant, you are an important member of the dental team. The care that you give the patient helps keep him or her healthy physically and mentally.

ODONTOLOGY

Odontology is the study of teeth. Teeth are **accessory** organs that help **masticate** food. There are two sets of teeth. They are the **primary** or **deciduous** (baby) teeth and the permanent teeth. When a baby is born it has 44 tooth buds. The tooth buds begin to **erupt** when the baby is about 6 months old. Deciduous teeth are the 20 baby teeth (primary teeth). Each tooth has a specific function in processing food and acting as a guide for a permanent tooth.

When the child is between 5 and 12 years old, the deciduous teeth begin to fall out and the permanent teeth erupt through the gingiva/gums. Permanent teeth are the 32 adult teeth. The child who has some deciduous teeth and some permanent teeth has mixed **dentition.**

INTRODUCTION TO THE TEETH AND ORAL CAVITY

Teeth are identified by name, number, and the function they perform in the digestion of food. The following information teaches you how to identify teeth, where the teeth are located, and the anatomy of a tooth.

Face and Oral Cavity

When dentists examine patients they look at the face first. Dentists ask themselves:

■ Is the bone structure normal and balanced?

■ Do the skin and lips (labia) look healthy?

Next, the dentist does an oral examination (see Figure 24.1). This examination tells the dentist things about the patient's health and habits (for example, whether he or she practices good oral care). Often, a nondental disease shows up in the oral cavity first and is identified during the examination. The complete oral examination is one of the most important procedures that a dentist performs. As a dental assistant,

accessory
Helping.

masticate
Chew.

primary
First.

deciduous
Falling out (e.g., primary teeth fall out to make room for permanent teeth).

erupt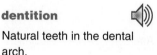
Push through.

dentition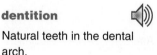
Natural teeth in the dental arch.

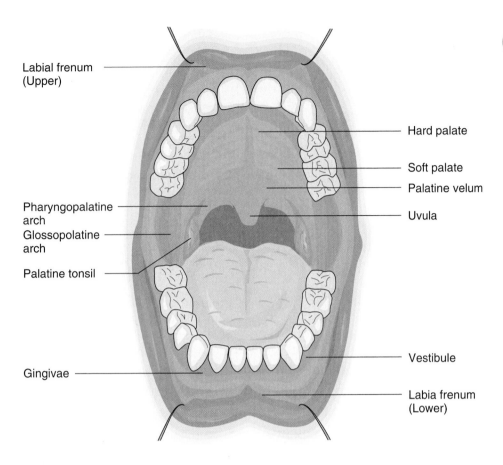

Figure 24.1

Mouth and oral cavity.

Labial frenum (Upper)

Hard palate

Soft palate

Palatine velum

Pharyngopalatine arch

Uvula

Glossopolatine arch

Palatine tonsil

Gingivae

Vestibule

Labia frenum (Lower)

you help the dentist during this examination and during **restorative** care. To assist the dentist, you need to know the following:

- Simple anatomy of the face and oral cavity
- Tooth numbers, parts, surfaces, and structures

Maxillary and Mandibular Arches

Refer to Figure 24.2, an illustration of the skull.

- **Maxilla.** The arched bone in the face where the roots of the upper teeth fit into the sockets (alveolus)
- **Mandible.** The arched lower bone (jawbone), where the roots of the lower teeth fit into the alveolus
- **Median line or midline.** Divides the teeth into left and right sides

restorative

To return to as close to normal conditions as possible.

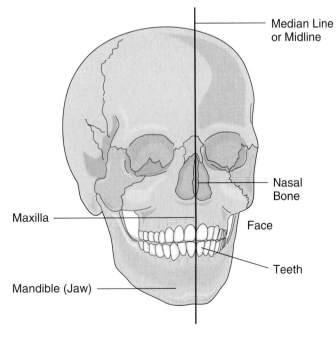

Figure 24.2

Skull.

Median Line or Midline

Nasal Bone

Maxilla

Face

Teeth

Mandible (Jaw)

Location of posterior and anterior teeth.

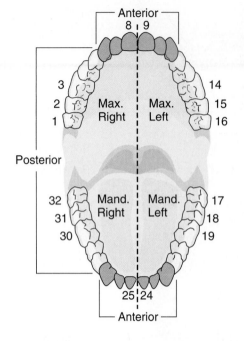

Placement and Function of Teeth

The following are the anterior teeth (see Figure 24.3):

- **Incisors.** Located in the very front of the mouth. Their thin cutting edge cuts food by biting pieces. They include the central and lateral incisors.

- **Cuspids/canines.** Located next to the lateral incisors. Their sharp points/cusps tear food that is too tough for the incisors to cut. Cuspids have the longest roots of all teeth.

The following are the posterior teeth (see Figure 24.3):

- **Premolars.** Located next to the cuspids/canines. They are also called *bicuspids* because the have two **cusps** for tearing and grinding.

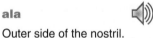

cusps

Pointed or rounded raised areas on the surface of the tooth.

- **Molars.** Located next to the bicuspids. These are the largest teeth in the mouth. They have broad grinding surfaces that grind down large chunks of food.

Identification of Teeth by Name and Location

There are 32 permanent teeth in the dentition (Figure 24.4). The following are the maxillary teeth:

2 central incisors in the center next to the midline.

2 lateral incisors next to the central incisors.

ala

Outer side of the nostril.

Universal method of identifying permanent teeth.

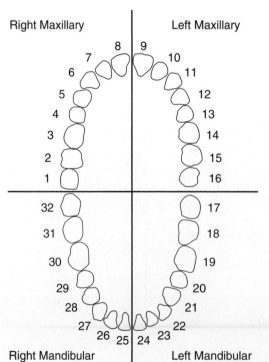

2 cuspids under the **ala** next to the lateral incisors.

2 first premolar/bicuspids next to the cuspids.

2 second premolar/bicuspids next to the first bicuspids.

2 first molars next to the second bicuspid.

2 second molars next to the first molar.

2 third molars or "wisdom teeth" in the back of the mouth. Not everyone has these molars. Some molars remain under the gingiva/gums line or in the alveolar bone and are often removed if the mouth does not have room for them.

The mandibular teeth:

2 central incisors in the center next to the midline.

2 lateral incisors next to the central incisors.

2 cuspids under the corner of the nose next to the lateral incisors.

2 first premolar/bicuspids next to the cuspids.

2 second premolar/bicuspids next to the first bicuspids.

2 first molars next to the second bicuspid.

2 second molars next to the first molar.

2 third molars or "wisdom teeth" in the back of the mouth. Not everyone has these molars. Some molars remain under the gingiva/gums line and are often removed if the mouth does not have room for them.

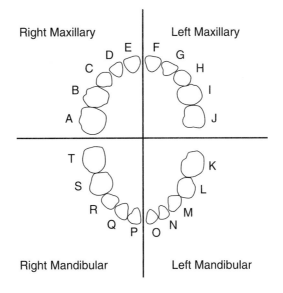

Right Maxillary   Left Maxillary

Right Mandibular   Left Mandibular

Figure 24.5

Universal method of identifying deciduous teeth.

There are 20 deciduous teeth in the dentition (Figure 24.5).

2 central incisors in the center next to midline

2 lateral incisors next to the central incisors

2 cuspids just under the ala wing of the nose

0 THERE ARE NO BICUSPIDS IN THE DECIDUOUS DENTITION

2 primary first molars

2 primary second molars

The mandibular arch:

2 central incisors in the center next to midline

2 lateral incisors next to the central incisors

2 cuspids just under the ala wing of the nose

0 THERE ARE NO BICUSPIDS IN THE DECIDUOUS DENTITION

2 primary first molars

2 primary second molars

Identification of Teeth by Letter and Number

One method of identifying teeth is the *universal method*. In this method, deciduous/primary teeth are identified by letter, and permanent teeth are identified by number.

When identifying deciduous teeth, begin lettering with the right second molar in the maxillary arch (see Figure 24.5). It is labeled A. Continue lettering from upper right to upper left, then lower left to lower right. The last molar on the right mandibular arch is labeled T.

When identifying permanent teeth, begin numbering with the right third molar in the maxillary arch (see Figure 24.4). It is numbered 1. Continue numbering from upper right to upper left, then lower left to lower right. The last third molar on the mandibular arch is numbered 32. A tooth that has not erupted or is missing is still counted.

⬤ ANATOMY OF THE TOOTH

The dental assistant works directly with the dentist. It is important to communicate with the dentist during **intraoral** procedures. You must know the anatomy of the tooth to communicate effectively with the dentist.

intraoral

Within the oral cavity.

Figure 24.6

Sections of a tooth.

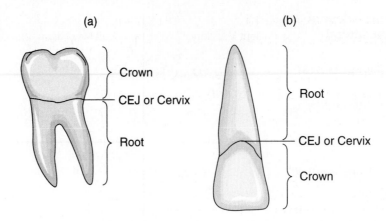

(a)

- Crown
- CEJ or Cervix
- Root

(b)

- Root
- CEJ or Cervix
- Crown

Sections of the Tooth

A tooth is divided into three main sections (see Figure 24.6):

- **Crown.** Covered with enamel. The enamel is the white part of the tooth that we can see in our mouth.
- **Cervix.** Neck of the tooth. It begins where the enamel stops and the **cementum** begins. Dentists call this the CEJ (cemento-enamel junction).
- **Root.** Covered with cementum, lies below the gingiva/gums. It holds the tooth in the bony sockets of the jaw. A tooth may have more than one root, depending on where it is in the mouth.
  - Mandibular molars have two roots. • Maxillary molars have three roots.

cementum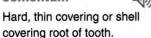

Hard, thin covering or shell covering root of tooth.

Parts of the Tooth

Each tooth has several parts (see Figure 24.7):

- **Enamel.** The hardest tissue in the body. It covers the crown section of the tooth. Enamel is a protective sheet made of calcium and phosphorus that protects the dentin of the tooth.
- **Dentin.** Harder than bone but softer than enamel. Dentin makes up the bulk of a tooth. It does not have nerves but it senses pain caused by **decay,** temperature, and chemical changes. Dentin may grow a second layer or wall of defense to try to keep decay from entering the pulp or nerve of the tooth.
- **Cementum.** The hard, thin covering or shell that covers the root.
- **Periodontal ligaments/periodontal membranes.** Small fibers that are anchored in the cementum and attached to the bone socket. They act as a shock absorber for the tooth and help the tooth withstand **functional stress.**
- **Pulp.** The soft tissue inside the hard wall of enamel and dentin. It has veins, arteries, and nerve tissue that nourish the tooth and sense pain.
- **Apex.** The very tip of each root. The blood vessels and nerves of the tooth enter through the **apical foramen** in the apex of the tooth.

decay

Breaking down; rot.

functional stress

Stress to tooth caused by its normal function (e.g., force of pressure when biting something hard).

apical foramen

Opening in the apex.

Tissues Around the Teeth

The structures that surround the teeth are also important. They are as follows:

- **Alveolar processes (bone).** Form the sockets that hold and support teeth in their position.
- **Gingiva/gums.** Cover the alveolar bone, protecting the tooth and deeper tissues from injury or infection.

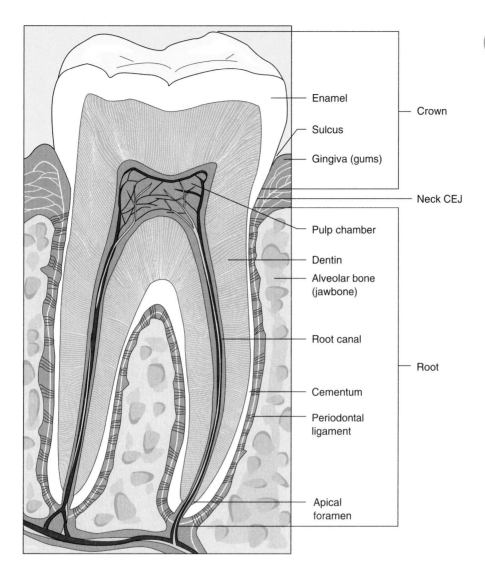

Figure 24.7

Parts of the tooth.

Enamel

Sulcus

Gingiva (gums)

Crown

Neck CEJ

Pulp chamber

Dentin

Alveolar bone (jawbone)

Root canal

Root

Cementum

Periodontal ligament

Apical foramen

■ **Gingival sulcus.** The open space between gingiva/gums and a tooth. This is the area where dental floss is applied to remove bacteria and food particles.

Surfaces of the Teeth

Dentists use terms that specify surfaces (sides of the tooth) to record information about the condition of each tooth. To chart conditions of the teeth, the dental assistant must know the crown surfaces. Each tooth has a crown and root. Each tooth also has four sides and a biting or chewing surface (see Figure 24.8).

■ **Anterior teeth.** Central and lateral incisors and the cuspids
■ **Posterior teeth.** Bicuspids and molars

The surfaces of the anterior teeth (see Figure 24.8) are called

■ **Labial.** Surface that touches the lips
■ **Lingual.** Surface facing toward the tongue
■ **Incisal.** Edge of the tooth that we bite with
■ **Distal.** Surface away from midline, toward the back
■ **Mesial.** Surface toward the midline

sulcus

Depression, groove, area where gingival tip meets tooth enamel.

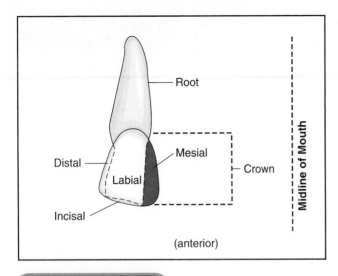

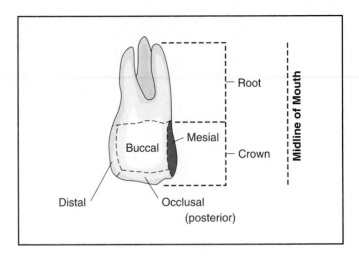

Figure 24.8

Surfaces of the anterior and posterior teeth.

The surfaces of the posterior teeth (see Figure 24.8) are called

■ **Buccal.** Surface that touches the cheeks
■ **Lingual.** Surface facing toward the tongue
■ **Occlusal.** Large chewing surface where food is ground
■ **Distal.** Surface away from midline
■ **Mesial.** Surface toward the midline

All teeth have mesial and distal sides that touch each other. The mesial side of one tooth touches the distal side of the tooth next to it. These sides are **proximal** to each other and are called proximal surfaces.

proximal

Nearest or next to.

CHARTING CONDITIONS OF THE TEETH

legal record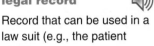

Record that can be used in a law suit (e.g., the patient chart).

Charting is an important responsibility. The chart is a **legal record.** Your charting must be neat, complete in detail, and correct. When charting the condition of a tooth, use abbreviations, symbols, and specialized forms. Dental offices may use different forms, but the basic guidelines are the same.

Dental Chart

Every patient has a dental chart. The dentist uses this chart for each visit. It provides a record for each dental visit (see Figure 24.9). The dental chart usually has three parts.

1. Personal information about the patient/client:
  • Name, address, phone number • Insurance coverage, billing address
  • Medical precautions such as allergies to medication, bleeding, etc.
2. Diagram of the teeth on which to chart/document
3. Other information:
  • Patient medical conditions affecting treatment • Radiographic history
  • Treatment given • Services performed • Estimated fee • Amount charges/ paid

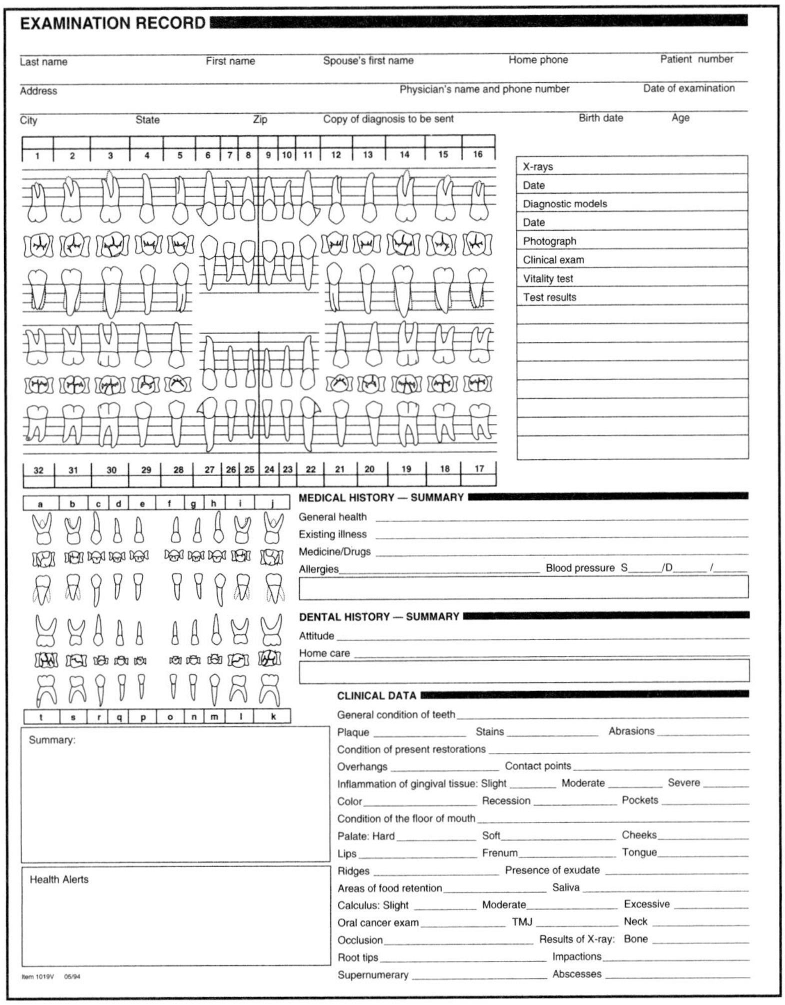

Figure 24.9

EXAMINATION RECORD

Last name First name Spouse's first name Home phone Patient number

Address Physician's name and phone number Date of examination

City State Zip Copy of diagnosis to be sent Birth date Age

| 1 | 2 | 3 | 4 | 5 | 6 | 7 | 8 | 9 | 10 | 11 | 12 | 13 | 14 | 15 | 16 |

| X-rays |
| Date |
| Diagnostic models |
| Date |
| Photograph |
| Clinical exam |
| Vitality test |
| Test results |

| 32 | 31 | 30 | 29 | 28 | 27 | 26 | 25 | 24 | 23 | 22 | 21 | 20 | 19 | 18 | 17 |

| a | b | c | d | e | f | g | h | i | j |

| t | s | r | q | p | o | n | m | l | k |

Summary:

Health Alerts

Item 1019V 05/94

MEDICAL HISTORY — SUMMARY

General health

Existing illness

Medicine/Drugs

Allergies Blood pressure S____/D____ /____

DENTAL HISTORY — SUMMARY

Attitude

Home care

CLINICAL DATA

General condition of teeth

Plaque Stains Abrasions

Condition of present restorations

Overhangs Contact points

Inflammation of gingival tissue: Slight Moderate Severe

Color Recession Pockets

Condition of the floor of mouth

Palate: Hard Soft Cheeks

Lips Frenum Tongue

Ridges Presence of exudate

Areas of food retention Saliva

Calculus: Slight Moderate Excessive

Oral cancer exam TMJ Neck

Occlusion Results of X-ray: Bone

Root tips Impactions

Supernumerary Abscesses

(a)

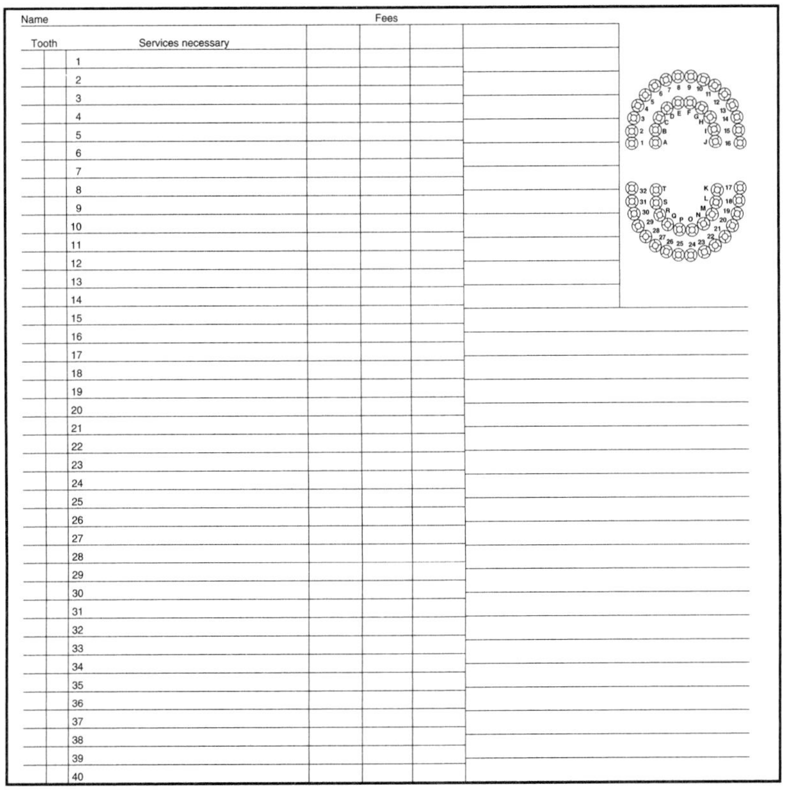

Name Fees

Tooth	Services necessary				
1					
2					
3					
4					
5					
6					
7					
8					
9					
10					
11					
12					
13					
14					
15					
16					
17					
18					
19					
20					
21					
22					
23					
24					
25					
26					
27					
28					
29					
30					
31					
32					
33					
34					
35					
36					
37					
38					
39					
40					

(b)

Dental chart. (Courtesy of SYCOM)

Charting Abbreviations

The following abbreviations apply to crown surfaces (see Figure 24.10):

M	mesial
La/F	labial facial
I	incisal
B, Bu/F	buccal/facial
D	distal
Lin, Li, L	lingual
O, Occ	occlusal
F	facial

Abbreviations in Table 24.1 are suggested terms, however it is important to use your dentist's terms if they are different.

Table 24.1 ■ Abbreviations

Abbreviation	Meaning	Abbreviation	Meaning
Abs	abscess	GO	Gold onlay
Adj	adjustment	GR	Gold restoration
Amal	amalgam	GT	Gingiva/gums treatment
Anes	Anesthetic	Imp	Impression
BWX	Bite-wing x-rays	Lido	Lidocaine
CA	Corrective appliance	Occ adj	Occlusal adjustment
C&B	Crown and bridge	OS	Oral surgery
cb	Cement base	PA	Preparatory appointment
CMX	Complete mouth x-rays	PFM	Porcelain fused to metal
Com	Composite	PL	Partial lower
Cr	Crown	POH	Personal oral hygiene instruction
Dent	Denture	POT	Postoperative treatment
Diag	Diagnosis	Prophy	Prophylaxis
DR	Denture repair	PU	Partial upper
DS	Denture service	Radiogr	Radiographs
Est	Estimate	RCT	Root canal therapy
Exam, Ex	Examination	Rem	Removable
Ext	Extraction	RR	Resin restoration
FGCr	Full gold crown	SM	Study models
Fix Br	Fixed bridge	SR	Silver restoration
FL	Full lower	ST	Sedative treatment
FM	Full mouth	Temp	Temporary
FT	Fluoride treatment	x-ray/X	x-rays
FU	Full upper	Xylo	xylocaine
GI	Gold inlay		

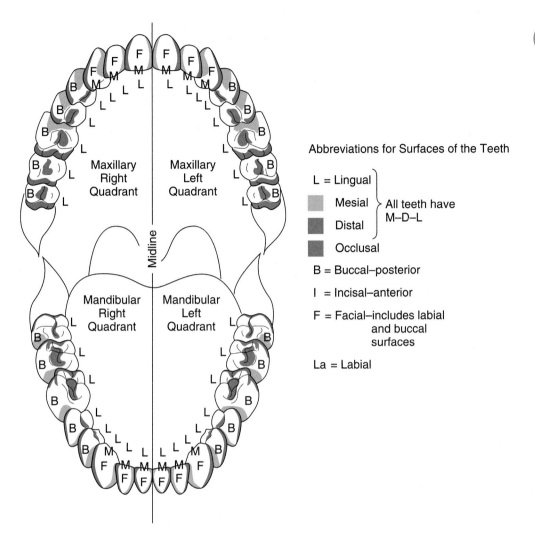

Figure 24.10

Abbreviations for the surfaces of the teeth.

Abbreviations for Surfaces of the Teeth

L = Lingual
Mesial ⎫
Distal ⎬ All teeth have M–D–L
Occlusal

B = Buccal–posterior

I = Incisal–anterior

F = Facial–includes labial and buccal surfaces

La = Labial

Types of Diagrams on Dental Charts

A dental chart has an anatomical or geometric diagram of the teeth.

- The *anatomical diagrams* of permanent and deciduous teeth (Figure 24.11) may show the crowns of the teeth, the crowns of the teeth and the root, or the crowns of the teeth and a small part of the root.

- The *geometric diagram* (Figure 24.12) is another type of diagram the dentist may use for charting. The teeth are identified by number and show all sides and the crown in a geometric drawing.

Charting Symbols

Basic symbols identify conditions of the teeth and procedures. There are many different ways to chart these conditions, required procedures, and completion of the necessary care. Examples of charting symbols are shown in Figure 24.13.

Match the listed conditions on pages 687 and 688 with the anatomical diagram in Figure 24.14 and the geometric diagram in Figure 24.15 on page 690. This will help you understand how to use charting symbols.

Figure 24.11

Anatomical diagram of the permanent and deciduous teeth.

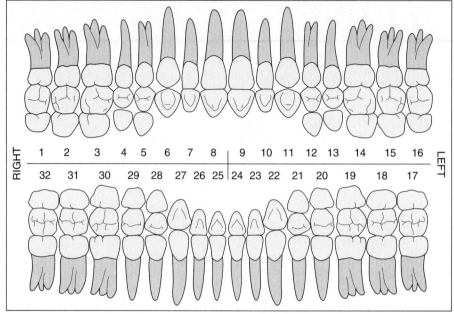

Anatomical Diagram of Permanent Teeth

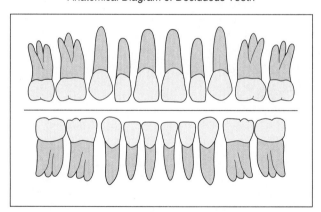

Anatomical Diagram of Deciduous Teeth

Figure 24.12

Geometric diagram of the teeth.

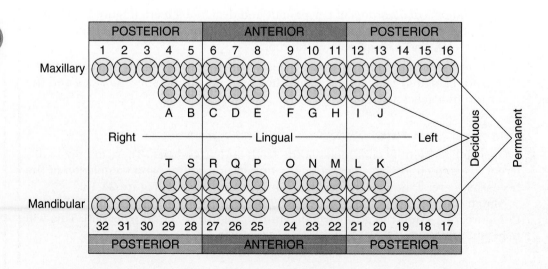

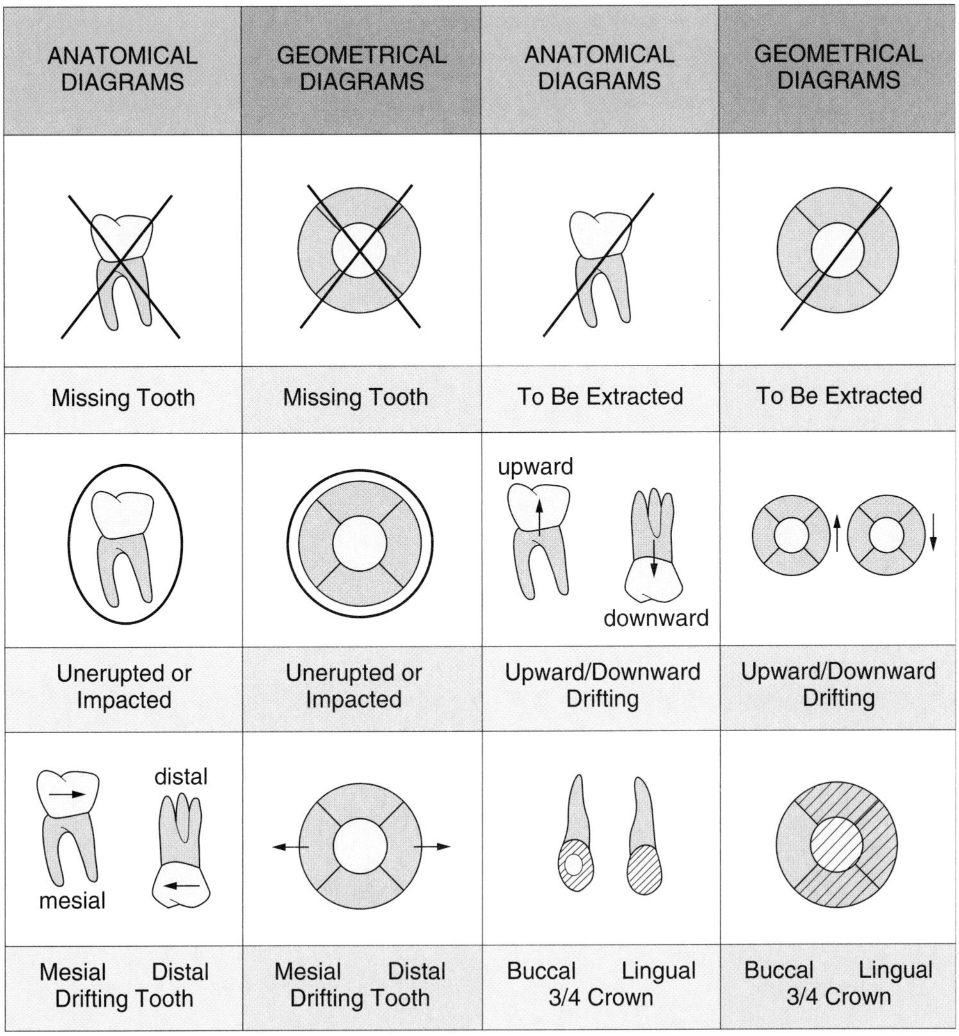

ANATOMICAL DIAGRAMS	GEOMETRICAL DIAGRAMS	ANATOMICAL DIAGRAMS	GEOMETRICAL DIAGRAMS
Missing Tooth	Missing Tooth	To Be Extracted	To Be Extracted
Unerupted or Impacted	Unerupted or Impacted	upward / downward Upward/Downward Drifting	Upward/Downward Drifting
distal / mesial Mesial Distal Drifting Tooth	Mesial Distal Drifting Tooth	Buccal Lingual 3/4 Crown	Buccal Lingual 3/4 Crown

Figure 24.13

Examples of charting symbols.

Tooth Number	Condition
2	Full gold crown bridge abutment (anchor tooth)
3	Pontic-fake tooth of bridge
4	Veneer with gold bridge abutment (anchor tooth)
8	Mesial decay
9	Mesial fracture
11	Distal decay
13	Full porcelain crown
16	Needs to be extracted
17	Impacted toward mesial
18	Buccal decay
19	Occlusal decay
20	Mod restoration already done filled in
24	Root canal
25	Periapical abscess (around the root)
29	Two occlusal pit decays

Figure 24.13

Examples of charting symbols (continued).

ANATOMICAL DIAGRAMS	GEOMETRICAL DIAGRAMS	ANATOMICAL DIAGRAMS	GEOMETRICAL DIAGRAMS
Full Crown	Full Crown	Porcelain Crown Fused to Metal	Porcelain Crown Fused to Metal
3/4 Crown Full Crown Fixed Bridge	Unerupted or Impacted	Fracture	Fracture
Abscess	Abscess	Root Canal	Root Canal

30   MO (mesiocclusal) decay

31   DO (distocclusal) decay

32   Missing

A common procedure is to use red and blue color codes on the chart. *Red* indicates that treatment is necessary. Use the following guidelines to chart conditions needing treatment.

- Outline fractures and dental **caries** in red.
- Use red for **impaction, abscesses,** overhanging margins, extractions, and periodontal pockets.
- Outline in red an old restoration that needs replacing and fill in with solid blue.

Blue indicates that the treatment is completed or that there is a condition that does not require treatment but must be watched carefully.

- Use blue to outline and shade amalgam restorations that are in good condition.
- Outline and draw diagonal lines in blue for gold restorations.
- Use blue to indicate missing teeth and root canals.

caries

Decay.

impaction

Any tooth that does not erupt when it should (e.g., tooth blocked by bone and/or tissue, keeping it under the surface of the gum).

abscesses

Pockets of pus in a limited area.

Figure 24.13

Examples of charting symbols (continued).

ANATOMICAL DIAGRAMS	GEOMETRICAL DIAGRAMS	ANATOMICAL DIAGRAMS	GEOMETRICAL DIAGRAMS
4 mm 4 mm	4 4		
Periodontal Pocket	Periodontal Pocket	Periodontal Abscess	Periodontal Abscess
Occ MOD Amalgam Restoration	Occ MOD Amalgam Restoration	D(III) MO(II) MI(IV) Composite Restoration	D(III) MO(II) MI(IV) Composite Restoration
Overhanging margin	Overhanging		

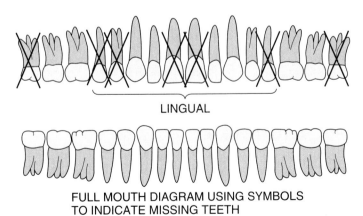

LINGUAL

FULL MOUTH DIAGRAM USING SYMBOLS TO INDICATE MISSING TEETH

- Outline tooth-colored restorations in blue (e.g., restorations that match the teeth).

Indicate a cavity (carie/decay) that covers more than one surface by writing, "Tooth #1 has an MO," which means a mesioocclusal cavity.

Learn the procedure that your dentist prefers.

Figure 24.14

Examples of charting an anatomical diagram.

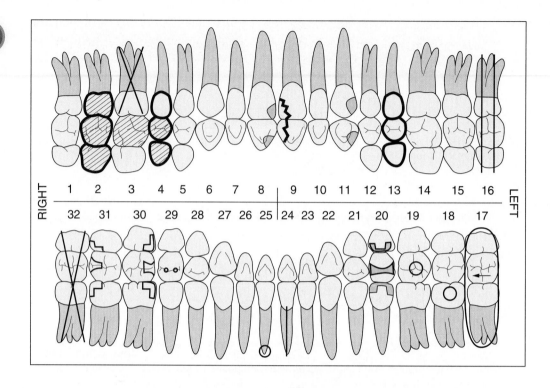

Figure 24.15

Examples of charting a geometric diagram.

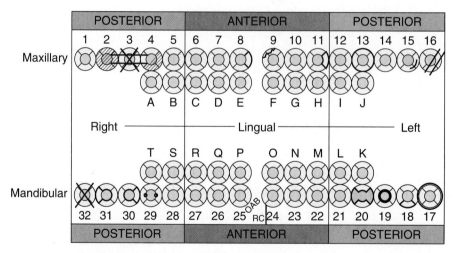

DENTAL EQUIPMENT

A dental treatment (operatory) room is designed and organized to ensure that the dentist and assistant perform procedures in a safe and time-efficient manner. Treatment room equipment includes the following:

- Dental chair
- Dental unit
- Operational light
- Mobile carts or cabinets
- Operatory stools
- X-ray machine and view box

The type of equipment varies depending on the office. As a dental assistant, you are responsible for learning how to use the various types of equipment. Dental equipment is costly and requires special care. It is important that you follow the manufacturers' cleaning and operating instructions.

Dental Chair

Parts of a dental chair are as follows (see Figure 24.16):

- The body of the chair includes the backrest, seat, and leg support.
- The armrest is usually movable.
- The headrest supports the patient's head and is movable.
- The control panel is on the side or back of the chair. Foot pedals are attached to base of chair or rest on the floor. These are used to move the chair into either a sitting or reclining (supine) position.
- The swivel lever is at the base of the chair, which allows the chair to rotate.

Dental Unit

A dental unit is attached to the dental chair or to a separate movable cart (Figure 24.16). The basic parts of a dental unit are as follows:

- Master switch/control for
  - Water and air • Handpiece
- Dental handpiece with burs or drills:
  - High speed • Slow speed
- Foot control (**rheostat**), which provides power to the handpiece.
- Air/water syringe to rinse and dry teeth.
- Oral **evacuation** system to **aspirate** saliva and drainage from the mouth. This system has two hoses attached to
  - A suction tip • A small saliva ejector
- Cuspidor, the bowl that patients spit into (modern offices use suction in place of a cuspidor).

rheostat
Control for flow of electric current.

evacuation
Removal.

aspirate
Remove substances.

Operational Light

The operational light is attached to the chair or the ceiling. It has handles to move the light. The light must focus on the site where the dentist is working.

Dental Mobile Carts or Cabinets

The dental cart/cabinet provides storage for a small number of sterile instruments, treatment trays, dental materials, and supplies. Large amounts of supplies are stored in areas away from the patient treatment room.

Operatory Stools

Operatory stools vary in design. There may be a footrest ring near the base on some stools, but all include the following:

- Padded seat
- Five casters at the base to prevent tipping
- Height-adjustment lever to position:
  - Dental assistant 4 to 6 inches above the dentist • Dentist stabilized below the assistant, with thighs parallel to floor when feet are flat on the floor
- Adjustable back support

Figure 24.16

(Photos courtesy of A-dec, Inc.) a. Dental unit; b. Chair; c. Air/water syringe; d. Mobile dental unit (note foot-controlled rheostat). e. Assistant's cart; f. and g. Operatory stools.

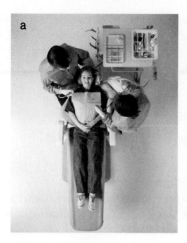
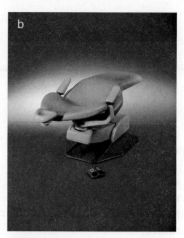
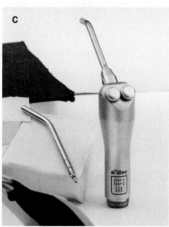
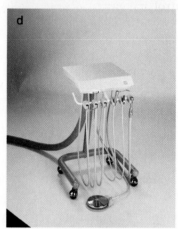
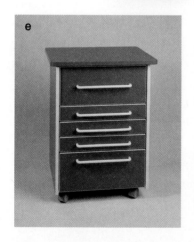
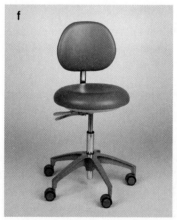
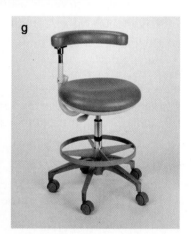

Radiology Machine

A radiology machine uses radiation to take x-rays. All radiology machines must operate according to state regulations to ensure safety. State regulations tell how to prevent **overexposure** to radiation and provide safety guidelines for machine operations. These regulations require the following:

- Registration of each radiology machine
- **Periodic** inspection of equipment to ensure safe operation
- A licensed person to operate a radiology machine

overexposure

Too much contact with radiation.

periodic

Occurring at regular intervals.

⬤ INFECTION CONTROL

Infection control guidelines exist to protect employees and patients against infectious viruses and bacteria. The Standard Precautions you follow depend on

- The potential for contact with blood
- The potential for contact with any body fluids
- The tasks that you perform

OSHA directs health care workers and their employers to follow specific guidelines to protect against infection (review Unit 1 of Chapter 12). As a dental assistant, you wear gloves, mask, and protective eyewear when assisting with or performing procedures. You are also required to wear a long-sleeve lab coat or top to protect against being scratched by an instrument. Table 24.2 helps you understand Standard Precautions and protective wear guidelines.

Infection control measures are necessary to prevent infecting other patients, yourself, and co-workers. Cleaning the treatment area is one way to control infection. Read the following Chapter 20 topics:

- Decontamination
- Preparation area

Table 24.2 ■ Standard Precautions: Examples of Tasks and Use of Protective Equipment

Task	Gloves	Gown	Mask	Eyewear
Controlling spurting blood	Yes	Yes	Yes	Yes
Controlling minimal bleeding	Yes	No	No	No
Oral or nasal suction	Yes	No	Yes	Yes
Handling/cleaning contaminated instruments	Yes	Yes	Yes	Yes

PROCEDURE 24.1 **CLEANING THE TREATMENT ROOM BETWEEN PATIENTS/CLIENTS**

RATIONALE

A properly cleaned area prevents the spread of infection. It also gives the patient confidence in the dental team.

ALERT: Follow Standard Precautions.

1. Wash hands.
2. Assemble equipment.
   a. Latex gloves or utility gloves
   b. Disinfectant solution
   c. Disposable towel
   d. Protective wear (see Table 24.2)
3. Put on protective wear.

4. Discard all disposable items.
5. Place soiled instruments in disinfectant container, and cover.
6. Spray/wipe disinfectant solution on all surfaces. Follow directions on disinfectant for the drying procedure.

PROCEDURE 24.2

PREPARING THE TREATMENT AREA FOR A PATIENT/CLIENT

RATIONALE

The dentist and dental assistant work together as an efficient team when the equipment is set up correctly. Time is saved and the patient feels secure in your care.

ALERT: Follow Standard Precautions.

1. Wash hands.
2. Assemble equipment.
   a. Procedure tray/instruments
   b. Plastic **barriers**
   c. Patient's chart
   d. Most recent x-rays
   e. Headrest cover
   f. Patient drape
   g. Alligator clips
   h. Two pairs of latex gloves
   i. Mask/safety shields or glasses
3. Open procedure tray or place instruments on treatment tray in the order of use, and cover.
4. Place all barriers on chair and handpieces.
5. Position patient chair in lowest position.

6. Raise armrest on patient-access side of chair.
7. Place chart for easy access by the dentist.
8. Display most recent x-rays on view box.
9. Place patient drape and alligator clips for easy access.
10. Use plastic barriers to cover:
    a. Handpiece and hoses
    b. Air/water syringes, tips, and hoses
    c. Suction hose and plastic tip
    d. Operative light handles
    e. X-ray tube head
11. Place latex gloves, mask, and protective glasses for easy access to dentist and dental assistant.

barriers   Items that prevent infectious material from contacting surface.

- Sterile wraps
- Monitoring effectiveness of sterilization

This information tells you how to clean, wrap, and sterilize instruments.

The treatment area must be clean and free of any items from the preceding patient. Prepare the room for the next client by doing the previous two procedures.

Clients may be nervous about seeing the dentist. The way you greet the patient and bring him or her to the treatment area helps set the atmosphere for that appointment. Once the treatment area is prepared for the patient, follow the steps below to admit and seat the patient.

PROCEDURE 24.3

ADMITTING AND SEATING A PATIENT/CLIENT

RATIONALE

Greeting patients in a positive manner and explaining what you want them to do help the patient relax. It is much easier to control discomfort and nervousness when the patient is comfortable and relaxed.

PROCEDURE 24.3 ADMITTING AND SEATING A PATIENT/CLIENT *(Continued)*

1. Greet patient by name. Verify that chart and patient's name match.

2. Say, "We are ready for you now, Mr./Mrs./Ms. _____, I'll show you to the examination room." (Keep the discussion pleasant; follow the dentist's instructions when answering questions. If you are unsure of an answer, instruct the patient to ask the dentist; for example, "Dr. _____ can answer that question when he/she comes in" or "Please ask Dr. _____ when he/she comes in.")

3. Show patient where to place personal items. (It's best to indicate a place for personal items within the patient's view.)

4. Seat patient and lower armrest.

5. Place patient drape over chest and secure with alligator clips.

6. Review and document patient's health history and current dental concerns.

7. Measure vital signs if required by dentist.

8. Provide patient with protective eyewear if necessary.

9. Wash hands.

10. Put on protective wear.

11. Notify dentist that patient is ready.

12. Adjust chair at time of examination/treatment. The patient's toes should be at the same level as his or her nose.

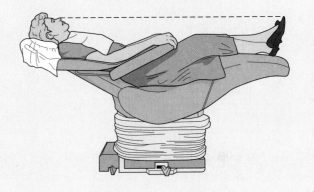

BASIC SETUP FOR DENTAL PROCEDURES

Always have the patient's chart, x-rays, and recently taken study models available when you set up the area. Be sure that you have pencils in all the colors that you may need.

The basic setup tray contains the following:

1. **Mouth mirror.** To reflect light to see the surfaces of the teeth; to inspect teeth, tongue, gingiva, and oral cavity; and for retraction (hold cheek back)

2. **Explorer.** To feel teeth for decay or other problems

3. **Cotton forceps.** To pick up gauze/cotton to dry areas of mouth/teeth

4. **Periodontal probe.** To check and measure sulcus area

5. **Gauze squares.** 4 × 4s/2 × 2s to dry and hold slippery tissues

6. **Suction tip/saliva ejector.** To keep mouth dry and structures visible

7. **Air/water syringe tip.** To rinse and dry

8. **Dental floss.** To check contacts between teeth

BASIC CHAIRSIDE ASSISTING SKILLS DURING DENTAL TREATMENT

There are specific guidelines that the dental assistant follows whenever he or she is assisting the dentist at chairside. These guidelines are as follows:

- Position light 36 inches away from mouth.

- Adjust the light to ensure that the area being worked on is always visible during treatment.

- Use the suction tip and air/water syringe as needed to ensure visibility.

- Pass instruments and materials as needed.

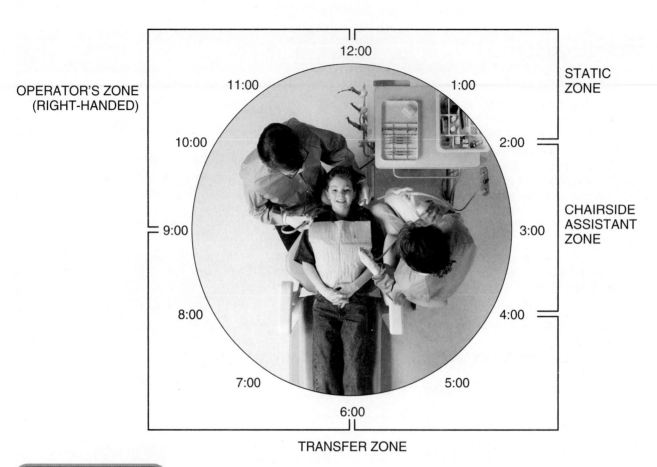

OPERATOR'S ZONE
(RIGHT-HANDED)

STATIC
ZONE

CHAIRSIDE
ASSISTANT
ZONE

TRANSFER ZONE

Figure 24.17

Clock positions/working zones. (Photo courtesy of A-dec, Inc.)

Instrument Transfer

Remember to pass instruments over the patient's chest and below the patient's chin. The positions of the dentist, dental assistant, and patient are compared to the positions of a clock. The patient's head is always at 12 o'clock. The right-handed dentist is usually at 9 to 11 o'clock. The dental assistant works between 2 and 3 o'clock. Familiarize yourself with the "clock" positions (see Figure 24.17).

ORAL EXAMINATION

During the oral examination, the dentist examines the face, joints, muscles, glands, tissue, and oral cavity with his or her fingers. This method of examination is called **palpation.** Next the dentist uses a mirror and explorer to check the teeth and gingiva/gums. The dentist examines each tooth, and the dental assistant uses symbols to draw needed services on the tooth chart. After a thorough examination, the dentist explains the findings and the recommended procedures.

palpation

Examine by feeling for unusual or abnormal conditions.

Pain Control

Controlling pain is an important part of patient care. There are different types of pain control.

■ An analgesic helps relieve pain or causes it to disappear. In dentistry the analgesia is often given in a gas and inhaled through a face mask. The advantages are that

PROCEDURE 24.4   ASSISTING DURING THE ORAL EXAMINATION

RATIONALE

The correct technique when assisting the dentist with an examination is essential for an efficient oral examination.

1. Seat and drape patient/client.
2. Wash hands.
3. Assemble equipment.
   a. Patient chart
   b. Pencils in colors you may need
   c. X-rays
   d. Current study models
   e. Sterile package with basic setup instruments
   f. Gauze
   g. Protective wear
4. Open sterile package and place on sterile field.
5. Put on protective wear.
6. Pass mouth mirror and explorer to dentist at same time. Use both hands to place mirror in dentist's left hand and explorer into right hand. (This is reversed if dentist is left-handed.)

• The patient feels relaxed and awake. • The medication is short acting and easy to control.

Other forms of analgesia are pills or injections that help **sedate** the patient. These are usually longer acting than gases. *Never leave a patient/client alone when he or she is sedated.*

- Local anesthetics take away feeling in a specific area. Local anesthetics are topical and **injectable.** The dentist often uses both.

   • Topical anesthetics such as lidocaine (Xylocaine) ointment are rubbed over the gingiva/gums and absorbed into the tissue. The surface tissue loses feeling. This lessens the discomfort of the injection. • Injectable anesthetic such as lidocaine (Xylocaine) is placed in the gingiva/gums tissue, either blocking a nerve or **saturating** the tissue around nerves.

The dentist decides which type of anesthetic to give the patient. When he or she orders an injectable anesthetic, the dental assistant prepares and passes the syringe to the dentist. The dental assistant selects the needle length depending on the site of injection. The dentist orders anesthesia for

- *Maxillary infiltration,* which requires a separate injection for each tooth. The anesthesia is injected near the nerve endings. It requires a 1-inch needle (see Figure 24.18a).

- *Mandibular nerve block,* which blocks the main nerve, causing several teeth to be free of pain. It requires a 1⅝-inch needle (see Figure 24.18b).

Anesthetic medication is available in narrow glass tubes called carpule/cartridges. The carpule/cartridge is placed into an aspirating syringe. Follow the steps in the procedure "Loading and Unloading a Carpule/Cartridge in an Aspirating Syringe."

sedate
Calm.

injectable
Medication given by needle.

saturating
Soak.

Figure 24.18

Injection sites for anesthesia.

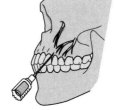
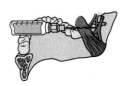
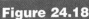

(a) Maxillary infiltration   (b) Mandibular nerve block

PROCEDURE 24.5

PROCEDURE 24.5 | LOADING AND UNLOADING A CARPULE/CARTRIDGE IN AN ASPIRATING SYRINGE

RATIONALE

Correct loading and unloading of a syringe ensures that there is no contamination of the needle. It also ensures that the dentist will not have a problem when using it.

1. Wash hands.
2. Assemble equipment. (Keep syringe and medication out of patient's view to prevent anxiety.)
   a. Lidocaine carpule
   b. Aspirating syringe
   c. Sterile needle
   d. Alcohol wipe
   e. Protective wear
3. Inspect the carpule for
   a. Large bubbles (more than 2 mm), which are usually caused by freezing. **Do not use.**
   b. Bulging/protruding plunger, which means either
      (1) The cartridge was left in a chemical disinfectant solution too long. **Do not use.**
      (2) The cartridge was frozen. **Do not use.**
   c. Cracks and chips, which can cause a cartridge to break during injection. **Do not use.**
   d. Expiration date. **Do not use after the last day of the month the medication expires.**
4. Put on protective wear.
5. Disinfect cap end of cartridge with 70% ethyl alcohol.
6. Pull piston/plunger all the way back on syringe.
7. Place plunger end of the cartridge into syringe at base of piston.
8. Move body of cartridge into syringe and gently secure in place by applying slight pressure to the plunger (harpoon).
9. Attach needle to syringe.
10. Loosen needle cover. **Do not remove it.**
11. Pass syringe to dentist. (See the procedure "Passing and Receiving the Syringe.")

To remove cartridge after the injection:

12. Draw cartridge back from needle and remove from syringe.
13. Remove needle according to office procedure and place in sharps container.
14. Disinfect syringe and sterilize.

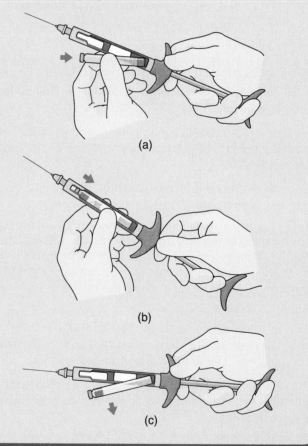

(a)

(b)

(c)

Passing the Syringe

Always pass syringe to the dentist below the patient's chin or behind the patient's head to help reduce his or her anxiety.

PROCEDURE 24.6

PASSING AND RECEIVING THE SYRINGE

RATIONALE

Following the same procedure for passing and receiving the syringe helps the dentist and the dental assistant to work together as a competent team.

ALERT: Follow Standard Precautions.

1. Hold syringe in your **dominant hand.**
2. Apply topical anesthetic to applicator, and hand it to dentist with your other hand.
3. Lay thumb ring/cradle of syringe at the dentist's thumb, making sure his or her fingers are in position to grasp the syringe before you release it.
4. Remove needle cap as you slide your hand away from syringe. Place cap on tray in position to slip used needle in place easily after injection.
5. Place your hand near patient's hands to prevent sudden movements from hitting syringe (especially important for new patients).
6. Observe patient before, during, and after injection for signs of fainting or allergic reaction.
7. Receive syringe by holding barrel, taking care to prevent needle sticks.
8. Recap needle by holding syringe with both hands and scooping cap into position on needle.
9. Carefully secure cap and remove needle.
10. Place needle in sharps container.
11. Loosen cartridge and place in sharps container.

dominant hand   Hand used for writing, eating, working.

PROCEDURE 24.7

INSTRUMENT EXCHANGE

RATIONALE

Instrument exchange is an important skill that allows the dentist and the dental assistant to work together as a competent team.

ALERT: Follow Standard Precautions.

1. Use thumb and forefinger of your left hand to pick up instruments from tray.
2. Stick out little finger.
3. Turn instrument and your hand **parallel** to instrument dentist is already holding.
4. Approach slowly.
5. Curl little finger around and pick up unwanted instrument. Squeeze instrument into your wrist.
6. Place new instrument into position between dentist's thumb and forefinger.
7. Turn used instrument with thumb and return it to tray in order of use.

parallel   Same direction and at a distance, so that two points do not touch.

⦿ ORAL EVACUATION/RINSING AND DRYING TECHNIQUES

When a tooth restoration such as removing decay and filling the tooth is necessary, the dentist uses instruments called handpieces. Handpieces, which hold small drills (burs) to cut and shape the tooth, operate at very high speeds. A small cutting device called a **rotary** cutting instrument (or bur) is placed in the end of the handpiece. Water comes out of the handpiece to cool the tooth because cutting (drilling) on the tooth creates heat that is painful.

The dental assistant picks up water and tooth debris with the high-volume evacuation tip. This tip is called an HVE, vacuum tip, suction, or aspirator (see Figure 24.19).

The plastic tip (usually disposable) is placed into the handle at the end of the suction hose. There are two ways to grasp the suction tip (see Figures 24.20 and 24.21):

1. Thumb-to-nose grasp

2. Pen grasp

CAUTION   Be gentle when using the suction tip in the patient's mouth to prevent injury to fragile tissue. Keep a good grasp to ensure constant control of the suction.

Proper placement and use of the suction tip save operating time and reduce by 80% the debris that flies out of the mouth during procedures (Figure 24.22).

The dental assistant usually sits on the left side of the patient and holds the suction tip in his or her right hand. Reverse this if working with a left-handed dentist.

rotary
Move in a circular fashion.

Figure 24.19

HVE, vacuum tip.

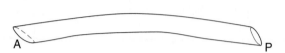

Figure 24.20

Thumb-to-nose grasp.

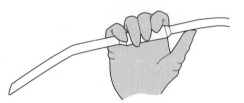

Figure 24.21

Pen grasp.

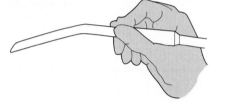

Figure 24.22

Placement of suction tip during a procedure.

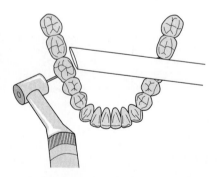

PROCEDURE 24.8 HIGH-VELOCITY EVACUATION

RATIONALE

Correct placement and evacuation of debris maintains a clear area for the dentist to repair the tooth. It also assists in preventing choking or discomfort for the patient.

ALERT: Follow Standard Precautions.

PROCEDURE 24.8 — HIGH-VELOCITY EVACUATION (Continued)

1. Wash hands.
2. Assemble equipment.
   a. Long-sleeved lab coat
   b. Gloves
   c. Eye protection
   d. Mask
   e. Suction tip
3. Put on protective wear.

4. Grasp HVE (suction tip) according to area of mouth to suction.
5. Position tip before dentist places handpiece and mirror into position.
6. Place beveled edge parallel to buccal or lingual side of tooth being treated.
7. Keep tip close to treated tooth to pull debris and water over tooth into tip.

PROCEDURE 24.9 — AIR-WATER SPRAY OR TRIPLEX SYRINGE

RATIONALE

The dental assistant keeps the teeth in the area the dentist is working on clean and dry. Teamwork provides efficient care and reduces the time required for dental work and also reduces the time the patient is in the dental chair for treatment.

ALERT: Follow Standard Precautions.

1. Wash hands.
2. Assemble equipment.
   a. Gloves
   b. Gown/lab coat
   c. Eye protection
   d. Mask
   e. Air/water syringe and tip
   f. Plastic protective covers for hoses
3. Put on protective wear.

4. Test syringe by pressing
   a. "A" to spray a stream of air
   b. "W" to spray a stream of water
   c. "A" and "B" to combine water and air in a spray
5. Place air/water tip near opening of oral cavity and aim at surfaces to be rinsed. Position suction tip close to water spray.
6. Immediately dry area with air, allowing dentist to continue treatment. (Avoid spraying directly into a surgical wound and use short burst of air.)

PROCEDURE 24.10 — COMPLETION OF TREATMENT AND PATIENT/CLIENT DISMISSAL

RATIONALE

Helping the patient after the treatment is finished is essential for the patient's well-being. It protects his or her safety and ensures that the patient feels cared for as an individual.

1. Fold client drape to collect debris as you remove alligator clip and drape.
2. Return patient to sitting position. (Place hand on patient's shoulder and caution him or her not to stand up too fast, allowing time to balance.)
3. Lower chair to a safe height.
4. Check area to see that patient collects all belongings.

5. Escort patient to reception desk.
6. Chart completion of procedures.
7. Wash hands.
8. Perform the procedure "Cleaning the Treatment Room Between Patients/Clients."

STUDY MODELS

Study models or casts of teeth, gingiva/gums, and soft tissues provide the structure necessary to make dentures, partial dentures, bridgework, and other corrective/prosthetic devices. An impression of these structures is made before making a model. The impression creates a mold to pour plaster/stone material into. The study model is made when the plaster/stone dries and is removed from the impression/mold. There are four steps to follow:

alginate

Material for making impressions.

1. Make an **alginate** impression of the mandibular/lower teeth first, then of the maxillary/upper teeth. The maxillary impression procedure may cause gagging, so it is best to take it second.

2. Make a wax bite impression. A wax bite shows the relationship of the occlusal (touching) surfaces of the maxillary and mandibular teeth.

3. Mix the plaster.

4. Pour into impression mold, and trim.

To make a study model, take each step in the following procedures.

PROCEDURE 24.11

PREPARING TO TAKE ALGINATE IMPRESSIONS

RATIONALE

Proper fit is essential for the well-being of the patient, and preparing alginate impressions correctly ensures that the dental prosthesis will fit properly.

ALERT: Follow Standard Precautions.

1. Wash hands.
2. Assemble equipment.
   a. Gloves
   b. Protective eyewear
   c. Mask
   d. Gown
   e. Basic setup (see "Basic Setup for Dental Procedures")
   f. Alginate powder
   g. Rubber bowl
   h. Measuring scoop (with alginate powder)
   i. Water measure (with alginate powder)
   j. Water at room temperature
   k. Spatula (shaped like a beaver's tail)
   l. Impression trays
   m. Round pencil-like strips of beading wax
   n. Plastic drape
   o. Clock/watch
3. Seat and drape client. Leave seat in upright position while taking impressions, to minimize gagging.
4. Ask patient if he or she has ever had an impression taken.

5. Explain what you are going to do, including what the patient will feel/experience.
6. Put on protective wear.
7. Remove any removable items (bridge, loose crown, dentures, etc.) from patient's mouth, rinse, and place on paper towel.
8. Rinse patient's mouth with water syringe.
9. Fit impression trays (upper and lower) by placing a tray size you think will fit in patient's mouth. (The correct size will not stretch lips.) The teeth must be in center of tray, not touching tray sides.
10. Rinse and dry selected trays.
11. Apply beading wax around edge of each tray to form impression edge and prevent pressure on gingiva/gums tissue (vestibule).
12. Place prepared trays on covered treatment tray ready for use.

Mixing–Loading Trays
13. Verify whether alginate is fast set or regular set. Fast or regular set determines length of time alginate takes to mix and become firm in patient's mouth.

14. Follow mixing directions on alginate container.

    a. Place measured room-temperature water into rubber bowl.

    b. Place measured alginate powder into bowl.

    c. Mix water and powder until powder is completely wet.

    d. Hold bowl sideways in your **nondominant hand.** Holding spatula in your dominant hand, mix by rubbing mixture against sides of bowl in a figure-eight motion until creamy smooth.

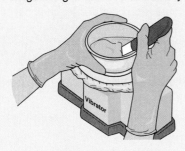

15. Load mandibular tray with a spatula, as you would frost a cake. Be sure to fill tray without leaving air bubbles.

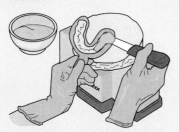

16. Wipe and smooth surface of alginate mixture with wet gloved finger before placing tray in patient's mouth.

17. Stand in front of patient.

18. Instruct patient to open mouth just enough to allow tray to be placed in mouth.

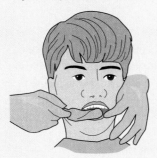

19. Insert tray into mouth one side at a time.

20. Line up tray handle with patient's midline (nose).

21. Press back of tray over molars.

22. Press onto front teeth, while easing lip away from impression material.

23. Instruct client to lift tongue; at same time press down, **seating** impression material around teeth and gingiva/gums.

24. Hold tray in position until alginate is firm enough to stay in shape or to set. (Alginate directions will give the approximate time period.)

25. Feel alginate to see if it holds its shape, before removing tray.

26. Run your gloved index and middle fingers along labial edge of tray to release seal around teeth when alginate is set.

27. Lift front of tray first, then lift back.

28. Turn tray sideways and remove from mouth one side at a time.

29. Rinse and suction patient's mouth.

30. Gently rinse impression with water and spray with disinfectant.

31. Display impression for dentist to inspect.

32. Place in plastic bag for a minimum of 10 minutes before pouring plaster/stone to make model.

33. Load maxillary tray as described in steps 13 and 14.

34. Provide patient with tissue to blot moisture if necessary.

35. Instruct patient to breathe through his or her nose and slightly lean forward once tray is in place.

36. Stand behind patient.

37. Instruct patient to open mouth just enough to accept tray.

38. Insert tray one side at a time and position over teeth.

39. Center tray by placing handle in line with patient's nose.

40. Press impression material over back teeth first.

41. Press over front teeth while easing lip away from impression material.

42. Press tray in place, seating impression material over gingiva/gums line.

43. Allow client to lean slightly forward and to breathe through the nose.

44. Hold tray in place until alginate is set (see step 24).

45. Follow steps 26 to 32 to complete procedure.

46. Remove protective wear.

47. Wash hands.

nondominant hand   Hand that is not used for writing or other tasks.

seating   Putting firmly in place to prevent moving.

PROCEDURE 24.12

REGISTERING A WAX BITE

RATIONALE

Registering a wax bite verifies the midline and occlusion alignment.

1. Wash hands.
2. Assemble equipment.
    a. Bowl of warm water
    b. Wax bite wafer (thin, U-shaped)
    c. Lab knife
    d. Protective wear
3. Explain what you are going to do.
4. Put on protective wear.
5. Trim back edges of wax to fit patient's mouth if necessary.
6. Place wax in warm water to soften.
7. Grasp wax so that U shape can be placed in mouth to align with U shape of teeth.
8. Instruct patient to open mouth.
9. Place wax in position over lower teeth.
10. Instruct client to bite down on wax hard enough to make an impression but not enough to bite through wax. Ask the patient to hold the bite.
11. Spray air onto wax to gently cool.
12. Ask patient to open mouth when cool.
13. Gently remove wax, being careful not to bend or tear impression.
14. Gently rinse wax and spray with disinfectant.
15. Mark patient's initials in upper right corner of wax impression.
16. Place wax impression with alginate impressions.
17. Remove protective wear and wash hands.

PROCEDURE 24.13

PREPARING AND POURING PLASTER/STONE INTO IMPRESSIONS TO MAKE CASTS

RATIONALE

Carefully preparing and pouring plaster/stone impressions ensures correct fit of a prosthesis. Improper fit requires additional appointments and more stress to the patient.

1. Wash hands.
2. Assemble equipment.
    a. Modeling plaster/stone
    b. Scale or measuring device for plaster
    c. 100-mL graduated cylinder
    d. Rubber bowls/flexiboles
    e. Plaster spatula
    f. Vibrator
    g. Impressions
    h. Wax paper/glass slab/tile square
    i. Scale
3. Place 45 to 50 mL of water into bowl.
4. Measure 100 g of plaster.
5. Mix plaster powder into water by pouring a slow, steady stream of powder and stirring carefully.
6. Mix until material looks like sour cream.
7. Hold mixing bowl on vibrator for approximately 2 minutes, allowing bubbles to rise to surface.
8. Remove bowl from vibrator and mix ingredients with spatula again.
9. Secure impression in your hand by holding tray handle.
10. Rest impression tray on vibrator.
11. Secure impression tray to keep from falling.
12. Scoop plaster/stone mixture with spatula.
13. Pour small portions of plaster/stone from spatula into one end of impression.
14. Watch plaster/stone vibrate into each tooth form.

PROCEDURE 24.13 | PREPARING AND POURING PLASTER/STONE INTO IMPRESSIONS TO MAKE CASTS *(Continued)*

15. Turn impression tray as you gradually fill each tooth form with plaster/stone.

16. Remove impression tray from vibrator when all tooth forms are filled with plaster/stone.

17. Pour plaster to fill remainder of impression tray.

18. Use spatula to smooth and fill total impression tray.

19. Form a ½-inch-thick round patty on a glass slab or tile. The patty must be the size of the impression tray.

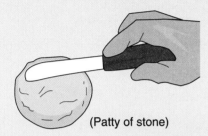

(Patty of stone)

20. Turn impression tray filled with plaster/stone onto patty. Keep tray level with countertop.

21. Inspect to ensure that plaster/stone impression and base are joined together. Make sure that edge of impression tray is not covered with plaster.

22. Flatten inside area of tray where the tongue normally is when placing mandibular impression on base.

23. Allow at least 29 to 60 minutes for plaster/stone to set/harden.

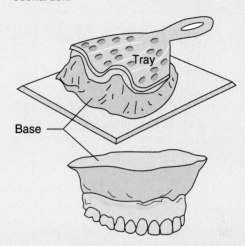

24. Hold plaster/stone model and impression tray under running water.

25. Gently slide plaster/stone model out of impression tray.

26. Dispose of impression material.

27. Clean trays if they are reusable.

PROCEDURE 24.14 | TRIMMING STUDY MODELS

RATIONALE

Trimming models the same way each time ensures that the dental lab will be able to make a prosthesis that fits correctly.

1. Wash hands.

2. Assemble equipment.
   a. Protective eyewear
   b. Laboratory knife
   c. Model trimmer
   d. Bowl of water

3. Soak models in water at least 5 minutes. (Wet models are easier to trim and do not break as easily.)

4. Put on protective eyewear.

5. Turn on model-trimmer water.

6. Allow time for water to moisten grinding wheel.

Safety precaution: Hold model securely with steady pressure against grinding wheel. Always keep fingers away from wheel.

7. Place base of model against grinding wheel to smooth and level surface. The base must be at least ½-inch thick and parallel to biting surface of teeth.

8. Place heel of mandibular model against wheel and trim to approximately ¼ inch behind third molar.

9. Hold heel at a 90° angle (perpendicular) to the base.

PROCEDURE 24.14 | TRIMMING STUDY MODELS *(Continued)*

10. Measure maxillary model against mandibular model and trim to match.
11. Trim side of
    a. Maxillary model at a 63° angle to heel.
    b. Mandibular model at a 55° angle to heel.
    c. Keep edge of models between ¼ and ⅜ inch of bicuspids.
12. Trim heel points to ½ inch to a 125° angle to heel.
13. Mark by making a small cut on the
    a. Maxillary model on each side of cuspid and central incisors, to form a point.
    b. Mandibular model to form an arc at cuspids.
14. Clean trimmer according to manufacturer's instructions.
15. Clean area and return equipment to its storage area.
16. Wash hands.

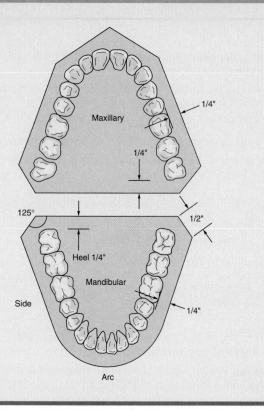

PROCEDURE 24.15 | CAVITY PREPARATION

RATIONALE

Correct assistance during cavity restoration prevents delay and ensures that the restoration is completed smoothly and without complications.

ALERT: Follow Standard Precautions.

1. Wash hands.
2. Assemble equipment.
    a. Gloves
    b. Gown
    c. Protective eyewear
    d. Mask
    e. Anesthetic solution
    f. Aspirating syringe
    g. Lidocaine ointment
    h. Cotton rolls
    i. Basic procedure tray
    j. Restoration instruments
    k. Suction tips
    l. Air/water tips
    m. Handpieces and burs
3. Prepare anesthetic syringe.
4. Put on protective wear.
5. Position yourself, suction, and water/air devices for easy access.
6. Perform suction, rinsing, and drying procedures as needed during restorative process. This is referred to as "keeping the operating field clear."

NOTE When you learn to prepare materials to line and fill the cavity, you may begin performing these duties.

ASSISTING DURING BASIC RESTORATIVE PROCEDURES

Restoring a tooth to a healthy state is a frequently performed procedure in a dental office. The dental assistant is very important in this procedure. Be certain to learn your dentist's preferences. It is important to become familiar with the materials that your dentist uses in these procedures. Always read all product directions carefully when preparing to assist with restorative procedures. Be prepared to provide the dentist with all materials and equipment needed during a procedure. (See procedures 24.4 through 24.9.)

ORAL HYGIENE

Human teeth are meant to last a lifetime. Remember that enamel is the hardest tissue in the body. Why, then, do we lose teeth? The bacteria that live in everyone's mouth cause disease. There are two main reasons why we lose teeth:

■ Disease of the gingiva/gums, periodontal tissues, and/or the alveolar process (bony socket)

■ Holes in the enamel and/or dentin (cavities)

Proper toothbrushing and flossing plus good nutrition can help prevent disease and destruction (review Chapter 10).

Dental assistants explain and demonstrate proper toothbrushing and flossing techniques to their patients. The instruction must be clear and meet each patient's needs (for example, working around a bridge). Correct flossing and brushing helps

■ Remove **plaque**

■ Prevent bad breath (halitosis)

■ Prevent periodontal infection

■ Prevent bleeding gingiva/gums

plaque
Soft deposit of bacteria and bacterial products on teeth.

TEACHING ORAL HYGIENE

Your dentist may ask you to use disclosing tablets or solution to show the client that there is plaque in the mouth. The disclosing tablets are usually red and stain the plaque to help the patient see the areas where plaque has formed. Patients can see that even when they think plaque is removed, it may not be. This is a very good way to help patients understand that correct brushing and flossing are important.

There are several types of brushing techniques. Use the technique your dentist prefers. The Bass technique is a common one.

Common abbreviations for charting patient education:

■ **OHI.** Oral hygiene, complete cleansing of oral cavity

■ **TBI.** Toothbrushing instruction

■ **DFI.** Dental floss instruction

Flossing removes the plaque from the **interproximal surfaces** (between teeth). It removes plaque and food. Flossing cleans areas where brushing cannot reach. Correct flossing is very important because tooth decay often begins on the interproximal surfaces.

interproximal surfaces
Sides between teeth.

DISCLOSING TABLET/SOLUTION

RATIONALE

Use a disclosing tablet/solution to show patients that they are or are not cleaning their teeth properly and to help teach them proper cleaning technique.

1. Wash hands.
2. Put on gloves.
3. Assemble equipment.
   a. Disclosing tablets or solution
   b. Toothbrush recommended by dentist
   c. Mirror
   d. Cup
   e. Towels
   f. Protective wear if required
4. Explain why brushing/flossing is important.
   a. To prevent disease
   b. To prevent halitosis
   c. To prevent bleeding gingiva/gums
   d. For total body health

5. Follow directions for preparing disclosing tablets/solution.
6. Ask patient to swish solution around in mouth and spit solution into container.
7. Have patient rinse mouth.
8. Have patient look at teeth in mirror.
9. Explain that red areas are plaque.
10. Explain that this plaque must be removed to keep the mouth healthy. The best way to remove it is by toothbrushing and flossing. All surfaces of the teeth must be brushed carefully.

BASS TOOTHBRUSHING TECHNIQUE

RATIONALE

Correct dental flossing is essential for healthy teeth and gums. Explaining the importance of correct flossing and showing a patient good technique help protect against dental problems.

1. Wash hands.
2. Assemble equipment.
   a. Tooth model (if using a model for teaching)
   b. Protective wear (if brushing patient's teeth or if there is contact with saliva)
   c. Toothbrush
3. Explain importance of toothbrushing.
4. Demonstrate correct brushing using model or on patient.

NOTE Put on gloves if demonstrating on patient.

   a. Place soft brush on upper right molars (maxillary).
   b. Position brush at 45° angle to teeth.
   c. Gently move bristles into gingival sulcus.
   d. Move brush in short strokes at least 10 to 20 times, keeping brush in place (wiggle-jiggle motion).
   e. Move brush to next two or three teeth and repeat until all buccal/labial surfaces are brushed.

NOTE Place brush in vertical or horizontal position for anterior teeth.

   f. Repeat technique beginning at upper right molars until all maxillary teeth are brushed.
   g. Use short, vibrating motion to scrub occlusal surfaces.
   h. Repeat this procedure for lower teeth (mandibular).
5. Ask client if he or she has any questions.
6. Remove and clean equipment.
7. Remove protective wear.
8. Wash hands.
9. Chart TBI (toothbrushing instruction).

PROCEDURE 24.18 | **DENTAL FLOSSING**

RATIONALE

Correct dental flossing is essential for healthy teeth and gums. Explaining the importance of correct flossing and showing a patient good technique help protect against dental problems.

1. Wash hands.
2. Assemble equipment.
   a. Tooth model (if using a model for teaching)
   b. Gloves (if flossing patient's teeth or if there is contact with saliva)
   c. Dental floss (waxed or unwaxed according to policy)
3. Explain importance of flossing.
4. Demonstrate correct flossing technique using model or patient.
   NOTE   Put on protective wear if demonstrating on patient.
   a. Cut floss 18 inches (measure from finger to elbow).
   b. Wrap floss around middle or index finger of both hands, leaving 1 to 2 inches between fingers.
   c. Stretch floss between fingers and gently guide floss in between teeth. *Do not snap floss;* it can damage gingiva/gums.
   d. Pass floss through **contacts** (where teeth touch) and wrap it around tooth in a C shape.
   e. Move floss up and down several times on sides of each tooth.
   NOTE   Make sure that floss goes beneath gingiva/gums into the sulcus.
   f. Unroll new floss from one hand and wrap used floss around middle finger of other hand.
   g. Repeat for each tooth until all teeth in maxilla and mandible are completed.
5. Explain that there may be some bleeding of the gingiva/gums the first few times the patient does this procedure.
6. Ask patient if he or she has any questions.
7. Remove protective wear.
8. Remove and clean equipment.
9. Wash hands.
10. Chart DFI (dental flossing instruction).

contacts   Place where surface of teeth touch.

DENTAL RADIOGRAPHS

Dental assistants must have special training before they can take radiographs of the mouth. (Call your state dental board or association for information.) As an entry-level dental assistant, you may mount dental radiographs after they are developed. To mount radiographs correctly, you need some basic information.

Dental radiographs are photographs of the teeth. The radiographs allow the dentist to see between the teeth, the pulp of each tooth, and the bone (for example, caries, metallic restorations, poorly fitted crowns, root end infection, **resorption** of alveolar bone). Radiographs allow the dentist to identify problems and make repairs before the problems cause further damage.

resorption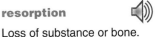

Loss of substance or bone.

Radiography Terminology

■ *Radiopaque* structures do not allow radiation to pass through. Enamel, metallic restorations, and dentin are radiopaque. They are very white on the film.

■ *Radiolucent* structures allow rays to penetrate through them. Pulp and caries are radiolucent. They are dark areas on the film.

■ *Periapical* films (PA) show two or three teeth and their surrounding bone structure (see Figure 24.23).

Figure 24.23

Periapical views.

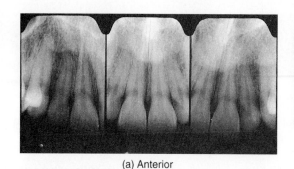

(a) Anterior

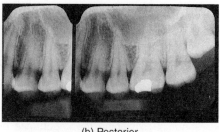

(b) Posterior

Figure 24.24

Bite wings.

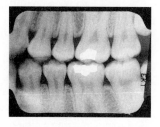 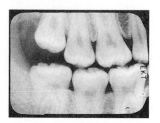

(a)   (b)

Figure 24.25

Occlusal view.

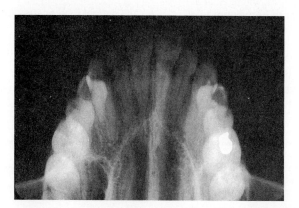

Figure 24.26

Panoramic survey.

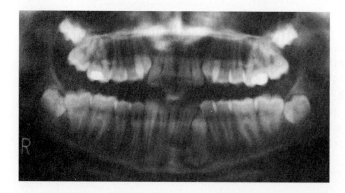

- *Bite wings* (BWX) show the crowns of the maxillary and mandibular teeth. These are often called the cavity detector films (see Figure 24.24).
- *Occlusal* (OCC) is a large film that shows the whole arch from the occlusal view (see Figure 24.25).
- *Panographic* (PANX) is a long film taken from outside the mouth (extra oral) by a special machine. It shows all structures and teeth (see Figure 24.26).

The radiographs serve as a guide that helps determine the treatment plan. After the radiograph is taken, it must be developed and mounted. Mounting film may be one of your duties.

Types of Mounts

Mounts come in different sizes. They may have 1, 2, 4, 7, 14, 16, 18, 20, and 28 windows. Bite-wing mounts have 2 or 4 windows. Common periapical mounts have 16 or 18 windows. When mounting films, you must remember the following:

- Periapical films show the crown and roots.
- Maxillary molars have three roots.
- Maxillary cuspids are the longest teeth in the mouth.
- Maxillary lateral incisors are larger than mandibular lateral incisors.

- Maxillary central incisors are larger than mandibular central incisors.
- Mandibular molars have two roots.
- Mandibular lateral incisors are wider than mandibular central incisors.
- The center of the mount is the median line.
- If the distal portion is on the right margin, it is the left-hand side of the dental arch.
- If the distal portion is on the left margin, it is the right-hand side of the dental arch.
- Dental film has a raised dot on a corner of the film.
- Place all films with the dot facing upward, which is a convex view.
- **Convex** is a facial surface view.
- Concave is a lingual surface view.
- A full-mouth series usually includes 14 periapical films plus two or four bite wings.

convex

Raised.

PROCEDURE 24.19 | MOUNTING DENTAL FILMS

RATIONALE

Correct mounting of dental films helps the dentist assess whether the patient needs treatment.

1. Wash hands.
2. Assemble equipment.
   a. Developed x-rays
   b. X-ray mounts
   c. View box
3. Turn on view box.
4. Lay out x-rays. (Make certain that raised dot is facing upward.)
5. Arrange film on view box before placing into mount.
6. Mount the two or four bite-wing films.

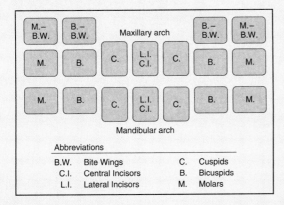

NOTE Bicuspid views are closest to the center of the mount.

7. Mount two central (CI) and lateral (LI) incisor films. Place mandibular films with roots downward and maxillary films with roots upward.
8. Mount the four cuspid (C) films. The two longest cuspids are maxillary teeth.
9. Mount the four bicuspid (BC) films.
10. Mount the four molars (M) films. The molars with three roots are the maxillary molars.
11. Review the anatomical charts to check mount for accuracy.
12. Turn off view box.
13. Clean and replace equipment.
14. Wash hands.
15. Record the following on patient chart and dental x-ray mount:
    a. Patient's name
    b. Date x-rays were taken
    c. Name of person who took x-rays
    d. Dentist's name and address

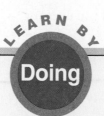

Doing

1. Complete Worksheets 2, 3, 4, 6, 9, and 10 as assigned.
2. Complete Worksheets/Activities 5, 7, 8, and 11 as assigned.
3. Practice all procedures.
4. Prepare responses to each item listed in Chapter Review—Your Link to Success at the end of this chapter.
5. When you are confident that you can meet each objective, ask your instructor for the unit evaluation.

Thinking Critically: Check Your Understanding

1. **Communication** Your office has long complied with OSHA guidelines and Standard Precautions. Mrs. Ricard is a new client and is clearly upset when you put on a mask, gloves, and protective eyewear. When you ask her what is causing her distress, she says, "I don't have AIDS and I certainly hope that you don't." What will you say to her to explain how modern dental offices practice infection control?

2. **Medical Terminology** An 8-year-old boy fell off of his bike and knocked his top two front teeth out. Using appropriate terminology and identifiers, write a description for a dental record of the dentition on this boy.

3. **Legal** Make a list of the legal and financial importance of clear and complete dental records.

4. **Patient Education** Describe what you would tell a patient about taking an alginate impression, including why it is necessary and how long it will take. Include instructions about how the patient will be positioned in the chair, how the patient should place his or her tongue, and how the patient should breathe.

5. **Computers** Describe ways computers are used in dental care.

6. **Case Study** You are preparing the instruments and aspirating syringe for a patient who is scheduled to have two teeth, numbers 5 and 31, extracted. Using medical terminology, describe the size of the needles you will prepare for each anesthesia injection and where you will place the topical anesthesia.

Portfolio Connection

Once you attain competence as a dental assistant, ask for permission to copy an example of your charting. (Remove all patient identifiers.) Place this copy in your portfolio as evidence of your skills. Place a copy of your on-site trainer's evaluation in your portfolio.

Write a paper describing your doubts and realizations and the barriers that you were able to overcome during the dental assistant experience. For example, were you afraid that you couldn't learn to use the equipment? Describe the ways you plan to use the skills, information, and insights that you gained about people and about this job. This assignment must be in standard report format.

Portfolio Tip

Keep a pocket notebook with you at all times to jot down any tips for your personal portfolio section and any other helpful observations.

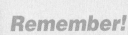 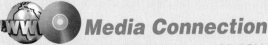

Remember! *Media Connection*

Use the Companion Website **www.prenhall.com/badasch** and the CD-ROM for additional interactive learning activities.

GLOSSARY

A

abbreviations Words that have been shortened.

abdominal thrust or **Heimlich maneuver** Forceful thrust on the abdomen, between the sternum and the navel, in an upward motion toward the head.

abrasive Compound used to rub away or scrape away another substance.

abreast Side by side.

abscesses Pockets of pus in a limited area.

absorption Passage of a substance through a body surface into body fluids and tissues (e.g., nutrients from digested food pass through the wall of the small intestine into the blood).

accessible Available to obtain.

accessory Helping.

accurate Exact, correct, or precise.

acids Substances that cause the urine to have an acid pH.

acquired Refers to a condition, disease, or characteristic that began after birth.

ADA American Dental Association.

adapt To change, to become suitable, to adjust.

adaptation Changing to work better.

adequate Enough, sufficient.

administrative Pertaining to processing, such as handling of paperwork, that assists in patient care and supports the physician.

admit To let someone in, take in.

adolescent Pertaining to the period of life between childhood and maturity.

aerobic Requiring oxygen.

agglutination Clumping together (e.g., red blood cells clump together).

aggressiveness Tendency to start fights and quarrels or to attack without reason.

airborne Particles that float in the air.

ala Outer side of the nostril.

alginate Material for making impressions.

alignment Keeping a resident in proper position.

alimentary canal Long muscular tube beginning at the mouth and ending at the anus.

alveolar-capillary Pertaining to air sacs in the lungs.

ambulation Walking.

amniotic fluid Liquid that surrounds the fetus during pregnancy.

amplify To increase or elevate a sound (e.g., the ossicles of the ear amplify sound waves).

amputation Removal of a body part.

anaerobic Able to grow and function without oxygen.

anesthesia Loss of feeling or sensation.

annoyance Irritation (e.g., to feel irritated with a co-worker or patient).

anorexia nervosa Loss of appetite with serious weight loss; considered a mental disorder.

antagonist Something that works against.

anterior Located in the front; opposite of posterior (e.g., the abdominal wall is anterior to the back).

antibiotics Substances that slow growth of or destroy microorganisms.

antibodies Substances made by the body to produce immunity to an antigen.

antigen Foreign matter that causes the body to produce antibodies.

antiseptic Substance that slows or stops the growth of microorganisms.

antitoxin Substance that provides immunity to a toxin.

anus Outlet from which the body expels solid waste.

apex Pointed end of something (e.g., the pointed end of the heart is called the apex of the heart).

apical foramen Opening in the apex.

apparatus Equipment needed to perform a task (e.g., blood pressure apparatus includes a blood pressure cuff and a stethoscope).

appendicular Pertaining to any body part added to the axis (e.g., arms and legs are attached to the axis of the body).

appropriate Suitable, correct.

arteriosclerosis Condition of hardening of the arteries.

artifacts Unwanted marks on an electrocardiogram.

asepsis Sterile condition, free from all germs.

aseptic technique Methods used to make the environment, the worker, and the patient as germ-free as possible.

aspirate Remove substances.

aspiration Withdrawal of a fluid.

asymptomatic Without visible symptoms.

atherosclerosis Condition of hardening of the arteries due to fat deposits that narrow the space blood flows through.

auditing Formal checking for correctness.

augmented Increased (e.g., augmented voltage leads show an increase in graph size).

auscultation Listening for sounds within the body.

autoclaves Sterilizers that use steam under pressure to kill all forms of bacteria on fomites (objects that pathogens live on and can transfer infection).

automated Method of lab testing that uses equipment to perform a series of steps, as compared to a manual method.

autopsy Medical procedure after death to determine the cause of death.

axial Pertaining to the central structures of the body (e.g., vertebrae, skull, ribs, and sternum).

axillary Referring to the armpit.

axis A center point that can be rotated around.

B

barriers Items that prevent infectious material from contacting surface.

baseline A number, graph, or indication to use as a guideline. A measurement taken at a later time may differ from the baseline, indicating a possible cause for concern.

biases Tendencies; prejudices.

biconcave Having a depressed surface on both sides.

bingeing Eating excessively.

biocular Having two eyepieces.

biohazard Substance that has potential to transmit disease.

birth defects Defects present at birth.

blood pressure Highest and lowest pressure against the walls of blood vessels.

boundaries Legal limits (e.g., you may know how to perform a task, but you may not do it because you are limited by your license, certification, registration, or rules and regulations).

bounding Leaping, strong, or forceful (e.g., a very strong pulse is a bounding pulse).

brittle Fragile, easy to break.

C

calcify To harden by forming calcium deposits.

calculated Figured out.

calibration Standard measure (e.g., each line on a thermometer or a ruler is a calibration).

calories Units of measurement of the fuel value of food.

capitation Payment to provide care for a set number of people.

carbon dioxide A gas, heavier than air; a waste product from the body.

cardiopulmonary Having to do with the heart and lungs.

caries Decay.

cartilage Tough connective tissue; forms pads at end of bones, is found in the nasal septum and external ear, and forms the major portion of the embryonic skeleton.

catheters Tubes inserted into body opening or cavity.

cell Smallest structural unit in the body that is capable of independent functioning.

cell membrane Thin, soft layer of tissue that surrounds the cell and holds it together.

Celsius Measure of heat; in medicine a Celsius thermometer is sometimes used to measure body heat. Also called centigrade.

cementum Hard, thin covering or shell covering root of tooth.

cerebrospinal fluid Liquid that flows through and around brain tissue.

cerebrovascular accidents (CVA) Complete or partial loss of blood flow to brain tissue caused by blood vessel spasms, intracranial bleeding, and/or obstruction of the blood vessels in the brain.

cervix Neck (e.g., the cervix of the uterus is the neck of the uterus).

characterized Distinguished by; refers to a trait or quality.

chronic Continuing over many years or for a long time (e.g., chronic illness).

chyme Creamy semifluid mixture of food and digestive juices.

cilia Hairlike projections that move rhythmically.

circulation Continuous one-way movement of blood through the heart and blood vessels to all parts of the body.

clammy Moist, cold skin.

classify To put like items together.

clumped Stuck together.

colitis Inflammation of the colon.

coma Deep sleep; unconscious state for a long period of time.

communicable Capable of passing directly or indirectly from one person or thing to another.

communication Act of exchanging information.

competent Capable or able to perform a skill or task.

complex Having two or more related parts.

comply To follow directions, do what you are asked to do.

components Parts or elements of a whole; an ingredient.

composed Formed by putting many parts together.

compromising Giving up something important.

concave Curved inward, depressed; dented.

concentrated Increased strength, strong solution.

conception Occurs when the male sperm fertilizes the female ovum and a new organism begins to develop.

concisely In a brief manner; to express in a few words.

confidential Private, personal, restricted, secret.

connective tissue Tissue specialized to bind together and support other tissues.

consecutive Following one after the other.

consistency Thickness.

constipation Infrequent or difficult emptying of the bowel.

contacts Place where surface of teeth touch.

contaminated Soiled, unclean, not suitable for use.

contingency Event that may occur but is not intended or likely to happen.

continuum Progression from start (birth) to finish (death).

contraceptives Items that serve to prevent pregnancy.

contract To shorten, to draw together; muscles shorten when you flex a body part.

contraction Drawing up.

contusion Condition in which the skin is bruised, swollen, and painful, but is not broken.

convents Establishments of nuns.

converse Talk, have a conversation.

convex Raised.

convey To say, tell, or express.

coordination State of harmonized action, such as eye and hand coordination.

coping Handling difficult situations.

corporal Bodily. For example, corporal punishment involves hitting or harming the body.

courteous Polite; considerate toward others.

crouch To stoop, using the large muscles of the legs to help maintain balance.

cusps Pointed or rounded raised areas on the surface of the tooth.

custodial Marked by watching and protecting rather than seeking to cure.

cycle Repeating steps (e.g., a wash cycle).

cylinder Long, narrow, circular container.

cystitis Inflammation of the urinary bladder.

cytoplasm All of the substance of a cell other than the nucleus.

D

debilitating Causing weakness or impairment.

decade Period of 10 years.

decay Breaking down; rot.

deciduous Falling out (e.g., primary teeth fall out to make room for permanent teeth).

decimal A number containing a decimal point.

decompose To decay; to break down.

decontamination Removal of unclean matter and living organisms.

defamatory Statement that causes injury to another's reputation.

defecation The pushing of solid material from the bowel.

deficiency Shortage (e.g., a deficient diet causes the body to function poorly because it is missing an important element).

deficient Lacking something (e.g., a deficient diet causes the body to function poorly because it is missing an important element).

definitive Clear, without question, exacting (e.g., when giving emergency care, each treatment should be done in a definitive manner).

dehydration Severe loss of fluid from tissue and cells.

delegates Gives another person responsibility for doing specific tasks.

delinquent Late.

dentition Natural teeth in the dental arch.

dentures False teeth.

designate To appoint or determine.

deteriorate Break down.

diabetes mellitus Condition that develops when the body cannot change sugar into energy; there is an insufficient amount of insulin, leading to an increased amount of sugar in the blood.

diagnosis Identification of a disease or condition.

diagnostic Pertaining to the determination of the nature of a disease or injury by examining (e.g., using x-ray and laboratory tests).

dialysis Process of removing waste from body fluids.

diarrhea Passage of watery stool at frequent intervals.

diastolic pressure Lowest pressure against the blood vessels of the body. It is measured between contractions.

digestion Process of breaking down food mechanically and chemically.

diluent Liquid added to powder that dissolves the powder.

disbursement Payment.

disinfection Process of freeing from microorganisms by physical or chemical means.

dismantles Takes apart.

disorientation State of being confused about time, place, and identity of persons and objects.

disoriented Being confused about time, place, or identity of persons and objects.

disposition Act of disposing of (e.g., a person desires that his or her monies be given to an organization after his or her death).

dissection Act or process of dividing, taking apart.

distal Farthest from the point of attachment.

distension Stretched out; bloated.

distribute To deliver.

diuretics Drugs that increase urine output.

diverticulitis Inflammation of the small sacs in the wall of the colon.

document Written record.

dressings Gauze pads that are used to cover a wound.

droplet A small drop of fluid.

duct Narrow, round tube that carries secretions from a gland.

dysfunction Impaired or abnormal functioning.

E

edema Swelling; abnormal or excessive collection of fluid in the tissues. Usually, the swelling is in the hands, ankles, legs, or abdomen.

efficiency Ability to accomplish a job with the least possible difficulty.

EKG/ECG Graphic record of the electrical currents produced by the heart.

elastic Easily stretched.

electrocardiograph Instrument that records electric currents produced by the heart.

elimination Process of getting rid of.

embryo Living human being during the first 8 weeks of development in the uterus.

embryonic Pertaining to the embryo.

emesis Vomit.

encephalitis Inflammation of the brain.

endometrium Interlining of the uterus.

endowments Gifts of property or money given to a group or organization.

enemas Solution introduced into the rectum.

ensure To make certain.

enterotoxin Poisonous substance that is produced in, or originates in, the contents of the intestine.

environment Surroundings we live in. Environmental disease can occur in any area around us (e.g., hospital, restaurants, public places, home, school).

environmental sanitation Methods used to keep the environment clean and to promote health.

enzyme Substance that causes a change to occur in other substances.

epidemic Disease that spreads rapidly among people.

epidermis Outer layer of skin.

epigastric Pertaining to the area over the pit of the stomach.

epilepsy Chronic disease of the nervous system.

episodes Events in a series.

epithelial Pertaining to covering of the internal and external organs of the body.

equilibrium State of balance.

equipment Instruments, machines, or items used to perform a task.

ergonomic Related to the study of the work environment.

erupt Push through.

essential Necessary (e.g., certain food elements are necessary for the body's functions).

estrogen Female hormone.

ethics Social values, conduct, description of what is right and wrong.

ethylene oxide Gas that kills living microorganisms.

evacuated Emptied out.

evacuation Removal.

excreted Thrown off or eliminated as waste material.

excretion Process of eliminating waste material.

exorcise To force out evil spirits.

expiration/exhalation Process of forcing air out of the body during respiration.

exploitation To use another person for profit or enjoyment.

exposed Left unprotected.

extemporaneous Completed with little preparation.

extract Identify and take out or emphasize.

extremities Arms, legs, hands, and feet.

F

facilities Places designed or built to serve a special function (e.g., hospital, clinic, doctor's office).

Fahrenheit Measure of heat; in medicine a Fahrenheit thermometer is often used to measure body heat.

familiar Known.

faulty Defective or imperfect.

feces Solid waste that is evacuated from the body through the anus.

feedback Information received as a result of something done or said.

fetus Infant developing in the uterus after the first three months until birth.

FICA Federal Insurance Contribution Act.

fixation Repair or fix.

flexibility Ability to bend easily.

flexible Able to bend easily.

flushed Showing reddening of the skin.

formula Accepted rule (e.g., a math formula and a baby formula are both guidelines or rules).

foster To develop; to promote; to stimulate.

fracture Broken bone.

frayed Worn or tattered (e.g., electrical cords may be worn, causing wires to be exposed).

friction Disagreement because of a difference of opinion.

functional stress Stress to tooth caused by its normal function (e.g., force of pressure when biting something hard).

functions Action or work of tissues, organs, or body parts (e.g., the heart's function is to pump blood).

G

gamma globulin Substance that acts as an antibody to increase immunity.

ganglia Mass of nerve tissue composed of nerve cell bodies. Ganglia lie outside the brain and spinal cord.

gastrointestinal Pertaining to the stomach and intestine.

gauge Standard scale for measurement.

generalized Affecting all of the body.

generic Major group (e.g., heart disease or skin disease).

geriatric Pertaining to old age.

germicidals Solutions that kill most bacteria.

gestures Motions of a part of the body to express feelings or emotions (e.g., nodding the head yes or no).

gravity Natural force or pull toward the earth. In the body, the center of gravity is usually the center of the body.

Greenwich time Standard time, a 12-hour clock.

gross pay Money earned before deductions are removed.

H

hazardous Dangerous.

heart block Interference with the conduction of the electrical impulses of the heart that is either partial or complete.

HEDIS Health Plan Employer Data and Information System; an organization that provides quality care guidelines.

Heimlich maneuver Forceful upward thrust on the abdomen, between the sternum and the navel.

hematoma Collection of blood beneath the skin.

hemoglobin Complex chemical in the blood; carries oxygen and carbon dioxide.

hemorrhage Large amount of bleeding.

heparinized Containing heparin, an anticoagulant.

hereditary Passed from parent to child.

heredity Characteristics passed from parent to child.

hernial Pertaining to projection through an abnormal opening in the wall of a body cavity.

holistic Pertaining to the whole; considering all factors.

homeostasis Constant balance within the body. This balance is maintained by the heartbeat, blood-making mechanisms, electrolytes, and hormone secretions.

hormones Protein substances secreted by an endocrine gland directly into the blood.

horseplay Rowdy behavior; acting inappropriately in a work environment.

host The organism from which a microorganism takes nourishment. The microorganism gives nothing in return and causes disease or illness.

hostility Unfriendliness; ill will toward another.

humidity Wetness, or moisture.

hydrotherapy Treatment that uses water therapy for disease or injury.

hypertension High blood pressure.

hypotension Low blood pressure.

I

idolizing Loving to excess.

ileitis Inflammation of the ileum (the lower three-fifths of the small intestine).

immunizations Substances given to make disease organisms harmless to the patient; may be given orally or by injection (e.g., tetanus, polio).

impaction Any tooth that does not erupt when it should (e.g., tooth blocked by bone and/or tissue, keeping it under the surface of the gum). Also, being tightly wedged into a part (e.g., fecal material wedged into the bowel that requires mechanical means to remove).

impatience Unwillingness to tolerate.

impending About to happen.

implement To accomplish; make it work.

impulses Measures of electrical activity to the heart tissue recorded on a graph.

incontinent Unable to control the bowel or bladder.

inferior Lower (e.g., one product is inferior in quality to another product).

infirmity Unsound or unhealthy state of being.

inflated To swell or fill up with air.

infuses Flows into the body by gravity (e.g., IV drips through a tube into the body).

ingestion By mouth.

initial First.

injectable Medication given by needle.

inoculation Instill, to put into the body.

inspiration/inhalation Process of breathing in air during respiration.

instruments Tools and measuring devices.

insulin Hormone secreted by the pancreas; essential for maintaining the correct blood sugar level.

insulin shock Condition caused by too much insulin.

interdisciplinary Involving two or more disciplines.

interproximal surfaces Sides between teeth.

interstitial Space between tissues.

interstitial fluid Liquid that fills the space between most of the cells of the body.

intoxication State of poisoning or becoming poisoned.

intracranial Inside the skull.

intraoral Within the oral cavity.

intravenously Directly into a vein.

invasive Entering the body.

involuntary Not under control (e.g., muscle twitching).

irregularities Different than normal.

irreversible Cannot be changed; condition will remain the same.

isolated Limited in contact with others.

IV poles Poles that raise and lower. IV solutions are hung on these poles.

K

kick buckets Metal buckets on wheels that can be kicked out of the way.

L

labeling Describing a person with a word that limits them (e.g., lazy, stupid).

laceration Wound or tear of the skin.

lacrimal Pertaining to tears.

lactation Body's process of producing milk to feed newborns.

lateral Relating to the sides or side of.

laxative Liquid or pill that causes evacuation of the bowel.

legal record Record that can be used in a law suit (e.g., the patient chart).

legible Capable of being read easily.

licensing Giving an agency or person permission to carry on certain activities and telling what they may not do as well as what they are authorized to do.

limb Arm, leg.

lipid Fat.

listlessness A state of being without energy.

localized Affecting one area of the body.

lumen Opening (e.g., opening in a tube or needle).

lymphocytes Type of white cell.

M

magnify Enlarge.

maintain Keep up.

malaise Weakness or discomfort.

malfunctioning Not working as it is supposed to.

malignant Cancerous.

mandates Commands, orders.

manual Book with guidelines.

masticate Chew.

maternal Relating to the mother or from the mother.

matures Becomes fully developed.

Mayo stands Adjustable, wheeled, small metal stands that hold equipment and supplies for many procedures.

mechanism Process or a series of steps that achieve a result.

meninges Lining of the brain.

meningitis Inflammation of the membrane covering the brain.

menstruation Cyclic deterioration of the endometrium.

metabolic Pertaining to the total of all the physical and chemical changes that take place in living organisms and cells.

metabolism The body's process of using food to make energy and use nutrients.

microns Units equaling one millionth of a meter.

microorganisms Organisms so small that they can only be seen through a microscope.

microscopic Too small to be seen by the eye but large enough to be seen through a microscope.

millimeters Measure of length.

minerals Inorganic elements that occur in nature; essential to every cell.

minute Exceptionally small.

misrepresentations Untruths; lies.

monasteries Homes for men following religious standards.

monocular Having one eyepiece.

monocytes Large single-nucleus white cells.

monogamous Having a sexual relationship with only one partner during a period of time.

mucosa Thin lining on the inside of the intestines.

N

neglect To ignore or not provide for.

nephron Functional part of the kidney that filters liquid waste.

net pay Money earned after deductions are removed.

neurological Pertaining to the nervous system.

neuron Nerve; includes the cell and the long fiber coming from the cell.

nondominant hand Hand that is not used for writing or other tasks.

noninvasive Not involving penetration of the skin.

nonpathogenic Not causing disease.

nosocomial infection An infection acquired while in a health care setting, such as a hospital.

nucleus The part of a cell that is vital for its growth, metabolism, reproduction, and transmitted characteristics.

nutrients Food.

O

obesity Extreme fatness; abnormal amount of fat on the body.

obligation Moral responsibility (e.g., to give the best possible patient/client care, to be on time for work).

observant Quick to see and understand.

observation Act of watching.

obsolete Out of date.

obstruction Blockage or clogging.

occult Hidden, unseen.

omission Neglect of duty.

opportunistic infections Infections that occur when the immune system is weakened. Common organisms that the body normally resists cause infection.

oral Referring to the mouth.

osseous Bonelike.

ossicles Three small bones in the middle ear: incus, stapes, and malleus.

outpatients Patients/clients who do not require hospitalization but are under a physician's care.

overexposure Too much contact with radiation.

ovum Female reproductive cell that when fertilized by the male develops into a new organism.

oxidation The mixing together of oxygen and another element.

oxygen Element in the atmosphere that is essential for maintaining life.

oxygenated Containing oxygen.

P

palpation Examine by feeling for unusual or abnormal conditions.

parallel Same direction and a distance, so that two points do not touch.

paralysis Loss of sensation and muscle function.

parasites Organisms obtaining nourishment from other organisms they are living in or on.

parasitic Pertaining to an organism that lives in or on another organism, taking nourishment from it.

parenteral Not in the digestive system (e.g., injections are parenterally administered).

pathogenic Disease causing.

Patient's/Client's Bill of Rights Document written by the American Hospital Association outlining expected patient/client rights while in a hospital.

penetrates Enters or passes through (e.g., a fractured bone passes through the skin).

periapical Around the apex (e.g., of the tooth).

pericardial fluid Liquid that surrounds the heart.

perineal Region between the vulva and anus in a female, or between the scrotum and anus in a male.

periodic Occurring at regular intervals.

peripheral Situated away from a central structure.

peristalsis Progressive, wavelike motion that occurs involuntarily in hollow tubes of the body.

peritoneal cavity Area of the body containing the liver, stomach, intestines, kidneys, urinary bladder, and reproductive organs.

peritoneal fluid Liquid in the peritoneal cavity.

personnel People who work in an establishment; a personnel office is where a worker goes to apply for a job.

phagocytes Cells that surround, eat, and digest microorganisms and cellular waste.

philosophy Theory; a general principle used for a specific purpose.

physiological Pertaining to normal body functions.

pigmented Colored areas of the body, e.g., iris of the eye, lips, moles, freckles.

plaque Soft deposit of bacteria and bacterial products on teeth.

plasma Colorless liquid part of the blood, consisting of water, nutrients, wastes, hormones, antibodies, enzymes, leukocytes, erythrocytes, and platelets.

pleural fluid Liquid that surrounds the lungs.

pneumonia Inflammation of the lungs.

pollutants Things that contaminate the air (e.g., smoke, smog).

polycythemia Condition of having too much blood.

polyps Small tumorlike growths.

porous Filled with tiny holes.

posterior Behind, to the rear, toward the back (e.g., the heel is posterior to the toes).

postmortem After death.

postural supports Soft restraints used to protect resident.

potential Possible.

pouch Small bag or sac.

predators Organisms or beings that destroy.

prejudge To decide or make a decision before having the facts.

prejudices Judgments or opinions formed before the facts are known.

prepaid Paid ahead of time.

prestige Influence obtained through success, wealth, or some other source.

preventable Able to be kept from happening.

primarily For the most part; chiefly.

primary First.

priorities Those things that are most important.

prioritize To put in order of importance.

progressive Moving forward, following steps toward an end product.

prohibit To not allow.

project To show or reflect.

prone Lying on the stomach.

prosthetics Artificial parts made for the body (e.g., teeth, feet, legs, arms, hands, eyes, breasts).

proteins Complex compound found in plant and animal tissues, essential for heat, energy, and growth.

protrusion Pushing through.

provider Physician, physician assistant, nurse practitioner.

proximal Nearest or next to.

prudent Careful or cautious.

psychiatric Pertaining to the mind.

psychological Pertaining to the mind.

psychotherapy Method of treatment using mental applications, such as hypnotherapy.

purging Causing oneself to vomit.

Q

quackery Practice of pretending to cure diseases.

R

radiopaque Shows as a white material when a fluoroscope x-ray is taken.

range of motion (ROM) Moving all joints of the body; can be active or passive.

rapport Harmony; a close relationship with another.

reagents Chemical substances that react to the presence of other substances in the blood and urine.

receptors Nerves that respond to stimuli.

recipient One who receives.

recognition Acknowledgment as being worthy of approval.

reconstituting Adding water to a powdered drug.

rectal Referring to the far end of the large intestine just above the anus.

refer To send to.

reflexes Result when a nerve is stimulated and an involuntary action occurs (e.g., touch a hot stove, and the muscles react involuntarily to move the fingers away).

regulate To control or adjust.

rehabilitation Process that helps people who have been disabled by sickness or injury to recover as many of their original abilities for activities of daily living as possible.

reimburse To pay back for something given or spent.

relevant Pertaining to, or having to do with, the patient/client.

rendered Given or provided.

replenish Refill or build up again.

reproduction Process that takes place in animals to create offspring.

resident Able to protect itself.

residual Left over.

resistance Ability of the body to protect itself from disease.

resorption Loss of a substance or bone.

responsibility One's answerability to an employer in areas such as dependability and honesty.

restorative To return to as close to normal conditions as possible.

restrict To keep within limits; to confine.

resultant Resulting from an action.

retention Keeping elements within the body that are normally eliminated (e.g., waste products such as urine and feces).

rheostat Control for flow of electric current.

rickettsiae Parasitic microorganisms that live on another living organism and cause disease.

rotary Move in a circular fashion.

S

sacral region The area where the sacrum is located; forms the tail end of the spinal column.

salmonella A rod-shaped bacterium found in the intestine that can cause food poisoning, gastroenteritis, and typhoid fever.

salutation A greeting (e.g., Dear Sir).

saprophytes Organisms that live on dead organic matter.

saturated Soaked; filled to capacity.

saturating Soak.

scattering Spreading in many directions, dispersing.

seating Putting firmly in place to prevent moving.

sebaceous Pertaining to fatty secretions.

secretion Producing and expelling a special substance (e.g., sebaceous glands secrete oil; salivary glands secrete saliva).

sedate Calm.

seizure Involuntary muscle contraction and relaxation.

self-esteem Belief in oneself.

semen Fluid from the testes, seminal vesicles, prostate gland, and bulbourethral glands. Contains water, mucin, proteins, salts, and sperm.

septic arthritis Bacterial inflammation of the joint caused by bloodborne bacteria carried from another place in the body.

serrated Sawlike notches.

sex cells Cells that allow reproduction to occur.

shocks Convulsion of muscles and extreme stimulation of nerves when an electric current passes through the body.

sloughed Discarded; separated from (e.g., to shed dead cells, as from the outer skin).

soluble Able to break down or dissolve in liquid.

solutions Two or more liquids mixed together.

specialties Fields of study or professional work (e.g., pediatrics, orthopedics, obstetrics).

specifications Exact way something should be done.

spermatozoa Male sex cells.

sphincter Circular muscle that allows the opening and closing of a body part (e.g., anus, pylorus).

sphygmomanometer Measuring device used to measure the pressure against the arteries of the body.

spirochetes Slender, coil-shaped organisms.

splints Firm object used to support an unstable body part.

spontaneous Occurring naturally without apparent cause.

spurts To force out in a burst; to squirt.

stability Ability to maintain a balance, both mentally and physically.

stamina Body's strength or energy.

stance The way you stand.

Standard Precautions Guidelines designed to reduce the risk of transmission of microorganisms from recognized and unrecognized sources of infection in the hospital.

sterility Absence of living organism or inability to produce offspring.

sterilized Made free from all living microorganisms.

stethoscope Instrument used to hear sound in the body (e.g., heartbeat, lung sounds, bowel sounds).

stimuli Elements in the external or internal environment that are strong enough to set up a nervous impulse.

stoma Opening, e.g., opening in abdomen in an ostomy.

structure Form in which the body is made.

subcutaneous Beneath the skin.

sufficient Enough.

sulcus Depression, groove, area where gingival tip meets tooth enamel.

superstitious Trusting in magic or chance.

supine Lying on the back.

suppository Bullet shaped mass inserted into rectum to stimulate bowel movement.

surgical Repairing or removing a body part by cutting.

susceptible Capable of being affected or infected (e.g., body can be attacked by microorganisms and become ill).

swathe Bandage.

syncope Fainting.

syndrome A number of symptoms occurring together.

systolic pressure Highest pressure against blood vessels. Represented by first heart sound or beat heard when taking a blood pressure.

T

terminal Last or ending.

terminology Specialized terms used in any occupation.

testicles Site of production of the male sex cell.

testosterone Male hormone.

therapeutic Pertaining to the treatment of disease or injury (e.g., physical therapy, radiology, diet, nursing).

tissues Group of cells of the same type that act together to perform a specific function.

tomography X-ray technique that produces film of detailed cross sections of tissue.

tone Firmness or tightness.

topical Surface of the body.

toxins Poisonous substances.

TPR Stands for "temperature, pulse, respiration."

traditional Customary beliefs passed from generation to generation.

translate To make understandable.

transmitting Causing to go from one person to another person.

trauma Damage to the body caused by an injury, wound, or shock; mental trauma occurs from emotional shock.

trend General direction or movement.

tuberculosis Disease caused by tubercle bacilli; may cause death if untreated.

24-hour time/military time Method of telling time by counting each hour consecutively for 24 hours (i.e., . . . 11, 12, 13, . . .).

U

ulcerations Open areas, or sores.

uniformity A state of being all the same; does not vary.

unoxygenated Lacking oxygen.

urethritis Inflammation of the urethra.

V

vaccine Dead or weakened organisms that stimulate the body to make antibodies.

value Importance, worth.

venipuncture Puncture of a vein.

vessels Tubes that carry fluid in the body.

viable Capable of living.

villi Tiny projections.

visibility Ability to see.

vital A must, essential.

vitality Ability of an organism to go on living.

vitamins Group of substances necessary for normal functioning and maintenance of health.

voluntary Under the control of the person (e.g., you voluntarily raise your arm; it does not rise automatically).

W

waste products Elements that are unfit for the body's use and are eliminated from the body.

Z

zygote Any cell formed by the coming together of two reproductive (sex) cells.

INDEX